The 10-Minute
Clinical Assessment

The 10-Minute Clinical Assessment

Second Edition

Knut Schroeder

MSc PhD DCH DRCOG DGM MRCP FRCGP CertMedEd
Honorary Senior Clinical Lecturer in General Practice
Centre for Academic Primary Care
University of Bristol
General Practitioner, Bristol

WILEY Blackwell　BMJ|Books

For Kiran and Rohan

Table of contents

Foreword

Being a GP is hugely rewarding but also incredibly complex. Patients can and do present themselves with a bewildering array of problems, and they expect their doctor to have the answer to everything straight away.

This variety is what makes general practice both satisfying and challenging, but it can be daunting for a recent graduate who is competent – but perhaps not completely confident.

Therefore, a guide like this is extremely valuable. It covers 154 selected clinical presentations from all the major clinical specialties that can be particularly challenging for people new to general practice. It contains references to the latest evidence and guidelines and tries to maintain a patient-centred approach throughout.

The target audience for this book is senior medical students and doctors starting their career in general practice, who may find the transition from full history and examination to the focused approach that we adopt in general practice difficult. It should also be helpful for candidates preparing for the CSA part of the MRCGP examination.

Even for experienced health professionals, this book will be extremely useful as a quick reference to have handy in the surgery. Because it is impossible to cover everything during a brief clinical assessment, the book tries to point out those areas that should be considered when faced with important and potentially tricky clinical presentations.

This guide is a highly valuable tool to use alongside the RCGP curriculum. It reflects a desire to improve patient care and the quality of general practice, a goal which should be applauded.

As someone who is passionate about general practice and GP education, I'm proud to recommend this book by Knut Schroeder as an excellent contribution to the genre.

Professor Steve Field FRCGP
Chairman, Royal College of General Practitioners

Preface to the 1st edition

Those of us who work in busy clinical settings often have to assess patients under considerable time constraints. This can be a challenge, particularly when faced with undifferentiated presentations such as 'headache', 'chest pain', 'weight loss' or 'dizziness'. *The 10-Minute Clinical Assessment* provides suggestions for a focused approach in such situations and covers a selection of important and frequently demanding or difficult clinical presentations – symptoms as well as conditions – from all the major clinical specialties.

Medical students, nurses and even doctors undergoing postgraduate training often get surprisingly little teaching and training on what to include in a focused history and examination. This book bridges the gap by highlighting important differential diagnoses, 'red flags' and key aspects to consider during clinical assessment, while also giving some indication as to *why* these might be relevant. Important clinical presentations are covered with reference to the latest evidence and guidelines, and traditional practice is challenged in areas where new evidence has emerged. The book takes a holistic approach and also emphasises issues that are important for patients, including their ideas, concerns, expectations and issues around quality of life.

This book aims to be an *aide memoire* for general practitioners, trainees in general practice, medical students, nurses and paramedics working in primary care settings. Hospital doctors might also find the book useful when patients under their care develop clinical problems that are outside their specialty interest or when working in the Accident & Emergency department. It has been designed to allow quick reference during busy clinical sessions and in exam preparation. Information is presented in a structured, condensed and hopefully easily accessible way.

The 10-Minute Clinical Assessment is based on experience gained from clinical practice, student teaching and examination, backed up by an extensive literature search and consultation with experts. Sections of the book have been 'field-tested' among general practitioners, trainee doctors, medical students and nurses. In addition, every section has been reviewed by expert readers from primary and secondary care, whose comments have been invaluable and have led to numerous improvements and alterations. Some of the chapters on chronic diseases and cancer have also been looked at by 'expert' patients.

The book is not meant to be prescriptive – clinical assessment is not a tick-box exercise! Each clinical encounter is different, has its own dynamic and needs to be tailored to the individual – taking a patient-centred and caring approach. Because it is impossible to cover everything during a brief clinical assessment, the book points out those areas that should be considered when faced with important and potentially tricky clinical presentations. It offers some of the 'essential pieces of a jigsaw puzzle' that can help with recognising the whole picture.

The book covers clinical assessment only and deliberately does not include investigation and management, which for symptom-based presentations will often depend on the outcome of the assessment. *The 10-Minute Clinical Assessment* therefore needs to be read in conjunction with larger textbooks, as well as books on consultation skills, physical examination and clinical diagnosis – assuming that readers will have had the relevant clinical teaching at the bedside.

It was tempting to include pictures, case studies and diagrams, but this would have made the book too bulky for use in day-to-day practice. There is some unavoidable overlap and repetition between some of the topics, but these are kept to a minimum and allow each chapter to be read alone and independently.

I hope that the book will give you a better understanding of:

- The issues that are important for patients.
- Which questions to ask and what to examine (and why!) during focused clinical assessment, especially when under time pressure.
- How to recognise 'red flags' and important disease patterns.
- The main differential diagnoses and risk factors for each presentation.
- How to exclude major and serious diagnoses quickly.
- How to reduce the potential for misdiagnosis.
- Which areas to explore in order to make informed decisions about patient management.
- What information to consider for inclusion in referral letters to specialists.
- Which clinical details are relevant when presenting history and examination findings to other colleagues.
- Which essential issues to cover when assessing patients during undergraduate finals or postgraduate clinical examinations.

I sincerely hope that you will find the format of the book and the information provided useful. Please feel free to contact me (k.schroeder@bristol.ac.uk) if you spot any errors or have suggestions for further improvements.

Knut Schroeder
Bristol

Preface to 2nd edition

This new 2nd edition of *The 10-Minute Clinical Assessment* continues to give you all the information you need to carry out an effective and focused clinical assessment in general practice.

We have fully revised all the chapters using the latest key references, including the latest guidance from the National Institute for Health and Care Excellence (NICE).

Based on feedback and suggestions, especially from medical students and general practitioners in training, we have also added the following three new chapters on topics that are right at the heart of general practice:

- **Focused Clinical Assessment.** Discover how to become more patient-centred, learn some useful tricks of the trade and explore how you can save time in the consultation without compromising on quality.
- **Useful Consultation Tools.** Find better ways of asking questions and – more importantly – getting patients to talk. Uncovering how you can become a more effective listener and explore sensitive topics under time constraints, this chapter is packed with tips for conducting more effective consultations.
- **Red Flags in General Practice.** Learn how to spot important warning signs of serious disease and how to make sense of red flags, and find useful advice on avoiding serious medical errors.

I hope not only that this book will help you provide excellent care for your patients, but also that it supports you in becoming a more effective, better and happier doctor.

Wishing you all the best for your career,

Knut Schroeder
Bristol
June 2016

About the author

Knut Schroeder is a practising NHS GP with over 20 years' experience (10 of these as a GP Principal) and Honorary Senior Clinical Lecturer in General Practice at the University of Bristol. He is passionate about teaching consultation skills to new generations of GPs, particularly around 'focused clinical assessment' and 'red flags'.

During his time as a full-time Consultant Senior Lecturer, he co-developed and delivered undergraduate and postgraduate courses on clinical diagnosis and evidence-based medicine. He was also responsible for the general practice part of the final-year examination for medical students at the University of Bristol for 2 years. He was a GP Trainer for 8 years and continues to teach medical students.

Knut has authored four books and co-written a number of book chapters, including *Sustainable Healthcare*, *Diagnosing Your Health Symptoms for Dummies* and two chapters of the *Oxford Textbook of Primary Medical Care*. He has written papers and articles published in international peer-reviewed journals and the GP press. Knut was Deputy Co-ordinating Editor for the Cochrane Heart Group for 4 years and has experience in writing and assessing systematic reviews of clinical literature.

Acknowledgements

I would like to thank Dr Gill Jenkins (part-time GP in Bristol, medical writer and broadcaster) for contributing to chapters in the obstetric, gynaecology and endocrine sections and for commenting on earlier versions of the manuscript.

Very special thanks go to Mary Banks, Simone Heaton and everyone else at Wiley-Blackwell for their tremendously kind support, encouragement, patience and professionalism.

Many thanks also to the doctors and nurses at the Stokes Medical Centre in Little Stoke, Bristol, for their comments and suggestions. I enjoyed the discussions!

Many general practitioners, hospital specialists, medical students, nurses, emergency care practitioners, paramedics and 'expert' patients have very kindly given up their time to read and comment on individual chapters or whole sections, or have contributed in other ways. I am particularly grateful to the following people (in alphabetical order) for their constructive criticisms and helpful suggestions, some of which have led to substantive changes:

Dr Andreas Baumbach, Dr Andrew Blythe, Dr Kate Boyd, Dr Simon Bradley, Dr Peter Brindle, Dr David Cahill, Dr Shane Clarke, Dr Mike Cohen, Dr Michelle Cooper, Mike Cox, Prof Paul Dieppe, Dr Lindsey Dow, Dr Ian Ensum, Dr Stuart Glover, Dr William Hamilton, Dr Michael Harris, Dr John Harvey, Dr Gayani Herath, Dr Rachel Hilton, Dr Rhian Johns, Dr James Jones, Dr David Kessler, Dr Tina LeCoyte, Prof Andy Levy, Dr Anne Lingford-Hughes, Dr Elaine Lunts, Dr Paul Main, Dr Kate Mather, Dr David Memel, Lionel Nel, Mr Desmond Nunez, Dr Jess O'Riordan, Dr Lucy Pocock, Dr Robert Przemioslo, Dr Jon Rees, Dr Rebecca Reynolds, Dr Hayley Richards, Dr Ginny Royston, Dr Trevor Thompson, Mr Derek Tole, Dr Antje Walker, Dr Jane Watkins, Dr Alastair Wilkins, Dr Philip Williams and Dr Wolfram Woltersdorf.

Finally, I would like to thank my wife, Dr Sharmila Choudhury, for her understanding, kind support and constructive comments during this project.

Selected useful resources

The following is a selection of resources that have been useful reference points during the preparation of this book and which provide excellent sources for further information:

1. The 10-Minute Consultation series in the *British Medical Journal*. Available from: http://www.bmj.com/specialties/10-minute-consultation (last accessed 29 April 2016).
2. Clinical Knowledge Summaries. cks.nice.org.uk.
3. National Institute for Health and Care Excellence (NICE). www.nice.org.uk.
4. PatientPlus articles. www.patient.co.uk.
5. People's Experiences at healthtalk.org. Available from: http://www.healthtalk.org/peoples-experiences (last accessed 29 April 2016).
6. The Rational Clinical Examination series in *JAMA*. Available from: http://jama.jamanetwork.com/collection.aspx?categoryid=6257 (last accessed 29 April 2016).
7. Scottish Intercollegiate Guidelines Network (SIGN). www.sign.ac.uk.

The focused consultation

Focused clinical assessment

Key issues

Practical points
- **Effective practice.** Conducting a focused clinical assessment provides a good basis for safe and effective clinical practice.
- **Time constraints.** Students and doctors working in general practice can find it difficult to perform an effective clinical assessment within short (e.g. 10–15 minutes) overall consultation times, which will often also include discussing a management plan, issuing prescriptions, ordering tests and writing case notes.
- **Strategies.** Various strategies exist to help assess patients in a focused yet patient-centred way.

Structuring the consultation

Preparation
- **Key thoughts.** Think about the key issues from the start of the consultation – or even before, if you know the reason for the patient's attendance. This will help you decide which issues to focus on during the consultation.
- **Practical points.** At the beginning of the consultation, make a mental list of the main points to bear in mind, such as red flags (ruling in and ruling out disease), possible differential diagnoses and diagnoses you do not want to miss.
- **Demographic variables.** Combine your medical knowledge with the likely prevalence of conditions in your work setting.
- **Risk factors.** Consider possible risk factors, such as alcohol, smoking and unhealthy diet(s).
- **Red flags.** Think about relevant alarm symptoms and signs that you might need to explore for a particular clinical presentation.
- **Stocking the room.** Make sure your consulting room is well stocked with essentials for the consultation (e.g. sampling bottles, stationery, thermometer covers, etc.), because having to leave your room to get these can waste valuable time.

History
- **Ideas, concerns and expectations.** Explore the patient's health beliefs, worries and understanding of their symptom(s) and condition(s), and what impact these have on their day-to-day life. Try to phrase your questions naturally (you can find useful phrases in the chapter on Useful Consultation Tools).
- **History of presenting complaint.** Focus initially on exploring issues around the presenting complaint and use relevant questions to rule in and rule out important diagnoses.

The 10-Minute Clinical Assessment, Second Edition. Knut Schroeder.
© 2017 John Wiley & Sons, Ltd. Published 2017 by John Wiley & Sons, Ltd.

- **Past and current medical problems.** Identify any comorbidities that might influence your diagnosis and management.
- **Medication.** Consider all medication, but especially any drugs that might be particularly relevant, such as oral anticoagulants (e.g. bleeding), nonsteroidal anti-inflammatory drugs (NSAIDs) (e.g. gastric problems) and steroids (e.g. immunosuppression).
- **Family history.** Does the patient have a significant family history that may be relevant?
- **Social history.** How does the clinical presentation fit into the patient's social context, including work, home life and social situation?
- **Review of previous investigations.** Check the results of any previous relevant investigations, because they may influence your assessment.

Examination

- **Ask permission.** Always ask patients' permission before you perform a physical examination, and offer a chaperone for intimate examinations, if appropriate. During the clinical assessment, stay sensitive to the patient's feelings, and be alert to nonverbal cues.
- **General assessment.** Quickly look for any obvious clues. Does the patient look unwell? Are there any obvious physical signs at first glance?
- **Vital signs.** Record important vital signs (e.g. pulse, blood pressure, temperature, respiratory rate, oxygen saturation in the periphery) to help in assessing the severity of the illness. Taking vital signs is also useful as a baseline for ongoing monitoring and for medicolegal reasons.
- **Focused physical examination.** Adopt a focused and selective approach, tailored to the findings from the history. Inspect, palpate, auscultate and check the function of relevant body areas and systems, as appropriate. You are looking for evidence that confirms or refutes your working diagnosis. Be curious and be prepared to reconsider your diagnosis when the findings are at odds with the history (e.g. hearing fine crackles in a patient with chronic obstructive pulmonary disease (COPD)).

The diagnostic process

Consider 'early triggers' in the consultation

- **Spot the diagnosis.** You may be able to recognise nonverbal patterns, such as skin conditions (e.g. atopic eczema) or a 'barking' cough (whooping cough), based on your previous experience or clinical knowledge.
- **Explore patients' self-labelling.** Patients may come with a self-diagnosis (which may or may not be correct), which can direct the diagnostic process.
- **Consider the presenting complaint.** The patient's initial statement (e.g. 'I have tummy pain' or 'I have a headache') can be used to direct your assessment.
- **Establish your working hypothesis.** Elements in both the history and the examination may trigger your working hypothesis. For example, thirst, feeling

unwell and looking tired in a young person may suggest the possibility of type 1 diabetes.

Strategies for narrowing down the possibilities

- **Rule out diagnoses.** Shortlist and rule out serious diagnoses based on what you consider to be likely causes of the presenting problem. This can also help to prevent clinical errors.
- **Assess in a stepwise fashion.** Assess patients based on the anatomical location of their problem or the suspected underlying pathological process. Clarify exactly where the problem is located, for example by asking them to point to the relevant body area.
- **Consider likelihood.** Use symptoms, signs and diagnostic tests to rule in or rule out likely and unlikely diagnoses. This requires you to know the degree to which a positive or negative result from your history, examination and bedside tests adjusts the probability of a given disease.
- **Recognise patterns.** Compare symptoms and signs with patterns you have seen in previous patients and cases you have read about – a common approach in general practice. This process relies on your memory of known patterns of disease. Remember that some conditions, such as myocardial infarction, brain tumour and depression, can present in various ways. Over time, you will build up a repertoire of these patterns and their variants.
- **Use clinical prediction rules.** Validated clinical prediction rules (e.g. the Ottawa ankle rules) represent a more formal version of pattern recognition.

Consider other strategies

- **Known diagnosis.** You can often rule out serious disease without further testing if a diagnosis is sufficiently certain (e.g. viral upper respiratory tract infection, viral wart, acne vulgaris).
- **Point-of-care tests.** Use appropriate point-of-care (bedside) tests to rule in or rule out a disease (e.g. blood glucose strip test, urine dipstick, oxygen saturation in the periphery). This can be useful in the presence of red flags and when a presentation or diagnosis does not fit any obvious pattern of disease.
- **Tests of treatment.** Use the response to treatment to refute or confirm a diagnosis (e.g. inhalers in nocturnal cough).
- **Tests of time.** Use the natural course of a disease to predict when the patient should improve (the 'wait and see' approach) (e.g. in suspected viral gastroenteritis or the common cold).
- **No label applied.** When you cannot arrive at a diagnosis, consider sharing your uncertainty with the patient and establish a 'safety net' by arranging appropriate clinical review, appropriate diagnostic tests or referral, as required.

Writing useful case notes

- **Concision.** Write concise yet comprehensive case notes and consider taking a structured approach (e.g. history, examination, impression and working diagnosis, management).

- **Thought process.** In addition to providing clinical details, give the reader a 'feel' for your thought processes and for how the consultation went.
- **History.** Record information relevant to the presenting complaint and underlying condition, including important positive and negative answers to direct questions.
- **Examination.** Include important positive and negative findings, in particular your general impression, the results of objective measurements (e.g. vital signs, size of skin lesions) and relevant 'system' findings (e.g. respiratory, cardiovascular or neurological findings).
- **Impression and diagnosis.** With the support of your findings, state your general impression and working diagnosis in clear and unambiguous terms. If you are uncertain about the diagnosis, say so, and mention any steps that you have taken to rule out serious disease.
- **Management.** Include any tests that you have arranged, what you have told the patient (including risks and benefits of any treatments), consent (including discussions around any procedures) (if applicable), treatment (including drug doses, prescription details and any other treatment), follow-up arrangements for tests and appointments and progress so far.

Summary of main principles

- **Apply focus.** Try to integrate your clinical and communication skills so that you can understand your patients' symptoms, physical signs and other important factors. Such factors include the impact of medical problems on patients' lives, their health beliefs and worries and their expectations about treatment.
- **Tailor your approach.** Remember that when serious illness is unlikely (absence of red flags, normal examination), you do not need to perform an exhaustive 'full' history and examination; it is preferable to tailor your approach to the clinical presentation (the clinical chapters in this book highlight the important aspects to consider for each clinical presentation).
- **Acknowledge problems.** Directly acknowledge and respond to patients' concerns.
- **Take a holistic approach.** Take a holistic and structured approach when gathering information. Apply your understanding of human diseases, while staying person-centred.
- **Gather data systematically.** Take a well-organised history and gather data methodically to create a solid foundation upon which to base your physical examination and from which to make clinical judgements.
- **Prioritise.** Try to establish early on in the consultation whether a patient has multiple problems they wish to talk about, so that you can prioritise accordingly.
- **Make use of consultation models.** Learn about the various consultation models that exist to help you structure and manage your consultation (you can find some useful summaries and starting points at the Bradford Vocational Training Scheme website, www.bradfordvts.co.uk).

Key references and further reading

1. Fahey T, van der Lei J. Producing and using clinical prediction rules. In: *The Evidence Base of Clinical Diagnosis: Theory and Methods of Diagnostic Research* (2nd edition). Knottnerus JA, Buntinx F (eds). Wiley-Blackwell BMJ Publishing, Hoboken, NJ; 2008.
2. Heneghan C, Glasziou P, Thompson M et al. Diagnostic strategies used in primary care. *BMJ* 2009;338:b946.
3. Schroeder K, Chan W-S, Fahey TP. Focused clinical assessment. *InnovAiT* 2011;4(1):41–48.

Useful consultation tools

Key thoughts

Practical points
- **Focused assessment.** Various consultation and communication techniques can help you perform a concise yet comprehensive clinical assessment in primary care.
- **Question types.** Open questions, especially at the beginning of the consultation, are useful in getting an overview of a clinical problem. Direct questioning can help establish further details.
- **Body language.** Be aware of your conscious and unconscious movements and postures, which convey your attitudes and feelings, beyond what you express with words.

History-taking

Introducing yourself
- **Initial contact.** Stand up, gently smile, establish good eye contact (without staring) and consider shaking hands with your patient, if you feel it is appropriate.
- **Greeting.** Greet and welcome the patient, using their name and language appropriate to the context (e.g. 'Good morning, Mrs Gupta, nice to meet you' or 'Hello, Mr Jones'.
- **Introduction.** Unless the patient knows you, clearly introduce yourself using your professional title and surname (e.g. 'Hello, my name is…'). Some people think that calling yourself 'Dr' emphasises hierarchy, while introducing yourself with your first and second names suggests equality and partnership. In any case, make it clear to the patient what your professional role is.
- **Acknowledging others.** Greet anyone who accompanies the patient, and establish their relationship to the patient, if it is unclear. Avoid making assumptions.

Opening the consultation
- **Listening.** You can start the consultation by saying nothing and actively listening, adopting an interested and welcoming posture. Many patients will start talking spontaneously and tell you why they have come to see you.
- **Open questions.** Starting with open questions can help find the main reason for the patient's attendance. Examples are, 'What would you like to talk about today?' and 'What brought you here today?'.
- **Probing questions.** A second open (probing) question or 'soft command', such as, 'Can you tell me a bit more about this, please?' or 'Is there anything else that

The 10-Minute Clinical Assessment, Second Edition. Knut Schroeder.
© 2017 John Wiley & Sons, Ltd. Published 2017 by John Wiley & Sons, Ltd.

you'd like to tell me?', will help explore the nature of the presenting problem and the patient's agenda.

- **Story.** The 'story' of the patient's complaint can be established by asking questions like, 'Could you tell me how it all started?', 'When were you last well?', 'How long has this been going on for?' and 'Tell me more about....'. Keep the flow going by asking, 'And what happened then?', 'What did you do when...?' and 'This is interesting. Can you explain it to me in a bit more detail?'.

- **The golden minute.** For the first minute or two (the 'golden minute'), allow the patient to tell their story in their own words, without interrupting them unnecessarily. Make sure you listen attentively, because patients will often direct you to the correct diagnosis!

- **Patient agenda.** Try to pick up cues about the patient's agenda (which may not initially be obvious), as well as their worries and emotions. It is easy to underestimate the significance of seemingly trivial or simple reasons for consultation.

- **Observation.** Be alert to any body signals the patient sends out (e.g. tone of voice, raised eyebrows, blushing, fidgeting).

- **Encouragement.** Encourage patients to keep talking by maintaining appropriate eye contact, leaning slightly forward, giving them your full attention and saying 'Mmh', 'Yes' or 'Sure' every now and then.

- **Concerns.** Patients often worry about the possibility of a serious underlying condition, such as cancer. Explore whether there are particular reasons why the patient is concerned (e.g. reading a newspaper article, diagnosis of cancer in a friend or relative, the presence of risk factors such as smoking).

- **Avoidance of leading questions.** Try not to use leading questions, such as, 'You haven't passed any black tarry stools, have you?'.

History of the presenting complaint

- **Closed questions.** Closed questions are useful for collating and clarifying further details about the patient's problem (e.g. 'Where exactly does it hurt?', 'When exactly did you first notice your symptoms?', 'What were you doing when your pain started?').

- **Selective questioning.** Let further questions, following possible diagnostic lines, be guided by the probabilities of underlying conditions.

- **Effect on life.** Explore how symptoms have affected the patient's life (e.g. 'How has this pain affected your daily life?', 'Is there anything that you can't do because of your symptoms?', 'How are things at home?').

- **Open-mindedness.** Avoid making immediate assumptions and having preconceived ideas about the problem and possible underlying diagnoses.

- **Patient cues.** Avoid changing the topic when a patient presents important information that needs further exploration (e.g. Patient: 'Yesterday, I bled so much that I stained my sofa, which was very embarrassing.' Doctor: 'So, tell me: have you lost any weight?').

- **Patient-centredness.** Continue to be led by what the patient wants to talk about, and show flexibility. Strive to let the consultation progress fluently and logically.

- **Natural manner.** Avoid interrogating the patient by using formulaic phrases or questions that sound unnatural. Being natural will allow them to speak openly.

Ideas, concerns and expectations
- **Important health beliefs.** Make sure you explore the patient's health beliefs, preferences and understanding – their 'ideas, concerns and expectations' (ICE). Try to avoid formulaic questions or questions that sound 'scripted', such as, 'What worries you?'. Sometimes, stating what other people have felt in the patient's situation can help (e.g. 'When my friend John was diagnosed with depression, he...').
- **Ideas.** Explore the patient's ideas with questions like, 'Have you had any thoughts about what might be causing your symptoms?', 'Have you had any ideas about what might be going on?' or 'What do you think may be happening with you?'.
- **Concerns.** Ask about the patient's worries and concerns (e.g. 'Is there anything in particular about your symptoms that's worrying you?', 'What do you think is the worst thing that your symptoms might mean?').
- **Expectations.** Find out what the patient expects from the consultation (e.g. 'Have you had any thoughts about what we might be able to achieve today?').
- **Dealing with ICE.** Make sure you pick up and deal with the patient's ICE later in the consultation, to demonstrate that you take them seriously and that you will take them into account when considering management options.

Asking direct or sensitive questions
- **Explain your questions.** Consider warning the patient before you ask a series of closed questions (e.g. 'Would it be OK if I asked you a few specific questions about your symptoms now?', 'Just so that I can get a better idea of what might be going on and to rule out a serious problem, I'd like to ask you some more questions. Would that be OK?', 'Is it OK if I asked you a more sensitive/personal/private question now?').
- **Clarify details.** Ask the patient to explain any 'jargon' (e.g. 'What do you mean by diarrhoea/dizziness/constipation?'). Go back if necessary, by saying, 'Is it OK if, just to clarify things, we go back a little and talk about...again?'.
- **Show empathy.** Consider making reflective statements when it is appropriate (e.g. 'This must be very difficult for you', 'You seem quite anxious/angry/upset about this', 'You seem to find it quite hard to talk about this', 'This must be a very difficult situation for you').
- **Ask the patient.** Ask the patient what question they would like you to ask next, then ask it. Or, after summarising your findings, ask, 'Is there anything important that you think I've missed out?'. Such questions can help reveal issues that are particularly important to your patient.
- **Frame the consultation.** Try to reframe the consultation by using the patient's own language before you move on to discuss the management plan.

Key references and further reading

1. Kenny D. Some key suggested phrases for consultations. Available from: http://damiankenny.co.uk/listofphrases.doc (last accessed 29 April 2016).
2. Khan I. *Focused Clinical Assessment in 10 Minutes for MRCGP.* Radcliffe Publishing, London; 2012.
3. Schroeder K, Chan W-S, Fahey TP. Focused clinical assessment. *InnovAiT* 2011;4(1):41–48.

Red flags in general practice

Key thoughts

Practical points

- **Definition.** Red flags are alarm or warning symptoms, signs and diagnostic test results that suggest a potentially serious underlying disease.
- **Diagnosis.** Being able to spot red flags can help with ruling in and ruling out serious diagnoses, such as cancer, myocardial infarction or stroke.
- **Test.** Red flags can be regarded as 'diagnostic tests', in that their presence or absence can help adjust the probability of serious diagnoses.
- **Call to action.** In primary care, further investigation or referral is often required when red flags are present.

Red flags in context

- **Duration.** Symptoms that are usually harmless and are often caused by self-limiting illnesses, such as cough, tiredness or diarrhoea, can develop into red flags when they last longer than expected (approximately 4–6 weeks) (e.g. in patients with cancer). Be suspicious when symptoms are progressive (e.g. worsening breathlessness or abdominal pain).
- **Associated features.** Interpret red flags in the context of the history, because their significance depends on the circumstances in which they develop.
- **Demographics.** Take demographic characteristics such as age into account when interpreting red flags, because some diagnoses (e.g. certain cancers, myocardial infarction) are more common in later life.
- **Clinical signs.** The presence or absence of additional clinical features provides important contextual information when considering serious underlying conditions and associated red flags. Checking and monitoring vital signs, such as pulse rate, respiratory rate, blood pressure, temperature and oxygen saturation in the periphery, can often yield useful clues.

Spotting and interpreting red flags

The role of red flags

- **Clinical practice.** Identifying and interpreting red flags is an important part of clinical practice.
- **Over-interpretation.** Wrongly over-interpreting the significance of a red flag can lead to over-referral and may increase patient anxiety.
- **Missing red flags.** Not spotting or ignoring red flags may result in missed diagnoses or, in the worst case, death.

The 10-Minute Clinical Assessment, Second Edition. Knut Schroeder.
© 2017 John Wiley & Sons, Ltd. Published 2017 by John Wiley & Sons, Ltd.

- **Referral.** The presence or absence of red flags can help decide whether a referral needs to be immediate, urgent (within 2 weeks) or routine.
- **Early disease.** In the early stages of conditions such as cancer, symptoms can be nonspecific and difficult to spot. Be vigilant to the early warning signs, such as loss of appetite, weight loss, malaise, lethargy, fever or sweats, generalised itching, shortness of breath, bone pain and lymphadenopathy.

Reasons for missing red flags

- **Lack of attention.** Beware of paying too much attention to other findings and ruling out a serious diagnosis prematurely. This can happen easily if a patient presents with two or more different problems at the same time.
- **Lack of knowledge.** It is easy to miss red flags when you are unaware of their significance for the underlying diagnosis.
- **Not listening.** Avoid missing clues by listening carefully to the patient's story. Do not rush. Avoid suppressing evidence that does not seem to fit.
- **Follow-up.** Make sure you reassess a patient if the working diagnosis does not fit. A useful rule of thumb is to perform a full review (perhaps together with a colleague), arrange further investigation or refer to a specialist if the patient's symptoms persists after two alternative diagnoses have been considered.

Useful techniques for identifying red flags

- **Open questions.** Use open questions and start generally (e.g. 'What can I do for you?'), before engaging in further open probing (e.g. 'Can you tell me more about your symptoms and how they started?', 'Is there anything else that you think may be important?', 'What happened then?').
- **Reasons for consulting.** Establish the reason why the patient has come, then explore all their presenting symptoms in detail.
- **Vigilance.** Be vigilant to the presence of red flags at all times, and actively search for important 'hidden' red flags: in defiance of their name, red flags are not always obvious!
- **Symptom combinations.** Be aware of important symptom combinations that may suggest serious underlying disease (e.g. older age AND tiredness AND weight loss AND rectal bleeding may suggest bowel cancer).

Key references and further reading

1. Hamilton W. The CAPER studies: five case-control studies aimed at identifying and quantifying the risk of cancer in symptomatic primary care patients. *Br J Cancer* 2009;101:580–586.
2. Hamilton W, Peters TJ. *Cancer Diagnosis in Primary Care.* Churchill Livingstone Elsevier, Oxford; 2007.
3. National Institute for Health and Care Excellence (NICE). Suspected cancer: recognition and referral. NICE guidelines [NG12]. June 2015. Available from: http://www.nice.org.uk/guidance/ng12 (last accessed 29 April 2016).
4. Schroeder K, Chan W-S, Fahey TP. Recognising red flags in general practice. *InnovAiT* 2011;4(3):171–176.

Undifferentiated and miscellaneous presentations

Suspected cancer

Key thoughts

Practical points

- **Diagnosis.** Diagnosing cancer early on clinical grounds alone can be difficult. It is important to think about the possibility of cancer if symptoms are unusual or persistent. A number of cancers may present with typical features.
- **Referral.** Early diagnosis of cancer will in many cases improve the prognosis. Symptoms and signs of cancer should prompt urgent referral for further investigation and management.

RED FLAGS

- Unusual symptom patterns
- No improvement of symptoms over time
- New-onset alarm symptoms (e.g. haematuria, haemoptysis, dysphagia or rectal bleeding)
- Three or more consultations for the same problem

History

Ideas, concerns and expectations

- **Ideas.** Explore the patient's knowledge and beliefs about cancer – there are many myths about the disease.
- **Concerns.** Patients often worry about the possibility of cancer. Explore any particular reasons why the patient is concerned (e.g. reading a newspaper article, diagnosis of cancer in a friend or relative, the presence of risk factors such as smoking).
- **Expectations.** What does the patient expect in terms of investigation and treatment?

History of presenting complaint

- **Onset.** Symptoms of cancer usually start gradually and develop over weeks and months.
- **Progression.** Aggressive tumours may grow and spread rapidly.
- **Severity and quality of life.** How severe are the symptoms and how far do they affect the quality of life? Are there any activities that the patient cannot do anymore?
- **Context.** How do the symptoms fit into the context of the patient's life?

The 10-Minute Clinical Assessment, Second Edition. Knut Schroeder.
© 2017 John Wiley & Sons, Ltd. Published 2017 by John Wiley & Sons, Ltd.

Nonspecific symptoms

- **Weight and appetite.** Progressive, unintentional and unexplained weight loss with or without reduced appetite may indicate cancer, particularly if there is no other obvious physical or psychological cause.
- **Nausea and vomiting.** These are particularly common with upper gastrointestinal cancers.
- **Tiredness.** Fatigue is a common nonspecific symptom of many cancers (especially haematological ones), but may also be due to iron-deficiency anaemia caused by, for example, gastrointestinal tumours.
- **Fever and night sweats.** Particularly common with haematological cancers.
- **Lymphadenopathy.** Swollen lymph nodes are commonly due to infection, but may also be caused by lymphoma or metastatic disease.
- **Infections.** Cancer may affect the immune system, which increases the risk of concomitant and recurrent infections.

Risk factors for cancer

- **Smoking.** Smoking is linked to various cancers, particularly lung, bladder and cervix cancer.
- **Age.** Many cancers become more common with age.
- **Toxins.** Ask about drug use, as well as industrial and occupational exposures. Certain chemicals are risk factors for bladder cancer. Alcohol and chronic hepatitis may lead to liver cancer. Asbestos exposure may cause lung cancer.
- **Previous cancer.** Always ask about a past history of cancer, as this increases the risk of recurrence.

Lung cancer

- **Cough.** A chronic, persistent and treatment-resistant cough is a common presenting symptom.
- **Haemoptysis.** This is an important symptom in smokers or ex-smokers over the age of 40.
- **Hoarseness.** This may occur if the recurrent laryngeal nerve is affected.
- **Other chest symptoms.** Ask about chest pain, shortness of breath and shoulder and arm pain (Pancoast tumour).
- **Underlying respiratory problem.** Ask about any unexplained changes in existing symptoms if there is an underlying chronic respiratory problem such as asthma or chronic obstructive pulmonary disease (COPD).

Upper gastrointestinal cancer

- **Gastrointestinal symptoms.** Important symptoms are unexplained upper abdominal pain in conjunction with weight loss (with or without back pain), chronic gastrointestinal bleeding, dyspepsia, dysphagia and persistent vomiting.
- **Jaundice.** The presence of jaundice should raise concern, particularly if it is associated with other gastrointestinal symptoms.
- **Anaemia.** Unexplained iron-deficiency anaemia suggests possible upper or lower gastrointestinal cancer.

Lower gastrointestinal cancer
- **Rectal bleeding.** Fresh blood dripping into the toilet pan is common with haemorrhoids. Rectal bleeding raises the possibility of cancer if it is associated with a change in bowel habit to looser stools (without anal symptoms), as well as in patients aged over 40. Any rectal bleeding in patients over the age of 60 is suspicious. Blood mixed with stool is suggestive of a higher lesion.
- **Change in bowel habit.** Looser stools and/or increased stool frequency persisting for 6 weeks or more and without anal symptoms are suggestive of malignancy, particularly in patients over the age of 40 and/or if associated with rectal bleeding.

Breast cancer
- **Breast lump.** Consider breast cancer if a lump persists after the next period, presents after the menopause or enlarges.
- **Family history.** There may be a positive family history.
- **Past history.** Ask about a past history of breast cancer.
- **Skin changes.** Ask about nipple distortion, nipple discharge (particularly if blood is present) and unilateral eczematous skin changes that do not respond to topical treatment.

Gynaecological cancer
- **Post-menopausal bleeding.** This should raise suspicions if the woman is not on hormone replacement therapy, continues to bleed 6 weeks after stopping therapy or is taking tamoxifen.
- **Vaginal discharge.** Women with vaginal discharge should be offered a full pelvic examination, including visual assessment of the cervix.
- **Vague, unexplained abdominal symptoms.** Bloating, constipation, abdominal pain, back pain and urinary symptoms may all suggest ovarian cancer (particularly in women over 50 years of age), although benign causes are much more common.
- **Intermenstrual bleeding.** Ask about any persistent intermenstrual bleeding and alterations in the menstrual cycle. Is there postcoital bleeding?
- **Vulva.** Any unexplained vulval lump or bleeding vulval ulceration is suspicious.

Urological cancer
- **Urinary symptoms.** In men, ask about lower urinary tract symptoms such as hesitancy, poor stream and haematuria. Is a recent prostate-specific antigen (PSA) result available? Recurrent or persistent urinary tract infection, particularly if associated with haematuria, may suggest cancer.
- **Testicular mass.** Any swelling or mass in the body of the testis is suspicious.
- **Penis.** Signs of penile carcinoma include progressive ulceration in the glans, shaft or prepuce of the penis. Lumps within the corpora cavernosa can indicate Peyronie's disease.

Haematological cancer

- **General symptoms.** Consider haematological cancer if there are symptoms such as night sweats, bruising, fatigue, fever, weight loss, generalised itching, breathlessness, recurrent infections, bone pain, alcohol-induced pain or abdominal pain, either alone or in combination.
- **Back pain.** Spinal cord compression or renal failure may occur with myeloma and will require immediate referral.

Skin cancer

- **Non-healing skin lesions.** Any non-healing keratinising or crusted tumour larger than 1 cm with induration on palpation should raise suspicion of skin cancer.
- **Sun exposure.** Ask for details about previous sun exposure and frequency of sunburns.
- **Features of melanoma.**
  - Change in size.
  - Change in colour.
  - Irregular shape and borders.
  - Irregular and dark pigmentation.
  - Largest diameter 7 mm or more.
  - Change in sensation/itching.
  - Bleeding.

Head and neck cancer

- **Lumps.** Any unexplained lump in the neck of recent onset or a previously undiagnosed lump that has changed over a period of 3–6 weeks is suspicious. Also of concern are unexplained and persistent swellings of the parotid or submandibular gland.
- **Pain.** An unexplained persistent sore or painful throat or other pain in the head or neck for more than 4 weeks may suggest underlying cancer, particularly if associated with otalgia and normal otoscopy.
- **Ulcers.** Any unexplained mouth ulcer, mass or patches of the oral mucosa persisting for more than 3 weeks are suspicious, particularly if there is associated swelling or bleeding.
- **Thyroid swelling.** Any solitary nodule increasing in size, a history of neck irradiation, a family history of endocrine malignancy, unexplained hoarseness or voice changes, cervical lymphadenopathy or lumps in prepubertal patients or patients over 65 years of age raise the possibility of thyroid cancer.
- **Other symptoms.** Unexplained loosening of teeth or hoarseness persisting for more than 3 weeks requires further investigation or referral. Heavy drinkers and smokers over the age of 50 are especially at risk.

Brain tumour

- **Headaches.** Look out for features of raised intracranial pressure (e.g. vomiting, drowsiness, posture-related headache), pulse-synchronous tinnitus or other neurological symptoms, including blackout and change in personality or cognitive function. Any headache that is worse in the morning and gets progressively worse or changes its character should raise suspicions.

- **Central nervous system (CNS) symptoms.** Consider the possibility of brain tumour if there is progressive neurological deficit, new-onset seizure, mental change, cranial nerve palsy or unilateral sensorineural deafness.

Features suggestive of metastasis
- **Brain.** Ask about new and persistent headaches, fits or any change in personality (see also section on Brain Tumour).
- **Bone.** Bone pain due to malignancy is often intermittent at first and then becomes constant. It commonly keeps patients awake at night. Pathological fractures may occur.
- **Liver.** Metastases may not cause any symptoms. Features can include anorexia, fevers, nausea, jaundice, right upper quadrant pain, sweats and weight loss.
- **Skin.** Skin lesions may present as new nodules or as non-healing ulcerative lesions.

Social history
- **Home.** Ask about the patient's family circumstances and support network. Are home life and hobbies affected by any of the symptoms?
- **Work.** Are there any problems with work? Ask about exposure to carcinogens, including asbestos, which is a risk factor for lung cancer and mesothelioma.

Review of previous investigations
- **Full blood count.** A recent full blood count showing unexplained anaemia with haemoglobin of <11 g/dl in men and 10 g/dl in women suggests the possibility of cancer. A blood film may suggest haematological cancer.
- **Inflammatory markers.** Raised plasma viscosity or C-reactive protein (CRP) suggests a general inflammatory response.
- **PSA.** A raised PSA can indicate prostate cancer, particularly if values have been rising and if there are associated urinary symptoms.
- **Chest X-ray.** Look for opacities suggesting primary lung cancer or metastases. Pleural effusion and slowly resolving consolidation can be signs of lung cancer.
- **Smear test.** In women, check results from the last smear test. Does the patient take part in a screening programme?
- **Mammogram.** In women, are results from a previous mammogram available?
- **Barium enema, colonoscopy or gastroscopy.** Ulcerative colitis and polyposis coli increase the risk of colorectal cancer.

Examination

General
- **General condition.** Look for evidence of muscle wasting and assess general nutritional status.
- **Finger clubbing.** This may indicate primary or secondary lung cancer.

Vital signs
- **Temperature.** Raised temperature can occur with some cancers or if there is associated infection.
- **Respiratory rate.** Stridor and tachypnoea are late signs of lung cancer.

Skin
- **Inspection.** Look for evidence of metastasis, such as nodules and other new or non-healing lesions.

Head and neck
- **Sclerae.** Look for jaundice (biliary obstruction, liver involvement).
- **Palpate lymph nodes.** Cervical or supraclavicular lymphadenopathy may be present in cancers such as lung cancer and lymphoma. Lymph nodes that persist for 6 weeks or more, increase in size, are >2 cm in size, are widespread and are associated with splenomegaly ± weight loss may indicate haematological cancer.
- **Face and neck swelling.** Facial swelling with fixed elevation of jugular venous pressure can indicate superior vena cava obstruction (advanced cancer).

Chest
- **Lungs.** Listen for any chest signs that might be caused by lung cancer (e.g. bronchial breathing, monophonic wheeze).
- **Breasts.** In women, consider checking the breasts for lumps. Consider cancer in women of any age if there is a discrete hard lump with or without fixation or skin tethering. Is there any nipple distortion or obvious discharge?

Abdomen
- **Palpation.** Search systematically for an epigastric (e.g. stomach cancer) or right-sided (e.g. colon cancer) lower abdominal mass.
- **Liver and spleen.** Liver metastases may be impossible to detect clinically. Hepatosplenomegaly may occur with haematological cancers.
- **Rectal examination.** A rectal examination is important in the work-up of any patient with unexplained symptoms relating to the lower gastrointestinal or urogenital tract. Important features are inflammatory or obstructive lower urinary tract symptoms, erectile dysfunction, haematuria, lower back pain, bone pain and weight loss (especially in the elderly). A palpable intraluminal rectal mass suggests cancer of the rectum. A pelvic mass outside the bowel is more suggestive of urological or gynaecological cancer. In men, assess the size, consistency and regularity of the prostate gland.

Vaginal examination in women with symptoms suggestive of cancer
- **Inspection.** Look for any obvious vulval ulceration.

• **Pelvic examination, including speculum assessment.** This should be performed in all women who present with alterations of the menstrual cycle, intermenstrual bleeding, postcoital bleeding, post-menopausal bleeding or vaginal discharge. Search in particular for any adnexal or uterine masses, the presence of vaginal discharge and signs of cervical cancer.

Lower limbs
• **Leg swelling.** Cancer is a risk factor for deep venous thrombosis.

Key references and further reading
1. Hamilton W, Peters TJ. *Cancer Diagnosis in Primary Care.* Churchill Livingstone Elsevier, Oxford; 2007.
2. Jones R, Latinovic R, Charlton J, Gulliford M. Alarm symptoms in early diagnosis of cancer in primary care: cohort study using General Practice Research Database. *BMJ* 2007;334:1040–1044.
3. National Institute for Health and Care Excellence (NICE). Suspected cancer: recognition and referral. NICE guidelines [NG12]. June 2015. Available from: http://www.nice.org.uk/guidance/ng12 (last accessed 29 April 2016).
4. Okkes LM, Oskam SK, Lamberts H. The probability of specific diagnoses for patients presenting with common symptoms to Dutch family physicians. *J Fam Pract* 2002;51:31–36.

Weight loss

Key thoughts

Practical points
- **Diagnosis.** Weight loss is a common presentation that, if unexplained, raises the possibility of underlying pathology.
- **Prognosis.** Unexplained and persistent weight loss is an important presenting symptom of cancer.

Possible causes
- **Gastrointestinal.** Intentional dieting, malnutrition, malabsorption (e.g. coeliac disease), oral problems, inflammatory bowel disease, parasitic bowel infections.
- **Eating disorders.** Anorexia nervosa, bulimia.
- **Drugs.** Many drugs cause anorexia and resulting weight loss.
- **Malignancy.** Particularly colorectal, lung and haematological cancer, as well as tumour spread due to metastases.
- **Infection.** Acute viral infection, human immunodeficiency virus (HIV), tuberculosis (TB).
- **Endocrine/metabolic.** Hyperthyroidism, diabetes mellitus.
- **Mental health.** Depression, stress, alcohol or drug misuse, life events (e.g. bereavement, divorce), dementia.
- **Chronic disease.** Chronic organ failure (e.g. liver, kidneys).

RED FLAGS

- Unexplained and/or rapid weight loss
- Symptoms suggestive of malignancy
- Eating disorders
- Depression
- Abnormal blood tests
- Abnormal physical examination
- Night sweats
- Fever
- Lymphadenopathy
- Past history of cancer

The 10-Minute Clinical Assessment, Second Edition. Knut Schroeder.
© 2017 John Wiley & Sons, Ltd. Published 2017 by John Wiley & Sons, Ltd.

History

Ideas, concerns and expectations

- **Ideas.** What does the patient think is causing the weight loss? Has the patient always lost weight in certain situations?
- **Concerns.** Worries about the possibility of cancer or diabetes are common.
- **Expectations.** Diagnosis of an underlying cause, exclusion of cancer and help with weight gain are common reasons for consultation.

History of presenting complaint

- **Context.** Ask how the weight loss fits into the context of the patient's life.
- **Quality of life.** Ask how the weight loss has affected the patient's quality of life.
- **Onset.** Find out when the weight loss began and whether it has been associated with an acute illness, such as gastroenteritis or pneumonia.
- **Degree of weight loss.** Try to quantify the degree of weight loss by comparing actual weight with previous readings. A loss of 5–10% of body weight suggests significant weight loss. Find out over what period of time the weight loss has occurred. Weight loss tends to be fairly rapid if it has a malignant cause and is accompanied by loss of appetite (although appetite may also be increased).
- **Lifestyle changes.** Ask about any changes in lifestyle that might be responsible for the weight loss, such as a change in exercise, a change in job towards more manual work or a change in diet. In teenagers and younger adults, consider the possibility of an underlying eating disorder, such as bulimia or anorexia nervosa.
- **Mental health.** Depression and anxiety are common causes of weight loss, particularly in the elderly. Ask about recent life events, such as bereavement, divorce, relationship problems or job loss, all of which may lead to reduced appetite.
- **General systemic symptoms.** Ask about lethargy, night sweats, loss of appetite, malaise and generalised lymphadenopathy, which may be symptoms of underlying cancer or other systemic disease (e.g. TB, HIV). Excessive thirst may be a symptom of new-onset diabetes.
- **Gastrointestinal symptoms.** Ask about any change in bowel habit, abdominal pain, abdominal swelling and rectal bleeding. Patients with dyspepsia or constipation may avoid eating for fear of exacerbation of symptoms. Weight loss in association with upper abdominal pain and jaundice may be due to pancreatic cancer.
- **Chest symptoms.** Ask about cough and shortness of breath, which may be caused by respiratory infection or, less commonly, lung cancer. In women, ask about any new breast lumps.
- **Urinary symptoms.** Consider the possibility of chronic urinary infection or prostate cancer if there are persistent lower urinary tract symptoms such as voiding difficulties or frequency of urine. Polyuria may suggest new-onset diabetes.
- **Endocrine symptoms.** Tremor, sweating, diarrhoea and increased sensitivity to heat may be due to hyperthyroidism.

- **Skin.** Ask if any moles have changed recently. Malignant melanoma spreads early and may go undiagnosed for a long time.
- **Additional unexplored issues.** Ask if there are any other problems or issues that you have not covered but which might be important.

Past and current medical problems
- **Cancer.** Consider the possibility of recurrence if there is a past history of cancer.
- **Anaemia.** Previous unexplained anaemia could be due to unidentified malignancy.
- **Thyrotoxicosis.** Previously treated thyrotoxicosis may recur even if the patient has received carbimazole or radiotherapy in the past.

Medication
- **Polypharmacy.** This is a common reason for loss of appetite and may interfere with taste perception, particularly in the elderly.
- **Antidepressants.** Some antidepressants may cause loss of appetite. Sedatives may affect eating habits.
- **Diuretics and laxatives.** Overuse may lead to weight loss.

Social history
- **Home.** Has weight loss affected home life in any way?
- **Work.** Has there been any effect of weight loss on the ability to work?

Alcohol, smoking and 'recreational drugs'
- **Alcohol.** Excess alcohol intake may lead to appetite suppression and alcoholic liver changes. Depression may result in increased alcohol consumption.
- **Smoking.** Lung and stomach cancer are more common in smokers. Heavy smokers may also have a poor diet, leading to malnutrition.
- **Drug misuse.** Consider the possibility of drug misuse, particularly in younger people.

Review of previous investigations
- **Full blood count.** Iron-deficiency anaemia may be a feature of nutritional deficiency, bowel cancer or occult bleeding. Macrocytosis suggests possible malabsorption or alcohol misuse.
- **Inflammatory markers.** Plasma viscosity may be raised in infection, inflammation or malignancy.
- **Blood glucose.** Is there evidence of underlying diabetes mellitus?
- **Liver and renal function.** Look for evidence of organ failure.
- **PSA.** A raised PSA may point towards prostatic cancer in men.
- **Abdominal ultrasound.** Is there evidence of structural liver or gall bladder disease?
- **Chest X-ray.** Look for evidence of infection and lung cancer (however, a negative chest X-ray does not exclude malignancy in all cases).

Examination

General
- **General condition.** Does the patient look unwell? Cachexia, pallor or jaundice may suggest underlying malignancy. Is there evidence of self-neglect?
- **Lymphadenopathy.** Check for localised or generalised lymphadenopathy.
- **Weight.** Measure weight using accurate scales and compare current weight with any previous readings.
- **Mental state.** Consider a mental state examination if there is dementia, depression and/or eating disorder.

Vital signs
- **Temperature.** Temperature may be raised in infection, severe inflammation or, occasionally, in malignancy.
- **Pulse.** Consider anxiety, infection or anaemia if there is tachycardia. Atrial fibrillation or tachycardia may be caused by hyperthyroidism.
- **Blood pressure.** Check for postural hypotension. Low blood pressure may be present in anorexia nervosa.

Skin
- **Finger clubbing.** This may be present in lung or liver conditions.

Head and neck
- **Eyes.** Look for signs of anaemia and jaundice.
- **Lymph nodes.** Check for lymphadenopathy.

Upper and lower limbs
- **Muscle wasting.** Consider malnutrition, neurological disease or cancer if there is muscle wasting.

Chest
- **Lungs.** Check for signs of infection and cancer (e.g. focal bronchial breathing, monophonic wheeze).
- **Breasts.** In women, consider breast examination for any lumps. Check both axillae for lymphadenopathy.

Abdomen
- **Organs.** Palpate all the major organs for organomegaly.
- **Masses.** Check all areas for any masses or tenderness.
- **Digital rectal examination.** If indicated, check the rectum for any mucosal lesions. In men, assess the prostate for size and consistency.

Bedside tests
- **Urinalysis.** Check for haematuria, proteinuria, glucosuria, nitrites and leucocytes.

Key references and further reading
1. Hamilton W, Peters TJ. *Cancer Diagnosis in Primary Care*. Churchill Livingstone Elsevier, Oxford; 2007.
2. Hernández JL, Riancho JA, Matorras P, Gonzáles-Macías J. Clinical evaluation for cancer in patient with *involuntary weight loss without* specific symptoms. *Am J Med* 2003;114:631–637.
3. Huffman GB. Evaluating and treating unintentional weight loss in the elderly. *Am Fam Physician* 2002;65:640–650.
4. National Institute for Health and Care Excellence (NICE). Suspected cancer: recognition and referral. NICE guidelines [NG12]. June 2015. Available from: http://www.nice.org.uk/guidance/ng12 (last accessed 29 April 2016).

Tiredness

Key thoughts

Practical points

- **Diagnosis.** Tiredness is a common presentation. It rarely occurs due to physical causes. A structured approach to clinical assessment helps to avoid missing any serious organic or psychological conditions, which usually present with additional symptoms and signs.

Possible causes

- **Mental health/lifestyle.** Lack of sleep, young children, working long hours, stress, depression, alcohol and other substance misuse, primary sleep disorder.
- **Idiopathic.** Chronic fatigue syndrome, primary fibromyalgia.
- **Infective.** Postviral fatigue, HIV, TB, syphilis.
- **Anaemia.** Iron deficiency (e.g. menorrhagia), vitamin B12/folate deficiency, pregnancy, malignancy.
- **Respiratory.** Obstructive sleep apnoea, COPD.
- **Organ failure.** Renal, heart or liver failure.
- **Endocrine/metabolic.** Diabetes mellitus, hypothyroidism, hyperthyroidism, Addison's disease (rare), vitamin D deficiency.
- **Drugs.** Sedatives, beta blockers, antidepressants, etc.
- **Malignancy.** Haematological and other cancers.
- **Connective tissue disorders.** Rheumatoid arthritis, polymyalgia rheumatica, myasthenia gravis.
- **Other.** Coeliac disease, systemic lupus erythematosus (SLE), motor neurone disease.

> **RED FLAGS**
>
> - Constitutional features such as weight loss, loss of appetite, fevers, night sweats and lymphadenopathy (serious disease, malignancy)
> - Depression
> - Abnormal physical examination
> - Pain anywhere in the body
> - Disabling tiredness
> - Polyuria and polydipsia (diabetes)

The 10-Minute Clinical Assessment, Second Edition. Knut Schroeder.
© 2017 John Wiley & Sons, Ltd. Published 2017 by John Wiley & Sons, Ltd.

History

Ideas, concerns and expectations
- **Ideas.** What does the patient think might be wrong? This may give important clues about the possible underlying cause.
- **Concerns.** Worries about cancer or 'never getting better' are common.
- **Expectations.** Patients may expect a miracle cure, or just want reassurance that nothing major is wrong with them. What are the patient's attitudes to different treatment options?

History of presenting complaint
- **Context.** How does the symptom of tiredness fit into the context of the patient's life?
- **Quality of life.** Chronic tiredness can be very disabling and may severely impact on the quality of life. Explore the impact of symptoms on daily activities.
- **Description of symptoms.** What does the patient mean by being 'tired'? Differentiate between sleepiness, tiredness, lack of energy and muscle weakness. Chronic fatigue syndrome usually presents with profound physical and cognitive fatigue and exhaustion, which is different from day-to-day tiredness.
- **Onset.** Acute onset is common after viral infection. Chronic development of symptoms may suggest stress, depression or an organic cause.
- **Depression.** Ask about mood, appetite, memory, concentration, energy and suicidal thoughts. Tiredness may in itself cause depressive symptoms. Cognitive impairment, such as poor concentration, memory problems and difficulties with word finding or multiple tasks, may occur in chronic fatigue syndrome.
- **Muscle symptoms.** Muscle aches and pains are common in chronic fatigue syndrome. Consider polymyositis if there is muscle weakness, particularly of the proximal muscle groups. Has climbing stairs or combing hair become more difficult?
- **Malaise.** Flu-like malaise can occur in chronic fatigue syndrome, as well as in organic conditions.
- **Bleeding.** Chronic bleeding may cause iron-deficiency anaemia. Ask in particular about any rectal bleeding, menorrhagia, haematemesis, haematuria or easy bruising.
- **Sleep disturbance.** Is lack of sleep a problem? Ask about early-morning wakening, unrefreshing sleep, hypersomnia and disturbed sleep/wake cycle. Has a sleep partner reported snoring and episodic apnoea (sleep apnoea syndrome)?
- **Digestive problems.** Irritable bowel syndrome often coexists with chronic fatigue syndrome. Ask about indigestion, nausea, flatus, bloating and loss of appetite, alternating constipation and diarrhoea, abdominal cramps and any food intolerance.
- **Exercise.** Tiredness is usually related to exercise in chronic fatigue syndrome, with bursts of activity followed by periods of enforced inactivity ('rollercoaster').
- **Other symptoms.** Ask about weight loss, pains, swollen lymph nodes, fever, headache, loss of appetite, night sweats and sore throat (infection, chronic

inflammation, malignancy). Consider bowel cancer, coeliac disease or other gastrointestinal disorders if there is rectal bleeding or persistent change in bowel habit. Cold intolerance, hair loss, weight gain and constipation may point towards hypothyroidism. Shortness of breath may indicate lung or cardiac conditions.

- **Diet.** Poor diet can lead to iron- or vitamin (B12, folate)-deficiency anaemia, which may present with tiredness.
- **Foreign travel.** Ask about any recent foreign travel (tropical infectious diseases). Has the patient been exposed to TB, or is there a past history of the disease?
- **Additional unexplored issues.** Are there any other problems or issues that you have not covered which might be important?

Past and current medical problems
- **Significant past illnesses.** Ask about any chronic or acute conditions that might be relevant (e.g. heart failure, diabetes, endocrine disorders).

Medication
- **Drugs causing tiredness.** Many drugs can cause tiredness, particularly sedatives, antidepressants, antiepileptics and beta blockers. Have any new drugs been started recently that might be responsible?

Family history
- **Chronic disease.** Ask about a family history of relevant conditions, such as diabetes or cardiovascular disease (CVD).

Social history
- **Home.** How has tiredness affected home life? Are there any activities that the patient cannot do due to feeling tired?
- **Domestic and marital relationships.** Have relationships at home been affected? Lack of libido can lead to marital problems.
- **Work.** Has work been affected? How many days have been taken off sick?

Alcohol, smoking and recreational drugs
- **Alcohol.** Excessive alcohol intake may lead to chronic tiredness and irritability via fragmented sleep. Is there a reason for the patient's drinking more alcohol (e.g. stress)?
- **Smoking.** Heavy smoking is a risk factor for lung cancer, COPD and heart disease, all of which may present with initial tiredness. Tiredness may be the only presenting feature in heart failure.
- **Recreational drugs.** Opioids and other recreational drugs are common causes for tiredness.

Review of previous investigations
- **Full blood count.** Look for anaemia. Microcytosis would suggest iron deficiency, whereas macrocytosis may point towards vitamin deficiency (B12/folate), alcohol

misuse or hypothyroidism. A raised white cell count suggests infection or severe inflammation. A raised platelet count may occur in inflammatory conditions, occasionally in infections and sometimes in cancer. Eosinophilia is a rare but useful clue for Addison's disease (rare), if the patient does not suffer from atopy or parasitic infection.

- **Inflammatory markers.** A raised plasma viscosity or CRP may indicate infection, inflammation or malignancy.
- **Infectious mononucleosis.** Glandular fever can cause tiredness for weeks or months.
- **Liver and renal function.** Check these for any evidence of organ failure. Hyponatraemia may occur with Addison's disease (rare).
- **Glucose.** New-onset diabetes mellitus commonly presents with tiredness.
- **Thyroid function.** Look for evidence of hypo- or hyperthyroidism.
- **Bone profile.** Calcium disorders can present with tiredness. An abnormal bone profile may also be due to malignancy.
- **Creatine kinase.** This may be raised in polymyositis and other muscle disorders.
- **Autoimmune screen.** Has rheumatological disease been tested for in the past? Check if there has been a previous test for coeliac disease (antibodies to tissue transglutaminase).
- **Chest X-ray.** This may show signs of infection, heart failure or malignancy.
- **Electrocardiogram (ECG).** Look for evidence of cardiac hypertrophy and arrhythmias.

Examination

General

- **General condition.** Does the patient look unwell or depressed? Cachexia and pallor may suggest serious disease (e.g. TB, HIV, malignancy). Are there signs of dehydration?
- **Lymphadenopathy.** Cervical or generalised lymphadenopathy suggests infection or malignancy.
- **Signs of liver disease.** Look for jaundice, scratch marks, palmar erythema, spider naevi and injection marks.

Vital signs

- **Temperature.** Raised temperature suggests infection or inflammation.
- **Pulse.** Check rate and rhythm. Atrial fibrillation commonly causes tiredness.
- **Blood pressure.** Blood pressure may be low in Addison's disease (rare). Check for a difference in lying and standing blood pressure (postural hypotension).
- **Respiratory rate.** Tachypnoea may be due to anaemia, infection, heart failure or malignancy.

Skin

- **Colour.** Pale skin suggests anaemia. Is there a yellow tinge, which could indicate hepatic or renal failure?

- **Hair.** Look for evidence of hair loss or thin hair, which can occur in metabolic disturbances (particularly thyroid disease).
- **Nail beds.** Pallor suggests anaemia. Look for splinter haemorrhages (endocarditis – rare).

Head and neck

- **Eyes.** Check conjunctivae for signs of anaemia and sclerae for jaundice. Exophthalmos may rarely be seen in thyroid disease.

Chest

- **Heart.** Check for evidence of atrial fibrillation, cardiomegaly and valvular heart disease.
- **Lungs.** Examine for signs of infection and airway obstruction. Poor air entry suggests emphysema. Basal crackles may be heard in heart failure.

Abdomen

- **Organs.** Hepatomegaly may rarely be found in liver disease, malignancy and rheumatological conditions. Check the spleen for associated splenomegaly.
- **Swelling and masses.** Check all areas for any masses and tenderness. Is there ascites?
- **Rectal and vaginal examination.** If appropriate, check for signs of malignancy and other sources of bleeding (e.g. haemorrhoids). Prostate and bowel cancer should be considered in older men. Consider gynaecological cancers if there are any masses or unusual vaginal bleeding.
- **Genitals.** Check the testes and penis (older men) for evidence of cancer.

Lower limbs

- **Oedema.** Mild leg oedema is common in the elderly. Consider underlying causes, such as heart failure, liver failure, renal impairment and treatment with calcium antagonists.

Bedside tests

- **Urinalysis.** Check for signs of urinary infection, renal disease and diabetes.
- **Blood glucose.** A glucostix test may show hyper- or hypoglycaemia.

Key references and further reading

1. Association for Myalgic Encephalomyelitis. www.afme.org.uk.
2. Carruthers BM, Jain AK, De Meirleir KL et al. Myalgic encephalomyelitis/chronic fatigue syndrome: clinical working case definition, diagnostic and treatment protocols. *J Chronic Fatigue Syndr* 2003;11:7–115.
3. Hamilton W, Peters TJ. *Cancer Diagnosis in Primary Care*. Churchill Livingstone Elsevier, Oxford; 2007.
4. National Institute for Health and Care Excellence (NICE). Chronic fatigue syndrome/myalgic encephalomyelitis. NICE guidelines [NG53]. August 2007.

Available from: http://www.nice.org.uk/Guidance/CG53 (last accessed 29 April 2016).
5. National Institute for Health and Care Excellence (NICE). Suspected cancer: recognition and referral. NICE guidelines [NG12]. June 2015. Available from: http://www.nice.org.uk/guidance/ng12 (last accessed 29 April 2016).
6. National Institute for Health and Care Excellence (NICE). Tiredness/fatigue in adults. Clinical Knowledge Summaries. 2015. Available from: http://cks.nice.org.uk/tirednessfatigue-in-adults (last accessed 29 April 2016).

Dizziness

Key thoughts

Practical points

- **Diagnosis.** Dizziness is a common symptom. It may result from both vestibular and nonvestibular causes. Postural hypotension, benign positional paroxysmal vertigo, vestibular neuronitis and Menière's disease are common. Rarely, serious underlying causes such as acoustic neuroma, multiple sclerosis, tumours or encephalitis need to be considered. Sometimes, no underlying cause can be found.

Possible causes

- **Infection.** Acute viral infection, severe systemic infections.
- **Intoxication.** Alcohol and drug misuse.
- **Ear, nose and throat.** Benign paroxysmal vertigo, vestibular neuronitis, Menière's disease, middle ear disease, ototoxic drugs.
- **Psychogenic.** Hyperventilation (anxiety, depression).
- **Drugs.** Diuretics, selective serotonin reuptake inhibitors (SSRIs).
- **Cardiovascular.** Postural hypotension (pregnancy, elderly), arrhythmias, aortic stenosis.
- **Endocrine/metabolic.** Hypoglycaemia, hyponatraemia, Addison's disease.
- **Neurological.** Vertebrobasilar insufficiency, migraine, multiple sclerosis, epilepsy.
- **Space-occupying lesion.** Acoustic neuroma, CNS tumours.
- **Trauma.** Head injury, surgical.
- **Other.** Systemic disease, carbon monoxide poisoning.

RED FLAGS

- Ear discharge
- Acute trauma
- Suspected cancer
- Progressive symptoms
- Disability and loss of confidence
- Neurological symptoms

The 10-Minute Clinical Assessment, Second Edition. Knut Schroeder.
© 2017 John Wiley & Sons, Ltd. Published 2017 by John Wiley & Sons, Ltd.

History

Ideas, concerns and expectations
- **Ideas.** People with vertigo or dizziness often think that their symptoms are due to a brain tumour or stroke.
- **Concerns.** Dizziness can be very distressing, and patients often fear that their quality of life will be permanently reduced.
- **Expectations.** Explore the patient's expectations with regard to further investigation and treatment.

Common presenting symptoms
- **Vertigo.** Vertigo is an illusion of movement or rotation, commonly caused by vestibular disease. Patients often describe this as the room spinning or as them spinning in space. Vertigo may also be caused by conditions affecting the cervical spine or vertebrobasilar arteries (not usually rotatory and often transient). Associated nausea and vomiting are common. Lack of true vertigo makes a vestibular cause less likely.
- **Imbalance.** A feeling of unsteadiness or 'drunkennesss' (dysequilibrium) and postural discoordination with a fear of or actual falling can indicate both vestibular and nonvestibular disease. To maintain balance, vision, vestibular sensation and proprioception need to be adequate.
- **Faintness.** Faintness can range from lightheadedness to loss of consciousness and is usually not vestibular in origin. A vague description of 'muzzy' or 'fuzzy' head or a pressure inside or outside the head is unlikely to have a vestibular cause.
- **Loss of consciousness.** Regular loss of consciousness in association with dizziness makes a serious cause more likely.

History of presenting complaint
- **Context.** How does the onset of dizziness fit into the context of the patient's life? Are there any obvious reasons for the development of symptoms?
- **Quality of life.** Dizziness symptoms can be very disabling and may severely affect quality of life. Which day-to-day activities are mainly affected?
- **Description of dizziness.** If sensations are described in a vague or nonspecific way (e.g. 'It feels like I am going to pass out'), a nonvestibular or general medical disorder is more likely. 'I feel unsteady on my feet' suggests dysequilibrium. If 'the room spins around me', vertigo is likely.
- **Onset.** Sudden onset of severe vertigo associated with nausea and vomiting suggests vestibular neuronitis. If, in addition, there is hearing loss and tinnitus, involvement of the rest of the labyrinth is likely (labyrinthitis). Symptoms usually improve gradually over a couple of weeks. Further mild attacks may occur over the next few months. This is important for the patient to know, so that they can avoid situations in which loss of balance might be dangerous.
- **Duration.** Vertigo lasting only a few seconds that is associated with certain movements suggests benign paroxysmal positional vertigo. Symptoms become

less severe with repeated stimulation without other otological symptoms or signs, and are usually first noticed on waking. In Ménière's disease, episodes last for minutes to hours, and in vestibular neuronitis, days to weeks.

- **Mental health.** Anxiety is common in association with dizziness. Symptoms such as a feeling of impending doom, déja-vu, claustrophobia or derealisation suggest a mental health problem, rather than a vestibular cause. Check for symptoms of depression or stress.
- **Ear symptoms.** Consider chronic suppurative otitis media or cholesteatoma if there is purulent ear discharge or ear pain. In both these conditions, erosion of the labyrinth may be a complication. Vertigo associated with unilateral hearing loss, tinnitus, aural fullness and vomiting suggests Ménière's disease. Hearing usually returns between attacks, which can last anything from 30 minutes to 12 hours and occur in clusters. Always consider the possibility of acoustic neuroma if there is unilateral hearing loss or tinnitus. Vertigo is a late feature of this condition.
- **Nausea and vomiting.** Nausea and vomiting are common problems in association with dizziness and may make it impossible for the patient to take oral medication.
- **Trauma.** A fracture of the temporal bone due to head injury may involve the labyrinth. Barotrauma can cause rupture of the round or oval windows, leading to vertigo, hearing loss and tinnitus. Bloodstained or clear discharge due to cerebrospinal fluid (CSF) leak may suggest temporal bone injury after trauma. Perilymph leakage may occur after middle ear surgery, resulting in vertigo and hearing loss.
- **Precipitating factors.** Reduced blood flow in atheromatous vertebral arteries associated with cervical spondylosis and loss of proprioception in spinal degenerative disease may cause an illusion of movement when the neck is moved rapidly or hyperextended. In contrast to vestibular problems, this effect is usually caused by movement and is transient.
- **Visual problems.** Poor vision can cause balance problems. It is important that patients are formally assessed by an optician or ophthalmologist if there is any associated visual loss.

Past and current medical problems
- **Ear disease.** Ask about previous ear disease and surgery involving the ears or other parts of the head.
- **Chronic conditions.** Are there any chronic conditions, such as heart, lung or neck problems, that may contribute to or exacerbate dizziness?

Medication
- **Vestibular sedatives.** Have these already been prescribed for treatment of vertigo? Buccal, rectal or intramuscular preparations may need to be considered if the patient cannot take oral medication due to nausea and vomiting. Extrapyramidal adverse effects may occur, particularly in young people and the elderly, in whom long-term use should be avoided.

- **Sedatives.** Sedatives and hypnotics may affect balance, particularly in conjunction with alcohol.
- **Aminoglycosides.** Given at high doses or over prolonged periods of time, aminoglycosides may cause ototoxicity and balance problems.

Other treatments
- **Vestibular rehabilitation.** Vestibular rehabilitation programmes can help with vestibular compensation in vestibular disorders.

Social history
- **Home.** Have the symptoms caused any significant problems with coping at home?
- **Work.** Has work been affected? Is a sick note needed?

Alcohol, smoking and recreational drugs
- **Alcohol.** Acute and chronic alcohol misuse commonly leads to balance problems.

Review of previous investigations
- **Full blood count.** Anaemia may lead to dizziness. A low mean corpuscular volume (MCV) suggests iron deficiency. Consider alcohol misuse, hypothyroidism or vitamin B12/folate deficiency if there is macrocytosis.
- **Renal function.** Check for hyponatraemia and renal disease.
- **Liver function.** Abnormal liver tests may be caused by excess alcohol consumption.
- **Blood sugar.** Look for evidence of diabetes.
- **ECG.** Look for any underlying arrhythmia.
- **Echocardiography.** This is helpful for excluding structural heart lesions (e.g. aortic stenosis).
- **Electroencephalogram (EEG) and computerised tomography (CT) of the head.** These may have been arranged in the past for investigation of possible epilepsy.

Examination

General
- **Gait and balance.** Does the patient walk steadily when coming into the room? Ataxia rather than vertigo is one of the main findings in cerebellar disease. Check heel-to-toe walking.
- **Hyperventilation.** If you suspect psychogenic dizziness, ask the patient to hyperventilate. This will reproduce the symptoms immediately.

Vital signs

- **Pulse.** Check the pulse for any arrhythmia. Rarely, central lesions may cause bradycardia.
- **Blood pressure.** Check lying and standing blood pressures (postural hypotension).
- **Temperature.** Consider infection if the temperature is raised.
- **Respiration rate.** There may be mild tachypnoea in anxiety and hyperventilation syndrome.

Cerebellar function and balance

- **Romberg's test.** In recent vestibular lesions, the patient may sway to one side when standing with the feet together, arms by the side and eyes closed. Remember that a positive test is not specific for vestibular lesions.
- **Unterberger's test.** Suspect a cerebellar lesion if the patient moves a metre forward or backward or if they turn more than 30° when asked to march on the spot with arms outstretched to the front and eyes closed.

Head and neck

- **Neck movement.** Do specific neck movements bring on symptoms?
- **Otoscopy.** Exclude suppurative middle ear disease. Look for impacted wax and evidence of cholesteatoma.
- **Rinne and Weber test.** If indicated, these can help distinguish between sensorineural and conductive hearing loss.
- **Fistula test.** Pressure on the tragus may induce vertigo if there is an abnormal connection (fistula) between the middle ear and the vestibular labyrinth.
- **Cranial nerves.** Look particularly for nystagmus in both the horizontal and vertical planes (make sure that you move your finger slowly). Nystagmus may indicate benign postural vertigo. Nystagmus at lateral gaze >30° is normal. Any nystagmus that is vertical or changes direction is suggestive of a central lesion. Check eye movements, corneal reflex and facial movements.
- **Fundi.** Check for papilloedema (raised intracranial pressure).
- **Carotids.** Bruits may suggest carotid artery disease.
- **Dix–Hallpike manoeuvre.** This can be useful for diagnosing benign paroxysmal positional vertigo and other causes of positional nystagmus. This manoeuvre is contraindicated if the patient has cervical spine problems (see box).

DIX–HALLPIKE MANOEUVRE

- Explain the procedure, stressing that the patient will not fall. Have a sick bowl ready.
- Position the patient sitting upright on the examination couch, just far enough away from the head end to allow the head to be lowered over it.
- Hold the head firmly and turn it in the horizontal plane towards the ear being tested until it is positioned at 45° to the shoulders.

- Next, lay the patient backwards until the head is 30° below the horizontal edge of the couch.
- While still holding the head, look for nystagmus and ask if this movement causes vertigo. In a positive test, the nystagmus will usually be rotatory and directed to the undermost ear (i.e. the side of the affected vestibular organ).
- If after 30 seconds there is no vertigo or nystagmus, return the patient to the upright position and look again for nystagmus, while asking about vertigo.
- If the test is negative after 30 seconds, repeat the same manoeuvre on the opposite side.

Chest
- **Heart.** Listen for aortic stenosis and other abnormalities and confirm the heart rate.

Limbs
- **Neurology.** Assess tone, power, sensation, coordination and reflexes. Loss of sensation may give a feeling of dizziness or unsteadiness. Any abnormalities may point towards a central cause. In the absence of dysdiadochokinesis, significant cerebellar disease is unlikely.
- **Vascular.** Check peripheral pulses and capillary refill.
- **Feet.** Any ulcers or fungal infections may suggest underlying diabetes mellitus.

Bedside tests
- **Urinalysis.** Check for glucose, as diabetes may cause dizziness (autonomic neuropathy, dehydration, changes in blood sugar).

Key references and further reading
1. Froehling DA, Silverstein MD, Mohr DN, Beatty CW. Does this patient have a serious form of vertigo? *JAMA* 1994;271:385–388.
2. Hanley K, O'Dowd T. Symptoms of vertigo in general practice: a prospective study of diagnosis. *Br J Gen Pract* 2002;52:809–812.
3. Hanley K, O'Dowd T, Considine N. A systematic review of vertigo in primary care. *Br J Gen Pract* 2001;51:666–671.
4. Kanagalingam J, Hajioff D, Bennett S. Vertigo: 10-minute consultation. *BMJ* 2005;330:523.
5. National Institute for Health and Care Excellence (NICE). Vertigo. Clinical Knowledge Summaries. 2010. Available from: http://cks.nice.org.uk/vertigo (last accessed 29 April 2016).
6. National Institute for Health and Care Excellence (NICE). Vestibular neuronitis. Clinical Knowledge Summaries. 2011. Available from: http://cks.nice.org.uk/vestibular-neuronitis (last accessed 29 April 2016).
7. National Institute for Health and Care Excellence (NICE). Meniere's disease. Clinical Knowledge Summaries. 2012. Available from: http://cks.nice.org.uk/menieres-disease (last accessed 29 April 2016).

Chronic pain

Key thoughts

Practical points
- **Diagnosis.** Many patients suffer from pain that persists even without significant tissue damage. Management can be difficult and requires a structured physical and psychological assessment.
- **Impact.** It is important to establish the impact of pain on physical and mental well being and to assess treatment response.

Possible causes
- Inflammation.
- Infection.
- Trauma.
- Ischaemia.
- Cancer.

> ### RED FLAGS
>
> - Unexplained weight loss, fever or night sweats
> - Systemic illness
> - History of violent trauma
> - Associated depression and poor social contacts
> - Reduced activity with avoidance behaviour
> - History of cancer, drug misuse or HIV infection
> - Immunosuppression or systemic steroids

History

Ideas, concerns and expectations
- **Ideas.** What does the patient think is causing the pain? What are the patient's beliefs about the pain? What is the patient's attitude towards any underlying diagnoses? How much does the patient know about the cause(s) of their pain and its management? Has any educational material been provided? Is the patient aware of self-help strategies?
- **Concerns.** Explore any fears in relation to the pain. Anxiety and depression can lower the pain threshold.
- **Expectations.** What has been the response to help in the past? Are expectations about the effectiveness of treatments realistic?

The 10-Minute Clinical Assessment, Second Edition. Knut Schroeder.
© 2017 John Wiley & Sons, Ltd. Published 2017 by John Wiley & Sons, Ltd.

History of presenting complaint
- **Context.** Ask about the circumstances at the time when the pain started, which might provide diagnostic clues. Was there any mental or physical trauma? How does the pain fit into the context of this patient's life?
- **Site.** The location of the pain may point towards a specific cause. Consider referred pain from other sites.
- **Character.** Nociceptive pain tends to be aching, sharp, dull or tender, whereas neuropathic pain is commonly described as burning or tingling.
- **Onset.** Did the pain start suddenly or gradually?
- **Severity.** How severe is the pain? Ask the patient to score the pain on a scale from 0 to 10, with 0 being no pain and 10 being the worst pain imaginable.
- **Progression.** Is the pain getting better, getting worse or staying the same? Worsening and constant pain should raise suspicions of a more serious underlying cause.
- **Precipitating factors.** Ask about precipitating and relieving factors. Pain may have been caused by an injury or disease. There may also be an increase in baseline sensitivity in response to an acute injury. Pain is said to be maladaptive if it continues beyond recovery from the original injury or disease.
- **Additional unexplored issues.** Ask if there are any other problems or issues that you have not covered which might be important.

Impact on the quality of life
- **Physical effects.** How does the chronic pain affect physical health and mobility? Is sleep affected?
- **Emotional effects.** How does the pain affect mental well being? Ask about symptoms of depression and anxiety.
- **Daily activities.** Ask details about the impact of the pain on the patient's daily activities, including routine tasks around the house, work and leisure.
- **Role functioning.** How does the patient cope with different roles in their life, such as being a partner, parent, carer or worker? What is the impact of pain on sexual function and relationships in general?
- **Social considerations.** Do social or financial problems result from the pain? Explore any problems in the family or problems with social isolation. To what extent is self-esteem affected?

Past and current medical problems
- **Treatable conditions.** Are there any potentially treatable underlying conditions (e.g. endometriosis, arthritis)?

Medication
- **Analgesics.** What drugs have been tried so far, and which have been most successful? Is there potential opioid overuse? Past treatment failures may be due to poor medication adherence, adverse effects or inadequate doses.
- **Over-the-counter medicines.** Consider oral and topical over-the-counter medications.

Other treatments
- **Complementary treatments.** Have complementary therapies been tried?
- **Other health professionals.** Have other health professionals, including hospital specialists, physiotherapists, massage therapists and acupuncturists, been involved in managing the pain? If so, has any treatment proved particularly effective?

Allergies
- **Analgesia.** Ask about allergies and intolerances to analgesics.

Social history
- **Family.** Enquire about family relationships and support networks. Is any additional help needed? Social isolation can have a negative impact on pain.
- **Physical activity and creativity.** How much does the pain affect the ability to exercise or follow other interests?

Review of previous investigations
- **Imaging.** Look out for any previous imaging results, including radiography, ultrasound and other scans.
- **Blood tests.** Have any recent blood tests shown abnormalities (e.g. signs of infection or inflammation)?

Examination

General
- **Identify a treatable cause.** One of the main aims of the physical examination is to identify a potentially treatable underlying cause.

Vital signs
- **Temperature.** Check the temperature if infection is a possibility.

Skin
- **Inspection.** Look for any obvious signs of trauma, infection or inflammation, as guided by the history.

Head and neck
- **Inspection.** Look for any obvious abnormalities, as guided by the history.
- **Movements.** Pain often leads to muscular tension and may lead to headaches and other secondary pains. Check movement of the cervical spine.

Other systems, as guided by the history

- **Inspection.** Look for obvious causes of pain.
- **Palpation.** Palpate the underlying structures and look for tenderness and increased temperature. Consider fibromyalgia if there is pain in relevant trigger areas.
- **Movement.** Check movement in all relevant joints.
- **Neurological.** Check sensation in relevant areas. Is there evidence of allodynia (pain caused by a stimulus that is not normally painful), dysaesthesia (abnormal and unpleasant sensation), hyperalgesia (increased response to painful stimulus) or paraesthesia (abnormal sensation)?

Key references and further reading

1. Carrington Reid M, Eccleston C, Pillemer K. Management of chronic pain in older adults. *BMJ* 2015;350:h532.
2. Hamilton W, Peters T. *Cancer Diagnosis in Primary Care*. Churchill Livingstone Elsevier, Oxford; 2007.
3. National Institute for Health and Care Excellence (NICE). Palliative cancer care – pain. Clinical Knowledge Summaries. 2015. Available from: http://cks .nice.org.uk/palliative-cancer-care-pain (last accessed 29 April 2016).
4. Royal College of Physicians, British Geriatrics Society and British Pain Society. *The Assessment of Pain in Older People: National Guidelines*. Concise Guidance to Good Practice Series, No 8. Royal College of Physicians, London; 2007.
5. Searle RD, Bennett MI. Pain assessment. *Anaesth Intensive Care Med* 2008; 9:13–15.

Sudden collapse and syncope

Key thoughts

Practical points
- **Diagnosis.** History and examination can identify a cause for syncope in about 40% of cases.
- **Prognosis.** If the patient is shocked or unconscious, clinical assessment should not delay resuscitation and initial management.

Possible causes
- **Cardiovascular.** Syncope, myocardial infarction, ruptured abdominal aortic aneurysm, heat exhaustion.
- **Respiratory.** Pulmonary embolus.
- **Neurological.** Stroke, epilepsy, subarachnoid haemorrhage.
- **Gastrointestinal.** Gastrointestinal bleed, pancreatitis.
- **Metabolic.** Hypoglycaemia, alcohol intoxication.
- **Other.** Anaphylaxis, ruptured ectopic pregnancy, testicular torsion, trauma, exposure to toxins, electric shock.

RED FLAGS

- Chest pain
- Shortness of breath
- Blood around the mouth
- Known drug misuse
- Animal bite
- Positive pregnancy test
- Headache
- Vomiting

History

Ideas, concerns and expectations
- **Ideas.** If the patient is conscious, ask what they feel is the reason for the collapse.
- **Concerns.** Sudden collapse can be very frightening, and many people describe a feeling of imminent death. Fears about further episodes of collapse in the future are common. People also get worried about implications for work, driving or family life.

The 10-Minute Clinical Assessment, Second Edition. Knut Schroeder.
© 2017 John Wiley & Sons, Ltd. Published 2017 by John Wiley & Sons, Ltd.

- **Expectations.** Consider asking about expectations with regard to further investigation and management. Many people expect extensive cardiac investigations or brain scans, even if these are not indicated.

History of presenting complaint

- **Patient's story.** What was the patient doing at the time of collapse? Find out what exactly happened.
- **Presyncopal symptoms.** Nausea and a feeling of warmth suggest vasovagal syncope. Ask about headache (subarachnoid haemorrhage), chest pain (myocardial infarction) and focal neurological deficits (stroke).
- **Previous episodes.** Any previous episodes and knowledge about past diagnosis will give important diagnostic clues.
- **Precipitating factors.** Did something bring on the collapse? Flashing lights may cause an epileptic fit.
- **Current illness.** Has the patient been unwell lately? If so, ask for specific details, with a view to possible differential diagnoses.
- **Blood loss.** Ask about any obvious blood loss. Consider ruptured ectopic pregnancy, gastrointestinal bleed, severe menorrhagia, ruptured aortic aneurysm and blood loss due to trauma.
- **Fluid loss.** Common causes for loss of body fluid include vomiting, profuse diarrhoea, major burns and fluid lost via sequestering into body spaces (e.g. in pancreatitis).
- **Cardiac problems.** Could there be a cardiovascular cause? Ask about a history of cardiac disease. Common cardiac problems include arrhythmias due to myocardial ischaemia or cardiac failure. Collapse during exercise suggests a cardiac aetiology, particularly if associated with chest pain, shortness of breath, palpitations and immediate onset with no warning. Consider ruptured abdominal aortic aneurysm if there are cardiovascular risk factors or if an aneurysm has been diagnosed previously.
- **Exposure to toxins.** Is there a history of liver or renal failure with accumulation of toxins? Ask about environmental or occupational exposure to toxins, if it is relevant.
- **Infection.** Consider septic shock if there is underlying infection. Have any drugs been taken?
- **Endocrine.** Consider diabetic ketoacidosis if there is a history of diabetes and the patient presents with vomiting, headaches, abdominal pain, thirst, reduced urine output and hyperventilation. Could this be hypoglycaemia due to insulin overdose or infection in diabetes? Collapse can rarely be a presenting feature of Addisonian (adrenocortical) crisis, diabetic complications such as ketoacidosis or hypoglycaemia, or hypothyroid crisis.
- **Heat exposure.** Consider heat exhaustion or simple faint if the patient was exposed to a hot environment or collapsed during or after excessive exercise.
- **Neurological.** Consider stroke if there is one-side weakness or speech problems. If there is sudden onset of a severe headache, subarachnoid haemorrhage is a possibility. Has there been a seizure?

Past and current medical problems
- **Medical problems.** Ask if there are any other medical conditions that have not already been covered, to ensure rarer conditions are not missed.

Medication
- **Current medication.** Consider drug-related causes (e.g. insulin overdose). Some drugs have adverse effects that can lead to fluid depletion. Consider NSAIDs (gastritis and bleeding peptic ulcer), diuretics (dehydration) and steroids (peptic ulcer with masked symptoms).
- **Diabetes.** If the patient is diabetic, ask about insulin and oral medication for the treatment of diabetes. Have there been any dose alterations? Has medication been taken as prescribed?
- **Prolonged QT interval.** Drugs such as erythromycin, quinine and major tranquillisers can prolong the QT interval.

Other treatments
- **Recent surgery.** Consider the possibility of a postoperative complication if the collapse follows a recent hospital discharge.

Allergies
- **Drugs.** Consider a drug reaction if there is a possibility of allergic shock.

Social history
- **Home life.** Ask about home life and whether there are any dependants for whom care will need to be arranged. Homelessness is a risk factor for many conditions that can cause collapse.
- **Recent travel.** Consider the possibility of a tropical disease if the patient has been abroad recently.

Alcohol and recreational drugs
- **Alcohol.** Ask about previous and current alcohol consumption.
- **Drugs.** Consider narcotics overdose and fluid/electrolyte disturbances in ecstasy misuse.

Examination

General assessment
- **Conversation.** If the patient speaks to you in a normal voice and responds logically, the airways are patent and the brain is perfused.
- **Airway, breathing and circulation (ABC).** Assess ABC first in any unconscious or shocked patient.
- **Mental state.** Check responsiveness to verbal commands and pain if there is reduced consciousness.

- **Mouth.** The breath may smell ketotic in diabetic ketoacidosis (rare). Look out for evidence of tongue biting, suggesting a fit.
- **Blood loss.** Are there traces of blood around the mouth, suggesting haemoptysis or haematemesis? Is there continuing blood loss?
- **Trauma.** Inspect the whole body from head to toe for any trauma, if relevant.

Vital signs

- **Temperature.** Consider sepsis if the temperature is raised.
- **Pulse.** Tachycardia is an early sign in collapse due to fluid depletion or heart failure. Severe postural dizziness or a rise in pulse of >30 bpm when standing suggests hypovolaemia. Supine hypotension and tachycardia may be absent if blood loss is less than a litre. Arrhythmias may suggest an underlying cardiac cause.
- **Blood pressure.** Blood pressure will be normal for a long time, and hypotension is a warning sign for an impending shock.
- **Respiratory rate.** This is increased in respiratory infection.

Skin

- **Hydration.** Dry mucus membranes and dry axillae suggest dehydration in patients presenting with vomiting, diarrhoea or decreased oral intake. Skin turgor in adults is an unreliable sign.
- **Perfusion.** Look for signs of underperfusion, such as pallor and cold peripheries. Is there evidence of bruising, jaundice, cyanosis, burns or perioral oedema? Look for local infection if the temperature is raised. Capillary refill time has no proven value in adults.
- **Blood stains.** Dried or fresh blood on the skin may give clues about any obvious previous or continuing blood loss.
- **Trauma.** Look for evidence of trauma, particularly fractures of limbs or the pelvis.
- **Rashes.** Purpuric rash occurs in meningococcal septicaemia.

Head and neck

- **Pupils.** Check pupil responses to light. Fixed dilated pupils indicate severe brain involvement. Consider opiate overdose in pinpoint pupils.
- **Cranial nerves.** Is there any obvious facial weakness, suggesting stroke? Ask the patient to put the tongue out.

Upper limbs

- **Hand squeeze.** This rapidly helps to assess the brain and spinal cord.
- **Reflexes.** Brisk reflexes may suggest upper motor neurone lesion.

Chest

- **Auscultation.** Check for crackles indicating heart failure. Are there any cardiac murmurs suggesting valve disease?

Abdominal examination

- **Palpation.** Is there a pulsating abdominal aortic aneurysm? Several litres of internal blood loss may occur before there is any visible sign of abdominal distension. Consider ruptured appendix or ruptured ectopic pregnancy if there is lower abdominal pain and tenderness.
- **Rectal examination.** Consider rectal and pelvic examination if rectal bleeding is a possibility.

Lower limbs

- **Toe movements.** If toe wiggling is possible, the spinal cord is grossly intact.
- **Reflexes.** Brisk reflexes may suggest upper motor neurone lesion. Upgoing plantars may indicate brain damage.

Bedside tests

- **Blood sugar.** Check blood or urine glucose with a dipstick. Hypoglycaemia or severe hyperglycaemia will be obvious.
- **Pregnancy test.** Do a pregnancy test if pregnancy is a possibility, as the outcome will be important for management.

Key references and further reading

1. Driscoll P, Skinner D. ABC of major trauma. Initial assessment and management – I: primary survey. *BMJ* 1990;300:1265–1267.
2. McGee S, Abernethy WB, Simel DL. Is this patient hypovolaemic? *JAMA* 1999;281:1022–1029.
3. National Institute for Health and Care Excellence (NICE). Transient loss of consciousness ('blackouts') in over 16s. NICE guidelines [CG109]. 2010. Available from: http://www.nice.org.uk/guidance/cg109 (last accessed 29 April 2016).
4. Reed MJ, Gray A. Collapse query cause: the management of adult syncope in the emergency department. *Emerg Med J* 2006;23:589–594.

Frequent attenders

Key thoughts

Practical points

- **Reason for consultation.** Psychological problems and worry about serious illness are common reasons why some patients consult frequently. Others may suffer from multiple illnesses or poorly controlled chronic conditions, for which frequent attendance may be entirely appropriate. Chronic and uncontrolled pain is another common reason.
- **Serious illness.** Patients who attend three or more times for the same (acute) problem may have an undiagnosed underlying illness or other unmet needs requiring further exploration.

Possible causes

- Worry or anxiety about underlying disease.
- Depression.
- Acute stress reaction.
- Multiple pathology.
- Uncontrolled chronic illness.
- Undiagnosed mental or physical illness, such as cancer.
- Somatisation disorder.
- Cognitive decline.
- Learning difficulties.

RED FLAGS

- Systemic symptoms, such as fever, malaise, weight loss, loss of appetite, sweats or lymphadenopathy
- Abnormal physical examination
- Multiple attendances for the same acute problem
- Anxiety and depression
- Abnormal blood tests
- Abnormal imaging results

History

Ideas, concerns and expectations

- **Ideas.** Try to find out what the patient believes to be the underlying problem. Explore knowledge and beliefs around any underlying illness and its treatment.

The 10-Minute Clinical Assessment, Second Edition. Knut Schroeder.
© 2017 John Wiley & Sons, Ltd. Published 2017 by John Wiley & Sons, Ltd.

- **Concerns.** Worries about serious illness, death or impending disability are common and are worth identifying and addressing.
- **Expectations.** Try to identify expectations, such as a desire for reassurance, symptom relief, reducing inconvenience, further investigation or referral. Are expectations unrealistic?

History of presenting complaint

- **Context.** Allow the patient time to tell you about their problem in their own words. How does the presenting complaint fit into the context of this patient's life?
- **Quality of life.** How is the quality of life being affected? Are there limitations to particular activities?
- **Review of systems.** Asking about important symptoms of all major systems is valuable for identifying diagnostic clues. Thorough questioning will also show that you take the patient's concerns seriously.
- **Inability to cope.** Some people seek medical help because they are temporarily unable to cope. This may be due to sudden stresses (e.g. bereavement, job loss), sudden severe illness or mental health problems (e.g. depression, learning disability).
- **Lack of knowledge.** Patients may be unaware of about the natural course of self-limiting minor illness. Some people believe that they need to seek medical help for even minor symptoms, rather than trying self-care to start with.
- **Loneliness.** Health professionals may provide the only social contact for some people, and loneliness may be the main reason for consulting.
- **Lack of diagnosis.** Many people who consult frequently may be concerned about a lack of diagnosis. They may have been told that 'nothing is wrong' with them, but continue to experience significant symptoms, such as pain, nausea or general malaise.
- **Pressure from others.** There may be underlying pressure from family, friends or an employer to seek medical help.
- **Dependent relationship.** You or your colleagues may have encouraged or fostered a dependent relationship with the patient.
- **Additional unexplored issues.** Ask if there are any other problems or issues that you have not covered. Deep-seated problems, such as involvement in crime, fear of sexually transmitted infection after an extramarital affair or abuse as a child, require trust between the patient and the practitioner before they can be discussed openly.

Review of previous investigations

- **Bloods.** Check which blood tests have been carried out so far and whether any have been abnormal.
- **Imaging.** Check any imaging results, such as X-ray, ultrasound and CT/MRI, if available.

Past and current medical problems
- **Significant past illnesses.** Ask, in particular, about chronic conditions and uncontrolled pain. How well are these managed and controlled?
- **Anxiety and depression.** These are common reasons for frequent attendance.
- **Trauma.** Some people are worried about possible sequelae from trauma, particularly if it involved the head or where there is a medicolegal dispute (e.g. road traffic accident).

Medication
- **Prescribed drugs.** Ask about any prescribed drugs, in particular anxiolytics and analgesia. Does the patient suffer from adverse effects that have not yet been addressed? Are there any worries or concerns about taking medication which have not yet been discussed?

Other treatments
- **Mental health.** Find out whether the patient has ever had treatment for mental health conditions, such as counselling or cognitive behavioural therapy.

Family history
- **Positive family history.** People with a positive family history for a particular disease (e.g. Alzheimer's, cancer, coronary heart disease, Huntington's chorea) may be worried that they will also develop it.

Social history
- **Home.** Has home life been affected in any way?
- **Domestic and marital relationships.** Are there any family or relationship problems?

Alcohol, smoking and recreational drugs
- **Alcohol.** Patients may be worried about increased alcohol consumption but be afraid to admit this. Explore past and present alcohol intake.
- **Recreational drugs.** Does the patient take any illicit drugs?

Examination

General
- **General condition.** Does the patient look unwell? Cachexia, pallor or jaundice may raise the possibility of underlying serious illness (e.g. cancer).
- **General inspection and examination.** Be guided by the history, but take care to check the major systems even if you do not suspect any major abnormality. It is difficult to reassure a patient that a physical cause is unlikely to be responsible for their symptoms if you have not performed a thorough examination.

Vital signs
- **Temperature, pulse, blood pressure and respiratory rate.** Check these for reassurance. Mild tachypnoea may occur in anxiety.

Skin
- **Skin lesions.** Scan the skin for any signs of injury, self-harm or liver disease.

Chest
- **Heart and lungs.** Check heart and lungs for any abnormalities. Many people find a normal auscultation reassuring.

Abdomen
- **Palpation.** Feel the abdomen for any masses or evidence of organomegaly. Is there any abnormal tenderness?

Bedside tests
- **Urinalysis.** Check for protein, glucose and blood.

Key references and further reading
1. Ellaway A, Wood S, Macintyre S. Someone to talk to? The role of loneliness as a factor in the frequency of GP consultations. *Br J Gen Pract* 1999;49:363–367.
2. Hodgson P, Smith P, Brown T, Dowrick C. Stories from frequent attenders: a qualitative study in primary care. *Ann Fam Med* 2005;3:318–323.
3. Little P, Dorward M, Warner G et al. Importance of patient pressure and perceived pressure and medical need for investigations, referral, and prescribing in primary care: nested observational study. *BMJ* 2004;328:444.
4. Reid S, Wessely S, Crayford T, Hotopf M. Medically unexplained symptoms in frequent attenders of secondary health care: retrospective cohort study. *BMJ* 2001;322:767–771.
5. Vedsted P, Christensen MB. Frequent attenders in general practice care: a literature review with special reference to methodological considerations. *Public Health* 2005/119:118–137.

Medication review and polypharmacy

Key thoughts

Practical points

- **Reason for consultation.** Patients may attend a medication review either because they have been invited as part of regular monitoring or because there are aspects of their medication that they wish to discuss with a health professional. A number of issues might be worth addressing routinely to optimise medication management.
- **Areas for exploration.** Try to identify any new medical problems that may need addressing or that put the person at risk. Check whether drugs are still indicated and whether current doses and frequencies are appropriate. Find out how effective the treatment is and whether there are any adverse effects. Also check whether medication is taken as prescribed (adherence).

RED FLAGS

- Anaphylaxis and other allergic reactions
- Adverse effects
- Significant nonadherence
- Lack of effect

History

Ideas, concerns and expectations

- **Ideas.** Does the patient know why their drugs are being prescribed? Try to identify the patient's health beliefs and attitudes to illness and its drug management.
- **Concerns.** Fears about experienced or expected adverse effects are common. Problems like erectile dysfunction and constipation may not be mentioned by the patient unless asked for, or may not be recognised as being adverse effects of a particular drug. People often fear they might get 'addicted' to medication.
- **Expectations.** Common reasons for consultation are adverse effects, lack of the desired effect or the need for reassurance that the management is correct. Effective drug treatment often requires patients to be actively involved in their management.

The 10-Minute Clinical Assessment, Second Edition. Knut Schroeder.
© 2017 John Wiley & Sons, Ltd. Published 2017 by John Wiley & Sons, Ltd.

Medication review

- **Quality of life.** Allow the patient time to tell you about their illness experience and medication. How is day-to-day life affected by any problems caused by the underlying illness or its management?
- **Indication and need.** Review the indication for each drug and check whether it is still needed. Is there a documented indication for each drug in the patient record? Check with the patient why individual drugs were started and continue to be prescribed. Are drug doses correct and appropriate? Have alternatives to drug treatment, such as physiotherapy or cognitive behavioural therapy, been considered and discussed? Check whether you and the patient agree what medication is being taken regularly. Are any medicines no longer required because the condition has improved or because treatment was only meant to be for the short term? Has new evidence, such as national guidance, been taken into account? Is the duration of therapy acceptable to the patient?
- **Adherence.** Ask questions like, 'Many people find it difficult to take their medicines regularly; how often do you not take all of your medication?' Try to find out whether nonadherence is intentional (e.g. due to certain beliefs, adverse effects) or unintentional (forgetfulness, containers difficult to open, difficulty in swallowing). Other common reasons for suboptimal adherence include fear of 'addiction' or of becoming habituated, forgetting to take a particular dose where there are too many to remember and a dislike for 'taking chemicals'. Are there any problems with reading the label or dosing instructions?
- **Effect.** Ask whether the patient feels the medicines are effective. Check the notes for relevant measures, such as blood pressure. If drugs are being used for symptomatic relief, is this adequate? Is an increase in dose or change of preparation needed?
- **Monitoring.** Does the patient take any drugs that need regular monitoring? Check with relevant drug sheets and guidelines (e.g. the US *Physician's Desk Reference* or the *British National Formulary* – www.bnf.org). Common tests used for monitoring are renal (e.g. angiotensin-converting enzyme (ACE) inhibitors) and liver (e.g. statins) function tests and full blood count (e.g. methotrexate).
- **Adverse effects.** Are there any drug adverse effects? Enquire about any symptoms and establish whether they are genuine adverse effects or whether there could be another underlying cause. It is easy to misinterpret a drug adverse effect as a new medical problem. Are there any contraindications, duplications or interactions that have not been taken into account?
- **New medication.** Is any new medication needed in view of the patient's current list of problems?
- **Evidence base.** Has there been any change in evidence since a drug was started? Check with the relevant prescribing guidelines if in doubt, and ensure that there have not been any recent relevant health warnings. Is there a need for additional investigations?

- **Cost-effectiveness.** Consider whether a switch from a branded to a generic preparation might be indicated. Are quantities aligned to avoid waste and help patients reorder medication in a single batch?
- **Simplification of drug regimen.** Can you simplify the drug regimen? Consider once-daily doses, if they are available and cost-effective. Ensure that the patient knows the importance of each drug. Is there duplication with other drugs that are being prescribed for the same indication?
- **Screening for risks.** Consider and address potential risks from taking medication (e.g. falls in older patients who take diuretics).
- **Prescribing errors.** Try to reduce the risk of prescribing errors by getting to know your patient. Review the notes if necessary, and make sure you know the drugs that you prescribe commonly. Check that you have calculated doses correctly and make sure that you record doses and quantities carefully on the script and in the case notes. Are the directions correct and practical?
- **Herbal and over-the-counter drugs.** Ask about any additional drugs that are being purchased over the counter or on the Internet. Do these have the potential to interact with currently prescribed drugs?
- **Drug allergies.** Has the patient developed any new allergies that have not yet been recorded?
- **Practical issues.** Does the patient have any problems receiving repeat prescriptions or obtaining a medication? Can the patient read the labels?
- **Additional unexplored issues.** Ask whether there are any other problems or issues that may need addressing.

Past and current medical problems
- **Significant past illnesses.** Ask whether there are any past or new illnesses that may be important but have not yet been documented?
- **Alcohol, smoking and recreational drugs**
- **Alcohol.** Alcohol and recreational drugs can interact with medications such as antidepressants and psychotics.

Examination

General
- **General condition.** Does the patient look unwell?
- **Examination.** Direct further examination based on findings from the history and the current problem list.

Key references and further reading
1. Drumbreck S, Flynn A, Nairn M et al. Drug-disease and drug interactions: systematic examination of recommendations in 12 UK national guidelines. *BMJ* 2015;350:h949.
2. Gallagher P, Ryan C, Bryne S et al. STOPP (Screening Tool of Older Person's Prescriptions) and START (Screening Tool to Alert doctors to Right Treatment). Consensus validation. *Int J Clin Pharmacol Ther* 2008;46:72–83.

3. Lewis T. Using the NO TEARS tool for medication review. *BMJ* 2004;329: 434.
4. Task Force on Medicines Partnership. *Room for Review. A Guide for Medication Review: The Agenda for Patients, Practitioners and Managers.* Medicines Partnership, London; 2002.

Medically unexplained symptoms

Key thoughts

Practical points
- **Diagnosis.** Medically unexplained symptoms are common and are potentially frustrating for both patients and health professionals. A good starting point is usually to identify and list the symptoms that the patient feels are most important and to assess the impact of these on their quality of life. Try to compare the risks of further investigation and 'medicalising' a problem with the likelihood of finding an undiagnosed physical cause.
- **Prognosis.** Patients may be at risk of harm due to over-investigation, as well as of a missed diagnosis.

Possible causes
- Stress.
- Depression.
- Anxiety.
- Irritable bowel syndrome.
- Chronic fatigue syndrome.
- Somatisation disorder.
- Fibromyalgia.
- Psychosis.
- Vitamin D deficiency.

RED FLAGS

- Systemic features (e.g. weight loss, loss of appetite, malaise, fever, sweats)
- Persistent and worsening symptoms
- Abnormal physical examination
- Abnormal blood tests

History

Ideas, concerns and expectations
- **Ideas.** Does the patient have any thoughts as to what might be wrong? This may give important clues to any underlying beliefs and possible diagnoses. What is the patient's model of illness?
- **Concerns.** Fears about undiagnosed cancer or other serious disease are common. Symptoms may prevent patients from taking part in certain activities. The

---

The 10-Minute Clinical Assessment, Second Edition. Knut Schroeder.
© 2017 John Wiley & Sons, Ltd. Published 2017 by John Wiley & Sons, Ltd.

lack of a specific diagnosis for what are genuine symptoms can cause significant anxiety and distress. Is the patient in any current dilemma or predicament?
- **Expectations.** Why has the patient come to see you? Find out what they expect in terms of assessment, investigation and further referral. A thorough assessment and reassurance is a common reason for consultation. Health professionals often feel challenged by having to try to explain some or all of a patient's symptoms.

History of presenting complaint
- **Context.** How do the symptoms fit into the context of the patient's life?
- **Quality of life.** Allow the patient time and opportunity to tell you about all of their symptoms in their own words (in more than one consultation, if necessary). How do the symptoms affect the activities of daily living?
- **History of presenting symptoms.** Identify and list all relevant presenting symptoms. Ask for details about onset, site, radiation, severity, character, progression, duration, associated features and relieving/exacerbating factors. This way, you will show that you take the patient seriously, and you may identify an undiagnosed abnormality. Encourage the expression of feelings and thoughts about the symptoms. Do they 'mean' anything for the patient? Show empathy and acknowledge that the perceived problem is 'real' for the patient.
- **Educational background.** There is some evidence that people presenting with medically unexplained symptoms have had fewer years of formal education than the general population.
- **Social background.** Has there been a lack of care or illness in childhood? Are there any psychosocial difficulties with regard to family, friends or work?
- **Mental health.** Ask about any symptoms of depression, such as low mood, lack of energy, poor concentration, suicidal thoughts, lack of appetite, feelings of being a failure and hopelessness. Has there been excessive stress or anxiety lately? Have there been any major life events?
- **Additional unexplored issues.** Ask the patient whether there are any other problems or issues that you have not covered but which might be important.

Systems review
- **General.** Ask about weight loss, tiredness, sleep problems, loss of appetite, malaise, loss of energy, night sweats, fever and swollen lymph nodes.
- **Cardiovascular system.** Ask about dyspnoea, chest pain, palpitations, peripheral oedema, calf pain and syncope.
- **Respiratory.** Ask about cough, sputum, haemoptysis, breathing, wheeze and pleuritic chest pain.
- **Upper gastrointestinal tract.** Ask about abdominal pain, loss of appetite, nausea, vomiting, dyspepsia and dysphagia.
- **Lower gastrointestinal tract.** Ask about diarrhoea, constipation, pain and rectal bleeding.
- **Urinary system.** Check for frequency, dysuria, haematuria, flow, pain and changes in urine volume.

- **Sexual history.** Ask about problems with sexual function and genitourinary symptoms.
- **Nervous system.** Ask about a family history of neurological conditions, fits, blackouts, paralysis, stroke, headaches and dizziness.
- **Musculoskeletal.** Ask about bone and joint pains or stiffness, gout, gait problems and disabilities.

Past and current medical problems

- **Significant past illnesses.** Does the patient suffer from chronic diseases, such as diabetes, CVD or respiratory conditions?
- **Trauma.** Has the patient suffered any physical or psychological trauma in the past?
- **Operations.** Has the patient had any significant previous operations?

Medication

- **Analgesics.** What is being taken, and at what dose? Are there any adverse effects or signs of overuse?
- **Psychotropic drugs.** Is the patient taking antidepressants or sedatives?
- **Herbal and over-the-counter drugs.** Ask for details about any medication purchased over the counter.

Family history

- **Significant conditions.** Is there any significant family history of any sort?

Social history

- **Home.** Who else is at home? Are activities of daily living affected by the symptoms? Are there any financial worries?
- **Domestic and marital relationships.** Does the patient have any close allies? Are there any family or relationship problems?

Alcohol, smoking and recreational drugs

- **Alcohol.** Ask for details about past and current alcohol consumption. Has this changed lately? Depression, anxiety and major life events are common reasons for an increase in alcohol consumption. Acute alcohol withdrawal can cause a multitude of physical symptoms.
- **Recreational drugs.** Illicit drugs and drug withdrawal may sometimes be responsible for medically unexplained symptoms, such as constipation and hallucinations.

Review of previous investigations

- **Full blood count.** Look for evidence of anaemia, infection or haematological malignancy.
- **Inflammatory markers.** These may be raised in infection, inflammation and cancer.
- **Liver and renal function.** Is there any evidence of organ failure?

- **Glucose.** Is there evidence of hyperglycaemia?
- **Thyroid function.** Hypo- or hyperthyroidism may present with nonspecific symptoms.
- **Other conditions.** Check whether tests for conditions such as HIV, coeliac disease, autoimmune disorders, syphilis and tuberculosis have been considered, requested or reported in the past.
- **Imaging.** Look out for any past imaging results.
- **Specialist involvement.** Check the notes for past involvement of any specialists. Check letters for relevant information.

Examination

General
- **General condition.** Does the patient look unwell? Cachexia, pallor or jaundice may raise the possibility of serious underlying disease.
- **General inspection and examination.** Be guided by the history, but check the major systems, even if you do not suspect any major abnormality. It is difficult to reassure a patient that a physical cause is unlikely to be responsible for their symptoms if they feel you have not examined them thoroughly.

Vital signs
- Temperature, pulse, blood pressure and respiratory rate. Check these for abnormalities and reassurance.

Skin
- **Skin lesions.** Scan the skin for any signs of physical disease (e.g. alcoholism, HIV), injury or self-harm.

Head and neck
- **Fundi.** Check the fundi for papilloedema if raised intracranial pressure is a possibility.

Chest
- **Heart and lungs.** Briefly check the heart and lungs for any abnormalities. Many patients will find a normal chest auscultation reassuring.

Abdomen
- **Organs and masses.** Feel the abdomen for any masses or evidence of organomegaly. Is there any tenderness?

Spine and limbs
- **Spinal assessment.** Check the spine and limbs for any abnormality if there is a history of back pain.

Bedside tests
- **Urinalysis.** Check for glucose, blood, protein, nitrites and leucocytes, and consider urinary tract infection, renal problems and diabetes if abnormal.

Key references and further reading
1. Brown RJ. Psychological mechanisms of medically unexplained symptoms: an integrative conceptual model. *Psych Bull* 2004;130:793–812.
2. Creed F, Barsky A. A systematic review of the epidemiology of somatisation disorder and hypochondriasis. *J Psychosomat Res* 2004;56:391–408.
3. Fischhoff B, Wessely S. Managing patients with inexplicable health problems. *BMJ* 2003;326:595–597.
4. Hatcher S, Arroll B. Assessment and management of medically unexplained symptoms. *BMJ* 2008;336:1124–1128.
5. Olde Hartman T, Lucassen P, van de Lisdonk E et al. Chronic functional somatic symptoms: a single syndrome? *Br J Gen Pract* 2004;54:922–927.
6. Royal College of Psychiatrists. Guidance for health professionals on medically unexplained symptoms. 2011. Available from: http://www.rcpsych.ac.uk/pdf/CHECKED%20MUS%20Guidance_A4_4pp_6.pdf (last accessed 29 April 2016).

Insomnia

Key thoughts

Practical points
- **Diagnosis.** Sleep problems are common and are mostly self-limiting. Most patients present with a change in their usual sleep pattern, which can cause considerable worry. Common causes are acute life events, stress, anxiety and depression.
- **Alcohol.** Many people with insomnia use alcohol to help them get to sleep, which may cause further sleep problems.
- **Physical problems.** Explore and address any physical problems leading to insomnia.
- **Drugs.** Drug misusers may present with 'sleep problems' to obtain a prescription for benzodiazepines.

Possible causes
- **Sleep habits.** Poor sleeping habits, shift work, daytime naps.
- **Mental health.** Family or work-related stress, depression, anxiety, nightmares.
- **Environmental.** Noise, temperature, snoring partner, small children, watching TV late at night, jet lag.
- **Substance misuse.** Alcohol, drugs, caffeine and other stimulants.
- **Medication.** For example, steroids, salbutamol, benzodiazepine withdrawal.
- **Physical.** Nocturia, pain, hot flushes, heart failure, respiratory problems, hyperthyroidism.

RED FLAGS

- Physical symptoms and signs
- Depression
- Suicidal ideation
- Alcohol or substance misuse

History

Ideas, concerns and expectations
- **Ideas.** What does the patient think is causing the sleep problem?
- **Concerns.** Try and identify any underlying concerns or worries that are keeping the patient awake at night. Worries about a damaging effect of lack of sleep on health are common.

The 10-Minute Clinical Assessment, Second Edition. Knut Schroeder.
© 2017 John Wiley & Sons, Ltd. Published 2017 by John Wiley & Sons, Ltd.

- **Expectations.** Why has the patient come to see you? Common reasons for consultation are a request for sleeping pills, treatment for depression and help with addressing family or work problems. Expectations may be unrealistic, as some people feel they have to sleep for at least 8 hours every night, even in old age.

History of presenting complaint
- **Context.** Allow the patient time to tell you about their sleep problems in their own words. What is the life context in which these problems are occurring?
- **Quality of life.** How do symptoms affect the activities of daily living? Excessive daytime tiredness may result from a sleep disorder.
- **Onset.** When did the sleep problems start? Short-term insomnia is often caused by acute life events, but may turn into long-term sleep problems if its lasts more than 6 months.
- **Type of sleep problem.** Find out whether the main problem is getting off to sleep, staying asleep or waking up early. Anxiety and worries often cause difficulties getting to sleep. Nocturia and other physical symptoms may wake a person during the night. Early-morning waking may be caused by depression.
- **Other symptoms.** Consider restless legs, nightmares and jerking limbs.
- **Timing.** Ask about when the patient goes to bed and wakes up. Daytime naps are a common reason for difficulties with sleep during the night.
- **Physical health.** Ask about any ongoing or new health problems. Chronic and uncontrolled pain can affect sleep. Does the patient feel generally well?
- **Mental and emotional health.** Are there any emotional problems? Most psychiatric conditions can cause problems with sleep, particularly if associated with mood changes or anxiety. Worries about not being able to get to sleep or not getting enough sleep may themselves cause sleep problems and lead to a vicious circle.
- **Stimulants.** Drinking alcohol, coffee, tea or other stimulants during the day or in the evening and engaging in heavy exercise later in the day can cause problems with sleep.
- **Self-help.** What has been tried so far? Ask about books, relaxation tapes, etc.
- **Sleep hygiene.** What are the routines around sleep? Is the bed comfortable? Is the blanket too hot or cold? Are bed times regular? Is the bedroom dark and sufficiently quiet? Does the patient lie tossing and turning in bed? Are lie-ins and daytime naps used to compensate for loss of sleep? Does the patient work in shifts?
- **Additional unexplored issues.** Ask whether there are any other problems or issues that you have not covered which might be important.

Past and current medical problems
- **Significant past illnesses.** Ask about any past or current medical conditions that may be relevant. Very high blood pressure may rarely cause agitation and sleep problems.

Medication
- **Hypnotics.** Have these been prescribed recently or in the past? Does the patient currently take sleeping pills?
- **Psychotropic drugs.** Ask about antidepressants and other psychotropic medication.
- **Steroids.** Steroids in higher doses may cause sleep problems.
- **Herbal and over-the-counter drugs.** Many people self-medicate initially when they have sleeping problems. Check whether any preparations have been bought over the counter, without prescription.

Other treatments
- **Psychotherapy.** Has the patient had psychotherapy or counselling in the past?

Social history
- **Home.** How has home life been affected? Are other family members a potential cause of sleep problems in terms of noise or relationship problems? Have tiredness or irritability due to lack of sleep affected relationships at home?
- **Work.** Has performance at work been affected by lack of sleep or adverse effects from taking hypnotics?

Alcohol, smoking and recreational drugs
- **Alcohol.** Ask for details about past and present alcohol consumption. Has there been a recent change in the amount and frequency of alcohol intake? If so, is there an obvious reason?
- **Smoking.** Smoking cessation may cause short-term sleep problems.
- **Recreational drugs.** Does the patient take any illicit drugs? Opioid withdrawal can lead to agitation and sleep problems. Ask about use of cocaine or other stimulants.

Review of previous investigations
- **Full blood count.** Blood tests are not usually required. Look for signs of anaemia. A raised MCV may suggest alcohol misuse.
- **Thyroid function.** Hyperthyroidism may cause sleeplessness.
- **Liver function tests.** Are there any alcohol-related changes?

Examination

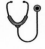

General
- **General condition.** Physical examination will often be normal. Does the patient look unwell or tired? Sweatiness and agitation may suggest alcohol or drug withdrawal.

Vital signs
- **Pulse.** Check for tachycardia or atrial fibrillation if hyperthyroidism is a possibility. Tachycardia may also occur in alcohol or drug withdrawal.
- **Blood pressure.** Rarely, severe hypertension may present with sleep problems.

Skin
- **Signs of liver disease.** Look out for signs of alcoholic liver disease (scratch marks, jaundice, palmar erythema, spider naevi) if there is a history of alcohol misuse.

Chest
- **Heart and lungs.** Check for heart and lung abnormalities, if suggested by the history.

Abdomen
- **Palpation.** Check for any abdominal masses or tenderness. Gastric reflux may cause nocturnal symptoms, but examination will usually be normal. An enlarged liver due to liver disease may cause jaundice and itching at night.

Limbs
- **Joints.** Look for joint swelling and tenderness, particularly if prompted by the history, which may suggest a rheumatological condition.

Key references and further reading

1. National Institute for Health and Care Excellence (NICE). Insomnia. Clinical Knowledge Summaries. 2015. Available from: http://cks.nice.org.uk/insomnia (last accessed 29 April 2009).
2. Ramakrishnan K, Scheid D. Treatment options for insomnia. *Am Fam Physician* 2007;76:517–526.
3. Sateia MJ, Nowell PD. Insomnia. *Lancet* 2004;364:1959–1973.
4. Silber MH. Clinical practice. Chronic insomnia. *N Engl J Med* 2005;353:803–810.
5. Wilson SJ, Nutt DJ, Alford C et al. British Association for Psychopharmacology consensus statement on evidence-based treatment of insomnia, parasomnias and circadian rhythm disorders. *J Psychopharmacol* 2010;24:1577–1600.

Irritability and 'stress'

Key thoughts

Practical points
- **Diagnosis.** Psychological causes are common (e.g. anxiety, depression), but symptoms may occasionally indicate an underlying physical disorder, such as hyperthyroidism.
- **Impact.** Carefully explore the impact that stress and irritability have on the patient's life.
- **Alcohol.** Always consider alcohol misuse, both as a cause of stress and as a 'self-treatment'.

Possible causes
- Anxiety.
- Depression.
- Stimulant overuse and withdrawal (e.g. caffeine, nicotine).
- Alcohol or drug problems.
- Medication use and withdrawal (steroids, SSRIs, benzodiazepines).
- Phobias.
- Work-related problems.
- Relationship problems.
- Sleep deprivation.
- Physical conditions (e.g. hyperthyroidism, menopause, cardiac arrhythmias).

RED FLAGS

- Weight loss
- Loss of appetite
- Fever
- Sweats
- Suicidal ideation

History

Ideas, concerns and expectations
- **Ideas.** What does the patient think is wrong?
- **Concerns.** Tense feelings can impair the quality of life of both the patient and those around them and may cause relationships to deteriorate. Worries about underlying physical illness are common. Suicidal ideas can be very frightening for people.

The 10-Minute Clinical Assessment, Second Edition. Knut Schroeder.
© 2017 John Wiley & Sons, Ltd. Published 2017 by John Wiley & Sons, Ltd.

- **Expectations.** Common reasons for consultation are a need for reassurance, further investigation and referral.

History of presenting complaint
- **Context.** How do the symptoms fit into the context of this patient's life? Ask for some idea of the story behind their symptoms.
- **Quality of life.** How is the quality of life being affected? Stress and irritability can be very distressing for both the patient and those around them.
- **Onset and progression.** Find out when the problems started and whether symptoms are getting worse.
- **External factors.** Life events and problems at work may cause or contribute to the development of stress-related symptoms. Talk about relationships with family members and people at work. Common occupational problems include excessive workload, shift work, general unhappiness with work and an unsympathetic or unreasonable boss. Are there any triggers in day-to-day life that make the symptoms worse?
- **Mental health.** Try to get an idea about the patient's usual mental state. Is there a history of anxiety or depression? Are there any symptoms or signs of psychiatric illness? Generalised anxiety disorder, depression, psychoses and phobias may all present as 'stress'. Are there any problems with sleep?
- **Physical symptoms.** Symptoms such as hyperventilation, palpitations, headaches and sweating may occur when the patient feels tense, rather than being caused by underlying pathology.
- **Drugs and alcohol.** Alcohol misuse and excessive intake of caffeine and nicotine can lead to tense feelings or may be used to relieve these feelings. A number of soft drinks contain considerable amounts of caffeine and may be responsible for such symptoms, particularly in younger people.
- **Withdrawal.** Symptoms may be caused by caffeine, nicotine or alcohol withdrawal. Emotional tension is seen when people suddenly stop taking antidepressants or anxiolytics, such as when they run out of medication or are being admitted to a residential home or for respite care.
- **General symptoms.** Excessive tiredness, weight loss, loss of appetite, malaise, fevers or swollen lymph nodes may indicate underlying physical problems.
- **Menopause.** Consider tension due to the menopause, if a woman has become amenorrhoic. Are there associated hot flushes?
- **Self-help.** What has been tried so far? Have self-help books, relaxation tapes, counselling or stress-management courses been considered or tried? Does the patient know how to access any of these?
- **Hyperthyroidism.** Ask about tremor, heat intolerance and palpitations.
- **Additional unexplored issues.** Ask whether there are any other important problems or issues which have not yet been addressed.

Past and current medical problems
- **Significant past illnesses.** In patients with hypertension, a very high blood pressure can cause tense feelings.

Medication

- **Antidepressants.** Have these been started or stopped recently? Feeling tense may occur in the first few weeks, particularly when starting or stopping SSRIs.
- **Other psychotropic drugs.** Stopping drugs like diazepam suddenly may cause agitation or a tense feeling.

Social history

- **Home.** How has home life been affected? Are relationships part of the problem, or are they suffering as a result of the problems around feeling tense?
- **Work.** Has work been affected in any way?

Review of previous investigations

- **Full blood count.** Look for signs of alcohol misuse, such as raised MCV or low platelets.
- **Inflammatory markers.** Check for evidence of infection or significant inflammation.
- **Thyroid function.** A normal test will exclude significant thyroid disease.
- **Liver function tests.** Alcoholism is an important cause to consider.
- **Reproductive hormones.** In women, could symptoms be due to the menopause?
- **ECG.** Is there evidence of atrial fibrillation or tachycardia, particularly in patients presenting with palpitations?

Examination

General

- **General condition.** Does the person look unwell? Cachexia or pallor may suggest underlying physical illness.
- **Alcohol.** Are there signs of alcohol abuse, such as palmar erythema, facial plethora or spider naevi?
- **Mental state.** Slow speech and movement, slouched posture and depressed facial expression may suggest underlying depression. Sweating, tremor, shakiness or agitation may be presenting features of generalised anxiety disorder. Consider performing a more formal mental state examination, if indicated by the history.
- **Hyperthyroidism.** Hyperthyroidism may cause weight loss. Look for other signs of hyperthyroidism, such as fine tremor, sweating or lid retraction.

Vital signs

- **Pulse.** Tachycardia and atrial fibrillation may occur with hyperthyroidism.
- **Blood pressure.** Agitation or feeling tense may cause blood pressure to rise or be caused by hypertension itself.
- **Respiratory rate.** Tachypnoea may occur with anxiety (hyperventilation).

Chest
- **Heart.** Check for arrythmias (e.g. atrial fibrillation).

Key references and further reading
1. Craig K, Hietanen H, Markova I, Berrios G. The irritability questionnaire: a new scale for the measurement of irritability. *Psychiatry Res* 2008;159:367–375.
2. Hogan C. Chronic stress: an approach to management in general practice. *Aus Fam Physician* 2013;42:542–545.
3. National Institute for Health and Care Excellence (NICE). Generalised anxiety disorder. Clinical Knowledge Summaries. 2015. Available from: http://cks.nice.org.uk/generalized-anxiety-disorder (last accessed 29 April 2016).
4. Reid J, Wheeler S. Hyperthyroidism: diagnosis and treatment. *Am Fam Physician* 2005;72:623–630, 635–636.

Domestic violence

Key thoughts

Practical points
- **Diagnosis.** Domestic violence can affect both women and, less commonly, men. It may present in different ways, from mental health problems to physical presentations. Begin by establishing the type of abuse (e.g. physical, sexual, emotional, financial or social).
- **Examination.** If indicated, physical examination should usually be performed by an examiner trained in documenting injuries from domestic violence.
- **Rapport and support.** Establish rapport, identify overall risk and risk factors, assess injuries and offer support.

Differential diagnosis
- Physical abuse.
- Emotional abuse.
- Sexual abuse.
- Financial abuse.
- Social abuse.
- Any combination of these.

Associated conditions
- Physical injuries.
- Depression.
- Alcoholism.
- Drug misuse.

Important risk factors
- History of abuse.
- Pregnancy.

RED FLAGS

- Suicidal ideation
- Depression
- Alcohol and drug misuse
- Bruises, injuries and burns
- Repeated terminations of pregnancy
- Sexually transmitted infection

The 10-Minute Clinical Assessment, Second Edition. Knut Schroeder.
© 2017 John Wiley & Sons, Ltd. Published 2017 by John Wiley & Sons, Ltd.

History

Ideas, concerns and expectations

- **Ideas.** What does the patient think is going on?
- **Concerns.** Concerns commonly focus around the patient's own health and the welfare of any children.
- **Expectations.** What does the patient expect from the consultation?

History of presenting complaint

- **Patient's own story.** Try to see patients on their own, as the presence of a partner or relative may hinder their ability to tell the whole story. Consider stressing that this is 'routine practice'. Allow patients plenty of time to tell their story in their own words. Denial is common, due to shame and embarrassment. Be aware that patients may not reveal the whole story in the first consultation. Male health professionals should consider having a female chaperone present. What is the context of the patient's life in which abuse has been taking place?
- **Domestic violence.** Consider the possibility of domestic violence and ask such questions as, 'Domestic violence is common: is this a problem for you?', 'Do you experience any abuse?' or 'Are you ever afraid of your partner?' Be sympathetic and direct, and assure the patient of their privacy and confidentiality. If a child is at risk, information may need to be shared. Be aware that abused women may feel humiliated, ashamed and frightened, and that they may blame themselves.
- **Safety.** Ask whether violence has escalated recently and whether there are any weapons in the house. In many countries, women can apply for a non-molestation order. Is there a plan in case things become dangerous? Women may feel more in control if they have a bag ready (including their personal documents) and know where they can go in an emergency.
- **Type of abuse.** Ask for details about any abuse and whether it is physical, emotional, financial or social. Has there been any sexual abuse?
- **Injuries.** Ask about bruises, burns and other injuries. When and how exactly did injuries occur?
- **Use of weapons.** Have any weapons been used against the patient?
- **Abusive partner or other perpetrator.** Where is the perpetrator now? Does he/she have any convictions for drugs or violence? Is the abuse getting worse? Has any injury been caused? Is the partner controlling or jealous? Is there denial? Is the patient allowed to talk freely? Have there been any punishments or sanctions from the perpetrator? Ask about current, previous or suspected stalking. Does this involve telephone calls or messages?
- **Pregnancy.** Is the patient pregnant, or has there been a recent child birth? Domestic violence often gets worse during pregnancy, as male partners may feel stressed about the new situation. Ask about any abuse, as women may be concerned about future child abuse and therefore keen to talk.
- **Previous problems in pregnancy.** Domestic abuse can lead to miscarriage, premature birth, low birth weight, fatal injury or intrauterine death. Ask about previous assaults during pregnancy.

- **Suicidal thoughts.** Are there any suicidal thoughts or plans? Consider any risks to children. Domestic violence may precede homicide.

___

Past and current medical problems
- **Abuse.** Did the patient grow up in an abusive household?
- **Injuries.** Have there been any injuries resulting from domestic violence in the past? Have these ever been reported, and to whom?
- **Mental health.** Sexual abuse is strongly correlated with mental health disorders in later life.

___

Social history
- **Indirect effects.** Ask about loss of friends or of the home, and any financial problems.
- **Relationships.** Consider asking about financial reasons for staying with the partner. Does the patient stay because of the children? Do they feel sorry for their abuser? Has there been or is there going to be a separation? If so, what has been the perpetrator's response? If separated, has there been any contact, and if so, how often?
- **Children.** What has been the impact on any children? Children can suffer behavioural and emotional problems. Are there any child contact issues? Are children being left alone with the abusive partner? Has the partner hurt or threatened to hurt any of the children? Are social workers or a child protection team involved?
- **Isolation.** Do any other factors contribute to social isolation? Consider disability, race, sexuality and the location of accommodation. Are religious convictions an issue, such as 'shame' or lack of family support? Ask about isolation from family and friends.
- **Housing.** Is the patient aware of local shelters and refuges?
- **Support.** Ask about knowledge of local support groups, hotlines and voluntary organisations. Are the police involved?
- **Job and income.** Has there been any loss of opportunity to work?
- **Legal help.** The police often have special officers dealing with domestic abuse. Some solicitors specialise in domestic violence.

___

Alcohol and drugs
- **Alcohol.** Ask about alcohol intake, including the intake of others in the household.
- **Drugs.** Are any other drugs being taken?

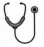

Examination

___

General
- **Initial screening.** Limit the first assessment to a general screening examination. Detailed examination should be carried out by an examiner with special training and expertise in assessing victims of domestic violence.

- **Appearance.** Does the patient try to conceal any injuries or minimise their extent (e.g. with clothing)? Do they appear anxious, depressed, frightened or distressed?

Skin
- **Bruises.** Check for bruises anywhere on the body.
- **Injuries.** Are there any obvious injuries to the head, face, neck, chest, breasts and abdomen? Multiple injuries at different stages of healing suggest the possibility of domestic violence. Are there different types of injuries? Look for burns, bruises and slap injuries. Be suspicious if injuries are unexplained or inconsistent with the patient's or another person's explanation.
- **Burns.** These may be caused by cigarettes or rope.

Key references and further reading

1. American Medical Association. Diagnostic and treatment guidelines on domestic violence. American Medical Association. 1992. Available from: http://www.ncdsv.org/images/AMA_Diag&TreatGuideDV_3-1992.pdf (last accessed 29 April 2016).
2. Department of Health. *Domestic Violence: A Resource Manual for Health Care Professionals.* Department of Health, London; 2000.
3. Hegarty K, Taft A, Feder G. Violence between intimate partners: working with the whole family. *BMJ* 2008;337:a839.
4. National Institute for Health and Care Excellence (NICE). Domestic violence and abuse: multi-agency working. NICE guidelines [PH50]. February 2014. Available from: http://www.nice.org.uk/guidance/ph50 (last accessed 29 April 2016).
5. Takey A. *Tackling Domestic Violence: The Role of Health Professionals.* Development and Practice Report 32. Department of Health, London; 2004.
6. Women's Aid. www.womensaid.org.uk.

Homelessness

Key thoughts

Practical points
- **Health needs.** Multiple morbidity is common among homeless people, who may have a variety of different health needs.
- **Diagnosis.** Try to identify any undiagnosed medical and psychological problems.
- **Prognosis.** Rough sleepers are more likely to develop serious health problems than the general population.

Associated conditions
- Drug and alcohol dependence.
- Mental illness (e.g. depression, anxiety, personality disorder, psychosis).
- Physical trauma.
- Adverse effects of taking illicit drugs.
- Infections.
- Skin problems.
- Respiratory illness.

RED FLAGS

- Alcohol or drug problems
- Mental health problems
- Risk of suicide
- Physical, sexual or emotional abuse
- Organic disease
- Relationship breakdown
- Unemployment
- Lack of education and qualifications
- Contact with the criminal justice system
- Financial problems

History

Ideas, concerns and expectations
- **Ideas.** Try to identify homeless people's beliefs and attitudes concerning their health. If there are symptoms, what does the patient believe to be the underlying cause?

The 10-Minute Clinical Assessment, Second Edition. Knut Schroeder.
© 2017 John Wiley & Sons, Ltd. Published 2017 by John Wiley & Sons, Ltd.

- **Concerns.** Worries about the future and financial concerns are common.
- **Expectations.** Help with alcohol or drug problems and management of acute infections are common reasons for consultation.

History of presenting complaint

- **Quality of life.** Allow the patient time to tell you their story in their own words. Identify the effect of problems on daily activities. Explore issues around the quality of life.
- **Personal background.** Are there any particular reasons why the patient has been marginalised? Age, gender, disability, ethnic background and sexual orientation may all contribute to people becoming homeless. What is the life context in which the patient has become homeless?
- **Housing status.** Find out details about the patient's current housing situation. There are different types of homelessness. 'Rooflessness' affects rough sleepers and victims of natural disasters or violence. 'Houselessness' concerns people living in temporary accommodation, such as hostels or foster homes. Other types include people living in inadequate accommodation, staying with others on a temporary basis or under threat of losing their accommodation.
- **General health-related problems.** Try to find out the main reasons for any health problems. Multiple morbidity is common, due to complications of illicit drug or alcohol misuse, exposure to other risk factors (see later) or delay in presentation to health services. Are there any particular problems with access to health care? Do offending and imprisonment play a role?
- **Mental health problems.** These are common, and include mental illness (depression, anxiety, personality disorder, psychosis). Dual diagnosis (mental health problems together with alcohol or drug misuse) is common. Agitation and paranoia may be caused by acute drug toxicity, alcohol overuse or withdrawal effects. Try to assess suicidal risk.
- **Alcohol and substance misuse.** Ask about previous and current alcohol intake. People may use drugs such as cocaine and heroin in combination. Are there risks from using unclean equipment for injection? Ask what and how much is being taken.
- **Nutrition.** Ask about food intake, as poor nutrition is common.
- **Infectious disease.** Hepatitis, HIV infection and tuberculosis are relatively common in homeless people. Ask about malaise, swollen lymph nodes, fever, cough, jaundice and weight loss.
- **Prostitution.** Does the patient get paid for sex? Sex workers are very vulnerable and are often subjected to physical, emotional and sexual abuse. There is an increased risk of sexually transmitted infection. Are condoms being used? Does the patient have access to effective contraception?
- **Physical trauma.** Homeless people are often vulnerable to physical attack and misuse.
- **Additional unexplored issues.** Always ask the patient whether there are any other problems or issues that you have not covered which might be important or which they would like to be addressed.

Systems review
* **Cardiac symptoms.** Ask about chest pain, shortness of breath and peripheral oedema. Cardiac problems may be caused by alcoholic cardiomyopathy.
* **Respiratory symptoms.** Chest infections are more common than in the general population. Toxic inhalation of cocaine or other drugs may lead to pulmonary inflammation and oedema (e.g. 'crack lung').
* **Neurological problems.** Neurological symptoms in the legs may be caused by peripheral neuropathy. Gait problems may suggest ataxia due to alcohol or cerebellar degeneration. Rarely, there may also be symptoms of Wernicke's encephalopathy or Korsakoff's psychosis. Have there been any alcohol-related seizures?
* **Gastrointestinal symptoms.** Gastritis, peptic ulcer, hepatitis, cirrhosis, pancreatitis, oesophageal varices and oesophageal carcinoma may occur due to alcohol misuse.
* **Metabolic problems.** Consider vitamin deficiency (in particular, thiamine). Obesity may be caused by poor diet, excessive alcohol intake and lack of exercise.
* **Skin infections.** Louse infestation, scabies and fungal infections are common. Fungal infections will increase the risk of cellulitis.
* **Legs and feet.** Ask about any foot or leg problems, such as leg pain, swelling and frostbite. Numbness may be caused by alcoholic neuropathy.
* **Mouth.** Does the patient suffer from toothache or other dental problems?

Past and current medical problems
* **Significant past illnesses.** Ask about any significant health problems, such as diabetes, respiratory problems and heart disease.
* **Vaccination.** Check the patient's current vaccination status, particularly against tetanus, influenza, pneumococcus and diphtheria, as well as hepatitis.

Medication
* **Chronic illness.** Is the patient taking prescribed medication for any chronic condition?

Family history
* **Significant illness.** Ask about a family history of significant illness, which may contribute to a person's becoming homeless (e.g. Huntington's chorea, Alzheimer's disease).

Social history
* **Housing.** Try and obtain detailed information on past and present housing.
* **Support.** Is support available from a partner, relatives or friends? Ask about the state of current relationships. Have outside agencies, such as social services, been contacted or involved in the past? What information has the patient received about how to contact people and agencies for further support? Are there any barriers, such as lack of confidence or illiteracy?

- **Finance.** Debts are common and can be an important factor in a person's becoming homeless.

Smoking
- **Smoking.** Smoking is more common in homeless people and may predispose to respiratory and cardiac problems.

Review of previous investigations
- **Full blood count.** Is there a history of anaemia? Raised MCV suggests alcohol misuse.
- **Liver function.** Abnormalities may suggest alcoholism or hepatitis.
- **HIV test.** Has the patient ever had a test for HIV?
- **Hepatitis.** What is the patient's immune status with regard to the various forms of hepatitis?
- **Chest X-ray.** Search for evidence of tuberculosis or other respiratory conditions.

Examination

General
- **General condition.** Does the patient look acutely unwell? Chest infections are common. Cachexia, malnutrition, muscle wasting, lymphadenopathy or reduced consciousness may suggest a more serious underlying illness.

Vital signs
- **Temperature.** Consider chest infection, HIV infection or tuberculosis if there is fever (although the temperature may be normal).
- **Blood pressure.** Hypertension is often undertreated.
- **Respiratory rate.** Check for tachypnoea (chest infection, cardiac disease).

Skin
- **Injuries.** Look for evidence of injuries or self-harm.
- **Infection.** Check the head for lice and the rest of the body for evidence of fungal infection or scabies.

Head and neck
- **Mouth.** Look for any obvious oral problems that might contribute to poor health or malnutrition.

Chest
- **Heart.** Check for any signs of heart disease (e.g. valve disease or cardiomegaly).
- **Lungs.** Assess for evidence of infection or fluid retention.

Abdomen

- **Masses.** A swollen abdomen may be due to ascites or malignancy. Check for organomegaly. Is there any tenderness?

Lower limbs

- **Skin and nails.** Foot trauma may occur as a result of walking long distances in inappropriate footwear. Oedema can be caused by venous stasis due to prolonged standing or sitting. The risk of frostbite is higher if there is underlying alcoholic neuropathy. Overgrown toenails are common. There may be a lack of hygiene and fungal infection due to prolonged wearing of unwashed clothing.
- **Neurovascular.** Check all leg pulses for evidence of peripheral vascular disease. Sensory and motor abnormalities due to alcoholic neuropathy are common.

Key references and further reading

1. National Institute for Health and Care Excellence (NICE). Alcohol – problem drinking. Clinical Knowledge Summaries. 2015. Available from: http://cks.nice.org.uk/alcohol-problem-drinking (last accessed 29 April 2016).
2. Shelter. http://england.shelter.org.uk/professional_resources.
3. Timms P, Balázs J. ABC of mental health: mental health on the margins. *BMJ* 1997;315:536–539.
4. Wright N, Tompkins C. How can health services effectively meet the health needs of homeless people? *Br J Gen Pract* 2006;56:286–293.

Paediatrics and adolescent health

The sick and/or feverish child

Key thoughts

Practical points

- **Diagnosis.** Feverish illness is commonly caused by acute viral infections. It is important not to miss serious conditions, such as meningococcal septicaemia or pneumonia, as symptoms and signs may be nonspecific in the early stages. Sick children can be worrying for both parents and health professionals.
- **Severity.** Assess and record temperature, conscious level, respiration rate, heart rate, capillary refill time and the state of hydration in every child that is unwell.
- **Management.** Thorough assessment will help decide whether a child needs to be admitted to hospital or if they can safely be managed in the community.

Possible causes

- **Infection.** Nonspecific viral illness, acute upper respiratory tract infection, gastroenteritis, otitis media, pneumonia, urinary tract infection or, rarely, meningitis, meningococcal septicaemia, septic arthritis or Kawasaki disease.
- **Toxic.** Accidental poisoning.
- **Allergy.** Food allergies (e.g. nuts), insect bites.
- **Trauma.** Accidental general trauma, head injury, non-accidental injury and child abuse.
- **Metabolic (rare).** Diabetic ketoacidosis, hypoglycaemia or an exacerbation of an inborn error of metabolism.
- **Shock (rare).** Septicaemia, hypovolaemia.

RED FLAGS

- Reduced level of alertness
- High fever unresponsive to antipyretic medication and lasting for longer than 5 days
- Petechial or purpuric rash
- Severe diarrhoea and vomiting
- Dehydration
- Increased capillary refill time >3 seconds
- Neck stiffness
- Bulging fontanelle
- Pale, mottled or ashen skin
- Blue lips or tongue
- Tachypnoea with chest indrawing
- Focal neurological signs

The 10-Minute Clinical Assessment, Second Edition. Knut Schroeder.
© 2017 John Wiley & Sons, Ltd. Published 2017 by John Wiley & Sons, Ltd.

History

Ideas, concerns and expectations
- **Ideas.** What do the parents/guardian believe to be the cause of the underlying illness?
- **Concerns.** Worries about meningitis and meningococcal septicaemia are common.
- **Expectations.** Parents may want to be reassured that there is no underlying serious illness. They may also expect a prescription for antibiotics, further investigation or hospital admission.

History of presenting complaint
- **Context.** Ask open questions and listen attentively to the child (if possible) and to what the parents have to say about their child's illness: they are the experts on their child, and may give important clues about possible underlying diagnoses.
- **Age.** Children under 3 months are at higher risk of serious bacterial infection.
- **Main symptoms.** In most cases, symptoms will point to a specific source of infection (e.g. cough, ear ache, sore throat, joint pains, urinary symptoms) or another cause of illness. Has there been any change in symptoms? Have new symptoms emerged? Urinary tract infections often present in a nonspecific way in young children. Poor feeding, lethargy, irritability, abdominal pain, urinary symptoms and offensive or bloodstained urine all point towards urinary tract infection.
- **Alertness.** Has the child been alert and responsive? Lethargy and drowsiness may indicate serious illness requiring hospital admission. If a child is semi- or unconscious, move straight on to assessing airway, breathing and circulation (ABC). A child that still plays and interacts with the environment is unlikely to be seriously ill.
- **Breathing.** Respiratory distress is likely if the child finds it hard to breathe due to chest infection or another cause. If the onset of shortness of breath is sudden and there is no fever or other pointer to infection, consider foreign-body aspiration. Stridor occurs in upper airway obstruction, which may occasionally be caused by laryngo-tracheobronchitis, croup, foreign body or acute epiglottitis (rare).
- **Fever.** Fever indicates infection, such as acute viral illness, gastroenteritis, otitis media, pneumonia, appendicitis, urinary tract infection or, rarely, meningitis, septic arthritis or epiglottitis. Any prolonged fever lasting for more than 5 days will usually require more detailed assessment and investigation and indicates an intermediate risk of serious infection. Has anything been tried to bring the fever down? Did the parents give antipyretics in adequate doses?
- **Rash.** Any non-blanching rash should raise suspicions of meningococcal septicaemia, particularly if the child is ill, if individual lesions are >2 mm in diameter, if there is neck stiffness and if the capillary refill time is ≥3 seconds. Facial petechiae are common, are often benign and are caused by coughing or vomiting.

- **Feeding.** Children who feed normally are less likely to suffer from serious illness. Failure to take oral fluids is of concern and may be a factor when deciding on whether to admit a child to hospital.
- **Diarrhoea and vomiting.** Dehydration is more likely if there is diarrhoea or vomiting associated with reduced fluid intake, particularly in young infants. In severe or prolonged cases, consider bacterial gastroenteritis due to pathogens that are prevalent in the area where the child lives. Vomiting is common and is usually caused by viral illness, but any bile-stained or prolonged vomiting is suggestive of more serious illness (e.g. sepsis, meningitis, abdominal pathology).
- **Pain.** Pain may be difficult to assess in younger children. Pain due to infection such as otitis media may be relatively easy to spot. If there is severe abdominal pain, consider appendicitis or, in rare cases, intestinal obstruction, Meckel's diverticulum or intussusception. Severe headache is common in acute viral illness but may potentially be caused by meningo-encephalitis.
- **Neurological features.** Consider serious illness if there are generalised fits, focal neurological signs or focal seizures. Photophobia should raise suspicions of measles (in susceptible children), meningitis or others causes of raised intracranial pressure.
- **Joint or limb swelling.** Consider septic arthritis or osteomyelitis in a child who has fever associated with joint or limb swelling, particularly if the child is not weight-bearing or not using the limb.
- **Trauma and injury.** Is there a history of trauma or burns? Ask in particular about head and abdominal injury. Has there been any significant bleeding?
- **Lumps.** Any new lumps >2 cm in size should raise suspicions.
- **Mucous membranes.** Consider Kawasaki disease if there is a fever of at least 5 days' duration in association with bilateral conjunctival injection, red mucous membranes, cervical lymphadenopathy, a polymorphous rash and skin changes in the extremities (e.g. peeling, oedema).
- **Allergies.** Has there been exposure to a known allergen, raising the possibility of anaphylactic shock?
- **Urine output.** In young children, ask whether nappies are still wet, as reduced urine output will indicate dehydration. Consider the possibility of new-onset diabetes mellitus if urine output has increased and there is increased fluid intake in a sick child (relatively rare).
- **Headache and neck stiffness.** Headache and neck stiffness may occur in nonspecific viral infections or tonsillitis. Significant neck stiffness indicates possible meningitis, particularly if associated with a fever, rash, reduced consciousness, vomiting or photophobia.
- **Foreign travel.** Consider malaria and other tropical infections if the child has recently returned from a malarial area.

Past and current medical problems
- **Significant past illnesses.** Serious illness is more likely if there are underlying conditions such as prematurity, asthma, diabetes, human immunodeficiency (HIV) infection or, less commonly, congenital heart disease, cancer, cystic fibrosis, immunodeficiency or inborn errors of metabolism.

- **Trauma.** Has there been any recent trauma that might contribute to the child's illness (particularly head injury)?
- **Operations.** Could this be a postoperative infection?
- **Immunisations.** Has the child been immunised as per the recommended schedule? Consider the possibility of measles, mumps, rubella, meningitis and epiglottitis in children who have not received appropriate immunisation and where uptake in the population has been suboptimal.
- **Immunodeficiency.** Any immunocompromised child is at higher risk of infection and serious illness. Consider immunosuppressant drugs, chemotherapy and immunodeficiency disorders (rare).

Medication
- **Analgesics and antipyretics.** What has been used so far, and in what dose? Has this been effective?
- **Antibiotics.** Have these been given? Check preparations and doses.
- **Steroids.** Steroids and immunosuppressants can increase the risk of infection and may mask symptoms such as abdominal tenderness.
- **Drug overdose.** Is there a possibility of accidental drug ingestion or overdose?

Allergies
- **Antibiotics and antipyretics.** Ask about allergies to any drugs that may be needed to treat the illness, particularly antibiotics and analgesics.

Family history
- **Significant diseases.** Ask about any relevant family history.

Social history
- **Home situation.** If the decision is to treat the child at home, can the parents be relied upon to seek medical advice immediately if the child becomes more unwell? Consider the attitude and reliability of the carers, telephone access, transport etc., as the clinical condition in children can change very quickly.

Review of previous investigations
- **Full blood count and inflammatory markers.** Blood tests are rarely required in children who are acutely unwell due to nonspecific viral infections.
- **Chest X-ray.** Useful for diagnosis of pneumonia but not usually required for most upper respiratory infections.
- **Urine microscopy and culture.** Look for signs of urinary tract infection.

Examination

General
- **General condition.** Start by observing the child and their interaction on the parent's lap, without touching. Examination without clothes comes later. Does the child look unwell?

- **Airway, breathing, circulation and disability (ABCD).** Assess ABCD. Defer further assessment until emergency medical care has been provided (if required).
- **Airways and breathing.** Stridor indicates upper airway obstruction. Nasal flaring and grunting suggest increased respiratory effort. Angioedema due to allergic reactions may cause lip and tongue swelling, which can lead to upper airway obstruction. Consider epiglottitis (rare) if there is drooling and inability to swallow, particularly if the child has not been involved in an immunisation programme. In an exhausted child (with or without raised intracranial pressure), respiratory effort can decline: this is a pre-terminal sign.
- **Activity and response.** Playful and cooperative children are unlikely to be seriously ill. Lack of interest in the surroundings, lack of eye contact or drowsiness should raise suspicions of serious underlying illness. Does the child respond to social cues? Is activity decreased? Is the child rouseable? Does the child smile? Is there weak, high-pitched or continuous crying?
- **Capillary refill time and hydration.** Look for evidence of dehydration and hypovolaemia, such as prolonged capillary refill time (>3 seconds), reduced urine output, dry mucous membranes, reduced skin elasticity, sunken fontanelle and sunken eyes. Important causes of dehydration are acute viral illness, diarrhoea and vomiting, burns, haemorrhage and diabetic ketoacidosis.

Vital signs

- **Temperature.** Fever is common with nonspecific viral illness and other infections, such as otitis media, tonsillitis and gastroenteritis. A high prolonged fever may suggest a serious underlying cause. Do not routinely use the oral or rectal route in children aged 0–5 years. A temperature of 38°C in children aged 0–3 months or 39°C in children aged 3–6 months indicates a high risk of serious illness. Preferably, use an electronic thermometer in the axila in children under the age of 4 weeks.
- **Capillary refill.** A reduced capillary refill time suggests more serious illness. Press on the big toe or a finger for 5 seconds and count how long it takes for the colour to return. Longer than 3 seconds suggests intermediate risk of severe infection, while longer than 4 seconds indicates possible shock.
- **Heart rate.** Tachycardia may be caused by high temperature, anxiety or serious illness. Bradycardia may rarely occur in shock or raised intracranial pressure (e.g. intracranial bleed, meningitis), or in pre-terminal children.
- **Blood pressure.** This can be difficult to measure in young children at first contact. Reduced blood pressure is a late sign in shock and indicates serious illness. Normal blood pressure values will depend on the age and sex of the child. Blood pressure tables are available at http://www.nhlbi.nih.gov/health-pro/guidelines/current/hypertension-pediatric-jnc-4/blood-pressure-tables.
- **Respiratory rate.** Consider pneumonia or serious illness if there is tachypnoea of more than 50 breaths per minute in children aged 6–12 months or more than 40 breaths per minute in those aged >12 months, or if the respiratory rate is more than 60 breaths per minute in a child of any age (see box). Nasal flaring or grunting may indicate respiratory distress or serious illness. Look for

any chest indrawing. Remember that respiratory effort can decline if the child gets exhausted or if there is raised intracranial pressure.

NORMAL HEART (HR) AND RESPIRATORY (RR) RATES

- **Infant.** HR 110–160 beats per minute, RR 30–40 breaths per minute.
- **1–2 years.** HR 100–150 beats per minute, RR 25–35 breaths per minute.
- **2–5 years.** HR 95–140 beats per minute, RR 25–30 breaths per minute.

Skin
- **Skin condition and colour.** Mottled, pale, cyanotic or cool skin occurs with impaired circulation. In septic shock, peripheries tend to be warm. Skin peeling suggests staphylococcal infection or Kawasaki disease.
- **Rash.** Any petechial or purpuric non-blanching rash in a febrile child should be treated with penicillin before undertaking further detailed assessment, as this may be caused by meningococcal septicaemia. In the early phases of the disease, the rash may be maculopapular, pink and blanching. Consider the possibility of Kawasaki disease in a child who has had a fever for a few days in conjunction with lymphadenopathy, conjunctivitis and inflamed lips and tongue. Is there any disease-specific rash indicating an infection such as scarlet fever, measles or chickenpox?

Head and neck
- **Pupil responses.** Fixed wide pupils or lack of pupil response indicates brain involvement (e.g. hypoxia, metabolic, trauma).
- **Fontanelle.** A bulging fontanelle in young children suggests serious illness.
- **Neck stiffness.** Consider meningococcal disease or meningitis if there is neck stiffness, particularly with a rash in an ill child.
- **Fundi.** Look for papilloedema, which may, in rare cases, indicate raised intracranial pressure.
- **Ear, nose and throat.** Look for otitis media, tonsillitis, pharyngitis and sinusitis. Koplik's spots may indicate measles (now rare in most countries). Look for central cyanosis in the mucous membranes, which is a serious sign and may suggest pneumonia or cardiovascular compromise.
- **Lymph nodes.** Cervical lymphadenopathy suggests acute upper respiratory infection or, rarely, Kawasaki disease or cancer.

Chest
- **Increased respiratory effort.** Look for intercostal recession and use of accessory muscles.
- **Chest expansion.** Look for asymmetrical or reduced chest expansion, particularly in conjunction with reduced air entry (e.g. pneumothorax, pleural effusion or pneumonia).
- **Wheeze.** Wheeze suggests obstruction of the smaller airways (e.g. bronchiolitis, asthma).

- **Crackles.** Inspiratory coarse crackles may be caused by bronchopneumonia. Bronchiolitis usually causes diffuse crackles. Wheeze may suggest bronchiolitis or asthma.
- **Heart.** Check for any murmurs and added sounds. Consider endocarditis and pericarditis. Cardiac complications may occur with Kawasaki disease.

Abdomen
- **Distension.** Intestinal obstruction may rarely result in a distended abdomen.
- **Tenderness.** Tenderness is common with many viral illnesses or constipation. Suprapubic tenderness may occur with urinary tract infection. Right iliac fossa pain may be caused by appendicitis. Guarding and rebound tenderness suggest peritonitis.
- **Hepatosplenomegaly.** This may indicate severe infection or other systemic disorder.
- **Groins.** Check the hernial orifices for strangulated hernias.
- **Testes.** Testicular torsion is important and not to be missed. It can present with lower abdominal pain and a tender testicle.

Upper and lower limbs
- **Tone.** Reduced or increased tone may occur in serious illness with involvement of the brain.
- **Swelling and tenderness.** If relevant, look for evidence of swollen joints or bones, which may rarely indicate septic arthritis or osteomyelitis.

Bedside tests
- **Blood glucose.** This will help rule out hypo- and hyperglycaemia.
- **Urine dipstick.** Check for signs of infection (blood, protein, leucocytes and nitrites).
- **Pulse oximetry.** Oxygen saturation will be reduced in severe cardiorespiratory compromise. Levels under 95% are abnormal, while levels under 90% suggest more severe hypoxia.

Key references and further reading
1. Baraff LJ. Management of fever without source in infants and children. *Ann Emerg Med* 2000;36:602–614.
2. National Institute for Health and Care Excellence (NICE). Fever in under 5s: assessment and initial management. NICE guidelines [CG160]. May 2013. Available from: http://www.nice.org.uk/guidance/cg160 (last accessed 29 April 2016).
3. Porter SC, Fleisher GR, Kohane IS, Mandl KD. The value of parental report for diagnosis and management of dehydration in the emergency department. *Ann Emerg Med* 2003;41:196–205.

Suspected meningococcal meningitis and septicaemia

Key thoughts

Practical points
- **Diagnosis.** A rash in a febrile child is a common reason for consultation in general practice.
- **Epidemiology.** Meningococcal disease is rare, but may present initially with symptoms very similar to those of nonspecific viral illnesses.
- **Red flags.** A high index of suspicion is important, especially if alarm symptoms are present.
- **Prognosis.** Meningococcal disease carries a poor prognosis if left untreated. Survivors may suffer reduced quality of life, neurological disability, amputation or other lifelong problems.

Differential diagnosis
- Unspecific viral illness.
- Viral meningitis.
- Meningococcal meningitis.
- Meningococcal septicaemia.

Important risk factors
- Contact with a case.
- Winter season.
- Outbreaks of influenza.
- Age under 5.
- Adolescence.

RED FLAGS

- High fever
- Purpuric or petechial non-blanching rash
- Neck stiffness
- Severe headache
- Photophobia
- Convulsions
- Limb pain
- Pale and mottled skin
- Cold hands and feet

The 10-Minute Clinical Assessment, Second Edition. Knut Schroeder.
© 2017 John Wiley & Sons, Ltd. Published 2017 by John Wiley & Sons, Ltd.

- Drowsiness
- Confusion
- Bulging fontanelle in children aged <12 months

History

Ideas, concerns and expectations

- **Ideas.** What do the parents or the child think is causing the symptoms? What do they understand about meningococcal disease? Would they know what to do if the situation got worse? Are they aware of red flag symptoms?
- **Concerns.** Parents are often very concerned when a child develops symptoms that may be caused by meningococcal disease, and it can be difficult to reassure them. Find out which symptom(s) they or the child are most worried about.
- **Expectations.** Parents may simply want reassurance, or they may expect you to arrange further investigation, referral or immediate hospital admission.

History of presenting complaint

- **Contacts.** Has the child or adolescent been exposed to meningococcal disease?
- **Prodromal symptoms.** Fever, nausea, vomiting, general malaise and lethargy are common prodromal symptoms of meningococcal disease but are nearly impossible to distinguish from those caused by benign and self-limiting viral illness. Prodromal symptoms in meningococcal disease may last up to 4 hours in young children and up to 8 hours in adolescents before more specific symptoms and signs develop. In meningococcal disease, symptoms usually develop quickly and the child may deteriorate rapidly.
- **Rash.** A rash typically appears about 8–9 hours after onset of the illness in babies and young children, and later in older children – though these timings may vary.
- **Symptoms in babies.** Meningococcal disease can be difficult to detect in babies and small infants. Symptoms may include poor feeding, irritability when being handled (in association with a high-pitched or moaning cry), vacant staring, poor responsiveness and lethargy.
- **Safety net.** Are the parents, carers or the patient sensible and are they capable of managing the situation? Do they know what to do and how to access health care and obtain medical help if the illness gets worse? Do they have access to a phone and will they easily be able to contact you or another health professional? Are there any problems with transport? Is appropriate help available out of hours, in case you decide not to admit to hospital?

Common presenting patterns

- **Septicaemia.** Ask directly about symptoms of septicaemia, not all of which may be present. In particular, consider fever, a rash anywhere on the body, limb or joint pains, cold hands or feet, pale or mottled skin, rigors, thirst, abdominal pain, diarrhoea, drowsiness, confusion and impaired consciousness. Death is usually due to cardiovascular failure.

- **Meningitis.** Symptoms of meningitis include headache, drowsiness, confusion and impaired consciousness. Neck stiffness, photophobia and a bulging fontanelle are important signs but may not always present in young children. Seizures may occur. Death may result from raised intracranial pressure.

Allergies

- **Antibiotics.** Ask about allergies to any antibiotics that may need to be given (especially penicillin).

Examination

General

- **General condition.** Children with meningococcal disease are likely to look unwell. Does the child maintain eye contact? Are they vomiting?
- **Mental state.** Adolescents or adults may appear aggressive or combative, or may behave in an odd way, which can easily be mistaken for alcohol or drug intoxication.
- **Hydration.** A sunken fontanelle indicates dehydration in young infants.
- **Signs in babies.** Look for abnormal tone on handling, which may be increased or decreased. Is there abnormal posturing? Poor responsiveness, lethargy, cyanosis and vacant staring may indicate serious underlying disease.
- **Conscious level.** Is the child drowsy, confused or not fully conscious? A child that continues to be playful and that is interested in the environment is less likely to be seriously ill. Assess whether the child is alert, responsive to voice only, responsive to pain or unresponsive.

Vital signs

- **Temperature.** There is usually a fever in meningococcal disease, but a normal temperature does not exclude serious illness.
- **Pulse.** Check for tachycardia.
- **Capillary refill.** A reduced capillary refill time suggests more serious illness. Press on the big toe or a finger for 5 seconds and count how long it takes for the colour to return. Longer than 3 seconds suggests intermediate risk of severe infection, while longer than 4 seconds indicates possible shock.
- **Respiratory rate.** Check for fast and laboured breathing (see box).

NORMAL HEART (HR) AND RESPIRATORY (RR) RATES

- **Infant.** HR 110–160 beats per minute, RR 30–40 breaths per minute.
- **1–2 years.** HR 100–150 beats per minute, RR 25–35 breaths per minute.
- **2–5 years.** HR 95–140 beats per minute, RR 25–30 breaths per minute.

Skin
- **Colour.** Look out for pale or mottled skin.
- **Rash.** Check for a rash anywhere on the body. Maculopapular rash is common with nonspecific viral illness. A non-blanching purpuric or petechial rash is suggestive of meningococcal disease, although a majority of children with petechial rashes will turn out not to have the disease. A purpuric rash may easily be confused with a bruise.

Head and neck
- **Neck stiffness.** This may indicate meningitis, but may not always be present in young children. Ask the child to kiss their knees, or check passive flexion if the child is not cooperative. The absence of neck stiffness does not exclude serious underlying illness.
- **Fontanelle.** In babies, a sunken fontanelle may be caused by dehydration, while a tense, bulging fontanelle may indicate raised intracranial pressure due to infection.
- **Conjunctivae.** Check the conjunctivae for a petechial rash.
- **Fundi.** Look for papilloedema and retinal haemorrhages.
- **Pupils.** Check pupil size and reaction.

Upper and lower limbs
- **Temperature.** Cold hands and feet may indicate severe underlying disease, although this sign is not very specific.
- **Limb or joint pain.** Look out for any limb or joint tenderness, which are easily misdiagnosed initially as fractures due to the intense pain.

Chest
- **Heart.** Check for any obvious murmurs.
- **Lungs.** Search for signs of respiratory infection.

Bedside tests
- **Oxygen saturation.** Hypoxia is present if oxygen saturation is <95% on air.

Key references and further reading
1. Brennan K, Somerset M, Granier S et al. Management of diagnostic uncertainty in children with possible meningitis: a qualitative study. *Br J Gen Pract* 2003;53:626–631.
2. Hart CA, Thompson AP. Meningococcal disease and its management in children. *BMJ* 2006;333:685–690.
3. Meningitis Research Foundation. Meningococcal meningitis and septicaemia: guidance notes. 2014 edition. Available from: http://www.meningitis.org/assets/x/50631 (last accessed 29 April 2016).
4. National Institute for Health and Care Excellence (NICE). Fever in under 5s: assessment and initial management. NICE guidelines [CG160]. May 2013.

Available from: http://www.nice.org.uk/guidance/cg160 (last accessed 29 April 2016).

5. National Institute for Health and Care Excellence (NICE). Meningitis (bacterial) and meningococcal septicaemia in children and young people. NICE quality standard [QS19]. June 2012. Available from: http://www.nice.org.uk/guidance/qs19 (last accessed 29 April 2016).

6. Thompson M, Ninis N, Perera R et al. Clinical recognition of meningococcal disease in children and adolescents. *Lancet* 2006;367:397–403.

Neonatal jaundice

Key thoughts

Practical points
- **Severity.** Mild jaundice in the first few days of life is physiological. Very high levels of bilirubin are toxic and can lead to encephalopathy (kernicterus). Jaundice is difficult to assess clinically, particularly in dark-skinned children.
- **Serious illness.** Consider infection or haemolysis if jaundice develops within the first 24 hours. Persistent jaundice lasting for more than 14 days may have pathological causes, such as infection, hypothyroidism, haemolysis or liver disease. Consider the possibility of congenital biliary atresia.

Possible causes
- Breast milk jaundice.
- Physiological jaundice.
- Infection.
- Hypothyroidism.
- Liver disease (e.g. neonatal hepatitis, biliary atresia).
- Haemolysis.
- Galactosaemia.

RED FLAGS

- Jaundice in the first 24 hours after birth
- Prolonged jaundice (>2 weeks)
- Severe jaundice
- Fever
- Poor feeding
- Poor weight gain
- Lethargy
- Irritability

History

Ideas, concerns and expectations
- **Ideas.** What do the parents believe to be the underlying problem?
- **Concerns.** Parents are often worried about the possibility of brain damage.
- **Expectations.** Parents will often expect further investigation or specialist referral, which may or may not be indicated.

The 10-Minute Clinical Assessment, Second Edition. Knut Schroeder.
© 2017 John Wiley & Sons, Ltd. Published 2017 by John Wiley & Sons, Ltd.

History of presenting complaint

- **Prematurity.** Premature babies are at higher risk of becoming jaundiced, due to the immaturity of the liver to process bilirubin. They are also more at risk of brain damage from a raised bilirubin than is a baby delivered at term.
- **Delivery.** A traumatic delivery that resulted in bruising, cephalohaematoma or internal bleeding may cause jaundice due to breakdown of haemoglobin into bilirubin.
- **Onset.** Early jaundice within 24 hours of delivery may indicate infection or haemolytic disease. Prolonged jaundice for more than 2 weeks can indicate serious underlying disease, such as biliary atresia.
- **Feeding.** Breastfeeding can lead to increased bilirubin levels, but the resulting jaundice is likely to settle without the need for investigation or treatment. Breastfeeding should be continued.
- **General well being.** If the child is alert, feeding well and generally healthy, the risk of serious illness is low. Fever, lethargy, feeding problems and irritability suggest a more serious underlying cause.
- **Urine and stools.** If a baby is jaundiced, stools and urine should always be inspected by a health professional. A baby's urine is normally colourless. Normal stools can be anything from yellow to green. A stools colour chart is available at www.yellowalert.org. Dark urine and pale stools suggest obstructive jaundice. If urine is offensive or cloudy, consider urinary tract infection. Jaundice associated with pale stools, yellow urine and bleeding tendency (due to impaired absorption of vitamin K) suggests biliary atresia, which is rare but is fatal if untreated. Delay in diagnosis may lead to irreversible cirrhosis and liver failure. Biliary atresia can be present even if the child appears to be thriving well in the short term. Check stools and urine yourself if possible, as parents' descriptions can be unreliable.
- **Hypothyroidism.** Look for the results of the heel prick test, which is usually performed about 1 week after delivery.
- **Weight.** If birth weight has not been regained after 10 days, consider referral for further investigation.
- **Dark skin.** Jaundice can be more difficult to spot in children with darker skin. Look for jaundice in the sclerae and have a lower threshold for checking split-conjugated and unconjugated bilirubin.
- **Complications.** If jaundice has been prolonged, look for evidence of brain damage (kernicterus) with symptoms of visual impairment, loss of hearing, cerebral palsy, seizures or learning difficulties.

Family history

- **Liver.** Ask about a family history of liver enzyme or other metabolic conditions which might lead to neonatal jaundice.
- **Blood group.** Is there a history of blood group incompatibility between the mother and previous children, such as rhesus incompatibility?

Social history

- **Home situation.** If the child is treated at home, can the parents be relied upon to report any change in the condition?

Review of previous investigations

- **Split bilirubin levels.** It is important to look at split bilirubin (i.e. both the conjugated (direct) and unconjugated (indirect) bilirubin) in all children in whom jaundice persists for more than 2 weeks after birth. The threshold for treating raised unconjugated bilirubin levels will depend on absolute bilirubin levels, the rate of increase in bilirubin concentration and the gestational age at delivery. In more severe cases, exchange transfusion may be needed. Breast milk jaundice is caused by unconjugated hyperbilirubinaemia. If the conjugated bilirubin is >20% of the total bilirubin, the baby needs to be referred immediately for further assessment and investigation.
- **Full blood count.** Is there evidence of haemolysis?
- **Direct Coombs test.** Use this to check for antibodies to red blood cells.
- **Liver function tests.** Abnormalities may indicate liver disease.
- **Urine culture.** Is there evidence of urinary tract infection?

Examination

General

- **Handling.** Poor handling and an increased muscle tone may result from neurotoxicity caused by jaundice.
- **General condition.** If the child is unwell, consider sepsis.
- **Dysmorphic features.** These may suggest a congenital abnormality.

Vital signs

- **Temperature.** Consider sepsis if there is fever, although the temperature may be normal.
- **Pulse.** Tachycardia may suggest infection or other serious underlying disease. There may be relative bradycardia in hypothyroidism.
- **Respiratory rate.** A raised respiratory rate may indicate respiratory infection or other serious illness.

Skin

- **Colour.** Is there obvious jaundice? This may be demonstrated by blanching the skin on the forehead, as jaundice often spreads from the head downwards. Serious illness is more likely if hands and toes are affected.

Head and neck

- **Sclera.** Look for evidence of jaundice.

Chest

- **Lungs.** Is there evidence of chest infection?

Abdomen

- **Liver and spleen.** Check for hepatosplenomegaly.

Bedside tests
• **Urine.** Examine blood, nitrites, leucocytes and protein to check for urinary tract infection.

Key references and further reading
1. Children's Liver Disease Foundation. www.childliverdisease.org.
2. Moerschel SK, Cianciaruso LB, Tracy LR. A practical approach to neonatal jaundice. *Am Fam Physician* 2008;77:1255–1262.

3. National Institute for Health and Care Excellence (NICE). Jaundice in newborn babies under 28 days. NICE guidelines [CG98]. May 2010. Available from: http://www.nice.org.uk/guidance/cg98 (last accessed 29 April 2016).
4. Venigalla S, Gourley GR. Neonatal cholestasis. *Semin Perinatol* 2004;28:348–355.

Faltering growth

Key thoughts

Practical points

- **Diagnosis.** Faltering growth is a common problem, with many possible causes. Be aware of possible underlying disease in a minority of cases. Faltering growth is defined as body weight consistently below the 3rd centile for age, progressive loss of weight to below the 3rd centile or a reduction in the expected rate of growth based on the appropriate growth chart.
- **Prognosis.** Identifying children who do not gain weight as expected may help to prevent short stature or poor academic performance when they get older.
- **Management.** Decide whether a child can be managed in the community or whether specialist referral is needed.

Possible causes

- **Non-organic causes.** Psychosocial causes, including reduced calorie intake (lack of food), difficult home circumstances, neglect and constitutional delay (variation of healthy development).
- **Organic causes.** Chronic severe asthma, chronic diarrhoea, intrauterine growth retardation, lactose intolerance, cow's milk protein intolerance, cystic fibrosis, coeliac disease, inflammatory bowel disease (e.g. Crohn's disease), chronic renal tract infection, genetic causes (e.g. Turner's syndrome or skeletal dysplasia), central nervous system (CNS) problems (such as cerebral palsy) and endocrine causes (growth hormone deficiency, Cushing's syndrome, hypothyroidism).

RED FLAGS

- Crossing two or more centiles downwards on the growth chart
- Weight below the 3rd centile
- Weight two centiles below the child's centile for height or length
- Underlying medical conditions
- Prolonged diarrhoea
- Social problems
- General malaise
- Physical or emotional abuse
- Abdominal pain

The 10-Minute Clinical Assessment, Second Edition. Knut Schroeder.
© 2017 John Wiley & Sons, Ltd. Published 2017 by John Wiley & Sons, Ltd.

History

Ideas, concerns and expectations
- **Ideas.** What do the parents or carers think is causing faltering growth?
- **Concerns.** Parents are often worried that their child is smaller than other children. Fussy eating is a common reason for concern.
- **Expectations.** Why does the child present now? What do the parents expect in terms of further investigation and management? Many parents will need reassurance only.

History of presenting complaint
- **Illness overview.** Encourage the child (if possible) and the parents to tell you in their own words about issues around growth.
- **Age.** Establish at what age the problems started. Most children considered small for gestational age will catch up within the first 2 years of life. Growth problems in infants are often a result of inadequate nutrition. Hormonal causes are more common in adolescents.
- **Weight and height.** Poor weight gain is common in faltering growth. Short parents often have short children. Look at the child's previous records in terms of height and weight to assess the growth pattern.
- **Diet.** Take a detailed dietary history. Is the infant breastfed or is formula milk being used? Find out whether the child snacks between meals, particularly with junk food. Is force being used for feeding? If the child is old enough, do the parents encourage self-feeding? Are there regular meal times? Is good eating behaviour rewarded? Excessive fluid intake of sweet drinks in particular can reduce appetite at meal times.
- **Insufficient calorie input.** There may be underfeeding if the child is of good health but not gaining weight in the absence of an organic cause. Breastfed babies may be slower to gain weight in the first few months. Do the parents prepare formula feeds correctly? Are there any physical or psychological problems with feeding (e.g. vomiting, regurgitation)? These may indicate gastrooesophageal reflux, especially in the first 6 months of life.
- **Physical neglect or abuse.** Faltering growth can result from abuse or neglect – consider this if there are inconsistencies in the history or if there is evidence of social problems. Has the mother been suffering from postnatal depression? Consider factitious disorders if the story changes or is inconsistent.
- **Diarrhoea.** Protracted diarrhoea can lead to weight loss and may potentially be caused by pancreatic insufficiency in cystic fibrosis or coeliac disease. In coeliac disease, stools are often offensive, bulky and floating. Symptoms only start once gluten-containing foods have been introduced into the child's diet. A dislike of biscuits is an early symptom.
- **Abdominal pain.** Abdominal discomfort after feeds suggests gastrooesophageal reflux. Painful abdominal distension may also occur with coeliac disease, lactose intolerance or cow's milk protein intolerance.

- **Recent gastrointestinal infection.** Immediate return to milk in an infant or young child after acute gastrointestinal infection may lead to lactose intolerance, which can persist for weeks or months. Symptoms include abdominal distension, diarrhoea (caused by osmosis), nappy rash due to acid stools and faltering growth.
- **Cow's milk protein intolerance.** This usually presents in children under 2 years of age, with bloody diarrhoea accompanied by mucus and malabsorption. Abdominal pain, growth retardation and vomiting may indicate allergic gastroenteritis. This can lead to anaemia and may be associated with eczema and allergy, as well as protein-losing enteropathy.
- **Fever and ill health.** Nonspecific viral illnesses or chronic infections (e.g. suppurative otitis media, tuberculosis (TB), HIV) may cause fever and affect growth. Crohn's disease is rare in childhood but may present with fever, general malaise, failure to thrive, arthritis and anaemia.
- **Development.** Ask whether expected milestones have been reached in terms of overall development, including speech, social and motor development.
- **Other physical symptoms.** Are there any other physical symptoms that might be important?

Past and current medical problems
- **Significant past illnesses.** Ask specifically about cardiac, renal, respiratory and endocrine disease, or any recent severe viral illness.
- **Perinatal history.** Ask about any problems in the mother's antenatal and postnatal period. Were there any complications around the time of the delivery?

Medication
- **Alginate preparations.** Alginate preparations are commonly used for the management of reflux. If prescribed, have these been taken, and are they effective?

Other treatments
- **Dietician.** Has the child ever been assessed and treated by a dietician?

Social history
- **Parental attitude.** Parental withdrawal or hostility can lead to growth problems in a child. Disappointment over the sex, growth or appearance of a child may lead to their rejection, with resulting growth problems. Was the child planned, or was this an unwanted pregnancy?
- **Home situation.** Are there any problems at home, for example, with finance, housing, relationships etc.?

Review of previous investigations
- **Full blood count.** Anaemia may be caused by malabsorption.
- **Inflammatory markers.** Plasma viscosity may be raised in infection or inflammatory conditions.

- **Urea and electrolytes.** Look for evidence of dehydration (raised urea) and renal problems.
- **Liver function tests.** A low albumin suggests malnutrition or liver disease.
- **Thyroid function.** Both hypo- and hyperthyroidism may cause faltering growth.
- **Urine culture.** This will identify underlying chronic urinary tract infection.
- **Coeliac antibodies.** Coeliac disease can easily be missed.
- **Stools.** If there is diarrhoea, has a stool culture been performed? Look for steatorrhoea or pallor.

Examination

General
- **General condition.** Does the child look well?
- **Muscle wasting.** Is there evidence of muscle wasting (e.g. wasted buttocks)?
- **Psychological impression.** Consider abuse or emotional deprivation if the child appears apathetic and emotionally detached. Does the child look unhappy, defiant or irritable? Is language development delayed? Is the child able to concentrate? How does the child interact with the parent or carer?
- **Physical signs.** Are there any obvious signs of neglect or abuse, developmental delay or physical illness?

Weight and height
- **Weight.** Consider the possibility of faltering growth in children who have a weight that is below the 3rd centile for their age and gender or that has crossed two or more centiles downwards. Diagnosing faltering growth can be difficult; a good way to do it is to keep looking at a child's growth chart over time. Compare with previous readings, if available, and plot on an appropriate children's growth chart (e.g. WHO Growth Standards, http://www.who.int/childgrowth/standards/en/).
- **Height.** A weight 2 centiles below the child's height and head circumference centiles indicates faltering growth and a need for further assessment. A reduced weight in a child of normal height suggests decreased calorie intake (e.g. feeding problems, malabsorption secondary to coeliac disease or Crohn's, poor relationship between mother and child).

Abdomen
- **Distension.** Abdominal distension may indicate coeliac disease.
- **Palpation.** Right iliac fossa tenderness may suggest appendicitis or Crohn's disease.
- **Perianal lesions.** Consider Crohn's disease if there are any perianal lesions.

Key references and further reading
1. Black MM, Dubowitz H, Hutcheson J et al. A randomized clinical trial of home intervention for children with failure to thrive. *Pediatrics* 1995;95:807–814.

2. Black MM, Dubowitz H, Krishnakumar A, Starr RH. Early intervention and recovery among children with failure to thrive: follow-up at age 8. *Pediatrics* 2007;120;59–69.
3. BMJ Best Practice. Failure to thrive. Available from: http://bestpractice.bmj .com/best-practice/monograph/747.html (last accessed 29 April 2016).
4. Krugman SD, Dubowitz H. Failure to thrive. *Am Fam Physician* 2003;68:879–884, 886.
5. Shields B, Wacogne I, Wright CM. Weight faltering and failure to thrive in infancy and early childhood. *BMJ* 2012;345:e5931.

Headache and migraine in children

Key thoughts

Practical points
- **Diagnosis.** Many headaches in children presenting in primary care are benign and self-limiting. Consider the possibility of intracranial complications after head injury.
- **Causes.** Rarely, serious causes such as tumour, intracranial bleed or meningitis may be responsible.
- **Action.** Acute severe headache is more likely to require urgent action than mild intermittent chronic headache.

Possible causes
- **Common.** Nonspecific viral infection, otitis media, sinusitis, psychological (e.g. problems at home or school), refraction error, migraine, post-traumatic.
- **Rare.** Meningitis, CNS tumour or haemorrhage, carbon monoxide poisoning.

RED FLAGS

- Vomiting
- Recent change in behaviour
- Reduced conscious level
- Convulsions
- Papilloedema
- Change in head circumference
- Prominent scalp veins
- Sun-setting eyes
- New or worsening squint
- Cranial nerve palsy
- Cerebellar signs
- Raised blood pressure with or without bradycardia

History

Ideas, concerns and expectations
- **Ideas.** What does the child or their parents think is causing the headache?
- **Concerns.** Parents are often concerned about the possibility of brain cancer or meningitis.

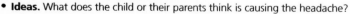

The 10-Minute Clinical Assessment, Second Edition. Knut Schroeder.
© 2017 John Wiley & Sons, Ltd. Published 2017 by John Wiley & Sons, Ltd.

- **Expectations.** Parents often come for reassurance or expect further investigation.

___

History of presenting complaint
- **Illness overview and context.** Ask the child and the parents to tell you in their own words about the headache and what it means to them. If the headache is chronic, how has day-to-day life been affected?
- **Onset and progression.** Is the headache acute or chronic? When did the headache start? Common infections (viral, otitis media) often cause headaches, but usually other symptoms are also present. Longstanding intermittent headache may be a result of migraine, particularly if there are attacks lasting between 1 and 72 hours.
- **Site.** Nonspecific headaches often affect the frontal region above the eyes. Migraine headaches are often unilateral.
- **Severity.** Most headaches in children will be mild or moderately severe. Very severe headache should raise suspicions of serious underlying disease. In migraine, the pain is often moderate to severe and of pulsating quality.
- **Trigger factors.** Stress (e.g. school problems, bullying, parental arguments) and sleep problems may precipitate tension headache. Chocolate, cheese and menstruation are possible trigger factors for migraine.
- **Aggravating factors.** Migraine headaches are usually made worse by exercise. Rarely, postural and early-morning headaches or those that get worse on straining or sneezing may be caused by raised intracranial pressure.
- **Associated symptoms.** Fever, malaise and respiratory symptoms suggest a nonspecific viral illness. Ask about dental problems. Consider meningococcal disease if there is a non-blanching rash. Nausea, vomiting, photophobia and focal neurological signs occur with migraines and with more serious underlying causes, such as meningitis or brain tumour. Visual problems may occur with migraine, meningitis or CNS lesions.
- **Precipitating factors.** Has any trauma or infection preceded the onset of headache? Has the child been exposed to any toxins?
- **General symptoms.** Rarely, weight changes, sleep problems, reduced levels of energy, night sweats and lymphadenopathy may indicate a systemic underlying cause or cancer.
- **Migraine.** Could the headache be due to migraine? Migraine without aura is most common. Migraine with aura occurs in around a quarter of children with migraine. Rarer forms are aura without headache, hemiplegic migraine, basilar migraine, ophthalmoplegic migraine and acute confusional migraine. Periodic symptoms may include abdominal migraine, cyclical vomiting and benign paroxysmal vertigo.

___

Past and current medical problems
- **Asthma.** A history of asthma is a contraindication to using beta adrenoceptor blockers for the prevention of migraine.
- **Cancer.** A past history of cancer raises the possibility of recurrence or metastasis.

- **Trauma.** Ask about any head trauma in the past 3 months.
- **Operations.** Have there been any major operations in the past?

Medication

- **Analgesics.** What has been tried so far, and what has been effective? Have there been any adverse effects? Have any herbal or over-the-counter drugs been taken? Is medication taken in the right dose and frequency? Could this be analgesic overuse headache?
- **Antiemetics.** These can be useful in the treatment of migraine, but may cause dystonia, particularly in young people.

Allergies

- **Drugs.** Are there any allergies to drugs that might be used for the treatment of the headache?

Family history

- **Migraine.** Migraine can run in families.

Social history

- **Home.** How has the headache affected home life? Have any new gas fires been installed (carbon monoxide poisoning)? Are there other people in the household with similar headaches?
- **School.** Has school performance been affected? Does the headache happen only on school days? Is the child being bullied at school?

Review of previous investigations

- **Full blood count and inflammatory markers.** These may have been performed in chronic headache for investigation of possible cancer.
- **Imaging.** Has the child had a brain scan for suspected intracranial pathology?

Examination

General

- **General condition.** If the child is unwell with reduced consciousness, consider a serious underlying cause.
- **Gait.** Unsteady gait may indicate cerebellar involvement in intracranial lesions.

Vital signs

- **Temperature.** If raised, consider self-limiting acute infection or, rarely, more severe infection such as meningococcal disease.
- **Pulse.** Tachycardia suggests severe pain or infection. Rarely, bradycardia may occur with brain tumours.
- **Blood pressure.** Raised intracranial pressure can lead to changes in blood pressure.

- **Respiratory rate.** Respiratory depression may occur with codeine overdose (analgesic overuse headache – rare in children). Tachypnoea may be a result of underlying infection or severe pain.

Skin

- **Rash.** Look for petechiae and purpuric rash if there is possible meningococcal disease.

Head and neck

- **Neck stiffness.** Consider meningitis if there is significant neck stiffness.
- **Photophobia.** Light intolerance occurs with migraine and is usually severe in meningitis.
- **Pupils.** Do the pupils react to light and accommodation? Abnormalities may suggest an intracranial lesion.
- **Fundi.** Papilloedema suggests raised intracranial pressure.
- **Ears and throat.** Look for evidence of upper respiratory infection and otitis media.

Chest

- **Lungs.** Is there any evidence of respiratory infection?

Limbs

- **Neurological assessment.** Check tone, power, sensation, coordination and reflexes if you suspect a CNS cause for the headache.

Key references and further reading

1. Abu-Arefeh I, Russell G. Prevalence of headache and migraine in schoolchildren. *BMJ* 1994;309:765–769.
2. Barnes N, James E, Millman GC. Migraine headache in children. *BMJ Clin Evid* 2006;15:469–475.
3. The International Headache Society. www.ihs-headache.org.
4. National Institute for Health and Care Excellence (NICE). Headaches in over 12s: diagnosis and management. NICE guidelines [CG150]. September 2012. Available from: http://www.nice.org.uk/guidance/cg150 (last accessed 19 April 2016).
5. Oleson J. The international classification of headache disorders. Cephalgia 2004;24(Suppl.):9–160.

Head injury in children

Key thoughts

Practical points

- **Diagnosis.** Identify any complications from head injury and consider the possibility of non-accidental injury.
- **Prognosis.** Assess severity and differentiate minor from serious head injury.
- **Management.** Evaluate whether a child can safely be managed at home or whether close observation in hospital or even referral to a neurosurgical unit is needed. Decide whether you should request an immediate computerised tomography (CT) of the brain and the cervical spine. Check for evidence of cervical spine injury.

RED FLAGS

- Reduced Glasgow Coma Scale (GCS) score
- Suspected open or depressed skull fracture
- Tense or bulging fontanelle
- Signs of basal skull fracture
- Fits
- Focal neurological deficit
- Vomiting
- Retrograde amnesia for more than 5 minutes prior to the impact
- Witnessed loss of consciousness lasting for more than 5 minutes
- Abnormal drowsiness
- Dangerous mechanism of injury
- Suspected non-accidental injury

History

Ideas, concerns and expectations

- **Ideas.** What do the parents or carers think is wrong?
- **Concerns.** Fears about possible brain damage are common.
- **Expectations.** Parents of children with minor head injury may expect admission to hospital or a brain scan, which in many cases will not be indicated.

History of presenting complaint

- **Context.** Allow the parents or carers time to explain in their own words what has happened. How have symptoms affected the child's activities to date?

The 10-Minute Clinical Assessment, Second Edition. Knut Schroeder.
© 2017 John Wiley & Sons, Ltd. Published 2017 by John Wiley & Sons, Ltd.

- **Mechanism of injury.** Find out exactly what has happened and at what times. Establish whether there has been a dangerous mechanism of injury. For example, did the child get struck by a motor vehicle? Was there a fall from a height or a high-speed injury from a projectile or an object? Establish whether there has been an axial load to the head, which may occur in rollover motor accidents, bicycle collisions or accidents involving motorised recreational vehicles.
- **Neck pain.** Any neck pain suggests possible injury to the cervical spine. Is there any other reason to suspect injury to the cervical spine?
- **Alertness.** Has the child been tired, drowsy or unconscious?
- **Focal neurological symptoms.** Ask about any focal neurological symptoms, such as problems with vision, hearing, swallowing, movements, muscle strengths, sensation or coordination. Any of these symptoms may suggest serious head or spinal injury.
- **Features of serious head injury.** A number of symptoms and signs may suggest serious head injury, including more than one episode of vomiting, seizures, open skull fracture, drowsiness, irritability, leaking of cerebrospinal fluid (CSF) from the nose or ears, severe headache and amnesia of events more than 5 minutes prior to impact.
- **Safety of cervical spine assessment.** Examination of the cervical spine will usually be safe if the child was involved in a simple rear-end motor vehicle collision, is sitting comfortably and has been walking around since the injury, if there is no midline tenderness of the spine and if there is delayed onset of neck pain. Immobilise the spine if there is a GCS <15 on initial assessment, focal neurological deficit, paraesthesia of the extremities or any other clinical suspicion of cervical spine injury.
- **Non-accidental injury.** Is there any indication to suggest that the child may have been subjected to non-accidental injury?
- **Head injury advice.** Check if any head injury advice has already been given, particularly if you plan to discharge the child home. An example from NICE is available at http://www.nice.org.uk/CG56.

Past and current medical problems
- **Clotting disorders.** A child with a history of bleeding or clotting disorders or who is currently taking anticoagulants is at higher risk of intracranial haemorrhage.
- **Chronic diseases.** Ask about any chronic diseases that might affect management (e.g. asthma, diabetes, epilepsy, congenital heart disease).

Medication
- **Analgesics.** Has any analgesia been given? If so, is pain adequately controlled?
- **Chronic diseases.** Ask about any regular medication and check for any drugs that might affect symptoms or management.

Allergies
- **Drugs.** Ask in particular about allergies to any drugs that may need to be used for the management of head injury, such as analgesics or antibiotics.

Social history
* **Home.** Children with head injury should only be discharged home if there is someone suitable to supervise and observe them.
* **Social background.** Is the child known to social services? Always consider the possibility of non-accidental injury, particularly if the story given by the parents or carer is vague and inconsistent with the injuries sustained.

Alcohol, smoking and recreational drugs
* **Alcohol.** In teenagers, has alcohol been involved in the injury? There is a higher risk of complications if there is alcohol intoxication.
* **Drugs.** Is there evidence of drug misuse, if you are dealing with a teenager? This may affect management with opioid analgesics and raises the possibility of their having been the victim of non-accidental injury, such as violent crime.

Examination

General

* **Level of consciousness.** Whenever giving the GCS score, always describe its four components (eye opening, verbal response, grimace response and motor response – full score details are available at www.glasgowcomascale.org). If the GCS is >8, this is an indication to involve an anaesthetist or critical care physician early. A deteriorating conscious level during or after the initial assessment suggests serious head injury. A child that is being assessed for discharge home needs to have a GCS of 15.
* **Screen for trauma.** Look for any evidence of other trauma, as suggested by the history. Copious bleeding into the mouth may require intubation.
* **ABC.** Ensure that airway, breathing and circulation (ABC) are adequate prior to further assessment.

Vital signs
* **Temperature.** Any fever may suggest a wound or an underlying infection.
* **Pulse.** Tachycardia may be caused by pain or by intravascular fluid depletion. Raised intracranial pressure may lead to tachycardia or bradycardia.
* **Blood pressure.** Raised intracranial pressure can lead to changes in blood pressure.
* **Respiratory rate.** A reduced respiratory rate or abnormal breathing patterns may occur in raised intracranial pressure.

Head and neck
* **Skull fracture.** Inspect the head for any signs of open or depressed skull fracture.
* **Ears.** Haematotympanum or leakage of CSF suggests fracture of the base of the skull. Also look for evidence of bruising over the mastoids (Battle's sign).

- **Nose.** Consider fracture of the base of the skull if there is leakage of CSF.
- **Eyes.** Look for periorbital ecchymosis (panda eyes), which may occur in fracture of the base of the skull. Check pupil size and reactivity, which may be abnormal in raised intracranial pressure.
- **Cranial nerves.** Check for any evidence of a focal neurological deficit.
- **Cervical spine.** If it is safe to do so (see History of Presenting Complaint), check for midline tenderness, which suggests possible cervical spine injury.
- **Neck rotation.** Check whether the child is able to actively rotate their neck to 45° to both sides.

Skin
- **Signs of injury.** Look for any signs of injury or clues that raise the possibility of non-accidental injury.

Upper and lower limbs
- **Movements.** Check for spontaneous limb movements. Is there any obvious asymmetry (suggesting a more serious brain injury)?

Chest
- **Inspection.** Look for any obvious chest injury. Are breathing patterns and depth of inspiration normal?
- **Lungs.** Check air entry to exclude pneumothorax. Percuss and listen to the lungs for any evidence of haemothorax.
- **Heart.** Are there any abnormalities that might pose an increased perioperative risk?

Abdomen
- **Inspection.** Look for any obvious injuries.
- **Palpation.** Feel for any masses and tenderness that might suggest intra-abdominal injury and bleeding.

Bedside tests
- **Blood oxygen saturation.** Check for evidence of hypoxia.

Regular observation
- **Documentation.** If the child is being observed, ensure that GCS (adult or paediatric), limb movements, blood pressure, respiratory rate, temperature, pupil size and reactivity, heart rate and blood oxygen concentration are recorded and documented at each assessment.

Key references and further reading
1. National Institute for Health and Care Excellence (NICE). Head injury: triage, assessment, investigation and early management of head injury in infants, children and adults. NICE guidelines [CG56]. September 2007. Available from: https://www.nice.org.uk/guidance/cg56 (last accessed 29 April 2016).
2. Smits M, Dippel D, De Haan G et al. External validation of the Canadian CT head rule and the New Orleans criteria for CT scanning in patients with minor head injury. *JAMA* 2005;294:1519–1525.

Suspected cancer in children and adolescents

Key thoughts

Practical points
- **Diagnosis.** Cancer is rare in children but should be considered in unusual presentations with unexplained or progressive symptoms. Missed or delayed diagnosis is common.
- **Unusual symptoms.** Consider cancer if symptoms are unusual or do not resolve as expected.

Important cancers in children and adolescents
- Leukaemia.
- Brain and CNS tumours.
- Bone tumours.
- Lymphoma.
- Soft-tissue tumours.

RED FLAGS

- Multiple consultations for the same unexplained problem
- Weight loss
- Sweats
- Malaise and fatigue
- Bone pains
- Unexplained chronic fever
- Progressive headache
- Neurological features

History

Ideas, concerns and expectations
- **Ideas.** What do the child and the parents believe to be the underlying problem?
- **Parental concerns.** Take parental concerns seriously. Parents are experts on their children, and persistent parental anxiety is a sufficient reason for a very careful and comprehensive assessment.
- **Expectations.** Ask about expectations with regard to further investigation, treatment and referral.

The 10-Minute Clinical Assessment, Second Edition. Knut Schroeder.
© 2017 John Wiley & Sons, Ltd. Published 2017 by John Wiley & Sons, Ltd.

History of presenting complaint

- **Context.** Ask open questions about the context in which symptoms started and the effect they have on the child and anyone around them.
- **Multiple presentation.** Consider serious underlying pathology if a child or young person presents three or more times with the same problem without a clear explanation for the symptoms.
- **General symptoms.** Nonspecific symptoms like malaise, pallor, profuse sweating, weight loss and lethargy may be caused by cancer. Excessive bruising or bleeding may be caused by leukaemia.
- **Lymph glands.** Acute lymphadenopathy is commonly caused by benign self-limiting infections. Chronically swollen lymph glands occur in metastatic disease or lymphoma and may indicate leukaemia if associated with petechiae and unexplained bruising.
- **Metastatic disease.** Think of possible metastatic disease if faced with:
  o Malaise.
  o Fatigue.
  o Bone pain.
  o Pallor.
  o Irritability.
  o Unexplained fever.
  o Respiratory symptoms and recurrent respiratory infections.
  o Haematuria.
  o Unexplained weight loss.
- **Bone pain.** Any chronic bone and back pain which is also present at rest may be caused by bone tumours, such as osteosarcoma or Ewing's sarcoma. Also consider bone cancer if there is unexplained and ongoing limp, particularly if associated with localised bone pain or swelling.
- **Shortness of breath.** Shortness of breath can be a presenting symptom of lymphoma, particularly if progressive and associated with petechiae and/or hepatosplenomegaly. A lack of response to bronchodilators is characteristic.
- **Alertness.** Ask whether there are periods when the child appears to have a reduced level of consciousness, which might raise the possibility of brain tumour.
- **Headache.** This can be a sign of raised intracranial pressure, particularly if associated with vomiting or if it occurs on waking.
- **Seizures.** These may be caused by a brain tumour, particularly if they are of new onset.
- **Behaviour.** Brain tumours can present with unexplained deteriorating school performance or developmental delays. Have there been any unusual mood swings or behavioural changes?
- **Extensor attacks.** These can be a symptom of CNS tumour in children under the age of 2.
- **Vomiting.** Persistent and unexplained vomiting can indicate CNS tumour.
- **Other neurological symptoms.** Ask about any focal motor and sensory symptoms and gait abnormalities, which may occur with brain tumours.

- **Eye symptoms.** Consider retinoblastoma in children under 2 when parents report an odd appearance in their child's eye or a new squint.
- **Head and neck symptoms.** Proptosis, persistent and unexplained unilateral nasal obstruction with or without discharge and/or bleeding and aural polyps or discharge all occur in sarcoma.
- **Symptoms of the genitourinary tract.** Ask about urinary retention, scrotal swelling and bloodstained vaginal discharge, which may be presenting features of sarcoma.
- **Children under 2 years of age.** The following symptoms and signs raise the possibility of cancer in children under 2:
  - Persistent vomiting.
  - New squint.
  - Bulging fontanelle.
  - Extensor attacks.
  - New-onset seizures.
  - Delay, arrest or regression of motor development.
  - Poor feeding and faltering growth (although these are more likely to be due to other causes).
  - Altered behaviour.
  - Malaise, pallor, bone pain, irritability, fever and respiratory symptoms (these may indicate metastatic disease).

Past and current medical problems
- **Down's syndrome.** Associated with leukaemia.
- **Neurofibromatosis.** Associated with CNS cancer.

Medication
- **Symptom relief.** What has been tried and what has been effective? Are there any adverse effects? Ask about both prescribed and over-the-counter medication.

Allergies
- **Analgesics and antibiotics.** Ask about allergies to any drugs that may need to be used for symptomatic relief or treatment of complications.

Family history
- **Cancers.** Some cancers run in families.

Social history
- **Home.** Ask for details about home life. Are there any problems the family or carers need help with?
- **School.** Are there any problems at school resulting from the illness?

Review of previous investigations

- **Full blood count, blood film and plasma viscosity.** These are often abnormal in leukaemia and metastatic disease.
- **Liver function tests.** These may become abnormal as a result of liver metastases.
- **Chest X-ray.** This may show a mediastinal or hilar mass in lymphoma.
- **Plain X-rays.** These may show lytic lesions in bone tumours.

Examination

General
- **General condition.** Does the child look unwell? Are there problems with coordination?

Skin
- **Nodules.** Any unusual skin nodules may indicate metastatic disease.
- **Rashes.** Look out for petechiae or bruising, which may occur with leukaemia and lymphoma.
- **Lymph nodes.** Lymph nodes in lymphoma are often non-tender, firm or hard, and are usually >2 cm in size. Check for axillary and supraclavicular node involvement, particularly in the absence of local infection or dermatitis.
- **Masses.** Examine any unexplained masses at any site. Be suspicious of masses deep to the fascia that are non-tender, progressively enlarging, >2 cm in size and associated with an enlarging regional lymph node. Check whether lesions are painful or deeply attached to the fascia.

Head and neck
- **Eye examination.** Look for a white pupillary reflex (leukocoria) indicating retinoblastoma. Check for papilloedema (raised intracranial pressure).
- **Cranial nerves.** Abnormalities are common in brain and CNS tumours. Look for squints (which may also occur in retinoblastoma), bulging eyes, abnormal eye movements and lack of visual following in children under 2.
- **Conjunctivae.** Look for pale conjunctivae. Anaemia in leukaemia is common and will often be obvious.

Abdomen
- **Liver and spleen.** Enlarged liver and spleen are features of leukaemia or lymphoma.
- **Masses.** Abdominal masses in infants younger than 1 year are often localised and may indicate neuroblastoma, Wilm's tumour or metastatic disease. In infants younger than 6 months, intra-abdominal disease can progress rapidly.
- **Bladder.** An enlarged bladder may be caused by urinary retention due to brain or spinal tumour.

Limbs

- **Motor function.** Check particularly for tone, weakness, sensation, coordination and reflexes in the upper and lower limbs. Any of these may be abnormal in brain and spinal tumours.

Key references and further reading

1. Hamilton W, Hajioff S, Graham J, Schmidt-Hansen M. Suspected cancer (part 1 – children and young adults): visual overview of NICE guidance. *BMJ* 2015;350:h3036.
2. Macmillan. http://www.macmillan.org.uk/Cancerinformation/Cancertypes/ Childrenscancers/Childrenscancers.aspx.
3. National Institute for Health and Care Excellence (NICE). Suspected cancer: recognition and referral. NICE guidelines [NG12]. June 2015. Available from: http://www.nice.org.uk/guidance/ng12 (29 April 2016).

Abdominal pain in children

Key thoughts

Practical points
- **Diagnosis.** Abdominal pain is common in children and is often caused by benign self-limiting illness. Consider more serious underlying causes in infants, if the pain is severe, if the child is unwell and if there are other significant features.
- **Investigation.** Unless there are alarm symptoms or pain is chronic, further investigation is not normally needed.

Possible causes in infants
- Functional.
- Gastroenteritis.
- Constipation.
- Infantile colic.
- Lactose intolerance.
- Rarely, intestinal obstruction (volvulus, intussusception, Hirschsprung's disease, incarcerated hernia).

Possible causes in older children
- Functional pain.
- Psychological causes (school, parental problems).
- Gastroenteritis.
- Constipation.
- Abdominal migraine.
- Accidental poisoning.
- Urinary tract infection.
- Mesenteric adenitis.
- Appendicitis.
- Pneumonia.
- Trauma.
- Rarely, diabetic ketoacidosis, sickle cell crisis, Henoch–Schönlein purpura.

Additional possible causes in adolescents
- Depression.
- Abdominal migraine.
- Functional dyspepsia.
- Irritable bowel syndrome.
- Inflammatory bowel disease.

The 10-Minute Clinical Assessment, Second Edition. Knut Schroeder.
© 2017 John Wiley & Sons, Ltd. Published 2017 by John Wiley & Sons, Ltd.

- Girls only: dysmenorrhoea, threatened abortion, pelvic inflammatory disease, ectopic pregnancy, eating disorders, imperforate hymen (rare).
- Boys only: testicular torsion.

RED FLAGS

- Severe pain
- Faltering growth
- Weight loss
- Signs of peritonism
- Significant vomiting
- Right iliac fossa or right upper quadrant pain
- Pain due to trauma
- Pain that wakes the child at night
- Fever
- Rectal bleeding
- Unexplained pain
- Gynaecological pain in adolescent girls (possibility of pregnancy)
- Abnormal physical examination

History

Ideas, concerns and expectations
- **Ideas.** What do the child and parents think is causing the pain?
- **Concerns.** Parents often worry about the possibility of problems at school, appendicitis or cancer. Parents can also get very anxious if the child is distressed or in pain.
- **Expectations.** Why does the child present now? Most parents will expect a thorough abdominal examination to rule out serious disease. Chronic abdominal pain may cause family distress, and parents may demand increasingly invasive and expensive investigations, which may or may not be appropriate.

History of presenting complaint
- **Context and quality of life.** Allow the child and parents to tell the whole story in their own words. If chronic, how has the pain affected day-to-day life or school? Have there been any school absences because of the pain?
- **Onset.** Intermittent mild abdominal pain is common and usually benign, particularly if there are other features of self-limiting viral illness. Always consider possible serious underlying causes if pain is severe, progressive and associated with other significant symptoms. Consider appendicitis if there is acute onset of central or right lower quadrant pain, particularly if there is associated anorexia, general malaise and low-grade pyrexia.

- **Progression.** Coeliac disease is a relatively common but frequently missed cause of recurrent and chronic abdominal pain. Failure to thrive and diarrhoea are additional features.
- **Periodicity.** Consider abdominal migraine if there have been three or more sudden episodes of intense acute midline abdominal pain lasting 2 hours to several days, with intermittent pain-free intervals of weeks or months.
- **Site.** Where is the pain? Right lower quadrant pain suggests possible appendicitis, particularly if the pain originally started in the centre of the abdomen. Dyspepsia is mainly felt in the epigastrium. Abdominal migraine and irritable bowel syndrome commonly present with central abdominal pain. Appendicitis may mimic other conditions, such as gastroenteritis, urinary tract infection and pelvic inflammatory disease.
- **Character.** Pain in appendicitis is often constant, with acute exacerbations. Cramp-like pain occurs with faecal impaction.
- **Exacerbating factors.** Movement tends to make pain worse if there is peritoneal irritation.
- **Relieving factors.** Irritable bowel syndrome often presents with central abdominal discomfort of at least 12 weeks' duration, which is relieved by defecation. There may be associated increased or decreased stool frequency and change in the form of stools, with no evidence of structural or metabolic abnormalities.
- **Diet.** Does the child eat a balanced diet?
- **Fever.** A raised temperature suggests infection, such as appendicitis, or severe inflammation, as in inflammatory bowel disease.
- **Vomiting.** Vomiting may occur in viral gastroenteritis, appendicitis, abdominal migraine or, rarely, in bowel obstruction or intussusception.
- **Constipation.** Constipation is a common cause of abdominal pain. Are stools hard and painful? Is the child drinking enough fluids? Symptoms of constipation may not always be reported, and overflow incontinence may present with soiling or diarrhoea.
- **Diarrhoea.** Acute diarrhoea will often be caused by gastroenteritis. Loose stools with mucus together with abdominal cramps and waking at night raise the possibility of inflammatory bowel disease. Ask about weight loss, nail changes (clubbing), tiredness, perianal fistulae and mouth ulcers. Diarrhoea may also suggest coeliac disease.
- **Rectal bleeding.** Rectal bleeding may indicate intussusception in young infants (rare) or inflammatory bowel disease in older children.
- **Headaches.** Headaches may occur in abdominal migraine. These are usually one-sided and may be associated with photophobia during attacks. An aura of visual, sensory or motor disturbances may precede migraine attacks, and there may be a family history of migraine.
- **Urinary symptoms.** Are there any urinary symptoms suggesting urinary tract infection?
- **School problems.** Are there any problems at school that might cause abdominal pain (e.g. bullying, exams, friendship problems)?

- **Trauma.** Injuries are a common cause of abdominal pain. Cycling accidents, such as falling on to the handle bar, may cause intra-abdominal injury. Always consider pancreatitis if there is upper abdominal pain following trauma that gets worse after meals.
- **Sexual history.** In adolescent girls, find out if they have been sexually active, as abdominal pain may be related to pregnancy. Obtain details about the last menstrual period, dates of any sexual intercourse and use of contraception. Consider sexually transmitted infection and tubal inflammation. Is there a possibility that the child has suffered sexual or other abuse?
- **Recent travel.** Ask if there has been any recent travel abroad and whether travel immunisation has been taken up. Traveller's diarrhoea is common and usually self-limiting. Rarely, consider conditions such as typhoid fever or malaria, which may present with abdominal pain.
- **General symptoms.** Ask about sleep, energy levels, night sweats, fevers and lymphadenopathy if there is a possibility of an underlying systemic cause.

Past and current medical problems
- **Anxiety and depression.** These can be linked to chronic abdominal pain and irritable bowel syndrome.
- **Operations.** Ask about any previous bowel or other surgery that might be relevant.
- **Diabetes.** Children with diabetes are at higher risk of infection. Rarely, diabetic ketoacidosis may present with abdominal pain and vomiting.

Medication
- **Laxatives.** Have these been taken regularly and in adequate doses, if there is constipation?
- **Contraception.** Ask sexually active girls about use of contraception.
- **Analgesia.** What has been taken? What has been effective? Also consider over-the-counter medication.
- **Steroids.** Use of oral steroids can mask abdominal symptoms and may cause a raised white blood cell count.

Allergies
- **Antibiotics.** These may be required for the treatment of infection.
- **Analgesics.** Ask about allergies to any medications that might be used for pain relief.

Family history
- **Bowel disorders.** Is there a history of inflammatory bowel disease or coeliac disease?

Social history
- **Home.** Who else is at home? Are there any problems with siblings or parents? Is there a new baby?

Alcohol and recreational drugs
- **Alcohol and drugs.** In adolescents, ask about recent alcohol intake and any drug use.

Review of previous investigations
- **Full blood count and inflammatory markers.** A raised white cell count and abnormal inflammatory markers suggest infection or severe inflammation. Anaemia may occur with inflammatory bowel disease or malabsorption.
- **Creatinine and electrolytes.** Look for evidence of renal disease and electrolyte abnormalities.
- **Liver function tests.** Abnormal tests may suggest liver involvement. Albumin may be low in malabsorption or inflammatory bowel disease.
- **Amylase or lipase.** Acute pancreatitis is rare in childhood, but consider traumatic pancreatitis after an injury to the abdomen. Serum amylase may not be raised until about 12 hours after the event.
- **Coeliac screen (anti-tTG).** Coeliac disease is frequently missed.
- **Stool culture and microscopy.** These may be positive in acute gastroenteritis.
- **Abdominal ultrasound.** This may be useful for the diagnosis of appendicitis or other intra-abdominal pathology.
- **Gynaecological swabs.** These may be relevant if the patient is sexually active and there is a risk of sexually transmitted infection.
- **Pregnancy test.** Always consider this in adolescent girls.

Examination

General
- **General condition.** Does the child look unwell?
- **Discomfort.** Consider giving analgesia prior to further assessment if the child is in a lot of pain.
- **Hydration.** Are there any signs of dehydration?
- **Height and weight.** Plot weight and height on a growth chart to assess development and record for future reference. Crossing of centiles is suspicious.

Vital signs
- **Temperature.** This may be raised in infection or severe inflammation.
- **Pulse.** This may be raised in infection, severe pain or anxiety.
- **Blood pressure.** This is usually normal unless the child is very unwell.
- **Respiratory rate.** This may be raised in respiratory infection or due to anxiety or pain.

Abdomen
- **Distension.** Abdominal distension may suggest constipation or coeliac disease.

- **Tenderness.** Carefully check for any tenderness in all areas, including the groins, loins and genitals. Is there any evidence of peritonism, such as guarding, rigidity or rebound tenderness? Right iliac fossa tenderness suggests appendicitis. Suprapubic tenderness may be caused by cystitis.
- **Masses.** In severe constipation, a loaded colon may be felt.
- **Swelling.** Check all relevant areas for hernias.
- **Bowel sounds.** Check carefully for the presence or absence of bowel sounds.
- **Rectal examination.** Only consider a rectal examination if you feel that the result might change your management. Tenderness on the right suggests appendicitis. Rectal examination may reveal faecal impaction. Perianal lesions may suggest Crohn's disease.
- **Genitals.** It is important not to miss testicular torsion in boys. The affected testicle will usually be tender, and referred pain may be present in the inguinal area. Rarely, an imperforate hymen can cause lower abdominal pain in girls.

Lower limbs
- **Obturator sign.** Pain on abduction and adduction of the flexed right knee may cause pain in appendicitis.

Bedside tests
- **Pregnancy test.** Perform this in all young girls in whom pregnancy is a possibility.
- **Urine dipstick.** This may suggest urinary infection or diabetes.

Key references and further reading
1. Berger MY, Gieteling MJ, Benninga MA. Chronic abdominal pain in children. *BMJ* 2007;334:997–1002.
2. Bundy DG, Byerley JUS, Liles EA et al. The rational clinical examination: does this child have appendicitis? *JAMA* 2007;298:438–451.
3. El-Matary W, Spray C, Sandhu B. Irritable bowel syndrome: the commonest cause of recurrent abdominal pain in children. *Eur J Pediatr* 2004;163(10): 584–588.
4. National Institute for Health and Care Excellence (NICE). Constipation in children. Clinical Knowledge Summaries. 2015. Available from: http://cks.nice .org.uk/constipation-in-children (29 April 2016).
5. Rasquin A, Di Lorenzo C, Forbes D et al. Childhood functional gastrointestinal disorders: child/adolescent. *Gastroenterology* 2006;130:1527–1537.
6. Rothrock SG, Skeoch G, Rush JJ, Johnson NE. Clinical features of misdiagnosed appendicitis in children. *Ann Emerg Med* 1991;20:45–50.
7. Walker LS, Lipani TA, Greene JW et al. Recurrent abdominal pain: symptom subtypes based on the Rome II criteria for pediatric functional gastrointestinal disorders. *J Paediatr Gastroenterol Nutr* 2004;38:187–191.

Hearing loss in children

Key thoughts

Practical points

- **Diagnosis.** Hearing loss is common in children. It is often caused by otitis media with effusion (glue ear) or ear wax. Further investigation and referral may be required if symptoms are severe and chronic, if there is no obvious cause or if there are any alarm features.
- **Causes.** Differentiate between conductive and sensorineural hearing loss.

Possible causes

- Otitis media with effusion (glue ear).
- Ear wax.
- Foreign body.
- Perceived hearing loss due to lack of concentration.
- Ear or craniofacial abnormalities.
- Ototoxic drugs.
- Prematurity.
- Rarely, Down's syndrome, congenital malformation, severe neonatal hyperbilirubinaemia, in utero infection such as toxoplasmosis or cytomegalovirus (CMV).

RED FLAGS

- Severe hearing problems
- Delayed speech and verbal comprehension
- Congenital or sensorineural deafness
- Parental concern
- Head trauma
- Postnatal infection, such as meningitis
- Recurrent or persistent otitis media with effusion for at least 3 months

---

History

Ideas, concerns and expectations

- **Ideas.** Ask what the parents believe to be the underlying problem.
- **Concerns.** Always consider parents' concerns about hearing seriously – they are usually right. Are the parents worried about speech problems or a possible need for a hearing aid?

The 10-Minute Clinical Assessment, Second Edition. Knut Schroeder.
© 2017 John Wiley & Sons, Ltd. Published 2017 by John Wiley & Sons, Ltd.

• **Expectations.** Parents often expect antibiotics or ear, nose and throat (ENT) referral for glue air, whereas 'watchful waiting' is usually indicated at the first instance if hearing loss is not severe and the child is managing well at school.

History of presenting complaint

• **Context.** Encourage the child and the parents to tell you about the hearing problems in their own words.
• **Hearing symptoms.** How did the parents or other people (e.g. teachers) first notice the hearing problems? In what types of situation do they become apparent (e.g. school, talking in groups, whispering, talking on the telephone)?
• **Onset.** When and how did the hearing problems start? Is hearing loss progressive?
• **Severity.** Does a baby respond to loud noises? What effect does the hearing loss have on communication within the family and at school?
• **Language and behaviour.** Hearing problems are an important cause of delays in speech development. Are there any difficulties with verbal comprehension? Have teachers commented on the child being withdrawn and not taking an active part in lessons? Does the child have any behavioural problems?
• **Pain and fever.** Deafness associated with pain and fever is likely due to otitis media. Is there any discharge?
• **Other ENT symptoms.** Ask about nasal discharge and congestion, snoring and mouth breathing (e.g. nasal polyps, adenoids), all of which can lead to blocked eustachian tubes and insufficient ventilation of the middle ear.
• **Smoky environment.** Smoky environments can contribute to hearing problems.

Past and current medical problems

• **Ear problems.** Ask about any previous ear problems, including operations and trauma.
• **Prenatal and perinatal history.** Ask the parents about any problems during pregnancy (e.g. infections such as rubella). Was the child delivered at term or premature? Were there any problems in the perinatal period, such as birth trauma, hypoxia, jaundice or infection?
• **Congenital malformation.** Are there any congenital birth defects which may be associated with hearing loss?
• **Infections.** Meningitis at any age can lead to sensorineural deafness.

Medication

• **Ototoxic drugs.** A number of drugs (e.g. aminoglycosides, vancomycin) can lead to sensorineural deafness, both in utero and after delivery.

Family history

• **Deafness.** Congenital sensorineural hearing loss may run in families.

Social history
- **Home.** What is the home setup? Do the hearing problems have any effect on the family? Is communication support required (e.g. use of sign language)?
- **School.** Ask about any school problems resulting from poor hearing. Is any special educational support needed?

Previous investigations
- **Hearing tests.** Look for results of neonatal and subsequent audiological tests. Most children aged 4–5 years are screened in school for hearing problems. Ask whether other tests, such as otoacoustic emissions, distraction testing, tympanometry performance testing or speech discrimination testing, have been performed in the past, depending on the child's age. Pure-tone audiometry is the gold-standard investigation in older children.
- **Magnetic resonance imaging (MRI) or CT scan.** These may be indicated for investigation of possible underlying causes.
- **Chromosomal studies.** These may rarely be performed to exclude particular genetic syndromes.

Examination

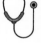

General
- **General impression.** If the child is unwell, consider acute otitis media or mastoiditis (rare).
- **Physical features.** Dysmorphic features suggest a possible genetic cause for the deafness.
- **Facial expression and speech.** Nasal speech, mouth breathing and adenoidal facies suggest enlarged adenoids with resulting glue ear.
- **Conversation.** Does the child lip read or fail to respond to speech?
- **Behaviour.** Look for any obvious behavioural abnormalities suggesting an associated or underlying mental health problem.

Vital signs
- **Temperature.** Fever suggests infection, such as otitis media.

Head and neck
- **External ear.** Look for any deformity or evidence of discharge. Is there tenderness on pressing the tragus or pain on pulling the pinna (infection)? Check the area behind the pinna for signs of mastoiditis.
- **Ear canal.** Look for any wax or foreign body. Discharge indicates perforation in otitis media or severe otitis externa.
- **Ear drum.** Look for evidence of infection or perforation. A dull or inflamed ear drum that does not move together with a fluid level or bubbles suggests otitis media.
- **Oropharynx.** Look for enlarged and inflamed tonsils (exudate).

- **Nasopharynx.** Are any polyps visible that might contribute to the development of glue ear?
- **Lymph nodes.** Enlarged and tender cervical lymph nodes suggest upper respiratory tract infection.

Hearing
- **Whisper test.** Quietly whisper two-syllable words appropriate to the child's age into the ear while gently placing and moving your finger on the tragus of the opposite ear to mask any noise. Then, ask the child to repeat the words.
- **Weber's and Rinne's tests.** If there is reduced hearing and the child is old enough, these tests will help differentiate between conductive and sensorineural hearing loss.

Key references and further reading

1. Isaacson JE, Vora NM. Differential diagnosis and treatment of hearing loss. *Am Fam Physician* 2003;68:1125–1132.
2. National Institute for Health and Care Excellence (NICE). Otitis media with effusion. Clinical Knowledge Summaries. 2011. Available from: http://cks.nice.org.uk/otitis-media-with-effusion (last accessed 29 April 2016).
3. Pirozzo S, Papinczak T, Glasziou P. Whispered voice test for screening for hearing impairment in adults and children: systematic review. *BMJ* 2003;327:967.

Childhood cough

Key thoughts

Practical points
- **Diagnosis.** Self-limiting upper respiratory infection is the most common cause. In chronic cough, consider asthma or, rarely, other chronic lung problems, such as cystic fibrosis.
- **Foreign body.** Always consider the possibility of foreign-body inhalation if onset is acute and presentation is unusual.

Possible causes
- Viral or bacterial upper respiratory tract infection.
- Post-infectious cough.
- Pneumonia.
- Croup.
- Bronchiolitis.
- Asthma.
- Tuberculosis in at-risk areas and populations.
- Psychogenic cough.
- Rarely, aspiration, foreign-body inhalation, whooping cough, bronchiectasis, cystic fibrosis, epiglottitis, immunodeficiency, swallowing problems.

RED FLAGS

- High fever
- Associated wheeze
- Shortness of breath
- Reduced activity and social interaction
- Reduced fluid intake and dehydration
- Faltering growth

History

Ideas, concerns and expectations
- **Ideas.** What do the child and parents think is causing the cough? Common self-diagnoses include asthma and pneumonia.
- **Concerns.** Many parents are worried that their child may die from a coughing fit, choking or vomiting. Concerns about the effects of disrupted nights due to night-time cough are also common, as are fears of chronic illness,

The 10-Minute Clinical Assessment, Second Edition. Knut Schroeder.
© 2017 John Wiley & Sons, Ltd. Published 2017 by John Wiley & Sons, Ltd.

such as asthma. Parents often worry that the child's lung may be damaged by a cough lasting for longer than a few days. Always take parents' concerns seriously.

- **Expectations.** Do the parents expect a prescription for antibiotics or do they just want reassurance? It is not unusual for coughs due to upper respiratory tract infection to last for 3 or 4 weeks, which is longer than most parents would expect.

History of presenting complaint
- **Context.** Allow the child and parents time to tell you about the cough in their own words.
- **Quality of life.** What have been the effects on day-to-day activities and quality of life for the child and the family as a whole?
- **Onset.** Infection is likely if the cough is associated with fever and symptoms of the common cold. Acute onset after choking suggests foreign-body inhalation – peanuts and small toys are common culprits. Recurrent choking may be caused by swallowing problems. Consider asthma if the cough is seasonal or has been present for a while.
- **Progression and duration.** Chronic cough in smaller children may be caused by bronchiolitis, prematurity or neonatal respiratory problems. Cough present from birth may suggest cystic fibrosis, particularly if associated with failure to thrive and gastrointestinal problems. Consider immunodeficiency or cystic fibrosis if there are multiple and recurrent respiratory infections. Neonates are usually screened for these conditions, so check the results of any neonatal screening tests.
- **Type of cough.** Consider croup if there is a barking cough with hoarseness and inspiratory stridor. Whooping cough usually presents with paroxysms of cough, which may lead to vomiting and episodes of apnoea. Asthma is associated with wheeze and shortness of breath, which usually responds well to a trial of inhalers, but nocturnal cough may be the only presenting feature.
- **Precipitating factors.** Ask if there has been a recent respiratory infection, such as the common cold, bronchitis, croup, bronchiolitis, whooping cough or pneumonia. Do the parents smoke?
- **Feeding.** Cough after feeding suggests gastrooesophageal reflux. Prolonged decreased food intake may suggest a more serious underlying illness.
- **Associated features.** Symptoms such as wheeze, shortness of breath, high fever, general malaise, reduced fluid intake and dehydration indicate a more severe illness. Ask about complications such as diarrhoea and ear ache. Rarely, drooling may suggest epiglottitis, particularly if associated with fever and general malaise in a child who has not been immunised against haemophilus influenzae type B (Hib).
- **Exacerbating and relieving factors.** Cough during exercise or in colder weather may be caused by asthma. Seasonal cough may also occur with asthma or allergic rhinitis. Psychogenic cough does not occur during sleep.

- **General symptoms.** Consider a more serious underlying cause if there is faltering growth, weight loss, night sweats, fever or generalised lymph node swelling.
- **Environmental exposure.** Pets, dust and cigarette smoke may all cause recurrent cough.

Past and current medical problems

- **Significant past illnesses.** Ask about any chronic lung conditions, previous infections and other illnesses, such as diabetes. Faltering growth and feeding problems may point towards reflux or cystic fibrosis (rare).
- **Immunisations.** Check whether the child has been fully immunised, particularly against *Bordetella pertussis* (whooping cough) and Hib infection (epiglottitis).

Medication and other treatment

- **Self-treatment.** Over-the-counter preparations are commonly used to treat acute cough in children, but there is little evidence for or against their effectiveness.
- **Antibiotics.** Has the child been taking any antibiotics lately?

Family history

- **Asthma.** Ask about a family history of atopy or asthma.
- **Tuberculosis.** Has the child been exposed to tuberculosis?

Allergies

- **Antibiotics.** Ask about allergies to penicillin or any other drugs that may need to be used should the cough not settle.

Social history

- **Home situation.** Ask about the home setup. Do the parents smoke? Is the central heating working? Is there sufficient ventilation, or is the air in the house very dry? Does the family have a pet?
- **Travel.** Have the child or the parents travelled or lived in countries with a high prevalence of tuberculosis, or has anyone visited the child who lives in these areas?

Review of previous investigations

- **Full blood count.** A raised white cell count suggests infection, and eosinophilia occurs in atopic disease.
- **Chest X-ray.** This may show signs of infection or inhaled foreign body.
- **Peak expiratory flow rate.** Previous measurements may be available in older children. Reduced and variable peak flow rates may indicate asthma, but children often have a poor technique.

Examination

General
- **General condition.** Does the child look unwell or pale? Are there signs of malnutrition or neglect? Is the child thriving?
- **ABC.** If the child is unwell and not very responsive, check ABC. Intercostal or subcostal recession and tracheal tug suggest respiratory distress.
- **Hydration.** Is there evidence of dehydration? Is the child sweaty?
- **Hands.** Finger clubbing may occur in cystic fibrosis (rare).

Vital signs
- **Temperature.** Is there any fever that suggests infection?
- **Pulse.** Check for tachycardia.
- **Respiratory rate.** Tachypnoea suggests respiratory compromise (e.g. chest infection, severe asthma, bronchiolitis). A normal respiratory rate makes severe asthma, hypoxia or pneumonia less likely.

Head and neck
- **Mouth and mucous membranes.** Look for evidence of central cyanosis, which would suggest serious illness and hypoxia.
- **Trachea.** Look for a tracheal tug and palpate for tracheal deviation, which may occur with foreign-body inhalation or pneumothorax.
- **Ears.** Impacted ear wax may rarely cause a vagal reflex cough (Arnold's ear-cough reflex).
- **Throat.** Look for evidence of tonsillitis or pharyngitis. Do not attempt to examine the throat if there is stridor, which may be caused by croup or, in rare cases, epiglottitis.

Chest
- **Wheeze.** Expiratory wheeze on auscultation may occur with asthma or bronchiolitis.
- **Crackles.** These may suggest chest infection, particularly if associated with general malaise and tachypnoea.
- **Air entry.** Is this present throughout both lungs and symmetrical?

Bedside tests
- **Peak flow.** If the child is old enough, measure peak expiratory flow rate, which can be useful for measuring diurnal variability and response to treatment in children with asthma. If possible, compare observed peak flow readings with expected peak flow values for the child's height.

Key references and further reading
1. Hay AD, Wilson AD. The natural history of acute cough in children aged 0 to 4 years in primary care: a systematic review. *Br J Gen Pract* 2002;52:401–409.

2. Margolis P, Gadomski A. Does this infant have pneumonia? *JAMA* 1998;279: 308–313.
3. National Institute for Health and Care Excellence (NICE). Cough – acute with chest signs in children. Clinical Knowledge Summaries. 2012. Available from: http://cks.nice.org.uk/cough-acute-with-chest-signs-in-children (last accessed 29 April 2016).
4. Smith SM, Schroeder K, Fahey T. Over-the-counter medications for acute cough in children and adults in ambulatory settings. *Cochrane Database Syst Rev* 2007;(3):CD001831.

Childhood wheeze

Key thoughts

Practical points
- **Diagnosis.** Wheeze is not always caused by asthma: there are other possible underlying causes. A priority is to identify those children who are seriously ill.
- **Reassurance.** Parents are often very concerned about wheeze. A thorough physical assessment will help reassure them if there is a benign underlying cause.

Possible causes
- Viral infection.
- Transient infantile wheezing.
- Gastrooesophageal reflux.
- Bronchiolitis.
- Asthma.
- Croup.
- Rarely, foreign body inhalation, tracheooesophageal fistula, ventricular-septal defect, recurrent aspiration, cystic fibrosis, developmental disorders, immunodeficiency, ciliary dyskinesia.

RED FLAGS

- Atypical or complex presentation
- Unable to feed
- Cyanosis
- Drowsiness
- Agitation
- Apnoea
- Increased respiratory effort
- Unclear diagnosis
- No response to treatment
- Faltering growth

History

Ideas, concerns and expectations
- **Ideas.** What do the parents think the underlying problem is? What does the wheeze mean to them? What ideas do they have about the likely consequences of wheeze?

The 10-Minute Clinical Assessment, Second Edition. Knut Schroeder.
© 2017 John Wiley & Sons, Ltd. Published 2017 by John Wiley & Sons, Ltd.

- **Concerns.** Parents are often concerned that wheeze indicates serious underlying illness (which may be entirely justified). They often fear that there is underlying asthma and worry about the implications of this diagnosis. Parents may worry that their child's chest may get damaged by wheeze.
- **Expectations.** Parents may expect you to diagnose straight away whether their child has asthma or not, which in clinical practice may be difficult and unrealistic.

History of presenting complaint

- **Context and meaning of wheeze.** Ask the child and the parents to tell you about the wheeze in their own words. Many think wheeze is just noisy breathing or a 'fruity' cough.
- **Effect on life.** What effects do the symptoms have on the child's life and on the family as a whole?
- **Severity.** Associated drowsiness, agitation, cyanosis, apnoea or inability to feed suggest serious illness that is likely to require hospital admission.
- **Age at onset.** Wheeze in infants and young children is often a result of transient infantile wheezing, a benign condition in which children are born with somewhat small airways (the 'happy wheezer'). The wheeze usually disappears spontaneously when the child grows. If symptoms have been present from birth, asthma is unlikely to be the main underlying cause.
- **Onset and pattern.** Wheeze starting a few days after the onset of a viral infection suggests viral wheeze. Wheeze following a general deterioration due to a respiratory infection is likely a result of pneumonia. Acute-onset wheeze in a previously well child suggests foreign-body inhalation or aspiration.
- **Cough.** An isolated cough is not usually caused by asthma. A persistent, productive cough is often caused by recurrent upper respiratory infections, but in rare cases may indicate immunodeficiency, cystic fibrosis, recurrent aspiration or tuberculosis.
- **Vomiting.** If there is vomiting, consider diagnoses other than asthma, such as gastrooesophageal reflux, which can cause wheeze through aspiration but may also cause wheeze independently.
- **Faltering growth.** Unless severe, asthma does not usually lead to faltering growth. If the child fails to grow, consider alternative underlying causes, especially gastrooesophageal reflux and cystic fibrosis.
- **Feeding.** Feeding problems and dysphagia increase the risk of aspiration, which can lead to infection and wheeze.
- **Crying.** Crying may sound abnormal in laryngeal or pharyngeal abnormalities.
- **Parental smoking.** Children of mothers who smoke are more likely to develop a wheezing illness, and childhood asthma is often made worse if parents smoke.

Important underlying conditions

- **Viral infections.** Recurrent viral-associated wheezing may occur in toddlers and slightly older children following a severe viral infection, especially bronchiolitis. These children are usually asymptomatic between episodes. It can be difficult to distinguish these symptoms from true asthma, as asthma can be triggered by viral infection. Viral wheeze tends to improve with time, whereas asthma may get worse in later childhood. Repeated viral infections may rarely indicate an underlying immune disorder.

- **Reflux.** If wheeze has been present from birth, think about the possibility of perinatal problems or reflux.
- **Asthma.** Diagnosing asthma in children can be difficult, and no gold-standard diagnostic tests exist. Diagnose asthma with caution in children under 1 year of age. Persistent symptoms of wheeze, noisy breathing and breathlessness together with a personal or family history of other atopic conditions, such as hay fever or eczema, supports the diagnosis. Symptoms in asthma are usually worse at night and early in the morning. Asthma tends to respond to inhaled bronchodilators and inhaled steroids. It is important to recognise asthma, as treatment can be very effective, but at the same time, children should not be wrongly labelled with this diagnosis if the wheeze has another cause.
- **Tuberculosis.** Has the child been exposed to tuberculosis?
- **Genetic conditions.** If the diagnosis is unclear or the presentation is unusual, consider rare genetic conditions such as cystic fibrosis, ciliary dyskinesia or tracheooesophageal fistula, which can all present with wheeze.

Past and current medical problems

- **Prematurity.** Wheeze is more common in babies with low birth weight or who were born prematurely. In the case of severe prematurity, the lungs may have suffered from assisted ventilation in the absence of surfactant.
- **Congenital heart disease.** Any deterioration of congenital heart disease, such as ventricular-septal defect, may present with wheeze.

Medication

- **Inhalers.** Good response to bronchodilators and steroids indicates asthma, whereas a lack of response makes a diagnosis of asthma much less likely, so long as the inhalers have been taken appropriately with use of a spacer. Check the dosage and frequency of inhaled steroids. High-dose inhaled steroids in children can cause complications such as cataract, osteopenia and adrenal suppression if used long-term. Parental counselling about potential adverse effects and the need to identify the lowest effective dose is therefore important.

Family history

- **Asthma.** A family history of asthma or other atopic disorders increases the risk of asthma in a child.
- **Inherited conditions.** Ask about other inherited conditions, such as cystic fibrosis, developmental abnormalities and neuromuscular disorders.

Social history

- **Home situation.** Ask for details about the domestic situation. Is housing adequate or is there damp and mould that might contribute to respiratory problems? Consider pets and other possible allergens.

Review of previous investigations

- **Peak flow.** Look for any previous peak flow readings in older children. Is there obvious seasonal or diurnal variation?
- **Chest radiography.** A chest X-ray may have been performed to look for infection or a suspected inhaled foreign body. In most cases of wheeze (including asthma), the chest X-ray will be normal.

Examination

General

- **General condition.** Does the child look unwell? Is the child floppy? Is there evidence of faltering growth?
- **ABC.** Check airways, breathing and circulation. In case of impairment, take the necessary action immediately before continuing with the assessment.
- **Alertness.** Is the child alert and interested in the environment?
- **Cyanosis.** Blue lips and tongue suggest hypoxia.
- **Stridor.** Inspiratory stridor does not usually occur with asthma – consider foreign-body inhalation, aspiration or another cause.
- **Finger clubbing.** This may occur in cystic fibrosis or bronchiectasis (rare).

Vital signs

- **Temperature.** Fever suggests infection.
- **Pulse.** Tachycardia suggests infection or respiratory distress. Bradycardia is a pre-terminal sign and suggests serious illness.
- **Capillary refill.** A delay of more than 3 seconds suggests hypoperfusion.
- **Respiratory rate.** Tachypnoea suggests serious underlying disease (see box).

NORMAL HEART (HR) AND RESPIRATORY (RR) RATES

- **Infant.** HR 110–160 beats per minute, RR 30–40 breaths per minute.
- **1–2 years.** HR 100–150 beats per minute, RR 25–35 breaths per minute.
- **2–5 years.** HR 95–140 beats per minute, RR 25–30 breaths per minute.

Skin

- **Eczema.** The presence of eczema increases the risk of wheeze being due to asthma.

Head and neck

- **Nose.** Nasal flaring suggests increased respiratory effort.
- **Throat.** Look for tonsillitis or pharyngitis (viral or bacterial infection). Do not examine the throat if there is a possibility of the wheeze being caused by epiglottitis (rare).
- **Ears.** Look for evidence of otitis media.

Chest

- **Chest expansion.** Look for use of accessory muscles and tracheal deviation (e.g. foreign-body inhalation).
- **Lungs.** Listen for crackles (e.g. chest infection, foreign-body inhalation). Is wheeze present, and if so, is it generalised? Make sure that breath sounds are audible in all lung areas.
- **Heart.** Listen for added sounds and murmurs that might indicate congenital heart disease.

Bedside tests

- **Peak flow and spirometry.** These are useful for measuring response to treatment and diurnal variability in children with asthma, but only if the child is cooperative and sufficiently old.
- **Pulse oximetry.** Oxygen saturation below 95% suggests moderate hypoxia, while levels below 90% indicate more serious illness.

Key references and further reading

1. British Thoracic Society, Scottish Intercollegiate Guidelines Network. *British Guideline on the Management of Asthma: A National Clinical Guideline.* May 2008. Available from: https://www.brit-thoracic.org.uk/document-library/clinical-information/asthma/btssign-guideline-on-the-management-of-asthma/ (last accessed 29 April 2016).
2. Cane RS, Ranganathan SC, McKenzie SA. What do parents of wheezy children understand by 'wheeze'? *Arch Dis Child* 2000;82:327–332.
3. National Institute for Health and Care Excellence (NICE). Asthma. Clinical Knowledge Summaries. 2013. Available from: http://cks.nice.org.uk/asthma (last accessed 29 April 2016).
4. Townshend J, Hails S, Mckean M. Diagnosis of asthma in children. *BMJ* 2007;335:198–202.

Constipation in children

Key thoughts

Practical points
- **Diagnosis.** The cause is usually functional, and investigations are rarely necessary in the initial management of constipation. Serious underlying causes are rare.
- **Quality of life.** Constipation can cause considerable distress for both child and parents, and may significantly interfere with their lives.

Possible causes
- Functional.
- Dietary (lack of fibre, inadequate fluid intake).
- Social problems.
- Psychological.
- Rarely, cystic fibrosis, cerebral palsy, lead poisoning, anatomical and neurological causes such as Hirschsprung's disease or spina bifida occulta.

RED FLAGS

- No passage of meconium in the first 24 hours
- Toothpaste-like stools
- Neurological abnormalities
- No or little response to adequate treatment
- Faltering growth
- Megarectum or megacolon

History

Ideas, concerns and expectations
- **Ideas.** Ask what the child and the parents understand about constipation and what might be causing it.
- **Concerns.** Parents can get very concerned about the child's bowel actions. There are often worries that even mild constipation can be harmful to the child and that there 'may be a blockage'. The perception of normal bowel movements can vary a lot – what do the parents think is 'normal'? Constipation in pre-school children can lead to extreme fear and avoidance of defecation. Parents often worry about the safety of giving laxatives.
- **Expectations.** Why is the child presenting now? Do the parents want treatment, reassurance or specialist referral?

The 10-Minute Clinical Assessment, Second Edition. Knut Schroeder.
© 2017 John Wiley & Sons, Ltd. Published 2017 by John Wiley & Sons, Ltd.

History of presenting complaint

- **Context.** Allow the child and the parents to tell the whole story in their own words. Is the child just starting school? Have there been any other significant life events?
- **Quality of life.** What effects do the bowel problems have on the day-to-day life of the child and the family as a whole?
- **Description.** What do the child or parents mean by 'constipation'? Are bowel movements infrequent or difficult, or both? Is there any associated pain or a feeling of incomplete evacuation? What is the consistency of the stool?
- **Onset.** Onset within the first month after birth suggests an organic cause, such as Hirschsprung's disease. Ask about any delay in the passage of meconium, faltering growth, persistent vomiting and episodes of severe diarrhoea. Potty training and school entry are common times for children to become constipated.
- **Frequency.** Normal stool frequency can vary considerably in children. Infants may have many dirty nappies a day, or may not pass stool for a few days. In older children, stools become firmer and, usually, more regular.
- **Duration.** Chronic constipation may lead to rectal distension, faecal retention, overflow and loss of sensory and motor function of the bowel.
- **Pattern.** Are problems with constipation present all the time or are they intermittent?
- **Potty training.** Disagreements between children and their parents can lead to faecal retention and constipation. Do the parents encourage use of the toilet after meals to maximise the gastrocolic reflex? Do they use positive reinforcement, such as star charts or whistles? Most children will be toilet-trained by the age of 4.
- **Schooling.** Many children avoid going to the toilet at school because of the smell, embarrassment or fear.
- **Diet.** Ask about food and fluid intake. Is the diet lacking in fibre? Does the child drink enough? Increasing fibre content in the diet and reducing excessive milk intake in toddlers are often helpful in the initial management.
- **Abdominal pain.** This may be caused by constipation, but consider other causes such as appendicitis or inflammatory bowel disease.
- **Pain on defecation.** Consider anal fissure if there is pain on defecation, which can be very distressing for the child and can lead to avoidance behaviour. In otherwise healthy infants under 6 months of age, episodes of straining lasting for about 10 minutes before the passage of soft stools (dyschezia) can be normal but may be mistaken for constipation.
- **Incontinence and soiling.** Faecal incontinence can be socially very upsetting for the child and needs to be taken seriously. Soiling can occur in the absence of constipation (encopresis) and may be associated with behavioural problems. Has normal stool ever been passed in socially unacceptable places? Overflow incontinence is an important cause not to miss.

- **Toxins.** Has the child been exposed to any toxins, such as old paints? Lead poisoning may lead to constipation.
- **Typhoid.** In countries where this is endemic, consider typhoid fever if the child has been exposed and has not been immunised. Typhoid fever can lead to initial constipation, followed by severe diarrhoea a few days later.
- **Other health professionals.** Has the child ever been seen by a dietician or a psychiatrist for behavioural therapy or biofeedback (rarely necessary)?

Past and current medical problems
- **Significant past illnesses.** Are there any significant past and previous medical problems?

Medication
- **Laxatives.** Have laxatives been used? If so, for how long, and were they effective? Were there any adverse effects? Were adequate doses used? Did the child take them? Many children appear resistant to treatment because adequate doses of laxatives have not been used consistently, and higher-than-standard doses are sometimes necessary. Treatment may need to be long-term and is generally safe.
- **Other medication.** Has any medication been given to the child that might cause constipation?

Family history
- **Inherited disorders.** Is there a family history of conditions such as Hirschsprung's disease (rare)?

Social history
- **Family stress.** Fear of defecation and avoidance behaviour can lead to severe stress in the child and the family as a whole. Ask about how everyone close to the child has been affected by any problems.
- **Social issues.** Ask about any problems with peer relationships.
- **School.** Have issues around constipation, such as soiling, led to any problems at school?

Review of previous investigations
- **Blood.** Occasionally, and in selected cases, tests such as a full blood count and ferritin may be useful.
- **Rectal biopsy.** This may be helpful if Hirschsprung's disease is suspected.

Examination

General
- **General condition.** Does the child look unwell?
- **Hydration.** Dehydration may lead to constipation.

Abdomen

- **Distension.** Does the abdomen look distended?
- **Palpation.** Faeces can sometimes be felt, predominantly in the left upper and lower quadrant ('loaded colon'). Check for organomegaly and any masses.
- **Anus.** Look for any anal fissures, tags or stenosis. Is there evidence of perianal infection or trauma?
- **Rectal examination.** Consider a rectal examination to distinguish between an empty rectum and a rectum full of faeces. Is there faecal impaction? If a rectal examination is needed, obtain verbal consent from the child and the parents, explain fully what you are doing and be sensitive in your approach.

Lower limbs and spine

- **Spine.** Look for any evidence of spina bifida and check lower-limb reflexes.

Key references and further reading

1. Auth MKH, Vora R, Farrelly P, Baillie C. Childhood constipation. *BMJ* 2012;345: e7309.
2. Baker SS, Liptak GS, Colletti RB et al. Constipation in infants and children: evaluation and treatment. *J Pediatr Gastroenterol Nutr* 1999;29:612–626.
3. Hyman PE, Milla PF, Benninga MA et al. Childhood functional gastrointestinal disorders: neonate/toddler. *Gastroenterology* 2006;130:1519–1526.
4. National Institute for Health and Care Excellence (NICE). Constipation in children and young people: diagnosis and management. NICE guidelines [CG99]. May 2010. Available from: http://www.nice.org.uk/guidance/cg99 (last accessed 29 April 2016).
5. Rasquin A, Di Lorenzo C, Forbes D et al. Childhood functional gastrointestinal disorders: child/adolescent. *Gastroenterology* 2006;130:1527–1537.
6. Rubin G, Dale A. Chronic constipation in children. *BMJ* 2006;333:1051–1055.

Childhood obesity

Key thoughts

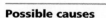

Practical points
- **Diagnosis.** Childhood obesity is becoming more common in many countries, and an unhealthy lifestyle is often responsible. In rare cases, consider the possibility of secondary obesity (e.g. genetic or endocrine).
- **Effect on daily life.** Find out how the child's and the family's life is affected and explore their physical, psychological and social needs.

Possible causes
- Psychological problems.
- Social problems.
- Poor diet and overeating.
- Lack of exercise.
- Rarely, endocrine or genetic disorders (e.g. hypothyroidism, Cushing's syndrome, Prader–Willi syndrome).

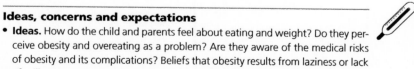

RED FLAGS

- Body mass index (BMI) above the 85th centile
- Serious comorbidity (e.g. orthopaedic problems, diabetes, depression)
- Height below the 9th centile, slow growth rate or a child who is unexpectedly short compared to their family members
- Severe and progressive obesity before the age of 2
- Late puberty (no signs of puberty at age 13 in girls or age 15 in boys)
- Precocious puberty (before 8 years of age)
- Severe learning disability
- Underlying medical conditions

History

Ideas, concerns and expectations
- **Ideas.** How do the child and parents feel about eating and weight? Do they perceive obesity and overeating as a problem? Are they aware of the medical risks of obesity and its complications? Beliefs that obesity results from laziness or lack of willpower are common and are worth addressing. Are there any distressing feelings of shame or embarrassment, either from the child or from the parents?

The 10-Minute Clinical Assessment, Second Edition. Knut Schroeder.
© 2017 John Wiley & Sons, Ltd. Published 2017 by John Wiley & Sons, Ltd.

- **Concerns.** Explore any concerns about body shape, future health and the effect of obesity on the child's self-esteem.
- **Expectations.** Explore the reason for the consultation and the child's and parents' expectations with regard to the outcome. Ask about their expectations for future management. Would they be ready to take part in a weight-management programme? How would the parents and child feel about adopting any lifestyle changes that would affect (and benefit!) the family as a whole? Are there any (unrealistic) expectations about how much weight the child should lose? Have expectations been influenced by the media, people around the child and family or other health professionals?

History of presenting complaint

- **Context.** Give children and their parents time to explain their views about the weight problem. Are there any particular problems or concerns that have led to their seeking medical help? Be sensitive, sympathetic and compassionate when you listen, as obese children and their parents may find it very difficult to talk about weight and appearance. Try to get an understanding of the family context.
- **Effect on life.** Ask open questions about how the child's and family's life may have been affected by overeating and increased weight. Are there tensions in the household? Is there bullying at school?
- **Onset.** At what age did the weight problems start (onset before 2 years of age may indicate a genetic cause)? Have there been any periods of weight loss? How and why may these have been achieved?
- **Dietary habits.** Find out about eating patterns and ask for details about the type and amount of food and drink being taken. Use objective and non-accusatory language, as this can be an emotive topic. Focus on behaviour (e.g. 'Do you find that eating is out of control at times?') rather than characteristics of the child (e.g. 'Do you lack willpower?'). Has the child ever binged on food? Consider the possibility of an underlying eating disorder. Often, the family attitude to food is indicative. Ask about how meals are taken. Is food prepared freshly, or does the diet contain mainly 'ready meals'? Are meals eaten in front of the television? Obesity is almost always caused by an imbalance between energy intake and expenditure. Sweet drinks often contain large amounts of calories.
- **Exercise.** Does the child exercise? How often, how much and in what form? Are there any problems when exercising, such as excessive shortness of breath, joint/muscle aches or chest pain? Explore attitudes and feelings around exercise to identify barriers to physical activity.
- **Mental health.** What is the child's mood like? Consider depression and low self-esteem, which can be factors in the development – or the result – of overeating and subsequent childhood obesity. Does the child have thoughts of self-harm?
- **Endocrine disorders.** Rapid recent onset of weight gain may indicate an endocrine disorder, particularly if the child was previously of normal weight and height. Also consider an endocrine cause if the child is relatively short and obese.

- **Type 2 diabetes.** Consider the possibility of underlying or complicating diabetes if the child suffers from tiredness, polyuria or polydipsia. Ask if there is a family history of diabetes.
- **Genetic causes.** If there are hearing and/or vision problems, learning difficulties or dysmorphic body features, consider genetic causes for obesity.
- **Attempts to lose weight.** Ask for details about any previous attempts to lose weight, including diets and weight-management programmes.
- **Bone and joints.** Muscle and joint pains are common in obese children, particularly in the hips, knees and lower back. Ask about any joint pain or swelling, and how this affects daily life. Proximal muscle weakness may be caused by steroid excess in Cushing's syndrome. Consider the possibility of slipped femoral epiphysis if there is hip or knee pain.
- **Oligomenorrhoea or amenorrhoea.** Consider polycystic ovaries if there are period abnormalities in older girls.
- **Sleep.** Sleep problems are common in obese children, and may affect eating patterns. Are there any breathing difficulties at night? Is there excessive daytime sleepiness?
- **Abdominal pain.** Right upper quadrant pain may occur as a result of gall stone disease. Ask about associated malaise, nausea and vomiting, particularly after food.
- **Rare comorbidities.** Severe headaches may point towards benign intracranial hypertension. Consider sleep apnoea if there are symptoms such as daytime sleepiness or snoring at night.
- **Involvement of other professionals.** Ask whether the child has already seen other professionals with regard to the weight problem (e.g. a practice nurse, health visitor, school nurse, community paediatrician, dietician or clinical psychologist). Are the child and parents aware of local support services, such as physical activity facilities, healthy eating and local parenting support groups?

Past and current medical problems
- **Feeding history.** Ask about birth weight and feeding history in early life.
- **Joint problems.** Ask about a history of joint problems, which may have occurred as a result of being overweight.
- **Diabetes.** Obesity is more common in children who are diabetic.
- **Genetic disorders.** Some genetic disorders may cause obesity.
- **Metabolic.** Consider hypothyroidism and adrenal problems.

Medication
- **Anticonvulsants.** Some anticonvulsants may lead to weight gain and obesity.
- **Steroids.** Systemic steroids can cause central obesity.

Family history
- **Genetic and endocrine conditions.** Diabetes, in particular, is an important disease to diagnose and treat. Is there a family history of polycystic ovaries?
- **Obesity.** Ask about levels of obesity in the closer family. Who else has weight problems?

- **Cardiovascular disease.** Is there a family history of cardiovascular disease, or risk factors such as hypertension or hyperlipidaemia?
- **Ethnic background.** People from certain ethnic groups (e.g. Afro-Caribbean, South Asian) are at higher risk of insulin-resistance syndrome and diabetes.

Social history
- **Home.** Are there any relationship problems between the parents? How does the child get on with siblings?
- **School.** Are there any problems at school? Ask about academic performance. Learning difficulties are common in some genetic syndromes.

Alcohol, smoking and recreational drugs
- **Alcohol.** Ask about alcohol consumption in older children, as alcoholic drinks can be high in calories and can pose health risks in themselves. Answers may not be very forthcoming if a parent is present.
- **Smoking.** Does the child smoke? Smoking increases the risk of cardiovascular problems in the future and has an appetite-suppressant effect. Stopping smoking should be encouraged, but may lead to short-term weight gain.

Review of previous investigations
- **Glucose.** Look out for previously raised glucose levels.
- **Cholesterol.** Cholesterol may be raised in obese children.
- **Luteinising hormone (LH) and follicle-stimulating hormone (FSH).** These are not usually required, but in some cases can be useful in adolescent girls.
- **Endocrine and genetic tests.** Endocrine and genetic tests (e.g. for hypothyroidism, Cushing's syndrome, genetic disorders) may already have been performed.

Examination

General
- **General condition.** Does the child look well and happy? Is there any obvious physical evidence of neglect or abuse? Does the child maintain eye contact and engage in conversation? How does the child interact with the parents or guardian?
- **Weight and height.** Measure weight, height and abdominal girth, and calculate the BMI percentile. Compare with previous readings, if available, and plot on an appropriate children's growth chart (e.g. WHO Growth Standards, http://www.who.int/childgrowth/standards/en/).
- **Truncal shape.** Truncal obesity may rarely suggest Cushing's syndrome.
- **Dysmorphic features.** These may rarely suggest genetic disorders, such as Prader–Willi syndrome.
- **Pubertal development.** This may be delayed, particularly if there are endocrine causes.

Vital signs

- **Blood pressure.** Use the appropriate cuff size (child cuff if <55 kg, small adult cuff if 55–110 kg, large adult cuff if >110 kg). For examples of normal blood pressure ranges by age and sex, see http://www.nhlbi.nih.gov/health-pro/ guidelines/current/hypertension-pediatric-jnc-4/blood-pressure-tables. Blood pressure may be raised due to systemic steroids or, rarely, because of an underlying endocrine disorder, such as Cushing's syndrome. Raised blood pressure is a risk factor for cardiovascular disease, particularly if associated with diabetes, severe obesity and lack of exercise. Rarely, hypothyroidism may cause bradycardia.

Skin

- **Hirsutism.** This may occur with Cushing's syndrome and polycystic ovaries.
- **Striae.** Physiological striae are common in adolescence. Deep-purple violaceous striae may be seen in Cushing's syndrome.
- **Acanthosis nigricans.** This may occur with insulin-dependent diabetes or insulin resistance (rare).

Head and neck

- **Face.** Look for facial plethora and moon face, which occur in Cushing's syndrome.
- **Eyes.** Check the fundi for papilloedema, which may suggest pseudotumour cerebri (very rare).
- **Throat.** Check for enlarged tonsils, which may occasionally contribute to sleep apnoea. Consider the presence of adenoids, which can easily be missed on routine inspection.

Abdomen

- **Palpation.** Briefly check for any obvious abdominal masses or organomegaly. Consider the possibility of pregnancy in adolescent girls.
- **Liver.** There may be hepatomegaly due to nonalcoholic steatohepatitis ('fatty liver').
- **Testes.** Testes of more than 3ml in volume suggest precocious puberty in boys below the age of 9. Consider delayed puberty if there is no testicular enlargement by the age of 15. Look for the presence or absence of pubic hair growth. Males with Prader–Willi syndrome usually have undescended testes.

Lower limbs

- **Hips and knees.** Look for any evidence of joint problems resulting from being overweight. Consider slipped upper femoral epiphysis if there is limited range of hip movement.

Bedside tests

- **Glucose.** Check blood glucose tests strips if you suspect diabetes.

Key references and further reading

1. Barlow S, Dietz W. Obesity evaluation and treatment. Expert Committee recommendations. *Pediatrics* 1998;102:E29.
2. Gibson P, Edmunds L, Haslam DW, Poskitt E. An approach to weight management in children and adolescents (2–18 years) in primary care. Royal College of Paediatrics and Child Health and National Obesity Forum. 2002. Available from: http://www.icid.salisbury.nhs.uk/ClinicalManagement/ChildHealth/Documents /ade314857b384fb88e9fd0d752ddcdedAapproachotweightmanagementinch ildrenazndadolescen.pdf (last accessed 29 April 2016).
3. Kipping RR, Jago R, Lawlor D. Obesity in children. Part 1: epidemiology, measurement, risk factors, and screening. *BMJ* 2008;337:a1824.
4. Lyznicki J, Young D, Riggs J, Davis R. Obesity: assessment and management in primary care. *Am Fam Physician* 2001;63:2185–2196.
5. National Institute for Health and Care Excellence (NICE). Weight management: lifestyle services for overweight or obese children and young people. NICE guidelines [PH47]. October 2013. Available from: http://www.nice.org .uk/guidance/ph47 (last accessed 29 April 2016).
6. National Institute for Health and Care Excellence (NICE). Obesity: identification, assessment and management. NICE guidelines [CG189]. November 2014. Available from: http://www.nice.org.uk/guidance/cg189 (last accessed 29 April 2016).
7. National Obesity Forum. www.nationalobesityforum.org.uk.
8. Summerbell CD, Waters E, Edmunds LD et al. Interventions for preventing obesity in children. *Cochrane Database Syst Rev* 2001;(1):CD001871.
9. World Health Organization (WHO). *Obesity: Preventing and Managing the Global Epidemic*. World Health Organization, Geneva; 1998.

Suspected child abuse and neglect

Key thoughts

Practical points

- **Diagnosis.** Child abuse is relatively common, but may go undetected in many cases. It is important to have a high index of suspicion and to be able to recognise symptoms and signs that may suggest child abuse (e.g. multiple fractures or fractures in unusual sites). If you suspect child abuse, try to see the child both alone and with their parents, with another health professional present, if possible.
- **Reporting.** One aim of the assessment is to gather evidence to decide whether an alleged incidence of child abuse needs to be reported and investigated further. Formal assessment needs to be carried out by a team experienced in the assessment of child abuse. Consider talking informally to other relevant health professionals or to child services, without mentioning a name, if you would like further advice. Evaluate the potential risk to the child from abuse – and from wrongly accusing someone of child abuse. Make sure you keep thorough notes, with details about the date, time, examination findings and explanations given.
- **Intervention.** If child abuse is detected in time, long-term physical and psychological consequences may be prevented by early intervention.

Forms of child abuse

- Physical abuse or non-accidental injury.
- Sexual abuse.
- Emotional abuse.
- Neglect.
- Factitious disorder by proxy (Munchausen syndrome by proxy).
- Any combination of these.

Risk factors

- **Parents.** Parental stress and relationship problems, unrealistic expectations placed on the child, unwanted pregnancy, mental illness, substance misuse.
- **Child.** Disability, premature birth, demanding or 'difficult' child, chronic illness.
- **Environmental.** Social deprivation, inadequate support network, poor or crowded housing, financial difficulties.

Differential diagnosis

- Epilepsy leading to multiple trauma.
- Increased bruising in haematological conditions.
- Birth marks (e.g. Mongolian blue spots).
- Osteogenesis imperfecta.

The 10-Minute Clinical Assessment, Second Edition. Knut Schroeder.
© 2017 John Wiley & Sons, Ltd. Published 2017 by John Wiley & Sons, Ltd.

RED FLAGS

- Danger to the child's health or life
- Physical injuries (e.g. fractures)
- Psychological problems
- Ongoing risk of abuse
- History of domestic violence
- Developmental delay
- Parental alcohol or drug problems

History

Ideas, concerns and expectations

- **Ideas.** What do the parents and the child think is happening? People seeking medical advice for an injury in a child may not suspect potential child abuse, particularly if it happens within the family.
- **Concerns.** Parents and children may be concerned about police and social worker involvement, as well as the potential for the child having to go into care. Parents may show an unusual lack of concern for a child's injury.
- **Expectations.** Parents may not expect further assessment and examination of the child. They may be reluctant to cooperate if the abuser is someone who is close to the child. What is the reason for consultation?

History of presenting complaint

- **Context.** Has the child disclosed that they are being abused? Allow the child and accompanying person(s) time to tell you the story in their own words. Open questions such as 'What happened?' are more helpful than leading questions like 'Did your father hit you?'. Be aware if the person accompanying the child is not the parent or guardian.
- **Consistency.** Be suspicious if the parents' or guardians' explanation of the injury does not match with the sustained injury or is inconsistent with the developmental stage of the child. Does the story change when repeated? Is the child's explanation different from that of the parents or another person?
- **Medical needs.** Are the medical needs of the child attended to? Has the mother attended antenatal appointments in the past? Is there any developmental delay?
- **Child left alone.** Is there evidence that the child is being left at home alone, with or without food? Does the child have to look after other children in the household because parents are absent or have alcohol or drug problems?

Common forms of abuse

- **Physical abuse.** Has there been a delay in the presentation of an injury? Are there any unexplained burns, recurrent injuries or fractures? Does the child or their parents try to keep skin covered in order hide injuries?

- **Sexual abuse.** Is the child overly affectionate? Is there chronic itching or pain around the genital areas? Are there mental health problems, such as self-harm, anorexia or depression? Has the child tried to run away from home? Has there been a recent change in personality? Has the child started to regress to behaviours of younger children, such as playing with discarded toys or thumb-sucking? Is there any fear of people the child knows well, such as a relative or a child minder? Is there regression to bed-wetting? Has the child suddenly started to draw pictures with sexually explicit content? Is there vaginal discharge or recurrent urinary infections in a girl under the age of 14?
- **Emotional abuse.** Be suspicious if there is a significant delay in development. Is there any evidence of a speech disorder or neurotic behaviour, such as hair-twisting, rocking or self-mutilation?
- **Neglect.** Is the child constantly hungry or tired? Does the child have any social relationships?

Past and current medical problems
- **Gestational age.** Prematurity is a risk factor for feeding problems and poor bonding with the mother.
- **Development.** Has the child developed normally to date? Any form of abuse may lead to behavioural problems.
- **Trauma.** Ask about any previous injuries to the child, particularly any poorly explained or unusual trauma, as well as fractures.
- **Recurrent attendances.** Recurrent consultations for the same condition or for other unusual problems raise the possibility of abuse or Munchausen by proxy syndrome.
- **Health visitor and social worker.** Ask whether there has been any contact with health visitors and social services. Is the child or a sibling on the 'special needs register'? Try to speak to other involved professionals to get a better picture of the family and the social situation.
- **Disability.** A child with a disability may be at higher risk of being abused.
- **Medical problems.** Any untreated or poorly controlled medical conditions, such as asthma, may suggest neglect.
- **Epilepsy.** Epileptic fits may potentially lead to multiple injuries.
- **Haematological disorders.** Rarely, thrombocytopenia and leukaemia may lead to increased bruising.
- **Fractures.** A number of bone conditions, such as osteomyelitis, rickets and osteogenesis imperfecta, may rarely increase fracture risk.

Social history
- **Domestic situation.** Problems in the parents' relationship and a general lack of support increase the risk of child abuse. If there is a male in the household, is he the father? Is there a history of domestic violence?
- **Parents' health.** Are the parents well in themselves, or do they suffer from chronic or acute physical or mental illness? Do the parents have an alcohol or drug problem?
- **Children.** Obtain details about other children in the household. How many are there? Is the mother pregnant? Is there a history of multiple pregnancies? Are

the other children well? Do any suffer from learning disabilities? The presence of sick children may increase the risk of abuse.

- **Social status.** Consider any employment or financial problems. Have other children been taken into care or been on the 'at risk' register?

Review of previous investigations

- **Full blood count.** This will exclude thrombocytopenia in case of severe bruising.
- **Clotting screen.** Extensive bruising may occur with abnormal clotting.
- **X-ray skeletal survey.** Look for past and present fractures that may suggest non-accidental injury. Be particularly suspicious of multiple rib fractures and fractures in children not yet walking.

Examination

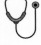

General

- **Parents.** How do the parents and child relate to one another? Do the parents allow the child to be examined? Do they overreact to the child's behaviour? Is there any obvious aggression towards the child? Do they have unrealistic expectations with regard to the child's behaviour?
- **Physical abuse.** Is there a fear of being touched? Does the child shrink back on physical contact? Is the child watchful of what you do, or even 'frozen'?
- **Neglect.** Is there evidence of poor personal hygiene? Are the clothes in a poor state?
- **Faltering growth.** Check weight and height, and plot these on the appropriate growth charts (e.g. WHO Growth Standards, http://www.who.int/childgrowth/standards/en/). Record the head circumference in smaller children.
- **Malnutrition.** Look for wasted muscles and the general condition of hair and skin.
- **Affect.** Children who suffer emotional abuse may appear emotionally flat and withdrawn.

Skin

- **Injuries.** It is good practice to fully undress the child, if they are brought in because of an injury. Is there any obvious bruising? Do bruises suggest finger marks through gripping or slapping? Be suspicious of bruises around the cheeks, eyes, ears and genitalia, especially in a non-mobile child. Any fractures in a child under 1 year of age or multiple fractures in any child are very suspicious. Do the injuries fit with the story? Are there any teeth impressions? Are there any burns suggestive of cigarette burns? Ligature injuries may present with red lines. Do older injuries coexist with newer ones?
- **Scalding.** Look for evidence of scalding, which may be found symmetrically on the buttocks or feet.

Head and neck

- **Mouth.** A torn frenulum of the upper lip may occur as a result of force feeding.

- **Fundi.** Check the fundi for evidence of retinal haemorrhages, which can result from vigorous shaking or head injury.
- **Scalp.** Check the scalp for any injuries or evidence of fractures. A raised fontanelle in an infant suggests raised intracranial pressure.

Abdomen

- **Genitals.** If there is suspicion of sexual abuse, leave further examination to a paediatrician with experience in the assessment of sexual abuse, so that the child does not have to go through multiple examinations.

Key references and further reading

1. Berkoff CM, Zolotor AJ, Makoroff KL et al. The rational clinical examination: has this prepubertal girl been sexually abused? *JAMA* 2008;300:2779–2792.
2. Carter YH, Bannon MJ. The role of primary care in the protection of children from abuse and neglect. Position statement. Royal College of General Practitioners, London; 2003.
3. Department for Education. What to do if you're worried a child is being abused. March 2015. Available from: https://www.gov.uk/government/publications/what-to-do-if-youre-worried-a-child-is-being-abused–2 (last accessed 29 April 2016).
4. Kemp AM, Dunstan F, Harrison S et al. Patterns of skeletal fractures in child abuse: systematic review. *BMJ* 2008;337:a1518.
5. National Institute for Health and Care Excellence (NICE). Child maltreatment: when to suspect maltreatment in under 18s. NICE guidelines [CG89]. July 2009. Available from: http://www.nice.org.uk/guidance/cg89 (last accessed 29 April 2016).

Nocturnal enuresis

Key thoughts

Practical points
- **Diagnosis.** Parents may have unrealistic expectations about when a child should become dry at night. Most children will be dry at night at around 7 years of age. If bed-wetting persists, consider emotional factors, nocturnal polyuria, bladder overactivity or lack of arousal from sleep.

Possible causes
- Functional.
- Psychological distress.
- Dysfunctional voiding.
- Urinary tract infection.
- Constipation.
- Rarely, urethral obstruction, diabetes mellitus, diabetes insipidus, epilepsy, acquired neurogenic bladder.

> **RED FLAGS**
>
> - Suspected underlying physical problem
> - Severe emotional distress
> - Persistent problems into adolescence
> - Daytime wetting

History

Ideas, concerns and expectations
- **Ideas.** Parents often suspect an organic cause for bed-wetting, such as kidney conditions, bladder disease, congenital defects or neurological problems.
- **Concerns.** Many parents are worried about the possible negative social and emotional effects of bed-wetting on their child. Nocturnal enuresis can affect whole families due to feelings of shame and embarrassment. Many children and parents have to build up courage to consult a health professional – and some may never present at all.
- **Expectations.** Some parents expect their children to stay dry through the night from an early age. The reason for consultation might be that the child is about to go on a school trip or has been invited to a sleepover party.

The 10-Minute Clinical Assessment, Second Edition. Knut Schroeder.
© 2017 John Wiley & Sons, Ltd. Published 2017 by John Wiley & Sons, Ltd.

History of presenting complaint

- **Context.** Encourage the parents and the child, using open questions, to give their side of the story about the problem. Give them plenty of time and be non-judgemental; this will help build rapport and trust. Tell the child that everything will be treated confidentially.
- **Quality of life.** How has the child's and their parents' life been affected by the bed-wetting?
- **Onset and pattern.** Has the child never been dry (primary enuresis) or did the child begin to wet the bed after at least 2 months of bladder control at night (secondary enuresis)? Charts can be useful in assessing the frequency of bed-wetting, identifying patterns and monitoring treatment.
- **Parental attitudes.** Are the parents supportive of their child or do they feel annoyed by the extra work (in terms of extra laundry), additional costs or smell? Are punishments being used to try to change behaviour?
- **Daytime toileting.** How often does the child visit the toilet during the day? Does the child have to rush without warning (urgency)? Daytime wetting is a problem that is likely to require further specialist input.
- **Daytime drinking.** Ask for details about the frequency and amount of fluid intake. Most children are not drinking enough. In particular, consider fizzy drinks and drinks like coffee and tea, which can have an effect on urinary output.
- **Toilet.** Is there easy access to a toilet at night? Is lighting sufficient? Is a night light being used? Is there a fear of the dark? Does the child sleep on a top bunk (this may prevent them from going to the toilet at night)?
- **Urinary symptoms.** Ask about signs of urine infection, such as dysuria, frequency or offensive urine.
- **Protection.** Are pull-ups being used? Is there a protective mattress?
- **Avoidance behaviour.** Has the bed-wetting led to avoiding sleepovers and school trips?
- **Bowel function.** Is the child constipated?
- **Psychological impact.** Ask whether the bed-wetting has affected the child's self-esteem and whether they feel 'different' from others. Such fears may make it more difficult for the child to spend nights away from home.

Common symptom patterns

- **Nocturnal polyuria.** Children with nocturnal polyuria do not usually show any urinary symptoms during the day. Bed-wetting is likely to occur early in the night, with large wet patches. A common cause is excess drinking at night. These children may respond to treatment with desmopressin.
- **Bladder overactivity.** Children with an overactive or small bladder often show urinary symptoms during the day. Bladder training may be helpful in these children.
- **Lack of arousal from sleep.** Difficulty in waking up and sleeping through even though the bed is wet are common. These children may benefit from an enuresis alarm if they are well motivated and if there is positive involvement from the family.

Medication

- **Treatment for enuresis.** Have any drugs been used for the treatment of enuresis (e.g. desmopressin, oxybutinin, amitriptyline)? What has been the effect of any such medications? Have there been any adverse effects?

Other treatments

- **Enuresis services.** Have any local enuresis services been involved in the management?
- **Enuresis alarm.** Has this been tried, in case of poor arousal from sleep? If so, how effective has it been?
- **Other treatments.** Have other options, such as star charts, waking the child from sleep to go to the toilet or restricting fluid intake, been tried?

Family history

- **Enuresis.** Is there a family history of enuresis or urinary problems (urological, renal)?

Social history

- **Domestic situation.** How has the bed-wetting affected home life? The atmosphere may have become more hostile and tense, which can affect the bedwetting adversely. Parents on low earnings or state benefits may find the additional costs of bed-wetting, in terms of laundry expenses, difficult to cope with.
- **Schooling.** Are there any school problems resulting from the bed-wetting? Is the child being bullied? Has the school nurse been involved?
- **Stresses.** Have there been recent stresses in the family, such as a new child, shifting house, financial or employment problems, marriage difficulties or other issues that might contribute to bed-wetting?

Review of previous investigations

- **Urine.** Has the urine been checked for infection?
- **Blood tests.** Blood tests are not always necessary. Full blood count, plasma viscosity (infection, inflammation) and renal function tests can be helpful for initial investigation but will in most cases be normal.

Examination

General

- **General condition.** Does the child look well?
- **Psychological appearance.** Does the child appear worried? Children often try and hide their true feelings and may want to appear indifferent, particularly if they have been unsuccessful in their attempts to overcome the problem.

Vital signs
- **Temperature.** Fever may indicate urinary tract infection. Urinary symptoms will often be present, but urinary infection may also be asymptomatic.
- **Blood pressure.** A raised blood pressure might rarely indicate renal disease.

Abdomen
- **Masses.** Examine the abdomen for any masses. The kidneys will usually not be palpable unless enlarged. Is there evidence of urinary retention in the form of a distended bladder? Is there evidence of constipation?
- **External genitalia.** If there is daytime wetting, look for any abnormalities such as hypospadias, which may be associated with further urogenital tract abnormalities.
- **Rectal examination.** Consider a rectal examination if there is a possibility of constipation.
- **Perianal sensation.** Check this if a neurological cause may be responsible for the bed-wetting.

Spine
- **Posture.** Does the spine appear normal? Look for evidence of spina bifida and other neural tube defects.

Lower limbs
- **Neurology.** Consider neurogenic bladder if tone, power, sensation, coordination and reflexes are abnormal.

Bedside tests
- **Urinalysis.** Check for haematuria and proteinuria (kidney disease). A test that is also positive to nitrites and leucocytes indicates urinary tract infection; this should be confirmed with a midstream urine microscopy and culture.

Key references and further reading
1. Butler RJ. Impact of nocturnal enuresis on children and young people. *Scand J Urol* 2001;163(Suppl.):39–47.
2. Butler RJ, Holland P. The three systems: a conceptual way of understanding nocturnal enuresis. *Scand J Urol Nephrol* 2000;34:270–277.
3. Butler RJ, Golding J, Northstone K. Nocturnal enuresis at 7.5 years old: prevalence and analysis of clinical signs. *BJU Int* 2005;96:404–410.
4. Education and Resources for Improving Childhood Continence (ERIC). www.eric.org.uk.
5. Glazener CM, Evans JH. Simple behavioural and physical interventions for nocturnal enuresis in children. *Cochrane Database Syst Rev* 2004;(2): CD003637.

6. National Institute for Health and Care Excellence (NICE). Bedwetting in under 19s. NICE guidelines [CG111]. October 2010. Available from: http://www.nice.org.uk/guidance/cg111 (last accessed 29 April 2016).
7. Touchette E, Petit D, Paquet J et al. Bedwetting and its association with developmental milestones in early childhood. *Arch Pediatr Adolesc Med* 2005;159:1129–1134.

Knee problems in children

Key thoughts

Practical points
- **Diagnosis.** Most knee pain in children is self-limiting and caused by trauma or overuse. Osgood–Schlatter disease is relatively common. Distinguish between true knee pain and referred pain from the hip or spine.
- **Red flags.** Consider more serious causes if alarm symptoms are present.

Possible causes
- Overuse.
- Trauma.
- Growing pains.
- Osgood–Schlatter disease (adolescents).
- Meniscal or cruciate ligament injury.
- Rarely, genu varum (bow legs), genu valgum (knock knees), referred pain from slipped upper femoral epiphysis or Perthes' disease, septic arthritis, osteomyelitis, bone tumours.

> **RED FLAGS**
>
> - Referred pain from the hip
> - Severe or constant pain
> - Inability to bear weight
> - Unexplained limp
> - Locking and giving way
> - Fever and malaise
> - Night pain
> - Unclear diagnosis

History

Ideas, concerns and expectations
- **Ideas.** What does the child and their parents believe to be the underlying problem?
- **Concerns.** Are there particular concerns about the effect of knee problems on schooling or other activities? Parents are often worried about a possible diagnosis of bone cancer.
- **Expectations.** Parents may have strong views about management and may request investigations and specialist referral, which in many cases will not be indicated.

The 10-Minute Clinical Assessment, Second Edition. Knut Schroeder.
© 2017 John Wiley & Sons, Ltd. Published 2017 by John Wiley & Sons, Ltd.

History of presenting complaint

- **Context.** Ask the child and parents open questions about the context in which the knee problems developed. Is the child a keen sportsperson?
- **Quality of life.** How has the knee pain affected day-to-day life? Consider home, school and sports.
- **Onset and progression.** Onset is usually acute in overuse and other trauma, as well as in infection (which is rare). Pain due to bone tumours develops gradually and gets worse over a period of weeks and months, but this is also rare.
- **Pain on movement and weight-bearing.** Pain that is worse on movement suggests trauma, overuse or, in rare cases, septic arthritis, which usually presents with additional symptoms, such as fever and malaise. Complete inability to bear weight suggests a possible serious underlying cause.
- **Anterior knee pain.** Consider chondromalacia patellae in teenage girls who complain of pain on walking up or down stairs or after prolonged sitting. This usually settles when the skeleton matures. In adolescent boys, localised swelling and tenderness over the insertion of the patellar tendon can be caused by chronic traction apophysitis to the tibial tubercle at the front of the knee (Osgood–Schlatter disease). Osgood–Schlatter disease and chondromalacia patellae are commonly caused by excessive or unaccustomed exercise.
- **Instability.** Consider meniscal or cruciate ligament damage if the knee feels unstable or gives way. If the knee feels particularly unstable when twisting or going downstairs, an anterior or, less commonly, posterior cruciate ligament injury is likely.
- **Fracture.** Consider a fracture if there is severe bony pain, tenderness and deformity after an injury. Be aware that bone tumours and osteomyelitis (both rare) predispose to fractures.
- **Lumps.** Any lump around the knee that is not resolving should raise suspicions of malignant sarcoma, even if the presenting complaint is trauma.
- **Night pain.** Episodic leg pain affecting the muscles and wakening the child from sleep is often a result of growing pains, but a tumour may need to be excluded. Growing pains are typically relieved by rubbing, usually do not last much longer than 30 minutes and disappear prior to waking up in the morning. Physical signs and raised inflammatory markers are usually absent.
- **Bone pain and swelling.** Consider rare bone tumours if there is constant and worsening bone pain and/or swelling that continues at rest or wakes the child at night. Consider rickets due to vitamin D deficiency if there is bone pain and tenderness in the legs, arms, spine or pelvis. This often leads to skeletal deformity, pathological fractures, dental problems, muscular weakness and impaired growth. Causes are usually dietary, but consider malabsorption, renal disease, liver problems and hereditary causes.
- **Soft-tissue swelling.** Consider soft-tissue sarcoma if there is an unexplained mass at any site of more than 2 cm in diameter which is growing, non-tender, deep to the fascia and associated with an enlarging regional lymph node.

Common symptom patterns

- **Genu varum (bow legs).** This involves outward curving of the tibia and internal torsion of the tibia, which usually resolves spontaneously. In severe cases, consider rickets or developmental disorders.
- **Genu valgum (knock knees).** These are usually benign if they affect both knees and are not associated with other orthopaedic abnormalities. They commonly occur in children aged 2–4 years. If they are severe and progressing, consider rickets.
- **Valgus injury.** This may be caused by the knee being pushed medially from the lateral side and is often the result of a football tackle or a hit by a car bumper. As a result, the medial collateral ligament can be stretched or ruptured.
- **Twisting injury.** Twisting injuries with the knee slightly flexed may lead to damage of the medial or, less commonly, the lateral meniscus. Common symptoms are intermittent swelling, locking and giving way.
- **Referred pain from the hip.** Knee pain in children may be referred pain from the hip. Consider Perthes' disease due to avascular necrosis of the nucleus of the proximal femoral epiphysis. In overweight, peripubertal and sexually immature boys, hip pain may suggest slipped upper femoral epiphysis. The resulting pain can be acute, chronic or acute-on-chronic, and early recognition is important.
- **Infection.** Knee pain may result from reactive arthritis in conjunction with a viral infection. In rare cases, consider septic arthritis, particularly in children under 5. Children will usually be systemically unwell and have a swollen, hot and tender joint, which is held very still. Fever, vomiting and headaches are common in older children, whereas younger ones may present with circulatory collapse. Skin infections, abscesses or surgery may lead to osteomyelitis, particularly in children with diabetes, immunodeficiency, sickle-cell disease or poor standards of living. Symptoms and signs are similar to those in septic arthritis, and include effusion of neighbouring joints. Osteomyelitis may result in septic arthritis, bone deformity, pathological fracture and chronic infection. In chronic cases, there may be discharge and pus from the sinuses, which may recur intermittently for years.

Past and current medical problems

- **Fractures.** Ask about any past trauma and fractures.
- **Arthritis.** This may occur in rubella, infectious mononucleosis, rheumatic fever or Henoch–Schönlein syndrome, or it may be one of the chronic forms of arthritis in childhood.

Medication

- **Analgesia.** What has been tried? What is effective? Have there been any adverse effects?

Allergies

- **Analgesics and antibiotics.** Ask about allergies to any treatments that might need to be used.

Other treatments
- **Physiotherapy.** Ask about the frequency and effect of any physiotherapy in the past.

Social history
- **Home.** Ask details about home circumstances.
- **Schooling.** Are there any school problems resulting from the knee problem?
- **Social life.** Has social life, including meeting friends and taking part in team sports, been a problem?

Review of investigations
- **Full blood count and plasma viscosity.** Raised white cell count and inflammatory markers suggest infection in rare cases.
- **X-ray.** This is useful in excluding slipped femoral epiphysis.
- **MRI or bone scan.** These can help detect osteomyelitis and other soft tissue or bony lesions.

Examination

General
- **General condition.** Does the child look unwell or toxic (infection)? Are there any indicators for neglect or abuse?
- **Walking.** Severe limping and the inability to bear weight suggest a more serious underlying cause.
- **Movement.** Is there protective muscle spasm, which may occur in injury or joint infection?
- **Pain.** Is the child in obvious pain? Consider giving analgesia prior to any further assessment and ensure that the child is as comfortable as possible.

Vital signs
- **Temperature.** Fever may suggest reactive arthritis due to viral infection. Consider the possibility of septic arthritis or acute osteomyelitis in rare cases.
- **Pulse.** Tachycardia may be the result of severe pain or infection.

Knee examination
- **Skin temperature.** Raised skin temperature over the affected joint suggests inflammation or, rarely, infection.
- **Tibial and torsional abnormalities.** Deformities and valgus knees may lead to patellar maltracking and subsequent subluxation, which can cause pain, particularly in girls. In boys, tenderness over the tibial tubercle may indicate Osgood–Schlatter disease.
- **Joint movement.** Does the knee move over the whole range?

- **Swelling.** Look for any bony swelling, which may indicate effusion or, in rare cases, osteomyelitis or tumour. Effusions in adjacent joints may also occur in osteomyelitis.
- **Collateral ligaments.** Palpate both medial and lateral collateral ligaments for tenderness. If they are tender after valgus injury, this suggests stretching or rupture of the medial collateral ligament.
- **Instability.** Check carefully for any instability suggesting ligamentous injury (collateral and cruciate ligaments).
- **Crepitus.** This may occur in chondromalacia patellae.
- **Hip rotation.** Check the internal and external rotation of the hip. If it is painful and reduced, this might be the cause of the knee pain. Always compare with the other side, but beware of bilateral disease.

Key references and further reading

1. Fischer S, Beattie T. The limping child: epidemiology, assessment and outcome. *J Bone Jt Surg* 1999;81:1029–1034.
2. Hamer A. Pain in the hip and knee. ABC of rheumatology. *BMJ* 2004;328: 1067–1069.
3. Mordecai S, Avis D. Evaluation of the limping child. *InnovAiT* 2011;4:319–324.

Hip problems in children

Key thoughts

Practical points
- **Diagnosis.** Transient synovitis and overuse injuries are common and are usually benign and self-limiting.
- **Prognosis.** Hip pain in children always needs to be taken seriously, as potential serious underlying causes will require urgent hospital assessment.

Possible causes
- **Any age.** Transient synovitis (irritable hip), overuse, trauma. Rarely, septic arthritis, osteomyelitis, juvenile rheumatoid arthritis, bone tumour, tuberculous arthritis.
- **Age under 5 years.** Developmental dysplasia of the hip, acute infective epiphysitis, infantile coxa vera.
- **Age 5–10 years.** Perthes' disease.
- **Age over 10 years.** Slipped upper femoral epiphysis.

> **RED FLAGS**
>
> - Severe pain
> - Inability to bear weight
> - Unexplained limp persisting for more than 5 days
> - Osteomyelitis
> - Fever and malaise
> - Night pain
> - Constant pain

History

Ideas, concerns and expectations
- **Ideas.** What does the child and their parents believe to be the underlying cause?
- **Concerns.** Parents are often worried about the possible diagnosis of bone cancer. Are there particular concerns about the effect of hip problems on schooling or other activities?
- **Expectations.** Parents may have strong views about management and will often expect further investigations and specialist referral, which in many cases will not be indicated.

The 10-Minute Clinical Assessment, Second Edition. Knut Schroeder.
© 2017 John Wiley & Sons, Ltd. Published 2017 by John Wiley & Sons, Ltd.

History of presenting complaint

- **Context.** Allow the child and parents to tell you about the hip problems in their own words.
- **Quality of life.** How has day-to-day life been affected (home, school, exercise)?
- **Onset and progression.** Onset is usually acute in trauma, overuse and infection. Bone tumours (rare) develop gradually and get worse over a period of weeks and months.
- **Delay in walking.** A delay in walking may raise the possibility of missed developmental dysplasia of the hip.
- **Trauma.** Ask for details about any injuries and consider the possibility of bone or cartilage damage.
- **Pain.** Pain that is worse on movement suggests overuse, trauma or infection. Other, more serious causes include Perthes' disease and slipped upper femoral epiphysis. Inability to bear weight is usually an indication for further investigation or referral. Pain is often referred to the knee in slipped upper femoral epiphysis, which presents typically in overweight, hypogonadal boys. Girls can also be affected.
- **Limping.** Hip disease in children often presents with a limp, and not necessarily with pain or a history of trauma. In children under 5 years of age, missed congenital dislocation of the hip is an important cause. In older children, limping and hip pain (and/or referred pain to the knee) may indicate Perthes' disease, particularly in boys aged between 5 and 10 years.
- **Recent upper respiratory infection.** Transient synovitis may occur after respiratory infections and presents with a unilateral and self-limiting limp, as well as with hip and/or knee pain, usually in boys aged 2–12 years.

Common symptom patterns

- **Congenital dislocation of the hip.** There is usually a delay in walking, a limp and a discrepancy in leg length in children aged <5 years.
- **Transient synovitis or irritable hip.** Children are not acutely unwell and can move the hip.
- **Perthes' disease.** This often occurs in boys aged 5–10 years and is associated with a limp or with hip or knee pain.
- **Slipped upper femoral epiphysis.** Pain is often referred to the knee and occurs in overweight hypogonadal boys between 10–15 years of age.
- **Septic arthritis.** This is rare but important, and not to be missed. The child will usually be ill and unable to walk. Pain prevents movement of the affected joint.
- **Other forms of arthritis.** Hip pain can be the presenting complaint in juvenile rheumatoid arthritis.

Past and current medical problems

- **Fractures.** Ask about any past trauma and fractures.
- **Arthritis.** This may occur in rubella, infectious mononucleosis, rheumatic fever or Henoch–Schönlein syndrome, or it may be one of the chronic forms of arthritis in childhood.

Medication
- **Analgesia.** What has been tried? What is effective? Have there been any adverse effects?

Allergies
- **Analgesics and antibiotics.** Ask about allergies to any treatments that might need to be used.

Other treatments
- **Physiotherapy.** Ask about the frequency and effect of any past physiotherapy.

Social history
- **Home.** Ask for details about home circumstances.
- **Schooling.** Are there any school problems resulting from the hip problem?
- **Social life.** Has social life, including meeting friends and taking part in team sports, been a problem?

Review of investigations
- **Full blood count and plasma viscosity.** A raised white cell count and inflammatory markers suggest infection (rare).
- **Plain hip X-rays.** Anteroposterior and lateral 'frog leg' views should usually be obtained for both sides, to allow comparison.
- **Ultrasound.** This may be useful for showing hip joint effusion.
- **MRI or bone scan.** These are rarely used, but may be useful for the detection of osteomyelitis, if the diagnosis is unclear or if surgery is being considered.

Examination

General
- **General condition.** Does the child look unwell or toxic (suggesting infection on rare occasions)? Are there any indicators for neglect or abuse?
- **Pain.** Is the child in obvious pain? Consider giving analgesia prior to any further assessment and ensure that the child is as comfortable as possible.
- **Movement.** Is there protective muscle spasm, which may occur in injury or joint infection?
- **Walking.** Severe limping and inability to bear weight suggest a more serious underlying cause, such as Perthes' disease or slipped upper femoral epiphysis.

Vital signs
- **Temperature.** This may be raised in reactive arthritis (viral infection), septic arthritis or acute osteomyelitis (all rare).
- **Pulse.** This is raised in severe pain and infection.

Hip examination

- **Inspection.** Look for symmetry of the skin creases in the thigh and buttock, and check whether both legs have the same length. Consider developmental dysplasia of the hip if skin creases over the thigh or buttocks are asymmetrical, if leg length is different, if there is reduced hip abduction in flexion (normally 90°) or if there is a reduced distance between the greater trochanter and the anterior superior iliac spine. In slipped upper femoral epiphysis, the affected leg may be externally rotated and shortened. In septic arthritis, the hip is often flexed, abducted and externally rotated.
- **Barlow's and Ortolani's tests.** In newborn children, consider performing Barlow's or Ortolani's tests if you suspect developmental dysplasia of the hip.
- **Palpation.** Tenderness over the anterior aspect of the hip is common in transient synovitis.
- **Movement.** Abduction, full extension and internal rotation are often restricted in transient synovitis, Perthes' disease and slipped upper femoral epiphysis.

Abdomen

- **Palpation.** Palpate the abdomen for tenderness if appendicitis is a possibility (can present with hip pain).

Key references and further reading

1. Gough-Palmer A, McHugh K. Investigating hip pain in a well child. *BMJ* 2007;334:1216–1217.
2. Hamer A. Pain in the hip and knee. ABC of rheumatology. *BMJ* 2004;328: 1067–1069.
3. Mordecai S, Avis D. Evaluation of the limping child. *InnovAiT* 2011;4:319–324.

Adolescent health problems

Key thoughts

Practical points
- **Identification of health problems.** Most adolescents do not have any medical issues, but they may engage in risky behaviours that can affect their health. Mental health problems are relatively common in adolescence and can cause a lot of suffering for the adolescent and their parents.
- **Quality of life.** Early recognition and support can dramatically improve the patient's (and their parents') quality of life.

Potential health risks and problems
- Risk-taking behaviour.
- Problems at home.
- Problems with education.
- Eating disorders.
- Lack of exercise.
- Drug and alcohol misuse.
- Mental health problems.
- Sexual problems and sexually transmitted infections.

RED FLAGS
- Suicidal thoughts
- Significant weight loss
- Involvement in crime
- Eating disorders
- Alcohol and drug use

History

Ideas, concerns and expectations
- **Ideas.** What does the patient and/or their parents believe to be the main problem? Why is the adolescent consulting now? If presenting with a specific condition, what are their ideas about possible causes?
- **Concerns.** Adolescents are often worried about confidentiality. Discuss issues around confidentiality early on in the consultation, particularly if there is a risk

The 10-Minute Clinical Assessment, Second Edition. Knut Schroeder.
© 2017 John Wiley & Sons, Ltd. Published 2017 by John Wiley & Sons, Ltd.

of significant harm through suicide or any form of abuse. Try to explain the importance and limitations of confidentiality to the parents as well.

- **Expectations.** Ask what expectations the adolescent or their parents have with regard to the outcome of the consultation.

History of presenting complaint

- **Communication.** Communication can be difficult with adolescents, who may find it hard to express themselves. They are often accompanied by a parent, who may describe their problem for them. Adolescents may also be reluctant to talk about any sexual problems, smoking or alcohol- or drug-taking in front of their parents. If possible, try to consult with adolescents alone and treat them as individuals. Allow time to discuss any problems around their family dynamics. Try to create a positive atmosphere by focusing on areas where they are doing well. Ask open questions initially, to find out more about their general health and the presenting problem, but be aware that communication can be difficult and that open questions may at times not work very well with adolescents. In those cases, simple, closed question with suggested multiple-choice answers in areas that are of interest to the adolescent can be helpful.
- **Context.** Ask the adolescent and/or their parents to describe any problems to you in their own words. Further questioning will be guided by the patient's story.
- **Quality of life.** How have day-to-day activities and quality of life been affected?
- **Education.** Ask questions like: 'Where do you go to school?', 'What do you like or not like about school?', 'What are your favourite topics?', 'What are you good at?', 'How do you get on with your teachers?' and 'What would you like to do after finishing school?'.
- **Home.** Ask for details about the home situation and who else shares the accommodation. Are there are concerns about safety at home or in the neighbourhood? Are there any problems with parents or siblings? Who would the patient choose to discuss any problems with?
- **Activities.** Ask questions like: 'What do you do after school and at weekends?', 'Do you play any sports?', 'Do you have any other interests?', 'Do you have a best friend or a group of friends?', 'Are you in any clubs or teams?', 'Do you read or watch a lot of TV?', 'Do you take part in Internet chat rooms?' and 'Do you listen to music a lot?'.
- **Eating disorders.** Ask questions like: 'Do you feel comfortable with your eating habits?', 'Do you ever think about losing weight?', 'Do you ever eat in secret?', 'Have you ever made yourself throw up to lose weight?' and 'Do you use any diet pills or laxatives?'
- **Drugs.** Adolescents may be more willing to talk about their friends than themselves. Ask questions like: 'Do any of your friends smoke or drink?', 'How do you feel about this?', 'Have you ever tried?', 'Have you ever used other drugs?', 'Have you ever used needles?', 'How much do you smoke, drink or use drugs?' and 'How do you manage to pay for drugs?'.
- **Mental health and suicide.** Ask questions like: 'Do you ever feel so low that you want to hurt yourself?', 'Have you ever tried to hurt or kill yourself?', 'Have

you ever run away from home?', 'Have you ever cut yourself intentionally?' and 'Do you often feel bored?'.

- **Sex.** Ask questions like: 'Do any of your friends have boyfriends or girlfriends?', 'Have you ever kissed anyone?', 'Have you ever had sex?', 'How many partners have you had?', 'Has anyone ever touched you in a way you did not want to be touched?', 'Has anyone ever forced you to do something sexually that you did not want to do?', 'Do you use condoms or any other form of birth control?', 'Have you ever suffered from a sexually transmitted infection?', 'Have you ever been pregnant?' and 'Have you ever received money or drugs for sex?'.

Past and current medical problems

- **Chronic diseases.** Chronic diseases are relatively uncommon in adolescents, but ask about conditions such as diabetes, asthma, epilepsy, cystic fibrosis and arthritis. Some adolescents resent having to take time out for health checks and to engage with services, particularly after they have left home. Adolescents with chronic health problems often generally resent being ill and therefore being different from their friends, which may make them rebel against diagnoses such as asthma and diabetes.
- **Acne.** Acne is common and can cause significant psychological distress.

Medication

- **Regular medication.** Ask whether any medication is being taken regularly. Are there any adverse effects?
- **Oral contraceptive.** Are there any problems with forgetting to take the pill?
- **Psychotropic drugs.** Ask about antidepressants and other psychoactive medication.
- **Over-the-counter preparations.** Ask about any herbal and over-the-counter drugs.
- **Acne treatment.** If relevant, ask what has been tried and whether treatment has been effective.

Social history

- **Parents.** If appropriate, consider asking questions like: 'What do your parents do for a living?', 'What are they like?' and 'Are there any new people in the home environment?'.

Examination

General

- **General condition.** Is there evidence of malnutrition? Is there obesity?
- **Specific examination.** Physical examination may not always be necessary and will be guided by findings from the history.
- **Mental state.** Does the patient look depressed? Is speech normal? Do they maintain eye contact? Are there any obvious behavioural abnormalities?

Skin

- **Signs of self-harm.** Look for any obvious signs of self-harm, such as cuts on the forearms.
- **Needle marks.** Are there any needle marks, suggesting intravenous drug misuse?
- **Acne.** Is there facial acne? Are the back and/or chest affected? Is there any scarring?

Key references and further reading

1. Cohen E, MacKenzie RG, Yates GL. HEADSS, a psychological risk assessment instrument: implications for designing effective intervention programs for run-away youth. *J Adolesc Health* 1991;12:539–544.
2. Goldenring MJ, Cohen E. Getting into adolescent heads. *Contemp Pediatr* 1988;5:75–90.
3. Goldenring JM, Rosen D. Getting into adolescent heads: an essential update. *Contemp Paediatr* 2004;21:64.
4. Laski L. Women's, children's and adolescents' health. *BMJ* 2015;351:h4119.
5. World Health Organization (WHO). Adolescents: health risks and solutions. Fact sheet no. 345. May 2014. Available from: http://www.who.int/mediacentre/factsheets/fs345/en/ (last accessed 29 April 2016).

Self-harm in teenagers

Key thoughts

Practical points
- **Diagnosis and prognosis.** Self-harm is relatively common among teenagers. Determine the severity of any physical injury, establish risk factors for suicide and explore the extent of current support systems. Overdoses of paracetamol are common and will require urgent management before more detailed psychological assessment can be carried out.
- **Rapport.** The first consultation after self-harm is crucial for building rapport. Always give adolescents the choice to have a friend, relative or advocate with them during the assessment.
- **Further management.** Any decisions about future management should be based on a comprehensive psychiatric, psychological and social assessment following on from the initial consultation.

Forms of self-harm
- Self-cutting.
- Self-poisoning.
- Attempted suicide.

> **RED FLAGS**
>
> - Current suicidal thoughts
> - Previous suicide attempts
> - Detailed plans of how to carry out self-harm
> - Suicide note
> - Depression, anxiety, psychosis or other mental illness
> - Feeling of hopelessness
> - Poor social support
> - Family history of self-harm or suicide
> - Child in care

History

Ideas, concerns and expectations
- **Ideas.** How does the patient feel about self-harm?
- **Concerns.** Does the patient feel vulnerable? Is there a tendency towards self-blame? Are there any school worries or relationship problems? Young people are

The 10-Minute Clinical Assessment, Second Edition. Knut Schroeder.
© 2017 John Wiley & Sons, Ltd. Published 2017 by John Wiley & Sons, Ltd.

often concerned about confidentiality: assure them that this will be maintained, but stress that information may need to be passed on to other professionals if necessary for quality of care or if the patient or others are at risk.

- **Expectations.** What does the patient expect in terms of further management? Ask about their views in terms of future involvement of other support services, as this may help to plan management.

History of presenting complaint

- **Context.** Ask open questions to find out how self-harm fits into the context of the patient's life and the story behind individual episodes. Give plenty of time to allow them to describe their feelings and what happened to them in their own words. Ask for details about what exactly happened and at what times.
- **Communication.** Silences are often a very active time for patients, allowing them to collect their thoughts. Be empathetic, respectful and supportive throughout.
- **Emotional state.** Ask, 'How do you feel about self-harm?' to explore their feelings about and understanding of self-harm. Self-cutting is often used to relieve mental pain, anxiety, tension or anguish. Take any inability to describe feelings or precipitating factors seriously, as this may indicate an increased risk of suicide. Try to take a full account of any emotional distress associated with an episode of self-harm.
- **Motivation.** Reasons for self-harm may vary for a single individual and each episode needs to be treated in its own right.
- **Overdoses.** Ask about current or previous overdoses of prescription and non-prescription medicines. Get details concerning the amounts and strengths of any medications taken in overdose. Has the patient vomited?
- **Self-cutting.** Self-cutting is particularly difficult to identify and treat. Apparently normal teenagers may be cutting themselves, as it may help them deal with emotional suffering. Common objects used include razor blades, pins, needles, glass and scissors. Assess the need for analgesia.
- **Other factors.** Enquire about any personal, cultural, religious or other factors that you will need to consider when further assessing the adolescent.

Suicide risk and red flags

- **Frequency of self-harm.** Repeated acts of self-harm increase the risk of suicide.
- **Mental illness.** Ask about symptoms of depression (e.g. hopelessness, guilt, loss of appetite, tiredness) and anxiety.
- **Risk of suicide.** Ask about previous suicide attempts, any recent broken relationships, social isolation and drug dependence.
- **Screening for high risk of suicide.** Asking screening questions may identify a high risk of suicide and depression in adolescents who have overdosed:
  - 'Have you had problems for more than 1 month?'
  - 'Were you alone in the house when you overdosed?'
  - 'Did you plan the overdose for more than 3 hours?'

o 'Are you feeling hopeless about the future: that things will not get much better?'

o 'Were you feeling sad for most of the time before the overdose?'

Past and current medical problems

* **Significant illness.** Ask about chronic conditions that may be relevant, such as diabetes and asthma. Adolescents may find it difficult to come to terms with a diagnosis of chronic disease. Is there a history of eating disorder?

Medication

* **Prescribed drugs.** Ask about any prescribed drugs that might interact with substances taken in overdose.

Social history

* **Family.** What is the family situation? Is the adolescent known to social services or living in care? Do the parents themselves suffer from mental illness or addictions? How good is communication between family members? Are the parents very critical? Do the parents show emotional warmth?
* **Abuse.** Consider asking about any past or current abuse, including emotional, physical and sexual abuse.
* **Other services.** Ask whether there are past or current links with other health professionals or services, including child and adolescent psychiatry, health visitors, social workers and any school staff. Try to obtain additional information from significant others and any health professionals who are involved.

Alcohol and drugs

* **Alcohol.** Ask about average and recent alcohol intake. Was alcohol involved prior to this episode of self-harm?
* **Drugs.** Consider illicit substance misuse and obtain details about past and current consumption.

Examination

General

* **General state.** Does the adolescent seem confused or unwell? Assess airway, breathing and circulation (ABC) and responsiveness if the patient is unwell. Assume mental capacity unless there is evidence to the contrary.
* **Level of consciousness.** Assess level of consciousness (e.g. Glasgow Coma Scale, GCS).
* **Mental state.** Is there obvious severe distress? Is the adolescent actively suicidal? Is there unusual behaviour? Does the adolescent maintain eye contact? Is speech normal? Is there evidence of psychosis?

- **Diagnostic clues.** Look for diagnostic clues about the type of self-harm. Are there empty bottles of tablets?
- **Jaundice.** Jaundice may indicate liver failure due to recent paracetamol overdose.

Vital signs

- **Temperature.** This may be below normal if the patient has been exposed to a cold environment.
- **Pulse.** Tachycardia may indicate anxiety or impending shock in medication overdose.
- **Blood pressure.** Check for postural hypotension.
- **Respiratory rate.** This may be reduced in opioid overdose or raised in overdose of central stimulants.

Ensure physical safety

- **Injuries.** Assess the extent of any physical injuries. Has an overdose been taken?
- **Risk of suicide.** Is the patient actively suicidal?
- **Risk of incomplete assessment.** Is there a risk that the patient might leave before the assessment is completed and treatment is provided?

Neurology

- **Pupils.** Miosis may indicate opioid overdose.

Key references and further reading

1. Kingsbury S. PATHOS: a screening instrument for adolescent overdose: a research note. *J Child Psychol Psychiatry* 1996;37:609–611.
2. National Institute for Health and Care Excellence (NICE). Self-harm in over 8s: short-term management and prevention of recurrence. NICE guidelines [CG16]. July 2004. Available from: http://www.nice.org.uk/guidance/cg16 (last accessed 29 April 2016).
3. National Institute for Health and Care Excellence (NICE). Self-harm in over 8s: long-term management. NICE guidelines [CG133]. November 2011. Available from: http://www.nice.org.uk/guidance/cg133 (last accessed 29 April 2016).
4. Royal College of Psychiatrists. Better services for people who self-harm – quality standards for healthcare professionals. February 2006. Available from: http://www.rcpsych.ac.uk/pdf/self-harm%20quality%20standards.pdf (last accessed 29 April 2016).
5. Webb L. Deliberate self-harm in adolescence: a systematic review of psychological and psychosocial factors. *J Adv Nurs* 2002;38:235–244.

Eating disorders

Key thoughts

Practical points
- **Diagnosis.** Eating disorders are relatively common and can severely affect a patient's quality of life, as well as their general health. Differentiate mainly between anorexia nervosa, bulimia and binge-eating, and assess the risk of physical harm.

Types of eating disorders
- Anorexia nervosa.
- Bulimia.
- Binge-eating.

Important risk factors
- Female gender.
- Perfectionism.
- Early menarche.

Potential complications of anorexia nervosa
- Anaemia.
- Hypokalaemia.
- Hypotension.
- Cardiac failure.
- Hypoglycaemia.
- Osteoporosis.
- Infections.
- Acute renal failure.

RED FLAGS

- BMI <18 kg/m^2
- Speed of weight loss >0.5 kg/week, or losing >10% of body weight
- Obsessive feelings about body image and food
- Physical, emotional and sexual abuse
- Dysfunctional family and parental problems
- Bereavement and major life events
- Self-harm

The 10-Minute Clinical Assessment, Second Edition. Knut Schroeder.
© 2017 John Wiley & Sons, Ltd. Published 2017 by John Wiley & Sons, Ltd.

History

Ideas, concerns and expectations

- **Ideas.** Assess the patient's attitude to eating and explore associated feelings.
- **Concerns.** Young people with eating disorders often do not see them as a problem, and it is the people around them who voice their concern. In anorexia nervosa, there is a distorted body image. Children and young people with bulimia or binge-eating disorder feel out of control with regard to their eating patterns.
- **Expectations.** What is the main reason for consultation? What are the expectations with regard to the outcome of the consultation?

History of presenting complaint

- **Context.** Ask open questions about the presenting problem and how it fits into the context of the patient's life. How is their daily life affected? Key to effective assessment is engaging the patient, as young people with eating disorders will often be less concerned than everyone else.
- **Screening questions.** If you suspect an eating disorder, consider asking the following questions: 'Do you think you have an eating problem?' and 'Do you worry a lot about your weight or appearance?'.
- **Presenting patterns.** Common presentations include young women with low BMI, menstrual disturbance or amenorrhoea, repeated vomiting, gastrointestinal problems or poor growth, as well as those consulting with weight problems who are not in fact overweight. Common eating disorders include anorexia nervosa and bulimia, which feature a morbid preoccupation with body weight and shape. Many young people wait for a long time before consulting a health professional.
- **Ideas about body image.** Is there a dread of fatness, which presents as an intrusive and overvalued idea? Consider questions like, 'How much would you like to weigh?', 'How do you feel about your weight?', 'Are you happy with your body?' and 'Do you believe yourself to be fat when others say that you are too thin?'. Younger children may find it difficult to give an account of their body image or fear of gaining weight. Ask about any pride or sense of achievement derived from losing weight.
- **Views of others.** Consider asking, 'Is anyone else concerned about your body weight or exercising?' and 'Does it annoy you if people ask you about this?'. There is reason for concern if an adolescent feels distressed about being asked about food intake and weight. Has the young person become more secretive and withdrawn? Do they find excuses for not taking part in family meals? Vomitus stuck to the toilet bowl, the sudden disappearance of food from the kitchen and laxatives hidden in the bedroom (as noticed by the parents) all point towards bulimia.
- **Type of eating disorder.** In anorexia, there is an intense fear of gaining weight, even if the patient is underweight. The experience of body shape or weight is disturbed, and this affects self-image excessively. In bulimia nervosa, recurrent bouts of binge-eating alternate with inappropriate compensatory behaviour to

prevent weight gain, such as use of laxatives, vomiting or fasting. Young people who binge-eat consume large amounts of food even if they are not hungry.

- **Diet.** Is there a preoccupation with food and diet? Are there any ritualistic patterns? Does the patient eat alone or with others? Chaotic or distorted eating behaviour is common in anorexia nervosa and bulimia.
- **Exercise.** Ask about the type and amount of any exercise.
- **Weight loss.** Has any weight been lost? Over what period of time? What are the patient's previous and current weights? Weight loss in children is more serious than in adults. During the adolescent growth spurt, maintaining weight can indicate deterioration. In bulimia, weight is usually normal.
- **Binge-eating.** Ask about any episodes of binge-eating. Consider questions such as, 'Do you feel you might have lost control over how much you eat?' and 'Does food dominate your life?'. Is anything being used to counteract binging? Ask, 'Do you make yourself sick because you feel too full?' Also ask about excessive exercise, dietary restrictions and use of laxatives.
- **Constipation.** Constipation is common in malnutrition as a result of reduced food intake, but may also be caused by slowed gastrointestinal motility. Ask about use of laxatives or purgatives.
- **Periods.** Amenorrhoea and other period disorders are common with eating disorders, but these are unreliable symptoms around the menarche.
- **Other physical symptoms.** Dry skin and hair, dizziness and feeling the cold are common in anorexia nervosa. Is there evidence of self-harm?
- **Mental health.** Ask about mood, withdrawal from leisure activities and low energy levels. Does the patient perform compulsive rituals?
- **Life events.** Have there been any recent significant life events, particularly around the start of the eating problems (e.g. bereavement, parental divorce, bullying at school, major illness)?
- **Other services.** Has the patient ever been seen by a mental health professional or in a specialist eating-disorders clinic?

Past and current medical problems

- **Cardiac problems.** Cardiac function may be compromised in patients with anorexia nervosa.
- **Diabetes mellitus.** Diabetic patients with anorexia will need very careful monitoring. About 1 in 10 girls with diabetes may also have an eating disorder.
- **Hyperthyroidism.** This may present with cold intolerance, anxiety or sleeping difficulties.
- **Inflammatory bowel disease.** Ask about gastrointestinal symptoms, including nausea, vomiting, abdominal pain and diarrhoea.

Medication

- **Laxatives.** Ask about the use of laxatives and purgatives, both prescribed and over-the-counter.
- **Drugs affecting cardiac function.** Care needs to be taken when prescribing drugs that may affect cardiac function in young people with anorexia nervosa.

Social history
- **Family.** Does the mother or any of the siblings have an eating disorder or mental illness? Have parents been overprotective or abusive? How have they looked after the family?
- **School or work.** Are there any problems with school or work as a result of the eating problems?

Alcohol and drugs
- **Alcohol.** Ask for details of any alcohol consumption and consider the possibility of alcohol dependence.
- **Drugs.** Are illicit drugs being taken? Drug addiction will complicate management and will need fuller assessment.

Review of previous investigations
- **Full blood count.** Look for evidence of anaemia.
- **Liver function tests.** Look for hypoalbuminaemia.
- **Bone profile.** Are there any abnormalities? Osteoporosis is a complication of anorexia nervosa but will not usually cause abnormal blood tests.
- **Renal and liver function.** Look for metabolic consequences of starvation.
- **Thyroid function tests.** Exclude hyperthyroidism.

Examination

General
- **General condition.** Does the patient look well? Physical examination is often normal in bulimia.
- **Dehydration.** Check skin turgor and mucus membranes for signs of dehydration.
- **Circulation.** Blue and mottled peripheries and a capillary refill ≥ 1.5 seconds may indicate poor circulation, although these are fairly weak signs.
- **Hands.** Look for callous formation or abrasions on the back of the hand or fingers due to self-induced vomiting over long periods of time (Russel's sign).
- **Breasts.** These may be shrunken in anorexia nervosa.
- **Puberty and sexual development.** There may be pubertal delay or arrest.

Vital signs
- **Pulse.** A raised heart rate may occur with anxiety, dehydration and severe weight loss. Bradycardia is common in anorexia nervosa, often due to the effect of increased exercise.
- **Blood pressure.** Blood pressure may be low in anorexia nervosa. Consider checking for postural hypotension if there are dizziness symptoms.

Nutrition

- **Nutritional status.** Try to identify signs of malnutrition. Some adolescents with eating disorders resist weighing and clinical examination and may cover up their body.
- **Check weight and height.** The BMI (kg/m^2) can be misleading in children and adolescents. Use appropriate BMI centile charts to determine underweight. A BMI equal to or below the 2nd centile indicates serious underweight. Reduced height may indicate growth retardation or short stature. Compare with previous readings, if available, and plot on an appropriate children's growth chart (e.g. WHO Growth Standards, http://www.who.int/childgrowth/standards/en/).

Skin

- **Body hair.** Look for thinning hair or lanugo hair.
- **Skin.** Look for dry skin. The skin may appear yellow due to carotenaemia and/or pale due to anaemia.

Head and neck

- **Eyes.** Petechiae on the sclerae may be caused by vomiting.
- **Parotid glands.** Parotid gland swelling occurs in malnutrition.
- **Teeth.** Dental caries may be caused by increased acid exposure due to repeated vomiting.

Key references and further reading
1. Luck A, Morgan JF, Reid F et al. The SCOFF questionnaire and clinical interview for eating disorders in general practice: comparative study. *BMJ* 2002;325:755–756.
2. National Institute for Health and Care Excellence (NICE). Eating disorders in over 8s: management. Nice guidelines [CG9]. January 2004. Available from: http://www.nice.org.uk/guidance/cg9 (last accessed 29 April 2016).
3. Nicholls D, Viner R. ABC of adolescence: eating disorders and weight problems. *BMJ* 2005;330:950.

Autism-spectrum disorder

Key thoughts

Practical points
- **Diagnosis and prognosis.** It is important to recognise an autism-spectrum disorder early in order to allow effective management. Early diagnosis will help avoid school problems and may help prevent depression as the child gets older.
- **Problems.** Find out what are the main problems in the child's life and in the lives of their parents, so that imaginative solutions can be explored.

Differential diagnosis
- Autism-spectrum disorder.
- Asperger's syndrome.
- Depression.
- Obsessive–compulsive disorder.
- Epilepsy.
- Attention-deficit hyperactivity disorder.
- Learning disability.
- Deafness.
- Emotional problems.

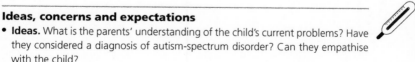

> **RED FLAGS**
>
> - Communication problems
> - Social problems
> - Behavioural problems
> - Developmental delay
> - Poor speech development
> - Any loss of social or language skills
> - Lack of pretend play
> - Little or no imagination

History

Ideas, concerns and expectations
- **Ideas.** What is the parents' understanding of the child's current problems? Have they considered a diagnosis of autism-spectrum disorder? Can they empathise with the child?

The 10-Minute Clinical Assessment, Second Edition. Knut Schroeder.
© 2017 John Wiley & Sons, Ltd. Published 2017 by John Wiley & Sons, Ltd.

- **Concerns.** Difficulty forming and maintaining relationships is often one of the major concerns of affected children and their parents.
- **Expectations.** Many parents of autistic children are desperate for a 'cure' for their child. Why is the child presenting now?

History of presenting complaint

- **Context.** Ask open questions about how problems started and how they fit into the context of the child's and the parents' lives.
- **Quality of life.** How is day-to-day life affected? What are the key problems?
- **Onset.** The typical age at which parents become concerned is around 18 months, but it can be much later.
- **Communication problems.** Children and adults with autism find it difficult to make sense of the world around them and to join in with everyday social interaction. The three main areas of difficulty include social interaction, social communication and imagination. Common problems include language delay, appearance of deafness, poor verbal communication and lack of response to verbal cues.
- **Social interaction.** Does the child appear indifferent to other people – especially other children? Do they ever initiate contact with other children? Do their methods of interaction with others appear odd or repetitive, or do they engage in inappropriate behaviours without attention to the responses they might evoke? Poor eye contact and a lack of social smiling are common, as is preferring to play alone.
- **Social communication.** Does the child enjoy communicating with others? Does the child talk at others rather than communicate with them? Autistic children often find it difficult to appreciate feelings or thoughts in others.
- **Imagination.** Children with autism struggle with playing imaginatively with toys or other objects and may instead focus on trivial or minor things around them.
- **Routines.** Autistic children often feel uncomfortable without routines and resist any changes to their routines. Repetitive behaviour patterns are characteristic.
- **Behaviour.** Tantrums, a lack of interest in things and unusual attachment to certain toys are common. Movement patterns may be odd, and resistance to change is common.
- **Coordination.** Are there any problems with handwriting or the use of cutlery?
- **Toddlers.** Does the child like being swung or bounced on a knee? Does the child enjoy imaginative play, such as 'peek-a-boo', hide-and-seek and 'pretend' games? Does the child come up and show the parents any objects?

Past and current medical problems

- **Significant past illnesses.** Ask about other significant illnesses in the past, particularly mental health problems.
- **Development.** Did the child reach developmental milestones at the right times?
- **Specialist input.** Have any specialist services been involved in the diagnosis and management of autism?

Family history

* **Autism.** Does autism run in the family?

Social history

* **Home.** Ask for details about the home situation and other members of the household. How are the family dynamics affected by the child's problems?
* **Pre-school and school.** How is pre-school or school performance affected? Are there any problems at school? Ask about classroom expectations, coping with change and support from peers.

Examination

General

* **Eye contact.** Does the child make eye contact? How does the child interact with the parents?
* **Physical problems.** Physical examination is usually normal in autistic children.

Response in toddlers

* **Pointing.** Does the child respond if you point at an object in the room and name it?
* **Imaginative play.** Using toys, does the child engage in imaginative play, such as pretending to eat or drink?
* **Language.** Ask a question like, 'Where is the door?' – does the child respond?
* **Building.** Can the child build a brick tower?

Key references and further reading

1. Baumer JH. Autism spectrum disorders, SIGN. *Arch Dis Child Educ Pract Ed* 2008;93:163–166.
2. Dover CJ, Le Couteur A. How to diagnose autism. *Arch Dis Child* 2007;92:540–545.
3. National Autistic Society. www.nas.org.uk.
4. National Institute for Health and Care Excellence (NICE). Autism in under 19s: recognition, referral and diagnosis. NICE guidelines [CG128]. September 2011. Available from: http://www.nice.org.uk/guidance/cg128 (last accessed 29 April 2016).

Cardiovascular

Chest pain

Key thoughts

Practical points

- **Diagnosis.** Chest pain is common and may indicate serious illness. Clinical signs can be unreliable, and more than one cause may coexist. Always consider the possibility of myocardial infarction, pulmonary embolism, dissecting aneurysm or pericarditis.
- **Risk factors.** Identify important risk factors for cardiac disease.
- **Prognosis.** The majority of chest pain seen in primary care is benign, but any acute chest pain not relieved by vasodilators within minutes needs to be regarded as a medical emergency. Myocardial infarction ('time is muscle'), pulmonary embolus, dissecting aneurysm and pericarditis can be life-threatening and will require immediate action. Any chronic, intermittent and stable chest pain is less likely to need urgent action.

Possible causes

- **Musculoskeletal.** Costochondritis, trauma.
- **Cardiovascular.** Ischaemic heart disease, aortic dissection, valvular disease.
- **Respiratory.** Pulmonary embolus, pneumothorax.
- **Gastrointestinal.** Gastrooesophageal reflux, oesophageal rupture.
- **Neurogenic.** Shingles.

Risk factors

- **Cardiac.** Smoking, hypercholesterolaemia, diabetes, hypertension, obesity, lack of exercise, family history, male gender, age.
- **Pulmonary embolism.** Recent surgery, immobilisation, deep venous thrombosis, pregnancy, trauma, obesity, malignancy, history of deep venous thrombosis or pulmonary embolism, oestrogen therapy.
- **Pneumothorax.** Tall stature, smoking, young male, chronic lung disease, Marfan syndrome, acquired immunodeficiency syndrome (AIDS), infection, drug use, trauma.
- **Aortic dissection.** Uncontrolled hypertension, atherosclerosis, Marfan syndrome, Ehlers–Danlos syndrome, valvular disease, coarctation of the aorta.

> **RED FLAGS**
>
> - Pain not relieved with nitrates
> - Pain on exercise
> - Nausea, vomiting and sweating

The 10-Minute Clinical Assessment, Second Edition. Knut Schroeder.
© 2017 John Wiley & Sons, Ltd. Published 2017 by John Wiley & Sons, Ltd.

- Severe pain and distress
- Pallor
- Tachycardia
- Tachypnoea
- Collapse
- Syncope

History

Ideas, concerns and expectations
- **Ideas.** What does the patient think is causing the pain? Many people with chest pain are afraid of wasting the doctor's or ambulance's time. They may not think or want to believe that chest pain may be due to a heart attack.
- **Concerns.** Undifferentiated and undiagnosed chest pain can cause great anxiety. Myocardial infarction can be very distressing, and fear of sudden death is common.
- **Expectations.** Common reasons for consultation are symptom relief, exclusion of serious disease and reassurance.

History of presenting complaint
- **Context.** Allow patients time to tell you about their chest pain in their own words.
- **Quality of life.** How is the quality of life being affected?
- **Onset, duration and progression.** What was the patient doing when the pain started? Chronic pain due to trauma or overuse is most likely to have a musculoskeletal cause. When was the first time the patient ever experienced this pain?
- **Severity.** The severity of cardiac pain can range from mild (e.g. silent infarct) to very severe. Acute onset of severe pain should always raise suspicions of myocardial infarction or pulmonary embolism. Any crescendo pain (increasing severity and/or frequency over recent weeks) will also need urgent action.
- **Type of pain.** Cardiac pain is often felt as a severe and pressing pain or bandlike chest tightness. Pleuritic pain tends to be worse on taking a deep breath. Musculoskeletal pain is often caused by injury or muscular strain, or is diagnosed by exclusion. Myocardial infarction may be painless ('silent infarct') in the elderly and in people with diabetes (diabetic neuropathy).
- **Location and radiation.** Cardiac pain tends to occur in the centre of the chest and may radiate to the left arm, shoulder and wrist, as well as the neck or jaw. Pancreatic and oesophageal pain often radiates to the back. Pain resulting from a pulmonary embolus may be felt centrally as tightness or as pleuritic chest pain closer to the chest wall. Pain in posterior myocardial infarction may radiate to the back, as may pain from a dissecting aortic aneurysm.
- **Character.** Cardiac chest pain is often described as squeezing, tight, burning or 'like a toothache', affecting an area rather than a point on the chest. In

contrast, pleuritic pain tends to be rather sharp and restricted to a smaller area. Patients with cardiac pain use the whole hand to locate the pain, rather than one finger.

- **Associated symptoms.** Shortness of breath, palpitations, syncope, nausea, vomiting and sweating in association with central chest tightness suggest myocardial ischaemia (angina, infarction). There may be feelings of strangulation or suffocation. Associated calf pain or tenderness indicates deep venous thrombosis and resulting pulmonary embolism. A blistery rash in association with a tingling pain suggests shingles as a cause for chest wall pain.
- **Exacerbating factors.** Pain worse on physical or emotional exertion may be cardiac or a result of pulmonary embolism. Angina is often worse after a large meal or when entering a cold environment. Pleuritic pain that is worse on breathing may be caused by pulmonary embolus or other conditions affecting the pleura. Oesophageal pain is usually worse after taking food. Psychogenic chest pain worsens during periods of anxiety or stress.
- **Relieving factors.** Angina pain usually improves with nitrates or rest. Pericardial pain is often relieved by leaning forward.
- **Risk factors for coronary heart disease.** Ask about hypertension, angina, diabetes, hyperlipidaemia and family or past history of cardiovascular disease, as well as lifestyle factors such as smoking, obesity, lack of exercise, poor diet and stress.
- **Mental health.** Anxiety and panic may cause chest pain or palpitations.
- **Contraindications for thrombolysis.** If there is a possibility of myocardial infarction and you may need to give thrombolysis yourself (e.g. in remote areas), check whether there are any contraindications to thrombolysis, such as recent haemorrhage/trauma/surgery, bleeding diatheses, aortic dissection, a history of cerebrovascular disease or severe hypertension.

Past and current medical problems

- **Cardiac history.** Ask about previous angina and myocardial infarction. Has the patient had any cardiac operations (e.g. stent or bypass surgery)? Some patients suffer from chronic chest wall pain without ischaemia after sternotomy.
- **Pulmonary disease.** Is there any history of pulmonary disease?
- **Systemic disease.** Check for a history of systemic disease (e.g. malignancy).

Medication

- **Analgesics.** Have any drugs been taken to treat the pain? Have they been effective? Are there any adverse effects?
- **Cardiac drugs.** Ask about any drugs that are currently being taken for treatment or prevention of cardiovascular disease (e.g. aspirin, nitrates, antihypertensives, digoxin, statins).
- **Oral contraceptive pill.** There is an increased risk of deep venous thrombosis and pulmonary embolus when taking the oral contraceptive pill, particularly in older or obese women who smoke.

- **Other medication.** List all other medication taken, including over-the-counter preparations.

Allergies
- **Aspirin.** Any allergy to aspirin is relevant, as this may need to be given as part of the early treatment of myocardial infarction.

Family history
- **Cardiovascular disease.** Ask in particular about a family history of heart disease.

Social history
- **Home.** If the chest pain is chronic, how has home life been affected? Are there any activities that the patient cannot do now due to the symptoms?
- **Work.** Has work been affected? Is the patient a heavy goods vehicle driver? If there is possible underlying heart disease, the patient may need to be advised to inform the relevant driving authorities.
- **Lifestyle.** Ask for details about dietary habits and exercise.

Alcohol, smoking and recreational drugs
- **Alcohol.** Check past and present alcohol consumption.
- **Smoking.** Record past and current smoking status and calculate the number of pack years (= (number of cigarettes smoked per day × number of years smoked)/20).
- **Drugs.** Cocaine and crack cocaine use may precipitate myocardial ischaemia.

Review of previous investigations
- **Full blood count.** Anaemia can exacerbate angina. A raised white cell count suggests possible infection.
- **Inflammatory markers.** Raised plasma viscosity or C-reactive protein (CRP) may suggest infection, severe inflammation or underlying malignancy.
- **Urea and electrolytes.** Check results for renal function as a baseline before starting any relevant cardiac or other medication.
- **Thyroid function.** Hyperthyroidism can cause anxiety and may worsen angina.
- **Creatine kinase or troponin.** Troponin is available as a near-patient test. Abnormalities may suggest myocardial damage.
- **Fasting lipids and glucose.** Look out for evidence of hypercholesterolaemia and diabetes.
- **Electrocardiogram (ECG).** Look out for any previous ECGs for comparison, and for any prior cardiac investigations. A resting ECG is normal in most people with angina.
- **Chest X-ray.** Are there any signs of underlying heart or lung disease on previous chest X-rays?
- **Cardiac investigations.** Has the patient ever undergone cardiac investigation, such as exercise testing, echocardiogram or angiography?

Examination

General
- **General condition.** Is the patient unwell, confused or anxious? Is the patient in pain or distress? Look for pallor and sweating, which may indicate severe underlying disease, such as myocardial infarction or pulmonary embolus.
- **Breathing.** Is there shortness of breath?

Vital signs
- **Temperature.** A raised temperature suggests infection.
- **Pulse.** Tachycardia may suggest infection, anxiety, myocardial infarction or pulmonary infection. Bradycardia may be caused by heart block due to myocardial infarction or other serious underlying disease.
- **Blood pressure.** Check blood pressure in both arms. High blood pressure may be caused by anxiety or hypertension. Hypotension or postural hypotension may be caused by cardiac disease and can be a sign of serious illness.
- **Respiratory rate.** A respiratory rate of <10 or >29 breaths per minute suggests serious disease.

Head and neck
- **Jugular venous pressure (JVP).** A raised JVP may be found in heart failure, pulmonary embolism or cardiac tamponade, or, if fixed, may be caused by superior vena cava obstruction.
- **Trachea.** Check for signs of tracheal deviation.
- **Cornea.** Look for a corneal arcus, which may suggest hyperlipidaemia.

Upper limbs
- **Fingers.** Check for finger clubbing, which may indicate underlying lung disease. Are there any tar stains from smoking?

Chest
- **Chest wall.** Feel for any chest wall tenderness, which may be caused by trauma but also occurs in myocardial infarction. Look for scars of previous thoracotomy (e.g. coronary artery bypass grafting, CABG).
- **Heart.** Check for signs of heart failure and dysrhythmia. Are there any murmurs or added sounds suggesting valvular disease? Aortic stenosis may lead to myocardial ischaemia. Listen for a pericardial rub. Gallop rhythm may be caused by heart failure.
- **Lungs.** Bilateral crackles suggest heart failure. Check for pleural effusions. Reduced chest expansion with hyperresonant percussion and absent or quiet breath sounds indicates pneumothorax. A pleural rub may be found in pulmonary embolism. Stony dullness with bronchial breathing or reduced breath sounds suggests pneumonia.

Abdomen
- **Palpation.** Check for any masses or tenderness, which may suggest intraabdominal pathology.

Lower limbs
- **Swelling.** Look for signs of venous thrombosis.

Key references and further reading

1. Cayley WE Jr. Diagnosing the cause of chest pain. *Am Fam Physician* 2005;72:2012–2021.
2. Chun AA, McGee SR. Bedside diagnosis of coronary artery disease: a systematic review. *Am J Med* 2004;117:334–343.
3. Flook N, Unge P, Agréus L et al. Approach to managing undiagnosed chest pain: could gastroesophageal reflux disease be the cause? *Can Fam Physician* 2007;53:261–266.
4. Hani MA, Keller H, Vandenesch J et al. Different from what the textbooks say: how GPs diagnose coronary heart disease. *Fam Pract* 2007;24:622–627.
5. National Institute for Health and Care Excellence (NICE). Chest pain of recent onset: assessment and diagnosis. NICE guidelines [CG95]. March 2010. Available from: http://www.nice.org.uk/guidance/cg95 (last accessed 29 April 2016).
6. Scottish Intercollegiate Guidelines Network (SIGN). Managing stable angina. Clinical guideline 96. February 2007. Available from: http://www.sign.ac.uk/pdf/sign96.pdf (last accessed 29 April 2016).
7. Swap CJ, Nagurney JT. Value and limitations of chest pain history in the evaluation of patients with suspected acute coronary syndrome. *JAMA* 2005;294:2623–2629.

Palpitations

Key thoughts

Practical points

- **Diagnosis.** 'Palpitations' can mean different things – find out what exactly is being talked about (usually, an awareness of faster and/or irregular heart-beating). The most common cause of palpitations is anxiety, but less common cardiac and other causes need to be excluded. Atrial fibrillation is an important independent risk factor for stroke.
- **Prognosis.** Palpitations are not associated with serious underlying disease in the majority of cases.
- **Reassurance.** Often, physical examination is not particularly helpful in establishing the diagnosis, but a thorough assessment can be invaluable in reassuring patients and showing that you take their symptoms seriously.

Differential diagnosis

- Extrasystoles.
- Sinus arrhythmia.
- Sinus tachycardia.
- Atrial fibrillation.
- Atrial flutter.
- Paroxysmal supraventricular tachycardia.
- Ventricular tachycardia.

Important risk factors

- Anxiety.
- Any risk factors for cardiovascular disease, particularly obesity.
- Family history of syncope, arrhythmia or sudden death.
- Hyperthyroidism.

RED FLAGS

- Previous myocardial infarction
- Abnormal ECG
- Chest pain
- Shortness of breath
- Syncope
- Signs of heart failure
- Heart rate over 140 beats per minute
- Abnormal physical examination

The 10-Minute Clinical Assessment, Second Edition. Knut Schroeder.
© 2017 John Wiley & Sons, Ltd. Published 2017 by John Wiley & Sons, Ltd.

History

Ideas, concerns and expectations
- **Ideas.** Can the patient offer a possible explanation for the palpitations?
- **Concerns.** Palpitations can be very worrying and will often be perceived as life-threatening. Patients may suspect a serious underlying condition, and such anxieties may exacerbate the symptoms.
- **Expectations.** A common reason for consultation is the need for symptom relief and reassurance. Patients may also expect urgent or immediate specialist referral or admission in severe cases, which may or may not be indicated.

History of presenting complaint
- **Context.** Allow patients time to tell you about their palpitations in their own words.
- **Quality of life.** How do the palpitations affect activities of daily living and quality of life?
- **Description of symptoms.** Palpitations may present as a subjective sensation of irregular, rapid or particularly noticeable and forceful heart beats. Feelings of anxiety may present as palpitations, as may musculoskeletal problems. Ask patients to try and tap out the perceived heart rhythm they are experiencing. Rarely, carotid bruits or tinnitus may be felt as palpitations. Older people are at higher risk of developing paroxysmal or persistent atrial fibrillation.
- **Onset and frequency.** When did the patient first notice the palpitations? How often do attacks occur? Sudden onset and cessation of symptoms suggests a true tachyarrhythmia.
- **Associated symptoms.** Underlying heart disease is more likely if there is associated chest pain, shortness of breath, fainting, nausea or sweating, and if palpitations wake the patient from sleep. Ask about dizziness and syncope.
- **Symptoms of anxiety.** Anxiety and depression may cause palpitations. Beta blockers and tricyclic antidepressants may be used for the treatment of anxiety or depression and may affect the heart rate.
- **Precipitating factors.** Does stress precipitate or exacerbate symptoms? Paroxysmal supraventricular tachycardia may occur suddenly ('switch on/switch off') without warning, whereas palpitations in association with atrial fibrillation may be present continuously. Sinus tachycardia usually occurs during physical exertion or emotional stress ('adrenergic'). Symptoms at rest, after exercise or after food are often benign 'vagal' palpitations.
- **Relieving factors.** Supraventricular tachycardia may stop with activities stimulating the vagal system, such as breath-holding, swallowing cold water, stooping and vomiting.
- **Lifestyle factors.** Ask about any recreational drugs, excessive alcohol intake, caffeine consumption and the use of slimming pills.

Past and current medical problems
- **Heart disease.** A personal history of heart disease makes a cardiac cause of the symptoms more likely. Also ask about risk factors for cardiovascular disease, such as smoking, hypertension, diabetes and hyperlipidaemia.

Medication

- **Antidepressants.** Antidepressants (e.g. selective serotonin reuptake inhibitors (SSRIs), tricyclics) commonly cause palpitations.
- **Antiarrhythmics.** Antiarrhythmics also have the potential to induce arrhythmias.
- **Arrhythmogenic drugs.** Calcium channel blockers, beta 2 agonists and nitrates may all cause palpitations.
- **Sedatives.** Anxiety and palpitations may result from withdrawal of sedatives, such as benzodiazepines.

Family history

- **Heart disease.** Check whether there is a family history of arrhythmia, sudden death or syncope, or any other form of heart disease. Also ask about a family history of risk factors for cardiovascular disease.

Social history

- **Home.** How has home life been affected? Some people develop a fear of leaving the house, resulting in social isolation.
- **Work.** Has work been affected?

Alcohol, smoking and recreational drugs

- **Alcohol.** Alcohol misuse may cause palpitations through direct toxic effects, anxiety or the development of alcoholic cardiomyopathy.
- **Smoking.** Record past and current smoking status and calculate the number of pack years (= (number of cigarettes smoked per day × number of years smoked)/20).
- **Recreational drugs.** In young people, ask about the use of illicit drugs, such as amphetamines, cocaine and ecstasy.

Review of previous investigations

- **Full blood count.** Anaemia may cause shortness of breath and sinus tachycardia.
- **Urea and electrolytes.** Electrolyte disturbances may cause or aggravate arrhythmias.
- **Thyroid-stimulating hormone (TSH).** Hyperthyroidism may cause atrial fibrillation.
- **ECG.** Look for arrhythmia and evidence of ischaemic heart disease. In patients on antiarrhythmics, ventricular tachycardia may be 'slow'.
- **24-hour ECG.** This can be useful for the detection of intermittent arrhythmias.

Examination

General

- **General condition.** Does the patient look unwell, anxious or depressed?
- **Signs of hyperthyroidism.** Look for exophthalmos, as well as warm and sweaty hands. A fine tremor may be noticed in the outstretched hands.

Vital signs

- **Pulse.** Feel the pulse for at least 30 seconds to increase the chance of detecting extrasystoles. Consider sinus tachycardia if there is a regular pulse of 100–140 beats per minute. In ventricular tachycardia, the rate may be much higher, at up to 220 beats per minute. Atrial flutter with 2 : 1 block usually has a rate around 150 beats per minute. Paroxysmal supraventricular tachycardia typically presents with rates of over 160 beats per minute. An irregularly irregular pulse indicates atrial fibrillation. Distinguish between fast and normal rates of atrial fibrillation.
- **Blood pressure.** Very high blood pressure may lead to a forceful heart beat, which may be felt by the patient.
- **Respiratory rate.** Hyperventilation may indicate anxiety.

Chest

- **Heart.** Check for a laterally displaced apex beat and feel for a parasternal heave. Confirm the heart rate and rhythm by auscultation. In atrial fibrillation, not all heart beats may be transmitted to the radial pulse, and fast atrial fibrillation can easily go undiagnosed. Murmurs may suggest structural heart disease.
- **Lungs.** Check for basal crackles indicating heart failure.

Legs

- **Oedema.** Check for peripheral oedema, which may occur as a result of cardio-vascular compromise.

Key references and further reading

1. Barsky AJ. Palpitations, arrhythmias, and awareness of cardiac activity. *Ann Intern Med* 2001;134:832–837.
2. Leitz N, Khawaja Z, Been M. Lesson of the week: slow ventricular tachycardia. *BMJ* 2008;337:a1955.
3. National Institute for Health and Care Excellence (NICE). Atrial fibrillation. NICE guidelines [CG180]. June 2014. Available from: http://www.nice.org.uk/guidance/cg180 (last accessed 29 April 2016).
4. Summerton N, Mann S, Rigby A et al. New-onset palpitations in general practice: assessing the discriminant value of items within the clinical history. *Fam Pract* 2001;18:383–392.

Cardiovascular risk assessment

Key thoughts

Challenges in assessment
- **Management.** Risk assessment tools estimating absolute coronary heart disease (CHD) or cardiovascular disease (CVD) risk are used to identify people at high risk for primary prevention. These tools help with making decisions as to whether lifestyle approaches or medications such as lipid-lowering drugs (e.g. statins) should be used.
- **Patient views.** Take account of patient preferences and needs in the decision-making process.

Risk factors used in the calculation of CHD and CVD risk
- Systolic blood pressure.
- Diabetic status.
- Smoking status.
- Gender.
- Age.
- Ratio of total cholesterol to high-density lipoprotein.
- Left-ventricular hypertrophy.

Groups of people in whom the use of charts is inappropriate (i.e. already high risk)
- Diabetes mellitus.
- Familial hyperlipidaemia.
- Pre-existing CVD.
- Chronic renal failure.
- Established hypertension and diabetes with target organ damage.
- Blood pressure persistently ≥160/100 mmHg.

Situations in which risk-assessment tools are likely to underestimate risk
- People from high-risk ethnic groups.
- Family history of premature CVD.
- Patients with impaired fasting glucose (6.1–6.9 mmol/l) who are not yet diabetic.
- Raised triglycerides.
- Women with premature menopause.
- Ex-smokers (classify ex-smokers as 'current smokers' for 5 years after quitting).
- Severe obesity (body mass index (BMI) >40 kg/m^2).

The 10-Minute Clinical Assessment, Second Edition. Knut Schroeder.
© 2017 John Wiley & Sons, Ltd. Published 2017 by John Wiley & Sons, Ltd.

Selected risk assessment tools
- **QRISK-2.** Based on the UK general practice population (www.qrisk.org).
- **ETHRISK.** Used in UK ethnic groups (http://www.epi.bris.ac.uk/CVDethrisk/CHD_CVD_form.html).

RED FLAGS

- 10-year CHD risk >15%
- Combined CHD and CVD risk of >10%

History

Ideas, concerns and expectations
- **Ideas.** How is the patient's own personal risk perceived? What is the patient's attitude to risk – are they a risk-taker? How does the patient feel about taking tablets for the rest of their life to try and prevent a cardiovascular event?
- **Concerns.** Are there fears about developing a heart attack or a stroke in the future? A positive family history or the presence of risk factors often gives rise to concerns.
- **Expectations.** Why has the patient come to see you? Reading a relevant newspaper article or knowing someone of the same age who has just had a cardiovascular event is a common reason for consultation.

History of presenting complaint
- **Symptoms.** Ask about any cardiovascular symptoms, such as chest pain, shortness of breath on exertion, nocturnal cough, leg swelling and intermittent claudication, as well as facial or limb weakness. Erectile dysfunction can be a presenting feature of cardiovascular disease.
- **Smoking.** Consider lifetime exposure to tobacco smoke and not just smoking status at the time of assessment. Record past and current smoking status and calculate the number of pack years (= (number of cigarettes smoked per day × number of years smoked)/20). Has smoking-cessation advice been offered? Categorise those who have given up smoking within the past 5 years as 'current smokers' for the purpose of using the charts.
- **Diabetes.** This is a common, important and modifiable risk factor. When was diabetes first diagnosed? The treatment goal should be normalisation of blood glucose levels.
- **Family history of CHD.** If a male first-degree relative aged <55 years or a female first-degree relative aged >65 years has died prematurely from CHD, this increases the risk by a factor of about 1.5.
- **High-risk ethnic group.** In people from the Indian subcontinent and those from Afro-Caribbean backgrounds, assume that the risk is 1.4–1.5 times higher than that predicted from the charts. Consider using a different calculator, such as ETHRISK.

- **Treated hypertension.** Unless pre-treatment levels are available, assume that CVD risk is higher than expected based on current levels of blood pressure.
- **Diet.** People on simvastatin should avoid grapefruit juice, because this can increase plasma concentration. Is the patient eating a healthy and balanced diet?
- **Obesity.** Obesity is an independent risk factor for CVD.
- **Exercise.** Regular aerobic exercise has an important effect on reducing the risk of morbidity and mortality from cardiovascular causes.
- **Alcohol.** Mild to moderate alcohol consumption reduces the risk of CVD, but drinking more than two units of alcohol per day increases the risk of death from cancer and liver cirrhosis.
- **Renal impairment.** Impaired renal function is an important risk factor, particularly in those with CVD and diabetes.

Past and current medical problems
- **CVD.** Ask about previous myocardial infarction, transient ischaemic attack and stroke.
- **Diabetes.** Is the patient known to be diabetic or is there evidence of impaired glucose tolerance?
- **Hyperlipidaemia.** Have lipids been raised in the past?
- **Liver problems.** Statins are contraindicated in active liver disease.
- **Hypothyroidism.** Hypothyroidism can lead to increased lipid levels. It is therefore important to manage hypothyroidism adequately before starting treatment with a statin.
- **Pregnancy.** Pregnancy is a contraindication for treatment with statins, and adequate contraception needs to be provided during treatment and for 1 month afterwards.
- **Porphyria.** Statins should be avoided in porphyria (which is rare), although rosuvastatin is thought to be safe.

Medication
- **Statins.** Has the patient taken statins in the past? Were there any problems?
- **Macrolide antibiotics.** Concomitant use of macrolide antibiotics such as erythromycin or clarithromycin should be avoided because of the risk of myopathy. If they need to be given, statins may need to be stopped temporarily.
- **Other interactions.** Statins can interact with a long list of drugs, including antifungals and warfarin.

Family history
- **Chronic disease.** Ask about a family history of hypertension, heart disease, diabetes and hyperlipidaemia, as these may affect risk calculation.

Alcohol, smoking and recreational drugs
- **Alcohol.** Statins need to be used with caution in people with a high alcohol intake.

Review of previous investigations

- **Renal function.** Check estimated glomerular filtration and electrolytes.
- **Liver function tests.** These should be carried out before and within 1–3 months of starting treatment and then at intervals of 6 months for 1 year, unless there are signs of hepatotoxicity, in which case they should be carried out sooner. Treatment should be discontinued if transaminases rise to and persist at three times the upper limit.
- **Lipid profile.** Look for previous cholesterol levels.
- **ECG.** Look for evidence of pre-existing cardiac disease on any previously taken ECG. Left-ventricular hypertrophy is a risk factor for cardiovascular events.

Examination

General

- Weight and height. Calculate BMI.

Vital signs

- **Pulse.** Check for evidence of atrial fibrillation.
- **Blood pressure.** Check for hypertension.

Chest

- **Apex beat.** Check for force and lateral displacement (hypertension, heart failure).
- **Heart sounds.** Check for any signs of valvular heart disease and confirm the peripheral pulse rate.

Bedside tests

- **Glucose.** Check blood glucose concentration using glucose stick to screen for diabetes.
- **Urine dipstick.** Check for proteinuria (renal disease).

Key references and further reading

1. British National Formulary. www.bnf.org.
2. Hippisley-Cox J, Coupland D, Vinogradova Y et al. Predicting cardiovascular risk in England and Wales: prospective derivation and validation of QRISK2. *BMJ* 2008;336:a332.
3. JBS-2: Joint British Societies' guidelines on prevention of cardiovascular disease in clinical practice. *Heart* 2005;91(Suppl. 5):v1–v52.
4. National Institute for Health and Care Excellence (NICE). Cardiovascular disease: risk assessment and reduction, including lipid modification. NICE guidelines [CG181]. July 2014. Available from: http://www.nice.org.uk/guidance/cg181 (last accessed 29 April 2016).
5. National Institute for Health and Care Excellence (NICE). CVD risk assessment and management. Clinical Knowledge Summaries. 2014. Available from:

http://cks.nice.org.uk/cvd-risk-assessment-and-management (last accessed 29 April 2016).

6. Scottish Intercollegiate Guidelines Network (SIGN). Risk estimation and the prevention of cardiovascular disease. Clinical guideline 97. February 2007. Available from: http://www.sign.ac.uk/pdf/sign97.pdf (last accessed 29 April 2016).

Hypertension

Key thoughts

Practical points
- **Diagnosis.** In most cases, persistently raised blood pressure is the result of essential hypertension. Rarely, consider secondary hypertension in young people if there are additional symptoms and in treatment resistance.
- **Prognosis.** Identify additional risk factors for CVD.

Differential diagnosis
- 'White-coat' hypertension.
- Essential hypertension.
- Pre-eclampsia.
- Rarely, renovascular disease, renoparenchymal disease, hyperaldosteronism, Cushing's syndrome, pheochromocytoma.

Risk factors

- Diabetes.
- Hyperlipidaemia.
- Established CVD.
- Smoking.
- Lack of exercise.
- Obesity.
- Age.
- Alcohol.
- Drugs, such as nonsteroidal anti-inflammatory drugs (NSAIDs) or steroids.
- Excessive stress.
- Pregnancy.
- Combined oral contraceptive pill.

RED FLAGS

- Features suggesting a secondary cause
- Accelerated hypertension (blood pressure >180/110 mmHg with signs of papilloedema and/or retinal haemorrhage)
- Proteinuria
- Visual symptoms (e.g. pituitary tumour)
- Lack of response to treatment
- Age <30 years

The 10-Minute Clinical Assessment, Second Edition. Knut Schroeder.
© 2017 John Wiley & Sons, Ltd. Published 2017 by John Wiley & Sons, Ltd.

History

Ideas, concerns and expectations
- **Ideas.** Many people are unaware of the risks of hypertension and see raised blood pressure as part of the normal ageing process. What are the patient's treatment preferences?
- **Concerns.** Worries about having a stroke or heart attack are common and may themselves raise blood pressure.
- **Expectations.** Opportunistic findings of high blood pressure at routine health checks or through home blood-pressure measurements commonly lead to a consultation.

History of presenting complaint
- **Blood-pressure readings.** Check previous blood-pressure readings and look for trends. Routine use of automated ambulatory blood pressure-monitoring or home-monitoring devices is not currently recommended in primary care.
- **Reasons for temporary rise of blood pressure.** Consider pain, anxiety, alcohol binge, white-coat hypertension and improper blood pressure measurement.
- **Risk factors for CVD.** Consider other risk factors for CVD, particularly smoking, diabetes, hyperlipidaemia, a positive family history and alcohol misuse. Calculate risk using one of the standard risk assessment tools. Assessment of overall risk is important, as this will affect the level of blood pressure at which to start treatment.
- **Cardiac symptoms.** Ask about symptoms of cardiovascular or cerebrovascular disease, including chest pain, shortness of breath, leg pain, intermittent dizziness, memory loss, slurred speech, episodic one-sided limb weakness and loss of vision.
- **Issues relevant to choice of drugs in antihypertensive therapy.** Thiazides are particularly indicated in the elderly or in Afro-Caribbean patients. If there is a history of angina or myocardial infarction, then a beta blocker should be considered. Heart failure, left-ventricular dysfunction or diabetic nephropathy calls for the use of an angiotensin-converting enzyme (ACE) inhibitor. Those with persistent dry cough due to ACE inhibitors may need an angiotensin II receptor antagonist instead. Calcium channel blockers are valuable in older people in whom a low-dose thiazide diuretic is contraindicated or not tolerated and in patients of African or Caribbean descent. Alpha blockers are commonly used in treatment-resistant hypertension and prostatism.
- **Contraindications for antihypertensive therapy.** Asthma, heart block and severe peripheral vascular disease are contraindications for treatment with beta adrenoceptor blockers. ACE inhibitors should not be used in renal artery stenosis and pregnancy. Thiazide diuretics can exacerbate gout. Rate-limiting calcium channel blockers should not be used in heart failure or heart block. Contraindications for alpha blockers are urinary incontinence and postural hypotension.
- **Lifestyle.** Ask about lifestyle, including smoking, exercise, alcohol, diet and salt intake. Has lifestyle advice been given?

- **Symptoms of severe hypertension.** Ask about any symptoms of severe hypertension, such as headaches, dizziness, chest pain, vertigo, malaise, visual problems, dyspnoea, claudication, sweating and tremors.
- **Secondary hypertension.** Consider secondary hypertension if there is raised blood pressure before the age of 30, a documented sudden onset or worsening of high blood pressure in middle age, malignant hypertension with diastolic blood pressure over 130 mmHg and end-organ damage, high blood pressure resistant to treatment with three antihypertensive agents at appropriate doses or renal impairment of unknown cause. Tetany, polyuria, muscle weakness and hypokalaemia may suggest hyperaldosteronism (Conn's syndrome). Possible signs of a rare pheochromocytoma include headache, palpitations, pallor and excessive sweating.

Past and current medical problems

- **Significant past illnesses.** Ask about previous myocardial infarction, angina, stroke, transient ischaemic attack, dementia, left-ventricular hypertrophy, heart failure, coronary angioplasty or bypass surgery, diabetes and renal disease.

Medication

- **Antihypertensives.** Does the patient already take blood pressure-lowering medication? Consider lack of adherence as a possible factor in treatment resistance. Are there any adverse effects? Sexual problems are common but may not be disclosed by the patient unless asked about.
- **Drugs causing raised blood pressure.** Ask about any drugs that may cause hypertension, such as NSAIDs, steroids, amphetamines, liquorice, caffeine, sympathomimetics, combined oral contraceptives and sodium-containing medications (antacids).
- **Indications for reducing cardiovascular risk.** Check whether aspirin and statins are indicated and prescribed.

Family history

- **Hypertension.** Ask about a family history of premature CVD (first-degree male relatives with CVD before 55 years or female relatives with CVD before 65 years). Is there a family history of secondary hypertension due to renal or endocrine disease (including diabetes)?

Alcohol, smoking and recreational drugs

- **Alcohol.** Ask for details about past and present alcohol consumption.
- **Smoking.** Record past and current smoking status and calculate the number of pack years (= (number of cigarettes smoked per day × number of years smoked)/20).

Review of previous investigations

- **Urea and electrolytes.** Abnormalities may suggest renal disease. Renal function needs to be checked before and after starting therapy with ACE inhibitors. Yearly checks should be performed in people with established hypertension.
- **Fasting glucose and lipids.** Check for diabetes and hypercholesterolaemia.
- **Thyroid function.** Hyperthyroidism may be associated with hypertension. Hypothyroidism is linked to diabetes and hyperlipidaemia.
- **ECG.** Look for evidence of left-ventricular hypertrophy.
- **Secondary causes.** If you suspect secondary hypertension, check whether any of the following investigations have already been performed: calcium, chest X-ray, renal ultrasound or computerised tomography (CT) scanning, intravenous urogram, renal arteriography, urinary free cortisol and 24-hour urinary vanillylmandelic acid (VMA) x3.

Examination

General
- **Obesity.** Check height and weight and calculate BMI. Truncal obesity may rarely be seen due to Cushing's syndrome.

Vital signs
- **Pulse.** The pulse volume may be large in aortic regurgitation.
- **Blood pressure.** Measure blood pressure in both arms. If the difference in readings is >20 mmHg, repeat the measurements. If it remains at 20 mmHg or more on the second measurement, use the arm with the higher readings for future measurements. If the clinic blood pressure is 140/90 mmHg or higher, take a second measurement. If the second measurement is significantly different from the first, take a third. Then record the lower of the last two measurements as the clinic blood pressure.

Skin
- **Striae.** Violaceous striae may rarely indicate steroid excess due to Cushing's syndrome.

Head and neck
- **Fundoscopy.** The role of fundoscopy in routine assessment of hypertension is limited, as microvascular changes such as retinal haemorrhages and exudates can only be reliably assessed with retinal photographs. Fundoscopy has a role in the emergency assessment of malignant hypertension to look for papilloedema (indicating raised intracranial pressure).

Chest
- **Apex beat.** Check for evidence of left-ventricular hypertrophy.
- **Lungs.** Listen to the lung bases for evidence of heart failure, which is a late complication of hypertension.

Abdomen
- **Liver.** The liver may be enlarged if there is associated right heart failure.
- **Kidneys.** Feel for enlarged kidneys.
- **Abdominal aorta.** This might be a good opportunity to screen for abdominal aortic aneurysm through palpation and auscultation.

Lower limbs
- **Peripheral pulses.** Check for evidence of peripheral vascular disease. Delayed or weak femoral pulses may rarely be found in coarctation of the aorta.
- **Oedema.** Leg oedema suggests heart failure or possible renal disease.

Bedside tests
- **Blood glucose.** Check for diabetes with a glucose test strip.
- **Urinalysis.** Look for evidence of proteinuria and haematuria.

Key references and further reading

1. British National Formulary. www.bnf.org.
2. JBS 3 Board. Joint British Societies' consensus recommendations for the prevention of cardiovascular disease (JBS3). *Heart* 2014;100:ii1–ii67.
3. National Institute for Health and Care Excellence (NICE). Hypertension in adults: diagnosis and management. NICE guidelines [CG127]. August 2011. Available from: http://www.nice.org.uk/guidance/cg127 (last accessed 29 April 2016).
4. van den Born B-JH, Hulsman CAA, Hoekstra JBL et al. Value of routine fundoscopy in patients with hypertension: systematic review. *BMJ* 2005;331: 73–76.

Atrial fibrillation

Key thoughts

Practical points

- **Diagnosis.** Atrial fibrillation (AF) is the most common sustained arrhythmia and occurs more frequently in advanced age. It may be completely asymptomatic but commonly presents with cardiac (e.g. palpitations) or unspecific symptoms, such as tiredness. Variants include paroxysmal, persistent and permanent AF. Always consider the possibility of myocardial infarction in acute onset of AF.
- **Prognosis.** AF is an important risk factor for embolic complications and may be diagnosed for the first time in conjunction with a stroke or heart failure. AF may also occur as a result of acute illness (e.g. pneumonia). In such cases, the prognosis is good, as AF will usually resolve after treatment of the primary problem.

Possible causes

- Coronary heart disease.
- Alcohol.
- Hypertension.
- Pneumonia.
- 'Lone' AF – no cause found.
- Hypertrophic or dilated cardiomyopathy.
- Hyperthyroidism.
- Pulmonary embolism.
- Rheumatic valvular heart disease (particularly mitral valve).
- Rarely atrial septal defect, pericarditis, myocarditis, congenital heart disease.

RED FLAGS

- Acute chest pain (myocardial infarction)
- Severe hypertension
- New onset of heart failure
- History of transient ischaemic attack (TIA) or stroke

History

Ideas, concerns and expectations

- **Ideas.** What does the patient know about the implications of untreated AF (risk of stroke) and the treatment involved? What are the patient's attitudes towards treatment with warfarin?

The 10-Minute Clinical Assessment, Second Edition. Knut Schroeder.
© 2017 John Wiley & Sons, Ltd. Published 2017 by John Wiley & Sons, Ltd.

- **Concerns.** Many people associate warfarin with rat poison and may be reluctant to take it as prescribed. Worries about developing a stroke are common.
- **Expectations.** Why has the patient come to see you? What are the expectations with regard to future management?

History of presenting complaint

- **Symptoms of AF.** Ask about palpitations, shortness of breath at rest or on exertion, chest pain or discomfort, syncope, fatigue and dizziness. Patients with known angina or heart failure may present with an acute exacerbation brought on by new onset of AF. A TIA or stroke may be the first presenting feature of AF resulting from an embolic complication.
- **Onset.** Consider urgent referral for cardioversion if the patient presents within 48 hours of onset of symptoms. Myocardial infarction may present with acute onset of AF.
- **Frequency.** Determine the presence, severity and frequency of symptoms. Is the diagnosis likely to be intermittent AF?
- **Circumstances.** When do symptoms occur? Are there any precipitating factors or activities? Ask about any relieving or exacerbating factors.
- **TIA and stroke.** Are there symptoms and signs indicating recent TIA or stroke?

SAF SCALE, CHA$_2$DS2-VAS$_c$ SCORE AND HAS-BLED

Assess risk factors for stroke, functional status and bleeding risk in AF at every visit (SAF Scale, CHA$_2$DS2-VAS$_c$ score, HAS-BLED, Combo Calculator) (Gage et al. 2004).

S	Symptoms: Palpitations, dyspnoea, dizziness, presycope or syncope, chest pain, weakness or fatigue, or other
A	Association: Is AF, when present, associated with the above symptoms?
F	Functionality: Do the identified symptoms associated with AF (or the treatment of AF) affect the patient's subjective quality of life?
C	Congestive heart failure
H	Hypertension or treated hypertension
A	Age >75 years
D	Diabetes
S2	Prior stroke or transient ischaemic attack (TIA)
H	Hypertension history
A	Abnormal renal function, abnormal liver function
S	Stroke history
B	Bleeding or predisposition
L	Labile INR [international normalised ratio] (<60% of time in therapeutic range)
E	'Elderly', age >65
D	Drugs predisposing to bleeding (antiplatelet agents, NSAIDs) and alcohol use

Past and current medical problems
- **Significant past illnesses.** Ask in particular about heart disease, hyperthyroidism and alcohol-related problems. Is there a history of angina?
- **TIA and stroke.** Is there a past history of TIA or stroke?
- **Cardioversion.** Have direct-current cardioversion or pharmacological conversion ever been performed or considered?

Medication
- **Anticoagulation.** Is the patient taking warfarin? Is monitoring adequate? Have there been any adverse effects, such as bleeding? Are there contraindications for anticoagulation?
- **Beta blockers and calcium antagonists.** Drugs such as beta blockers (e.g. atenolol or metoprolol) or calcium channel blockers (e.g. diltiazem or verapamil) are usually first-line treatments for rate control. Digoxin is effective only for rate control at rest, and is usually used second-line.
- **Antiarrhythmics.** Some patients with persistent AF will satisfy criteria for either an initial rate-control or a rhythm-control strategy (e.g. patients over the age of 65 who are also symptomatic), although the indications for each option are not mutually exclusive.

Social history
- **Home.** How have symptoms affected day-to-day life? Does the patient live alone? What is the level of independence?

Alcohol, smoking and recreational drugs
- **Alcohol.** Consider alcoholic cardiomyopathy if there is excessive alcohol consumption.
- **Smoking.** Check smoking status. Smoking may have contributed to the development of heart disease.

Review of previous investigations
- **Full blood count.** Look for anaemia.
- **Thyroid function.** Check for thyrotoxicosis.
- **Liver function tests.** These may be abnormal in excessive alcohol consumption.
- **Renal function.** Urea and electrolytes should be checked before certain cardiovascular drugs are started.
- **Coagulation screen.** This is required prior to starting anticoagulation.
- **ECG.** This may confirm the diagnosis, show the ventricular rate and suggest possible underlying structural heart disease.
- **Echocardiogram.** This may help to exclude mitral stenosis and will give an overall assessment of cardiac structure and function. Knowledge of left atrial size will help in estimating stroke risk.
- **Chest radiograph.** Look for heart size and pulmonary vascular pattern.

Examination

General
- **General condition.** Does the patient look unwell?

Vital signs
- **Pulse.** Check for an irregularly irregular pulse. Is there evidence of fast AF? Exclude an apex-radial deficit through cardiac auscultation.
- **Blood pressure.** Check for hypertension, which will increase the risk of stroke.

Head and neck
- **Jugular venous pressure.** Check for evidence of fluid overload due to heart failure.

Chest
- **Heart.** You may discover asymptomatic AF incidentally on auscultation. Is there auscultatory evidence of valvular disease, particularly the mitral valve? A displaced apex beat suggests cardiomegaly.
- **Lungs.** Check for basal crackles as evidence of heart failure.

Lower limbs
- **Oedema.** Leg swelling may suggest heart failure.

Key references and further reading
1. ACC/AHA/ESC 2006 guidelines for the management of patients with atrial fibrillation: full text. A report of the American College of Cardiology/American Heart Association Task Force on practice guidelines and the European Society of Cardiology Committee for Practice Guidelines. *Europace* 2006;8:651–745.
2. Dorian P, Cvitkovic SS, Kerr CR et al. A novel, simple scale for assessing the symptom severity of atrial fibrillation at the bedside: the CCS-SAF scale. *Can J Cardiol* 2006;22:383–386.
3. Gage BF, van Walraven C, Pearce L et al. Selecting patients with atrial fibrillation for anticoagulation: stroke risk stratification in patients taking aspirin. *Circulation* 2004;110:2287–2292.
4. Lane DA, Lip GYH. Use of the CHA2DS2-VASc and HAS-BLED scores to aid decision making for thromboprophylaxis in nonvalvular atrial fibrillation. *Circulation* 2012;126:860–865.
5. National Institute for Health and Care Excellence (NICE). Atrial fibrillation: management. NICE guidelines [CG180]. June 2014. Available from: http://www.nice.org.uk/guidance/cg180 (last accessed 29 April 2016).
6. New Zealand Guidelines Group (NZGG). *The Management of People with Atrial Fibrillation and Flutter*. New Zealand Guidelines Group, Wellington; 2005.

Heart failure

Key thoughts

Practical points

- **Diagnosis.** Heart failure is a condition brought on by left-ventricular systolic and/or diastolic dysfunction. Further investigation of the underlying cause is usually required. It is important to assess the severity of symptoms, look for precipitating factors and identify concomitant diseases. No symptoms or signs are sensitive or specific for the diagnosis of heart failure.
- **Prognosis.** The prognosis of heart failure can be worse than that of certain cancers. Try to anticipate complications.

Possible causes

- Angina pectoris or recurrent myocardial ischaemia.
- Arrhythmias, especially AF.
- Infections (e.g. pneumonia).
- Acute myocardial infarction.
- Anaemia.
- Alcohol excess.
- Iatrogenic (e.g. postoperative fluid replacement).
- Drugs (e.g. steroids, NSAIDs).
- Poor drug compliance (especially antihypertensive treatment).
- Thyroid disorders (e.g. thyrotoxicosis).
- Pregnancy.
- Pulmonary embolism.

RED FLAGS

- Acute pulmonary oedema
- Worsening symptoms
- Increasing weight gain due to fluid retention
- Valve disease
- Chest pain
- Symptomatic arrhythmia
- Pregnancy
- Anaemia
- Treatment resistance

The 10-Minute Clinical Assessment, Second Edition. Knut Schroeder.
© 2017 John Wiley & Sons, Ltd. Published 2017 by John Wiley & Sons, Ltd.

History

Ideas, concerns and expectations

- **Ideas.** The diagnosis of 'heart failure' may carry negative connotations, and the patient may think that death is imminent! Has it been explained to the patient what heart failure means?
- **Concerns.** Worries about reduced exercise tolerance are common. Consider asking about concerns regarding sexual activity.
- **Expectations.** Why has the patient come to see you? Relief of breathlessness and help with improving exercise tolerance are common reasons for consultation. Although symptoms can often be improved, return to a completely normal state is usually unrealistic.

History of presenting complaint

- **Context.** Allow the patient time to give a narrative account of their illness experience. How do symptoms of heart failure fit into the context of their life?
- **Quality of life.** How do symptoms affect activities of daily living and quality of life?
- **Main features of heart failure.** Ask about paroxysmal nocturnal dyspnoea (due to redistribution of excess fluid into the lung when lying down), breathlessness on exertion, tiredness, night-time cough and peripheral oedema. Patients may also complain of pink or brown sputum and wheeze (cardiac asthma). Only a small proportion of patients presenting in primary care with shortness of breath have heart failure.
- **Onset and progression.** When did the symptoms start? Has there been a recent deterioration? Are there any precipitating factors, such as intercurrent illness?
- **Severity.** Check what level of activity leads to symptoms, or whether symptoms are present at rest. How many pillows does the patient need to prop them up at night (orthopnoea)? Is there paroxysmal nocturnal dyspnoea?
- **Depression.** Screen for depression, which is common in people with heart failure and other chronic diseases.
- **Features suggesting alternative diagnoses.** Viral upper respiratory infection in a young patient with atopy suggests asthma rather than heart failure. Peak flow will be reduced and there is usually a good response to inhaled bronchodilators.
- **Associated symptoms.** Always ask about associated chest pain (myocardial ischaemia).
- **Diet.** Fluid restriction is often advocated to help with the control of symptoms in heart failure, but there is little evidence as to whether this is effective. Elderly patients may be at risk of dehydration and subsequent confusion if they follow this strategy too strictly. Salt intake should be restricted to <6 g daily.
- **Physical activity.** Patients with heart failure should engage in regular low intensity exercise.

- **Weight.** Patients with heart failure should be advised to weigh themselves at a set time each day. Any increase in weight of more than 1.5 kg over 2 days should be reported to a health professional.
- **End-of-life care.** Severe heart failure is a terminal disease. Establish the needs of the patient dying with or from heart failure. Consider discussing issues around sudden death and living with uncertainty.
- **Treatment resistance.** In patients who do not respond to treatment as expected, consider alternative diagnoses, check that the patient is prescribed – and takes – the correct treatment and look for perpetuating factors, such as salty foods or interacting drugs (e.g. NSAIDs).

Past and current medical problems
- **CVD.** Ischaemic heart disease, hypertension, diabetes and valvular disease are important underlying conditions.
- **Cardiovascular risk factors.** Check for diabetes and hyperlipidaemia.
- **Chronic disease.** Ask about a history of thyroid disease, malignancy, peripheral vascular disease, stroke, chronic obstructive pulmonary disease (COPD) and other systemic disease.
- **Immunisations.** Influenza and pneumococcal vaccination should be offered to all heart-failure patients.

Medication
- **ACE inhibitors.** These reduce mortality in patients with significant heart failure and may help with ventricular remodelling. Ask about adverse effects, such as cough and treatment-induced hypotension.
- **Beta blockers.** These should be considered in all patients with heart failure unless there is a contraindication, as there is evidence that they reduce all-cause mortality and cut hospital admissions due to worsening heart failure.
- **Aldosterone antagonists.** Low-dose spironolactone should be considered following specialist advice, as this drug can be beneficial in reducing mortality. Renal impairment and hyperkalaemia are contraindications. Has the patient received any other diuretic for treatment of acute heart failure?
- **Diuretics.** These are particularly useful if there is dyspnoea and ankle oedema.
- **Statins.** Many patients with ischaemic heart disease who have suffered a myocardial infarction or have a raised cardiovascular risk profile will already be taking a statin.
- **Digoxin.** Some patients with AF may already be taking digoxin, which also has positive inotropic effects.
- **Other drugs.** Check whether the patient is taking antiarrhythmics or vasodilators.
- **NSAIDs.** These may worsen heart failure.
- **Medication adherence.** Exacerbations and hospital admissions/readmissions are often caused by suboptimal medication adherence.
- **Important interactions.** Patients on warfarin should be advised to avoid cranberry juice. Grapefruit juice may interact with statins.

Social history
- **Home.** Ask how home life has been affected. Does the patient live alone? Is there a carer? What is the current level of independence? Are any services involved (e.g. social services, home care, meals on wheels)?

Alcohol, smoking and recreational drugs
- **Alcohol.** Excess alcohol consumption may cause alcoholic cardiomyopathy or direct toxic effects in the heart muscle.
- **Smoking.** Record past and current smoking status and calculate the number of pack years (= (number of cigarettes smoked per day × number of years smoked)/20). Has smoking-cessation advice been offered?

Review of previous investigations
- **Full blood count.** Look for anaemia.
- **Urea and electrolytes.** Check renal function as a baseline before starting treatment with ACE inhibitors or diuretics. Diuretics may lead to hyponatraemia.
- **Liver function tests.** These need to be monitored if the patient is taking a statin.
- **Fasting glucose.** Check for diabetes.
- **Thyroid function.** Hyperthyroidism may lead to AF.
- **B-type natriuretic peptide (BNP) and N-terminal BNP (N-BNP).** These tests are becoming increasingly available. Normal results make the diagnosis of heart failure unlikely. Abnormal tests in association with an abnormal ECG should prompt further investigation (e.g. echocardiography).
- **ECG.** Look for signs of ischaemia, infarction and ventricular hypertrophy. A normal ECG makes heart failure unlikely.
- **Chest X-ray.** Look for cardiomegaly, pleural effusions, diffuse patchy lung opacities and upper-lobe diversion. This may also be helpful in distinguishing an acute asthma attack from acute left ventricular failure.
- **Echocardiography.** Ideally, all patients with suspected heart failure should have an echocardiogram performed. This will provide information about the ejection fraction, the presence of left ventricular hypertrophy, valve function and wall-movement abnormalities and is the investigation of choice for the diagnosis of heart failure.
- **Peak flow.** A peak flow rate of <200 l/min is more likely due to a respiratory cause rather than to heart failure.

Examination

General

- **General condition.** Does the patient look unwell? Is there dyspnoea at rest? Cyanosis, restlessness and anxiety with a feeling of suffocation suggest acute pulmonary oedema. Breathing may sound bubbly, like a coffee machine. The patient may be sweaty and pale and will usually prefer to sit upright.

Vital signs
- **Temperature.** If suggested by the history, fever may point to pneumonia or other systemic infections, which may precipitate heart failure.
- **Pulse.** Tachycardia is an early sign and is more predictive in the diagnosis of heart failure than is raised blood pressure. Fast AF is an important cause of heart failure.
- **Blood pressure.** Hypertension is an important precipitating factor. Check lying and standing blood pressure for postural hypotension.
- **Respiratory rate.** Tachypnoea and laboured breathing may be present.

Head and neck
- **JVP.** An elevated JVP is an important sign but may be difficult to elicit.

Chest
- **Apex beat.** Search for a laterally displaced apex beat.
- **Heart sounds.** Listen for a third heart sound (gallop rhythm). This is an important sign. Listen for murmurs of aortic or mitral valve disease. It is impossible to assess ventricular function adequately by clinical assessment alone.
- **Lungs.** Listen for fine inspiratory basal crackles, which may suggest pulmonary oedema. Wheeze may indicate 'cardiac asthma'. Other causes of chest signs include infection, pulmonary fibrosis and bronchiectasis. Dull percussion and reduced breath sounds suggest pleural effusion, which often occurs on the right side first, before affecting both lungs.

Abdomen and back
- **Liver.** Tender or non-tender hepatomegaly is a common sign. Check for ascites.
- **Oedema.** Check for sacral and scrotal oedema.

Lower limbs
- **Skin temperature.** Peripheries will often feel cool.
- **Oedema.** Check for pitting oedema, which may also be caused by venous incompetence, obesity or hypoalbuminaemia.

Bedside tests
- **Urinalysis.** Check for proteinuria.

Key references and further reading
1. National Institute for Health and Care Excellence (NICE). Chronic heart failure in adults. NICE guidelines [CG108]. August 2010. Available from: http://www.nice.org.uk/guidance/cg108 (last accessed 29 April 2016).
2. Rutten FH, Moons KGM, Cramer M-JM et al. Recognising heart failure in elderly patients with stable chronic obstructive pulmonary disease in primary care: cross sectional diagnostic study. *BMJ* 2005;331:1379–1382.
3. Scottish Intercollegiate Guidelines Network (SIGN). Management of chronic heart failure. A national clinical guideline. SIGN guideline 95. February

2007. Available from: http://sign.ac.uk/guidelines/fulltext/95/index.html (last accessed 29 April 2016).

4. Thomas JT, Kelly RF, Thomas SJ et al. Utility of history, physical examination, electrocardiogram and chest radiograph for differentiating normal from decreased systolic function in patients with heart failure. *Am J Med* 2002;112:437–445.

5. Wang CS, FitzGerald JM, Schulzer M et al. Does this patient in the emergency department have congestive heart failure? *JAMA* 2005;294:1944–1956.

Peripheral vascular disease

Key thoughts

Practical points

- **Diagnosis.** The diagnosis can often be made clinically, and severity ranges from mild to severe. Intermittent claudication (pain in the leg muscles that improves at rest) is a marker of increased cardiovascular risk.
- **Prognosis.** Try to identify high-risk patients, as peripheral vascular disease carries an increased risk of morbidity and mortality. Early diagnosis and risk factor control are essential to reducing complications.
- **Quality of life.** The impact on a patient's quality of life and ability to work can be considerable.

Differential diagnosis

- Peripheral atherosclerosis.
- Nerve root compression.
- Spinal stenosis.
- Diabetic neuropathy.
- Arthritis.
- Phlebitic syndrome after deep venous thrombosis.
- Baker's cyst.
- Rarely myositis, arteritis.

Risk factors

- Smoking.
- Diabetes.
- Age.
- Hypertension.
- Hyperlipidaemia.
- Atrial fibrillation.
- Thrombogenic factors.

RED FLAGS

- Features of acute limb ischaemia, such as rest pain, pallor, pulselessness, paraesthesia and paralysis
- Suspected abdominal aortic aneurysm
- Severe intermittent claudication
- Skin cyanosis
- Muscle tenderness

The 10-Minute Clinical Assessment, Second Edition. Knut Schroeder.
© 2017 John Wiley & Sons, Ltd. Published 2017 by John Wiley & Sons, Ltd.

- Painful leg or foot ulcers
- Gangrene

History

Ideas, concerns and expectations
- **Ideas.** Many people with peripheral vascular disease think that their pain is caused by arthritis or is a normal part of ageing. These patients may delay seeing a health professional for a considerable time and present with late features of the disease.
- **Concerns.** Fears about losing a limb are common but usually unjustified. The risk of myocardial infarction or stroke is generally much higher, but this may not be appreciated. There may be worries about disability once people are unable to perform some of their daily activities.
- **Expectations.** Pain relief and help with increasing walking distance are common reasons for consultation.

History of presenting complaint
- **Context.** Allow the patient time to tell you about their leg pain in their own words. How do the symptoms fit into the context of this patient's life?
- **Quality of life.** How does the pain affect day-to-day life (consider home activities, work, leisure and social life)?
- **Intermittent claudication.** Classic symptoms include cramping muscle pain in the legs that occurs with the same degree on exercise and is relieved by rest. Consider other causes of leg pain, such as nerve root pain and spinal stenosis. In nerve root compression, the pain usually travels down the back of the leg and can be relieved by a change in position, such as leaning forward. In spinal stenosis, there may be additional motor weakness. Osteoarthritic pain is often worse on weight-bearing and is related to activity. Different conditions may coexist.
- **Severity.** Is there pain in either leg on running or walking or at rest? Does the pain ever start on standing or when sitting still? Does the pain get worse on hurrying or walking uphill/upstairs? Does the pain ever occur at ordinary pace on a flat level?
- **Site.** Pain usually affects the calves but may also be felt in the buttocks or thighs during exercise. The pain should only be felt in the muscle and not in the bone or joint.
- **Other symptoms.** The affected leg(s) may feel cold. In men, are there any problems with erections (an important and often early sign of peripheral vascular disease)?
- **Trauma.** Trauma or inadequate compression may lead to acute limb ischaemia.
- **Risk factors.** Smoking, hypertension, diabetes and hyperlipidaemia are important modifiable risk factors. Have these been addressed and are they being treated? Has the patient received smoking-cessation advice?

- **Management.** Does the patient avoid walking? Regular exercise (at least three times weekly) can improve the symptoms of intermittent claudication.
- **Surgery.** Has the patient ever had angioplasty or vascular bypass surgery?

Past and current medical problems
- **Significant past illnesses.** Ask in particular about risk factors for CVD, such as diabetes, previous myocardial infarction, hypertension and hyperlipidaemia.

Medication
- **Antiplatelet drugs.** There is good evidence that antiplatelet drugs reduce major cardiovascular events. They also reduce the risk of arterial occlusion and the consequent need for revascularisation.
- **Statins.** Statins reduce the risk of CVD and may improve the symptoms of claudication. Unless there is a contraindication, all patients with peripheral artery disease should be prescribed a statin.
- **Antidiabetics.** In people with diabetes, check whether glucose levels are controlled with current management and whether any medication is taken as prescribed.
- **Antihypertensives.** Good blood-pressure control reduces the risk of cardiovascular events, but the evidence is inconclusive with regard to peripheral artery disease.
- **Beta-adrenoceptor blockers.** Beta blockers are usually contraindicated in severe peripheral artery disease.
- **Symptomatic treatment.** Peripheral vasodilators such as cilotazol may improve walking distance but are often associated with adverse effects.

Allergies
- **Aspirin.** Ask about any allergies, particularly to aspirin or other drugs that may need to be used for the treatment of peripheral vascular disease, management of risk factors or treatment of complications.

Social history
- **Home.** How has home life been affected by the symptoms? Which activities have become difficult? Is further support needed?
- **Work.** Are there any problems at work?

Alcohol, smoking and recreational drugs
- **Alcohol.** Alcohol misuse may contribute to the development of peripheral vascular disease.
- **Smoking.** Smoking is by far the most important risk factor. Record past and current smoking status and calculate the number of pack years (= (number of cigarettes smoked per day × number of years smoked)/20). To what extent has smoking-cessation advice been offered?

Review of previous investigations

- **Full blood count.** Look for anaemia. A raised white count may suggest infection, complicating gangrene (if present).
- **Plasma viscosity.** This may be raised if there is underlying infection or arteritis (rare).
- **Fasting glucose and haemoglobin A1c (HbA1c).** Has the patient been checked for diabetes?
- **Fasting lipids.** Is there evidence of hypercholesterolaemia?
- **Liver function tests.** These need to be monitored during treatment with statins.
- **Urea and electrolytes.** Some antihypertensive drugs require monitoring of urea and electrolytes.
- **TSH.** Hypothyroidism may be associated with hyperlipidaemia.

Examination

General

- **General condition.** Suspect possible sepsis in patients with gangrene who are unwell.

Vital signs

- **Temperature.** Check for fever if there is the possibility of infected gangrene (rare).
- **Pulse.** Atrial fibrillation is a risk factor for acute ischaemia caused by a thrombotic event.
- **Blood pressure.** Check for hypertension.

Abdomen

- **Aortic aneurysm.** Palpate the abdomen for evidence of an abdominal aortic aneurysm. Listen for any bruits.

Lower limbs

- **Skin temperature and colour.** Skin on the peripheries is often cool in peripheral vascular disease. The skin colour may appear abnormally pink, red, blue or dusky purple. There may also be an absence of hair on the toes.
- **Capillary refill.** Consider any refill time of more than 5 seconds as abnormal, but be aware that this is a weak clinical sign.
- **Ulcers.** Severe ischaemia may cause ulcers around the tips of the toes, metatarsal heads, bunion areas and lateral malleolus. Ischaemic ulcers are usually painful and dry, whereas venous ulcers occur on the medial malleolus and tend to be painless. Look for any signs of gangrene.
- **Peripheral pulses.** Check the femoral, popliteal, tibialis posterior and dorsalis pedis pulses. Normal pulses do not rule out the diagnosis. Check also for any audible or palpable bruits.

Bedside tests

- **Ankle–brachial pressure index.** A low index of <0.9 supports the diagnosis, but a normal index does not rule it out. If the diagnosis is in doubt, an exercise ankle–brachial pressure index may be useful.

Key references and further reading

1. Bendermacher BL, Teijink JA, Willigendael EM et al. Symptomatic peripheral artery disease: the value of a validated questionnaire and a clinical decision rule. *Br J Gen Pract* 2006;56:932–944.
2. Cassar K. Clinical review: intermittent claudication. *BMJ* 2006;333:1002–1005.
3. Khan N, Rahim SA, Anand S et al. Does the clinical examination predict lower extremity peripheral artery disease? *JAMA* 2006;295:536–546.
4. Leng GC, Fowkes FGR. The Edinburgh claudication questionnaire: an improved version of the WHO/Rose questionnaire for use in epidemiological surveys. *J Clin Epidemiol* 1992;45:1101–1109.
5. National Institute for Health and Care Excellence (NICE). Peripheral artery disease: diagnosis and management. NICE guidelines [CG147]. August 2012. Available from: https://www.nice.org.uk/guidance/cg147 (last accessed 29 April 2016).
6. Scottish Intercollegiate Guidelines Network (SIGN). Diagnosis and management of peripheral arterial disease. SIGN guideline 89. October 2006. Available from: http://www.sign.ac.uk/pdf/sign89.pdf (last accessed 29 April 2016).

Respiratory

Shortness of breath

Key thoughts

Practical points
- **Diagnosis.** Shortness of breath is a common presenting symptom, and diagnosing the underlying cause can be challenging. Two or more underlying conditions may coexist.
- **Prognosis.** Exclude serious and potentially life-threatening causes that require urgent action, such as asthma attack, pulmonary embolism and myocardial infarction.

Possible causes
- **Respiratory.** Commonly, asthma, chronic obstructive pulmonary disease (COPD), respiratory infection (including pneumonia), pulmonary embolism. Others include lung cancer, tuberculosis (TB), pleural effusion, foreign-body inhalation, pneumothorax, interstitial lung disease (e.g. fibrosing alveolitis), bronchiectasis, lung/lobar collapse.
- **Cardiac.** Angina, myocardial infarction, arrhythmia, heart failure.
- **Other.** Anxiety and hyperventilation, anaemia, diabetic ketoacidosis.

Important risk factors
- Smoking.
- Risk factors for venous thromboembolism.
- Cardiovascular disease (CVD).
- Pre-existing lung disease.

RED FLAGS

- Tachypnoea
- Tachycardia
- Tracheal deviation
- Stridor
- Cyanosis
- Hypoxia
- Hypotension
- Confusion
- Use of accessory muscles
- Effortful breathing without effective air movement ('silent chest')

The 10-Minute Clinical Assessment, Second Edition. Knut Schroeder.
© 2017 John Wiley & Sons, Ltd. Published 2017 by John Wiley & Sons, Ltd.

History

Ideas, concerns and expectations

- **Ideas.** What does the patient believe to be the cause of the symptoms? Patients may find it difficult to make the link between shortness of breath and heart failure.
- **Concerns.** Worries about a serious underlying cause, such as heart attack or cancer, are common. Acute shortness of breath can be extremely frightening for patients and their families.
- **Expectations.** Common reasons for consultation are symptom relief and ruling out serious disease.

History of presenting complaint

- **Context.** Give the patient time to tell you the story behind their breathing symptoms and how they fit into the context of their lives.
- **Quality of life.** How does shortness of breath affect activities of daily living? The impact on quality of life is often considerable.
- **Breathing symptoms.** Shortness of breath is a feeling of being short of air and having to breathe faster and/or more deeply. Find out what exactly the patient means by 'shortness of breath'. This could be chest tightness, difficulty in breathing or chest pain that is restricting breathing. Is breathlessness present at rest or only on exertion? Is there orthopnoea at night? Ask about cough, sputum, haemoptysis and wheeze.
- **Onset.** Find out when and how quickly the symptoms developed. Breathlessness due to pneumonia usually develops over a few days. In pulmonary embolism, myocardial infarction and anxiety symptoms may develop quickly, whereas shortness of breath due to anaemia may take weeks or months to develop.
- **Severity.** The severity of the symptoms does not necessarily predict the severity of the underlying condition. Explore current exercise tolerance by finding out whether shortness of breath occurs at rest, on walking on a flat surface, when going uphill or only during more strenuous exercise.
- **Cardiac causes.** Ask about pointers to cardiac disease or myocardial infarction, such as central chest pain, nausea, vomiting, sweating and a history of CVD.
- **Associated symptoms.** Any leg swelling may be caused by deep venous thrombosis, an important risk factor for the development of pulmonary embolism. If present, ask about risk factors, including immobility, recent surgery and oral contraceptive pill.
- **General symptoms.** Ask about fever, weight loss, loss of appetite, night sweats and lymphadenopathy. Is the patient overweight?
- **Anxiety and hyperventilation.** Are there any particular stresses in the patient's life? Anxiety often leads to a feeling of shortness of breath. Consider hyperventilation if there is a combination of symptoms, such as chest pain or tightness, feeling tense, blurred vision, dizzy spells, tingling fingers, inability to breathe deeply, stiff fingers or arms, feeling anxious, cold hands or feet, tight feeling around the mouth and palpitations.

Past and current medical problems
- **Significant past illnesses.** Ask about any chronic conditions that might cause or exacerbate shortness of breath, such as CVD, asthma, COPD, emphysema, interstitial lung disease and anaemia.

Medication
- **Analgesics.** Nonsteroidal anti-inflammatory drugs (NSAIDs) may cause acute shortness of breath in patients with asthma.
- **Drugs causing pulmonary fibrosis.** Ask about drugs such as methotrexate and amiodarone, which may cause pulmonary fibrosis.
- **Inhalers.** If the patient has a chronic lung condition such as asthma or COPD, are inhalers being prescribed and taken regularly?

Allergies
- **Antibiotics.** Ask about allergies to antibiotics, in case these need to be prescribed for an underlying infection.
- **Aspirin.** Check whether the patient is allergic to aspirin if you suspect myocardial infarction.

Social history
- **Home.** How have symptoms affected home life and the ability to perform normal daily activities?
- **Work.** Has work been affected? Does work involve driving or handling machinery? Is there exposure to dusts, toxins or asbestos? Is a sick note needed?
- **Hobbies.** Consider psittacosis or allergic reactions if the patient is exposed to animals or poultry.

Alcohol, smoking and recreational drugs
- **Alcohol.** Ask about past and recent alcohol intake. Increased amounts of alcohol may suggest underlying stress or anxiety.
- **Smoking.** A long smoking history increases the risk of lung cancer, COPD and emphysema. Record past and current smoking status and calculate the number of pack years (= (number of cigarettes smoked per day × number of years smoked)/20). Has smoking-cessation advice been offered?
- **Recreational drugs.** Consider 'crack' lung or pneumonia in drug users.

Review of previous investigations
- **Full blood count.** Look for anaemia. A raised white cell count may suggest infection. Eosinophilia occurs in asthma, allergy or parasitic infections.
- **Inflammatory markers.** A raised plasma viscosity or C-reactive protein (CRP) may suggest infection or underlying malignancy.
- **Chest X-ray.** Is there any evidence of an underlying lung or cardiac cause for the symptoms? Overinflation suggests asthma, COPD or emphysema. Look for signs of pneumonia or TB in those at risk.

- **Electrocardiogram (ECG).** Look for arrhythmias and evidence of ischaemia. Tachycardia may be the only sign in pulmonary embolus.
- **Spirometry.** If shortness of breath is longstanding, has spirometry been performed?

Examination

General

- **General condition.** Does the patient look unwell? Is there dyspnoea at rest? Cyanosis suggests a more serious underlying cause, but it may not be obvious if there is underlying anaemia. Pallor may indicate anaemia. In carbon monoxide poisoning, the patient will appear to have a cherry-red skin colour. Is there evidence of lymphadenopathy?
- **Airway.** Is the airway clear or compromised? Is speech affected?
- **Breathing.** Is there laboured breathing with use of accessory muscles?
- **Mental state.** Are there signs of confusion or neurological symptoms? Is the patient alert and orientated?

Vital signs

- **Temperature.** A raised temperature suggests infection or, if mildly elevated, pulmonary embolism.
- **Pulse.** Tachycardia is common in association with shortness of breath. A fast heart rate may be the only sign in pulmonary embolus.
- **Blood pressure.** Blood pressure will often be normal. Consider hypertension and anxiety if blood pressure is raised. Hypotension may indicate impending shock.
- **Respiratory rate.** Tachypnoea will often be present and may suggest serious illness if severe (>30 breaths per minute).

Skin

- **Sweating.** Look for excessive sweating, which may indicate infection or myocardial infarction.

Head and neck

- **Jugular venous pressure (JVP).** A raised JVP may occur in heart failure. Alternatively, if fixed, it suggests superior vena cava obstruction, particularly if associated with neck and facial swelling.
- **Trachea.** Feel for a tracheal shift.

Upper limbs

- **Clubbing.** Look for finger clubbing, which may suggest underlying lung disease. Tar stains will be present in smokers.
- **Wrist flap.** In carbon dioxide retention, there may be a wrist flap when extending the arms.

Chest

- **Heart.** Is the apex beat displaced (cardiomegaly)? Are there any murmurs suggesting valve disease? A fourth heart sound may be heard in heart failure.
- **Lungs.** Look for breathing pattern and chest expansion. Percuss and auscultate all areas. Check for signs of infection and heart failure. Chest examination in pulmonary embolus may be entirely normal. Is there wheeze? Localised bronchial breathing may occur in pneumonia and lung cancer. Hyperresonance on percussion can be found in pneumothorax. Dull percussion may be caused by consolidation or pleural effusion.

Abdomen

- **Liver.** The liver may be enlarged in heart failure or by metastases from carcinoma.

Lower limbs

- **Ankle swelling.** Peripheral pitting oedema may suggest heart failure.
- **Calf swelling.** Consider pulmonary embolus due to deep venous thrombosis if there is unilateral calf swelling and tenderness.

Bedside tests

- **Pulse oximetry or arterial blood gases.** Hypoxaemia (SaO_2 <92% or PaO_2 <8 kPa), regardless of inspired oxygen concentration, indicates severe illness.

Key references and further reading

1. Huijnen B, van der Horst F, van Amelsvoort L et al. Dyspnoea in elderly family practice patients. Occurrence, severity, quality of life and mortality over an 8-year period. *Fam Pract* 2006;23:34–39.
2. National Institute for Health and Care Excellence (NICE). Breathlessness. Clinical Knowledge Summaries. 2010. Available from: http://cks.nice.org.uk/breathlessness (last accessed 29 April 2016).
3. Rees PJ. Respiratory diseases: symptoms and signs. *Medicine* 2003;31:1–6.
4. Zoorob RJ, Campbell JS. Acute dyspnea in the office. *Am Fam Physician* 2003;68:1803–1810.

Haemoptysis

Key thoughts

Practical points

- **Diagnosis.** Haemoptysis is a fairly common symptom in general practice and may be a presenting feature of respiratory infection, lung cancer, TB or pulmonary embolism. Try to distinguish between true haemoptysis (with coughing up of blood from below the larynx) and pseudohaemoptysis (bleeding from sites other than the oropharynx, e.g. the nose).
- **Prognosis.** Differentiating between benign and serious causes can be a challenge, but it is important to decide whether urgent referral to hospital is needed.

Possible causes

- **Respiratory.** Bronchitis and pneumonia, bronchiectasis, bronchial carcinoma, interstitial lung disease, lung abscess, TB, post-bronchoscopy, pulmonary embolism.
- **Cardiac.** Left ventricular failure, pulmonary hypertension (e.g. pulmonary embolism), mitral stenosis.
- **Ear, nose and throat.** Nose or pharyngeal bleeds.
- **Rare systemic causes.** Coagulopathy, platelet dysfunction or thrombocytopenia, Goodpasture's syndrome, systemic lupus erythematosus (SLE), Wegener's granulomatosis, Osler–Weber–Rendu disease (hereditary haemorrhagic telangiectasia).

Important risk factors

- Smoking.
- CVD.
- Underlying lung or systemic disease.
- Coagulation disorders.

RED FLAGS

- Severe blood loss
- Tachycardia
- Postural hypotension
- Systemic features, such as weight loss, fever and sweats
- Features suggestive of cancer

The 10-Minute Clinical Assessment, Second Edition. Knut Schroeder.
© 2017 John Wiley & Sons, Ltd. Published 2017 by John Wiley & Sons, Ltd.

History

Ideas, concerns and expectations
- **Ideas.** What does the patient think is causing haemoptysis?
- **Concerns.** Haemoptysis can be very frightening, and patients may fear they are going to die or that they have cancer.
- **Expectations.** Common reasons for consultation include reassurance and reaching a diagnosis.

History of presenting complaint
- **Nature of haemoptysis.** Try to find out whether the symptoms are the result of true haemoptysis. Is the blood being coughed up, or does it originate from the oropharynx (pseudohaemoptysis)? Are there clots, fresh red blood or just blood-stained sputum? Haematemesis and haemoptysis may be difficult to distinguish. Frequent nose bleeds which are worse in the supine position may present as haemoptysis. Throat or voice changes may suggest bleeding from the oropharynx. Other bruising or bleeding may suggest a coagulopathy.
- **Respiratory symptoms.** Association with respiratory symptoms makes underlying lung disease more likely. Ask about cough, shortness of breath, wheeze, pleuritic chest pain and sputum production, which all suggest infection or pulmonary embolism, particularly if onset is acute. The absence of respiratory symptoms does not rule out a respiratory cause.
- **Gastrointestinal symptoms.** Dyspepsia, heartburn, abdominal pain and other gastrointestinal symptoms may point towards an abdominal rather than respiratory cause. Because blood can be swallowed and then regurgitated, 'coffee grounds' vomit along with haemoptysis does not necessarily mean that the bleeding is gastrointestinal.
- **Constitutional symptoms.** Weight loss, malaise, fever, night sweats, lethargy, bruising and lymphadenopathy may suggest possible lung cancer or TB, particularly in people at risk.
- **Haematuria.** Very rarely, haemoptysis with associated haematuria may be caused by Wegener's granulomatosis or Goodpasture's syndrome.

Past and current medical problems
- **Respiratory problems.** Ask about any past or current chest problems, such as bronchiectasis, which can result in haemoptysis at any age. Other important lung conditions to consider are bronchitis, recurrent pneumonia, cancer, TB and mycetoma (rare).
- **Heart.** A number of heart conditions, such as left ventricular failure and mitral stenosis, can cause recurrent haemoptysis.
- **Thromboembolism.** Has the patient suffered from thrombosis or pulmonary embolism in the past? Risk factors include recent surgery or immobilisation, childbirth and taking the oral contraceptive pill.

Medication
- **Hormones.** Ask about the combined oral contraceptive pill and hormone-replacement therapy, as both increase the risk of pulmonary embolism.
- **Anticoagulants.** Anticoagulants increase the risk of haemoptysis, but usually there is an additional underlying cause.

Allergies
- **Antibiotics.** Ask about allergies to any antibiotics that may need to be used for the treatment of an underlying infection.

Family history
- **TB.** A family history or exposure to TB may be relevant.

Social history
- **Home.** Have symptoms affected home life in any way? Are usual activities limited?
- **Work.** Ask about any exposures at work that might cause lung disease, such as asbestos, silica and other dusts or chemicals.
- **Diet.** Consider scurvy due to vitamin C deficiency, particularly in elderly people with a poor diet.
- **Travel.** Has there been any travel to areas with a high prevalence of TB?

Alcohol, smoking and recreational drugs
- **Alcohol.** Heavy drinking may lead to coagulopathy due to alcoholic liver damage. Also consider the possibility of alcoholic gastritis or oesophageal varices.
- **Smoking.** Obtain details of past and present smoking habits.
- **Drugs.** Consider 'crack lung' in drug abusers.

Review of previous investigations
- **Full blood count.** Look for anaemia and a raised white cell count (infection, malignancy). Low platelets may lead to clotting problems (may be alcohol-related). Raised platelets may occur in lung cancer.
- **Inflammatory markers.** These may be raised in infection or malignancy.
- **D-dimers.** A negative test is useful for ruling out pulmonary embolism.
- **Chest X-ray.** Look for any signs of lung or heart disease.
- **ECG.** This may show signs of CVD.

Examination

General
- **General condition.** Does the patient look unwell? Cachexia and wasting may be caused by malignancy or TB.
- **Airway, breathing and circulation (ABC).** If the patient is unwell, proceed with checking ABC and resuscitation as appropriate.

Vital signs

- **Temperature.** A raised temperature suggests infection and may also occur with pulmonary embolism.
- **Pulse.** Tachycardia may be caused by infection, anxiety or blood loss and is an early (and sometimes the only) sign of pulmonary embolism.
- **Blood pressure.** Blood pressure will usually be normal. Hypotension may indicate impending shock. Hypertension may be found in underlying CVD or, very rarely, with renal involvement in Wegener's granulomatosis and Goodpasture's syndrome.
- **Respiratory rate.** Tachypnoea may result from pulmonary embolism, infection, lung disease or cardiac causes.

Skin

- **Purpura.** Rashes and purpura may rarely occur as part of a generalised bleeding disorder or due to malignancy.

Head and neck

- **Malar flush.** Red cheeks may occur in mitral stenosis or, rarely, as a 'butterfly rash' in SLE.
- **Neck swelling.** Neck oedema and swelling may be caused by superior vena cava obstruction due to lung cancer.
- **Nose and mouth.** Check for any abnormalities of the nose, mouth and gum. Telangiectasia may rarely suggest Osler–Weber–Rendu disease.

Upper limbs

- **Finger clubbing.** This is not a specific sign, but may indicate underlying lung disease, such as bronchiectasis, bronchial carcinoma or advanced TB. Also look for tar staining on the fingers.

Chest

- **Tenderness.** Localised tenderness of the chest wall suggests rib fracture, if indicated by the history.
- **Lungs.** Auscultation may reveal wheeze or crackles, which may indicate bronchitis, pneumonia or bronchiectasis. Diffuse, fine, late inspiratory crackles may be heard in interstitial lung disease, or, if affecting the lung bases, may be due to heart failure. Poor localised air entry together with dullness on percussion suggests lung collapse, likely due to obstruction caused by carcinoma or adenoma. There may also be localised wheeze on the affected side. A pleural rub may indicate pneumonia or pulmonary infarction due to pulmonary embolism.
- **Heart.** Are there any heart murmurs suggesting valve disease – particularly the low-pitched murmur of mitral stenosis (rare)?

Lower limbs

- **Swelling.** Leg swelling may result from peripheral oedema, suggesting a possible cardiac cause or complication. Also look for signs of deep venous thrombosis.

Bedside tests

* **Sputum examination.** Look at the sputum, if possible. Blood coughed up from the respiratory tract is usually bright red and frothy. Thick purulent sputum suggests infection. Spitting up of blood without any pus may occur as a result of cancer, TB or pulmonary infarction. Foul-smelling sputum may arise from an abscess. Pink and frothy sputum may be caused by pulmonary oedema. Consider testing for acidity – an acidic pH suggests haematemesis rather than haemoptysis.

Key references and further reading

1. Bidwell JL, Pachner RW. Hemoptysis: diagnosis and management. *Am Fam Physician* 2005;72:1253–1260.
2. Hamilton W, Sharp D. Diagnosis of lung cancer in primary care: a structured review. *Fam Pract* 2004;21:605–611.
3. Johnson JL. Manifestations of hemoptysis: how to manage minor, moderate, and massive bleeding. *Postgrad Med* 2002;112:101–106, 108–109, 113.
4. Jones R, Latinovic R, Charlton J, Gulliford M. Alarm symptoms in early diagnosis of cancer in primary care: cohort study using General Practice Research Database. *BMJ* 2007;334:1040.

Suspected lung cancer

Key thoughts

Practical points
- **Diagnosis.** Early diagnosis is difficult, as most symptoms of lung cancer can also be caused by common and benign causes. If lung cancer is suspected, assessment should include a search for metastases.
- **Prognosis.** Early diagnosis of lung cancer can improve the prognosis.

Differential diagnosis
- Recurrent upper respiratory infections.
- Pneumonia.
- COPD.
- Asthma.
- Tuberculosis.

Important risk factors
- Smoking.
- Family history of lung cancer.
- Increased age.
- Industrial dusts, especially asbestos.

RED FLAGS

- Persistent cough and/or breathlessness for more than 2 weeks without obvious cause
- Persistent systemic symptoms, such as unexplained weight loss, fatigue, loss of appetite, malaise
- Loss of desire for cigarettes
- Persistent haemoptysis
- Stridor
- Symptoms or signs suggesting metastasis (bone, liver, brain)
- Neck or facial swelling due to superior vena cava obstruction (late sign)
- Dysphagia
- Hoarseness
- Cervical or supraclavicular lymphadenopathy
- Chest X-ray suggesting pleural effusion, pleural mass or any suspicious lung pathology

The 10-Minute Clinical Assessment, Second Edition. Knut Schroeder.
© 2017 John Wiley & Sons, Ltd. Published 2017 by John Wiley & Sons, Ltd.

History

Ideas, concerns and expectations
- **Ideas.** What does the patient believe is causing the symptoms?
- **Concerns.** Worries about underlying lung cancer are common in smokers with a chronic cough and/or haemoptysis, but people may still present relatively late. The diagnosis of lung cancer can cause significant psychological trauma.
- **Expectations.** Why has the patient come to see you? Reassurance, diagnosing the underlying cause and symptom relief are common reasons for consultation.

History of presenting complaint
- **Quality of life.** Allow the patient time to tell you about their symptoms in their own words, and how they affect day-to-day life.
- **Current symptoms.** Ask which symptoms are most bothersome. When did the problems start? How did symptoms progress?
- **Cough.** Cough is often dry and persistent in lung cancer, whereas sputum production and response to antibiotic therapy indicate respiratory infection.
- **Chest and shoulder pain.** These may be caused by bony metastases or by a pressure effect of the tumour on adjacent nerves.
- **Shortness of breath.** Gradually worsening shortness of breath may also be caused by nonmalignant causes, such as heart failure or anaemia. Stridor may indicate compression of the trachea or larger central airways.
- **Haemoptysis.** Is any blood being coughed up? Ask for details about amount and appearance.
- **General symptoms.** Ask about weight loss, loss of appetite, tiredness, malaise, swollen lymph nodes, sweats and fevers, which are all indicative of cancer, especially if chronic and progressive.
- **Metastases.** Ask about bone pain and pathological fractures, which indicate bony metastasis. Neurological symptoms, headache, nausea, vomiting and personality changes can occur if the brain is affected. Right upper quadrant pain and jaundice may indicate liver metastases.

Past and current medical problems
- **Significant past illnesses.** Ask about chronic conditions that might affect prognosis, such as chronic lung problems (e.g. asthma, COPD, interstitial lung disease), diabetes and CVD.

Medication
- **Analgesics.** Have these been taken? Is any pain being controlled? Are there any adverse effects?

Allergies
- **Antibiotics.** Check for any allergies to antibiotics in case these are needed to treat infection.

Family history
- **Lung cancer.** There is an increased risk of lung cancer if there is a positive family history in first-degree relatives.

Social history
- **Home.** Has home life been affected by any symptoms? Are there any dependants? If lung cancer is likely, is there someone at home who is supportive and can help with care should the situation deteriorate?
- **Work.** Ask about exposures to relevant substances, such as toxic dusts and asbestos.

Alcohol, smoking and recreational drugs
- **Alcohol.** Explore past and current alcohol consumption.
- **Smoking.** Ask for a detailed smoking history, particularly in people over 40 years of age. Record past and current smoking status and calculate the number of pack years (= (number of cigarettes smoked per day × number of years smoked)/20).

Review of previous investigations
- **Full blood count.** Thrombocytosis is associated with lung cancer. Look for signs of anaemia.
- **Inflammatory markers.** Raised plasma viscosity or CRP may be found in chest infection and cancer.
- **Chest X-ray.** Check for pleural effusion or slowly resolving consolidation. Nearly a quarter of chest X-rays requested from primary care in lung cancer patients will be negative.
- **Lung function tests.** These may become abnormal in underlying lung cancer.

Examination

General
- **General condition.** Does the patient look unwell? Pallor and cachexia suggest serious underlying disease.
- **Gait and balance.** Consider brain metastases if gait is unsteady.
- **Mental state.** Brain metastases can cause changes in personality or memory.

Vital signs
- **Temperature.** Fever suggests infection but may also be raised in cancer.
- **Pulse.** Tachycardia indicates infection, or possibly heart failure, if suggested by the history. New-onset atrial fibrillation may occur in lung cancer.
- **Respiratory rate.** Significant tachypnoea suggests serious underlying disease or anxiety.

Head and neck
- **Raised JVP.** A fixed, raised JVP associated with a swelling of the head and neck indicates superior vena cava obstruction (late sign).
- **Throat.** Inspect the mouth and throat carefully if the patient presents with haemoptysis, as localised bleeding may be responsible.
- **Eyes.** Horner's syndrome suggests sympathetic nerve involvement (Pancoast tumour).

Chest
- **Lungs.** Chest signs may be absent, but check in particular for localised bronchial breathing, monophonic fixed wheeze and evidence of pleural effusion.

Abdomen
- **Liver.** Check for hepatomegaly, indicating possible liver metastases (difficult and often impossible to detect clinically).

Upper and lower limbs
- **Finger clubbing.** This may point towards lung cancer, but can have other respiratory and liver causes.
- **Neurology.** Check tone, power, sensation, reflexes and coordination if you suspect central nervous system (CNS) involvement.

Key references and further reading

1. Hamilton W, Sharp D. Diagnosis of lung cancer in primary care: a structured review. *Fam Pract* 2004;21:605–611.
2. National Institute for Health and Care Excellence (NICE). Lung cancer: diagnosis and management. NICE guidelines [CG121]. April 2011. Available from: http://www.nice.org.uk/guidance/cg121 (last accessed 29 April 2016).
3. National Institute for Health and Care Excellence (NICE). Lung cancer – suspected. Clinical Knowledge Summaries. 2012. Available from: http://cks.nice.org.uk/lung-cancer-suspected (last accessed 29 April 2016).
4. Patient UK. Lung malignancy. Available from: http://patient.info/education/lung-malignancy (last accessed 29 April 2016).
5. Stapley S, Sharp D, Hamilton W. Negative chest X-rays in primary care patients with lung cancer. *Br J Gen Pract* 2006;56:570–573.

Asthma

Key thoughts

Practical points

- **Diagnosis.** Asthma is common and can affect the quality of life considerably. Severe cases should be regarded as medical emergencies and are life-threatening. No single symptom or sign is diagnostic of asthma. Try to differentiate between intrinsic (later onset, not allergic, negative family history) and extrinsic (younger, allergic, positive family history) asthma.
- **Prognosis.** Assess the severity of asthma and the need for urgent action.

Differential diagnosis

- Postviral hyperreactivity.
- COPD.
- Lung cancer.
- Foreign body.
- Post-tracheostomy obstruction.
- Pneumothorax.
- Bronchiectasis.
- Cystic fibrosis.
- Left ventricular failure ('cardiac asthma').

Important risk factors

- Personal or family history of asthma or atopy.
- Smoking.
- Exposure to precipitating factors (10% of asthma has an occupational trigger).
- Viral infections in early childhood.
- Obesity.
- Inner-city environment.
- Socioeconomic deprivation.
- Learning difficulties.
- Nonadherence to treatment or monitoring.
- Mental illness.
- Social isolation.
- Severe stress.

RED FLAGS

- Inability to talk in full sentences
- Tachycardia

The 10-Minute Clinical Assessment, Second Edition. Knut Schroeder.
© 2017 John Wiley & Sons, Ltd. Published 2017 by John Wiley & Sons, Ltd.

- Tachypnoea
- Severely reduced peak flow (<50% recent best)
- Cyanosis
- Silent chest
- Hypotension
- Bradycardia
- Confusion

History

Ideas, concerns and expectations

- **Ideas.** What is the patient's understanding of asthma? Ask what they most 'hate' about their asthma. Worries about adverse effects of inhalers are common. Asthma may also wrongly be seen as a benign condition without life-threatening potential.
- **Concerns.** Symptoms of asthma can be very frightening.
- **Expectations.** Why has the patient come to see you? Symptom control and formal diagnosis are common reasons for consultation in new-onset breathing problems. People often present because they have run out of medication and are suffering from deteriorating symptoms. Low expectations are common regarding asthma treatment, but good control is achievable for the majority of patients.

History of presenting complaint
- **Quality of life.** Allow time for patients to tell you about their asthma in their own words, and how it affects their lives (e.g. school, jobs around the house, work). Are there any activities that the patient cannot do at present?
- **Respiratory symptoms.** Find out which respiratory symptoms are present or happen during an attack, including wheeze, shortness of breath, chest tightness and cough. Nocturnal cough may be the only symptom, particularly in children. In acute asthma, there is bronchospasm with increased secretions.
- **Onset and progression.** Find out when symptoms started and how they have progressed. Variable diurnal respiratory symptoms, such as wheeze and cough, suggest asthma rather than COPD. Peak flow dips naturally overnight, and the symptoms of asthma are often worse at night or early in the morning.
- **Severity.** Asthma can be life-threatening. Symptoms of severe asthma include the inability to talk in full sentences and severe breathlessness. Symptoms at night indicate more severe disease. Are there any problems with sleep? Has the patient ever been admitted to hospital because of asthma?
- **Intrinsic and extrinsic asthma.** Extrinsic asthma has identifiable triggers, classically starts in childhood and is associated with atopy and a positive family history. Intrinsic asthma, in contrast, has no specific triggers, typically starts in middle age, is not linked with atopy and has a negative family history.

- **Precipitating factors.** Ask about exercise, pets, stress, viral infections, drugs, occupational exposures, pollution, cigarette smoke and household allergens. Cold air may also bring on symptoms of asthma, but also consider angina if there is associated chest pain. Exacerbations may be seasonal at times of high pollen exposure. Consider work-related causes if symptoms improve at weekends or during holidays (10% of asthma).
- **Atopy.** Asthma is commonly associated with other atopic conditions, such as eczema, hay fever, urticaria and a general tendency to allergies.
- **Self-management plan.** In established asthma, has the patient discussed and agreed to a self-management plan with a health professional in the past? Has there been regular follow-up to monitor response to treatment and inhaler technique?
- **Urinary symptoms.** Chronic cough may cause urinary incontinence, which can be more troublesome than the cough itself. Be aware that patients may be too embarrassed to mention this unless asked.

Past and current medical problems
- **Chronic conditions.** Ask about any chronic conditions that might complicate management, such as diabetes and CVD.
- **Glaucoma.** Topical beta blockers used in glaucoma may exacerbate asthma.
- **Immunisation.** Check whether the patient has been immunised against influenza and pneumococcus.

Medication
- **Inhalers.** Is the patient already being prescribed inhalers? Find out which ones are being used and obtain details about prescribed doses and frequencies. How often are 'relievers' such as salbutamol being used? How often does the patient forget to take the inhalers – particularly 'preventers' such as inhaled steroids? Ask about the effectiveness of bronchodilators and inhaled steroids. Do they improve the quality of life? Does treatment need stepping up or down?
- **Drugs affecting asthma.** Certain drugs may exacerbate asthma. Ask in particular about beta blockers, aspirin and other NSAIDs. Angeotensin-converting enzyme (ACE) inhibitors may cause cough. Some drugs can cause pulmonary fibrosis (e.g. amiodarone, methotrexate).
- **Steroids.** Have courses of oral steroids been needed in the past? A therapeutic trial of steroids or bronchodilators can be a useful diagnostic tool.

Allergies
- **Antibiotics.** Ask about any allergies to antibiotics that may be needed for the treatment of infective exacerbations.

Family history
- **Atopy and asthma.** Ask about a family history of asthma and other atopic conditions.

Social history
- **Home.** How has home life been affected by the symptoms? Which activities are now limited? Are there any problems during exercise or sex?
- **Work.** Has work been affected by asthma? Has any income been lost? If relevant, ask about exposure to dust and volatile chemicals, which may cause or exacerbate symptoms.

Alcohol, smoking and recreational drugs
- **Smoking.** Consider COPD if there is a long smoking history. Smoking can exacerbate asthma. Also consider passive smoking. Record past and current smoking status and calculate the number of pack years ((number of cigarettes smoked per day × number of years smoked)/20). Has smoking-cessation advice been offered?

Review of previous investigations
- **Peak expiratory flow rate.** Look for previous results of peak-flow measurements. Is there a pattern or trend? A normal peak flow does not exclude asthma, and a low peak flow is not diagnostic, as it can be caused by COPD or poor technique. What are the patient's usual peak-flow readings? Have the readings shown reversibility on inhalation of beta agonists? Serial peak-flow readings can be useful in the diagnosis of asthma.
- **Spirometry.** Normal spirometry does not exclude asthma. A >15% improvement in forced expiratory volume in 1 second (FEV_1) following inhalation of a bronchodilator suggests reversibility.
- **Full blood count.** This is not needed routinely, but may show eosinophilia in asthma. Look for anaemia, which can also cause shortness of breath.
- **Chest X-ray.** This is not routinely performed and is usually normal in asthma. It may help to exclude other pathology if the diagnosis is unclear.

Examination

General
- **General condition.** Does the patient look unwell? Severe shortness of breath and inability to talk in full sentences suggest acute severe asthma. Pallor may suggest anaemia, which can also cause breathlessness. A normal physical examination does not exclude asthma. Is there obvious cyanosis?
- **Inhaler technique.** Unless the patient is acutely unwell, use the opportunity to check inhaler technique. Poor technique, which is common, may be the main reason for lack of response to treatment.
- **Peak flow.** Measurement of peak flow will help assess the degree of airflow limitation.

Vital signs
- **Temperature.** Consider respiratory infection if there is a fever.

- **Pulse.** Tachycardia suggests severe asthma or infection. In life-threatening asthma, there may be bradycardia. Tachycardia may also be caused by treatment with beta agonists.
- **Blood pressure.** This will usually be normal, but may be raised in severe asthma. Consider life-threatening asthma if there is hypotension.
- **Respiratory rate.** Tachypnoea suggests severe disease and may be the result of severe airflow obstruction, infection or anxiety.

Chest
- **Lungs.** Check for any wheeze, although this will not always be present, as the clinical signs of asthma can be variable. In very severe asthma or emphysema, there may be no wheeze and air entry will be reduced ('silent chest'). Basal crackles suggest heart failure, whereas focal crackles may indicate chest infection.
- **Heart.** Check for any signs of heart failure, such as cardiomegaly or a fourth heart sound.

Bedside tests
- **Pulse oximetry.** This is useful in detecting hypoxia (SaO_2 <95%).

Key references and further reading
1. British Thoracic Society (BTC) and Scottish Intercollegiate Guidelines Network (SIGN). British guideline on the management of asthma: a national clinical guideline. Revised January 2012. Available from: https://www.brit-thoracic. org.uk/document-library/clinical-information/asthma/btssign-guideline-on-the -management-of-asthma/ (last accessed 29 April 2016).
2. National Institute for Health and Care Excellence (NICE). Lung cancer: diagnosis and treatment. NICE guidelines [CG24]. February 2005. Available from: http://www.nice.org.uk/guidance/cg24 (last accessed 29 April 2016).
3. National Institute for Health and Care Excellence (NICE). Asthma. Clinical Knowledge Summaries. 2013. Available from: http://cks.nice.org.uk/asthma (last accessed 29 April 2016).
4. Pinnock H, Shah R. BMJ masterclass for GPs: asthma. *BMJ* 2007;334:847–850.

Chronic obstructive pulmonary disease

Key thoughts

Practical points

- **Diagnosis.** Consider the diagnosis in current or previous smokers over 35 years of age complaining of chest symptoms such as breathlessness, cough, wheeze, sputum production and frequent winter 'bronchitis' without features of asthma. COPD may also be present even if there are no symptoms. Have a high index of suspicion if there is a positive smoking or family history.
- **Prognosis.** Assess severity to estimate prognosis and to help decide on an appropriate management plan. In patients with established COPD, a lot can be done to improve symptoms.

Differential diagnosis

- Asthma.
- Congestive heart failure.
- Interstitial lung disease.
- Lung cancer.
- Bronchiectasis.

Important risk factors

- Smoking.
- Exposure to occupational dusts and chemicals.

RED FLAGS

- Shortness of breath at rest or with minimal exertion
- Haemoptysis
- Weight loss
- Raised JVP
- Oedema
- Cor pulmonale
- Hypoxia
- Severely reduced exercise tolerance
- Depression
- Need for oxygen therapy, pulmonary rehabilitation or surgery
- Under 40 years of age or family history of alpha-1 antitrypsin deficiency
- Rapid decline in FEV_1

The 10-Minute Clinical Assessment, Second Edition. Knut Schroeder.
© 2017 John Wiley & Sons, Ltd. Published 2017 by John Wiley & Sons, Ltd.

History

Ideas, concerns and expectations

- **Ideas.** Many smokers wrongly believe that nothing can be done about their symptoms or that it is too late to stop smoking. Does the patient know what to do in an exacerbation of COPD?
- **Concerns.** Worries about lung cancer or the need for oxygen treatment are common. Many people will feel guilty about their smoking and may not present because they are afraid that they will be advised to stop.
- **Expectations.** Common reasons for consultation are worries about lung cancer and reduced exercise tolerance.

History of presenting complaint

- **Context.** Allow the patient time to tell you about their problem in their own words.
- **Quality of life.** How is quality of life being affected by the symptoms?
- **Respiratory symptoms.** Ask in particular about any combination of shortness of breath, wheeze, chest tightness, cough, sputum production, reduced exercise tolerance and recurrent chest infections. COPD may be asymptomatic and should be considered in every current or former smoker, especially if there is a family history of COPD. Nocturnal symptoms are more common in asthma. Orthopnoea may suggest heart failure rather than COPD. Consider bronchiectasis if there is copious sputum production in connection with frequent chest infections and a history of childhood chest infection. Interstitial lung disease is a possibility if there is dry cough and a history of connective tissue disease. Think of opportunistic infections if there are risk factors for immunosuppression and fever. Could symptoms be a result of TB? Ask about weight loss, haemoptysis and risk factors for TB.
- **Exercise tolerance.** Which activities are limited by the symptoms? Ask about exercise tolerance when walking on a flat surface as well as up stairs or hills. Is breathlessness present at rest?
- **Exacerbations.** How frequent are exacerbations, and what tends to trigger them? Have there been any hospital admissions for COPD in the past? During exacerbations, there is usually an increase in cough and sputum production, with a change in sputum volume and colour to yellow or green, as well as increased breathlessness.
- **Weight loss.** Weight loss is an under-recognised symptom in advanced COPD and may also indicate possible lung cancer.
- **Mental health.** Ask about any symptoms of anxiety or depression, which may complicate management of COPD and other chronic illnesses.
- **Pulmonary rehabilitation.** Pulmonary rehabilitation can be effective in improving quality of life, dyspnoea, exercise capacity and psychological problems. Has this ever been offered to the patient?

Past and current medical problems

- **Significant past illnesses.** Ask about any other acute and chronic medical problems which might affect prognosis or management – in particular, other chronic lung problems, diabetes and CVD. Consider heart failure if there is a history of ischaemic heart disease.
- **Atopic predisposition.** Asthma is more likely if there is a history of eczema, urticaria or hay fever.
- **Immunisation status.** Check whether the patient has been immunised against influenza and pneumococcus.

Medication

- **Inhalers.** Ask about which inhalers are currently being prescribed (e.g. short- and long-acting beta$_2$ agonists, anticholinergics, steroids) and obtain details of doses and frequencies.
- **Theophylline.** This may be added in moderate to severe COPD that is not controlled with inhalers alone. There is a need to monitor plasma levels and drug interactions.
- **Antibiotics.** Have these been given lately for treatment of an acute exacerbation? Has a 'rescue' pack been considered for use at home in case of an infective exacerbation?
- **Steroids.** These are used for the management of acute exacerbations. Maintenance use of oral steroid therapy is not recommended, apart from in selected advanced cases in which steroids cannot be withdrawn after an acute exacerbation. Have bone protection and a home rescue pack been considered?
- **Methotrexate and amiodarone.** These drugs may cause interstitial lung disease, which can sometimes present in a similar way to COPD.

Allergies

- **Antibiotics.** Ask about allergies to any antibiotics that might need to be prescribed for infective exacerbations.

Family history

- **Asthma.** Asthma is more likely than COPD if there is a positive family history of asthma. Consider alpha$_1$-antitrypsin deficiency in rare cases if there is a family history or early onset of COPD.

Social history

- **Work.** Ask about previous and current exposures to dusts and chemicals that might cause respiratory problems. Have any days been missed at work due to the disease? Have there been any financial implications?
- **Home.** Is there any support at home? Have relationships with a partner and other people been affected? Are there any problems or worries with regard to sex?

- **Exercise and diet.** Has advice about diet and exercise been offered to obese people and to those with unhealthy lifestyles?

Alcohol, smoking and recreational drugs
- **Smoking.** Record past and current smoking status and calculate the number of pack years (= (number of cigarettes smoked per day $\times$ number of years smoked)/20). In a non-smoker, asthma is a more likely diagnosis. Has smoking cessation advice been offered?

Review of previous investigations
- **Spirometry.** Confirmation of airflow obstruction is needed to confirm the diagnosis of COPD, and spirometry is required in all patients in whom the diagnosis is suspected. Spirometry will also help estimate the severity of COPD and allows monitoring of changes over time, as well as of treatment effects. In COPD, FEV_1 is <80% of the predicted value, and the FEV_1/FVC is <70% of that predicted (see box). Reversibility testing may help distinguish between COPD and asthma if the diagnosis is genuinely unclear.
- **Chest X-ray.** This can help distinguish between COPD, lung cancer, interstitial lung disease and heart failure.
- **Peak-flow monitoring.** This will help to identify fluctuations of peak-flow readings, which might indicate asthma rather than COPD.
- **Full blood count.** Raised haemoglobin is likely to be caused by secondary polycythaemia in chronic hypoxia. Conversely, undiagnosed anaemia may be the cause of breathlessness and should be excluded. There may be a raised white cell count in infection. Eosinophilia may occur in asthma.
- **ECG.** This may be abnormal in cor pulmonale and heart failure.
- **Echocardiogram.** This may help confirm heart failure if the diagnosis is in doubt and will detect valve lesions such as tricuspid valve incompetence as a result of pulmonary hypertension and cor pulmonale. Right atrial and ventricular hypertrophy may also be visible, indirectly giving some indication of raised pulmonary artery pressure.
- **Alpha$_1$ antitrypsin.** This should be measured if COPD begins at a young age or if there is a positive family history to check for deficiency (rare).
- **Arterial blood gases.** These may be useful if resting oxygen saturation is <92% or, if appropriate, in the assessment of home or short-burst ambulatory oxygen therapy.

SEVERITY OF COPD (NICE)

- 50–80% predicted FEV_1 = mild
- 30–50% predicted FEV_1 = moderate
- <30% predicted FEV_1 = severe

Examination

General

- **General condition.** Physical examination can be entirely normal in mild disease. Cachexia and muscle wasting may indicate advanced disease or concurrent lung cancer.
- **Weight and height.** Measure weight and height to calculate body mass index (BMI), particularly if the patient appears underweight.
- **Muscle wasting.** Muscle wasting is common in COPD.
- **Cyanosis.** Look for peripheral and central cyanosis.
- **Breathing.** Pursed-lip breathing may be present in emphysema. Look out for use of accessory muscles and paradoxical movement of the lower ribs. Is there an audible wheeze? All these signs may be found in COPD but also with other chronic respiratory conditions.
- **Posture.** Severe kyphoscoliosis or obesity may lead to restrictive lung dysfunction.
- **Inhaler technique.** Take the opportunity to check inhaler technique – poor inhaler technique may be the main cause for treatment failure!
- **Peak flow.** Measurement of peak flow will help assess the degree of airflow limitation.

Vital signs

- **Temperature.** A fever may suggest infection, although a normal temperature does not rule this out.
- **Pulse.** Tachycardia may indicate infection, heart failure or significant hypoxia.
- **Respiratory rate.** Tachypnoea at rest indicates infection, more advanced disease, hypoxia or other underlying pathology.

Skin

- **Skin thickness.** Thin, paper-like skin and purpura is a side effect of long-term steroid use.

Head and neck

- **JVP.** If found to be raised, this may suggest development of cor pulmonale.

Upper limbs

- **Finger clubbing.** This is not a typical feature of COPD. If present, search for potential causes, such as bronchiectasis, lung cancer or idiopathic pulmonary fibrosis.

Chest

- **Hyperinflation.** A hyperinflated chest suggests emphysema. Look out for any paradoxical movement of the lower ribs. The apex beat may be absent on palpation, with loss of cardiac dullness on percussion.

- **Lungs.** Wheeze or quiet breath sounds are common in COPD. Fine basal crackles may suggest heart failure or, if more widespread, interstitial lung disease. Coarse crackles may indicate bronchiectasis.
- **Heart sounds.** Listen for loud P_2 heart sound, which may indicate cor pulmonale due to pulmonary hypertension. An early systolic murmur may be caused by tricuspid regurgitation.

Abdomen
- **Hepatomegaly.** The liver may be enlarged as a result of cor pulmonale.

Lower limbs
- **Peripheral oedema.** Pitting oedema may be present if there is cor pulmonale.

Bedside tests
- **Pulse oximetry.** Measure oxygen saturation to detect hypoxia due to advanced disease or polycythaemia and to assess the need for long-term O_2 therapy.

Key references and further reading
1. Currie GP, Legge JS. ABC of chronic obstructive pulmonary disease: diagnosis. *BMJ* 2006;332:1261–1263.
2. Fletcher CM, Elmes PC, Fairbairn AS, Wood CH. Significance of respiratory symptoms and the diagnosis of chronic bronchitis in a working population. *BMJ* 1959;2:257–266.
3. National Institute for Health and Care Excellence (NICE). Chronic obstructive pulmonary disease in over 16s: diagnosis and management. NICE guidelines [CG101]. June 2010. Available from: http://www.nice.org.uk/guidance/cg101 (last accessed 29 April 2016).

Suspected pneumonia

Key thoughts

Practical points

- **Diagnosis.** Spotting the early signs of pneumonia can be challenging and may require a high index of suspicion. Symptoms and signs can be nonspecific, especially in the elderly.
- **Prognosis.** Appropriate and timely treatment can reduce the need for hospital admission. Pneumonia may be a presenting feature of lung cancer, particularly in people at risk.

Differential diagnosis

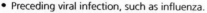

- Viral upper respiratory tract infection.
- COPD.
- Asthma.
- Left ventricular failure.
- Pulmonary embolism.
- Bronchiectasis.
- Lung cancer.
- Lung abscess.

Important risk factors

- Preceding viral infection, such as influenza.
- Young children and the elderly (age >65 years).
- Intravenous drug abuse.
- Hospital admission.
- Swallowing problems and aspiration.
- Diabetes.
- CVD.

RED FLAGS

- Tachypnoea <30 breaths per minute
- Raised urea >7 mmol/l
- Hypotension
- Confusion
- Immunosuppression
- Presence of risk factors

The 10-Minute Clinical Assessment, Second Edition. Knut Schroeder.
© 2017 John Wiley & Sons, Ltd. Published 2017 by John Wiley & Sons, Ltd.

History

Ideas, concerns and expectations
- **Ideas.** What does the patient believe is causing the symptoms?
- **Concerns.** Worries about possible underlying lung cancer are common. Many older patients think that pneumonia will be their final illness.
- **Expectations.** Why has the patient come to see you? Help with relieving shortness of breath or cough is a common reason for presentation.

History of presenting complaint
- **Context.** Allow the patient time to tell you about their chest symptoms in their own words.
- **Quality of life.** How do symptoms affect quality of life and activities of daily living?
- **Onset and progression.** Pneumonia often develops gradually over a few days. Rapidly worsening symptoms will require more urgent action.
- **Respiratory symptoms.** Symptoms suggestive of pneumonia include productive cough, sputum, shortness of breath and pleuritic chest pain.
- **Symptoms of cardiac disease.** Consider cardiac complications if there is central chest pain associated with nausea, vomiting and sweating.
- **Systemic symptoms.** Fever, malaise, sweating, shivers, lethargy and aches and pains are often present, but they may be absent in the elderly and those on steroids. Consider the possibility of lung cancer if these symptoms were present prior to the acute illness.
- **Additional unexplored issues.** Always ask the patient if there are any other problems or issues that you have not covered but which might be important.

Past and current medical problems
- **Lung disease.** Patients with underlying lung disease, such as COPD or lung cancer, are at increased risk of complications.
- **Significant past illnesses.** Diabetes, CVD and dementia may worsen the prognosis in patients with pneumonia.
- **Immunosuppression.** Always consider the possibility of chest infection in immunocompromised patients, including those with human immunodeficiency virus (HIV) infection.

Medication
- **Antibiotics.** Have any antibiotics already been used for this episode – either leftover tablets from a previous infection or new ones prescribed by another practitioner?
- **Statins.** Consider stopping statins during treatment with macrolide antibiotics such as erythromycin, due to potential interaction.

Allergies
- **Antibiotics.** Ask about any allergies to antibiotics.

Social history
- **Home.** Can the patient safely be managed in the community? What is their current level of independence? Are any carers involved?

Alcohol, smoking and recreational drugs
- **Alcohol.** Pneumonia is more common in people with alcohol problems.
- **Smoking.** Smoking increases the risk of underlying lung cancer and COPD, as well as of cardiovascular problems. Record past and current smoking status and calculate the number of pack years (= (number of cigarettes smoked per day × number of years smoked)/20).
- **Recreational drugs.** Consider chest infection and the possibility of lung abscess in intravenous drugs users.

Review of previous investigations
- **Full blood count.** A raised white cell count with neutrophilia will indicate infection. Anaemia poses a risk factor for cardiovascular complications and may contribute to the development of shortness of breath.
- **Inflammatory markers.** Plasma viscosity and CRP may be raised in infection or malignancy.
- **Urea and electrolytes.** A raised urea >7 mmol/l is a poor prognostic factor.
- **Chest X-ray.** This may show signs of consolidation. Look for bilateral or multi-lobe involvement, which indicates more severe disease.

Examination

General
- **General condition.** Does the patient look unwell? Cachexia, pallor, cyanosis and wasting may suggest underlying cancer, poor nutrition or other serious disease.
- **Mental state.** New-onset confusion and reduced cognition indicate severe disease.
- **Breathing.** Is there breathlessness at rest?

Vital signs
- **Temperature.** A raised temperature suggests infection, but normal temperature does not rule out pneumonia, particularly in the elderly.
- **Pulse.** Tachycardia may be caused by raised temperature and, if severe (>120 beats per minute), may indicate impending cardiorespiratory collapse.
- **Blood pressure.** Hypotension with a systolic blood pressure <90 mmHg or diastolic <60 mmHg indicates severe disease, impending shock and poor prognosis.
- **Respiratory rate.** Tachypnoea with a respiratory rate of >30 breaths per minute is a useful sign, indicating significant chest infection.

Chest

- **Lungs.** Chest expansion may be reduced on the affected side. Classic signs of pneumonia include focal crackles, tactile vocal fremitus and dullness on percussion. A pleural friction rub may be present. Elderly or immunocompromised patients may present without these signs even in relatively severe cases. Bilateral fine basal crackles may suggest heart failure, which may be precipitated or exacerbated by pneumonia.

Bedside tests

- **Pulse oximetry or arterial blood gases.** Hypoxaemia (SaO_2 < 92% or PaO_2 < 8 kPa), regardless of inspired oxygen concentration, indicates severe illness.

CRB score

- **Calculate score.** When you make a clinical diagnosis of community-acquired pneumonia, determine whether the patient is at low, intermediate or high risk of death using the CRB65 score (Lim et al 2003):
  - **Confusion.** Abbreviated Mental Test score ≤8 or new disorientation in person, place or time.
  - **Respiratory rate.** Raised respiratory rate at 30 breaths per minute or more.
  - **Blood pressure.** Diastolic blood pressure 60 mmHg or less or systolic blood pressure <90 mmHg.
  - **Age.** ≥65 years.
  - **Stratification.** 0 = low risk (<1% mortality risk), 1 or 2 = intermediate risk (1–10% mortality risk), 3 or 4 = high risk (>10% mortality risk).

Key references and further reading

1. British Thoracic Society. Guidelines for the management of community-acquired pneumonia in adults: update 2009. *Thorax* 2009;64:iii1–iii55.
2. Lim WS, van der Eerden MM, Laing R et al. Defining community-acquired pneumonia severity on presentation to hospital: an international derivation and validation study. *Thorax* 2003;58:377–382.
3. Metlay JP, Kapoor WN, Fine MJ. Does this patient have community-acquired pneumonia? Diagnosing pneumonia by history and physical examination. *JAMA* 1997;278:1440–1445.
4. National Institute for Health and Care Excellence (NICE). Pneumonia in adults: diagnosis and management. NICE guidelines [CG191]. December 2014. Available from: http://www.nice.org.uk/guidance/cg191 (last accessed 29 April 2016).
5. Wipf JE, Lipsky BA, Hirschmann JV et al. Diagnosing pneumonia by physical examination: relevant or relic? *Arch Intern Med* 1999;159:1082–1087.

Pleural effusion

Key thoughts

Practical points

- **Diagnosis.** A pleural effusion may be a chance finding in a patient presenting with shortness of breath. Usually, pleural effusions have to be fairly large in order to cause symptoms, and smaller effusions may be completely asymptomatic.
- **Prognosis.** The majority of causes of pleural effusion are relatively serious and will need further investigation.

Possible causes

- **Cardiac.** Left ventricular failure or mitral stenosis (rare), myocardial infarction (Dressler's syndrome).
- **Lung.** Parapneumonic effusion, malignancy, pulmonary infarction, TB, empyema.
- **Inflammatory.** Rheumatoid arthritis, autoimmune disease.
- **Other.** Hypoalbuminaemia, liver cirrhosis, peritoneal dialysis, breast cancer, hypothyroidism, ovarian hyperstimulation, pancreatitis, drugs, Meig's syndrome, postcoronary artery bypass graft.

Risk factors

- Smoking.
- Age.
- Occupational exposures (especially asbestos).
- Known systemic disease.
- TB.

RED FLAGS

- Severe breathlessness
- Systemic symptoms such as fever, night sweats and weight loss
- Past history of malignancy
- Risk factors for thromboembolism

History

Ideas, concerns and expectations

- **Ideas.** Small effusions may go unnoticed by the patient, who may think that nothing is wrong.

The 10-Minute Clinical Assessment, Second Edition. Knut Schroeder.
© 2017 John Wiley & Sons, Ltd. Published 2017 by John Wiley & Sons, Ltd.

- **Concerns.** Shortness of breath can be extremely frightening, and there may be fears about underlying cancer or heart disease.
- **Expectations.** Symptomatic relief and the desire to explain shortness of breath are common reasons for presentation.

History of presenting complaint
- **Context.** Allow the patient time to tell you about their symptoms in their own words.
- **Quality of life.** How do symptoms affect quality of life and activities of daily living?
- **Onset and progression.** Consider infection, cardiac causes or pulmonary embolus if onset is acute. Gradual onset is more likely with underlying malignancy, heart failure or TB.
- **Respiratory symptoms.** Pleural conditions may be asymptomatic. Breathlessness is an early symptom that often develops subacutely and gets progressively worse. Cough, sputum and haemoptysis may suggest underlying infection or malignancy. Ask about pleuritic chest pain, which suggests inflammation (e.g. infection, pulmonary embolism). If due to pulmonary embolism, symptoms will often appear worse than expected based on the size of the effusion, because of associated hypoxia.
- **Cardiac symptoms.** Are there any symptoms suggesting cardiac disease? Ask about chest pain, leg oedema, tiredness and underlying risk factors such as hypercholesterolaemia or diabetes.
- **Constitutional symptoms.** Ask about weight loss, loss of appetite, tiredness, night sweats and fevers, which may suggest serious underlying illness, such as malignancy or TB. Weight may have increased due to heart failure (fluid retention).
- **Associated symptoms.** Leg swelling may suggest deep venous thrombosis and subsequent pulmonary embolism.

Past and current medical problems
- **Chronic disease.** Check for CVD, liver failure, autoimmune conditions and renal disease, all of which may lead to pleural effusion.
- **Trauma.** Trauma may result in haemorrhagic effusions or empyema.
- **Infertility treatment.** Ovarian hyperstimulation as part of fertility treatment may present with pleural effusion.

Medication
- **Drugs causing pleural effusions.** Nitrofurantoin, phenytoin, amiodarone and methotrexate may all lead to pleural effusions. A useful website is www.pneumotox.com, which provides information on drug-induced lung conditions.
- **Antibiotics.** Have any antibiotics been taken to treat presumed infection?

Allergies
- **Antibiotics.** Ask about allergies to any antibiotics that may be needed to treat underlying infection.
- **NSAIDs.** Check for any allergies or contraindications to NSAIDs (e.g. asthma or peptic ulcer), which may need to be used for analgesia and to reduce inflammation. NSAIDs can also exacerbate heart failure and thereby contribute to the development of pleural effusions.

Social history
- **Home.** How has home life been affected? Which activities have been limited by symptoms?
- **Work.** Has work been affected? Have there been any exposures to toxic substances (especially asbestos) which might be implicated in the development of pleural effusion?
- **Travel.** Has there been any recent travel to an area with high prevalence of TB? Have there been any TB contacts?

Alcohol, smoking and recreational drugs
- **Alcohol.** Liver cirrhosis may lead to hypoalbuminaemia and can cause pleural effusion.
- **Smoking.** A positive smoking history increases the risk of underlying lung cancer. Record past and current smoking status and calculate the number of pack years (= (number of cigarettes smoked per day × number of years smoked)/20).

Review of previous investigations
- **Chest radiography**. Pleural effusions >200 ml will usually be visible on a plain chest X-ray. There may also be an indication of the underlying cause, such as heart failure, cardiomegaly, malignancy or pneumonia. Calcified pleural plaques indicate asbestos exposure and may therefore be seen in mesothelioma. Look out for apical and miliary opacities of TB.
- **Ultrasound**. This may help in localising the site of the effusion and the best spot for aspiration.
- **Pleural aspiration**. Has a pleural fluid sample been obtained and analysed? Straw-coloured fluid can be found in pneumonia, malignancy and heart failure. Bloodstained fluid indicates trauma, malignancy or infarction. Purulent fluid suggests empyema. Consider anaerobic infection if the fluid has an offensive smell.
- **Full blood count.** Anaemia may suggest underlying chronic disease or malignancy. A raised white cell count with neutrophilia indicates infection.
- **Inflammatory markers.** Raised plasma viscosity or CRP may indicate infection, inflammation or malignancy.
- **Creatinine and electrolytes.** These are useful in establishing renal function. Sodium levels may be low in heart failure.
- **Liver function tests.** These may be abnormal and show hypoalbuminaemia in alcoholic liver disease and cirrhosis.

Examination

General
- **General condition.** Does the patient look unwell or very breathless? Is there cyanosis or pallor, suggesting serious underlying disease?

Vital signs
- **Temperature.** A raised temperature is suggestive of infection, severe inflammation or pulmonary embolus.
- **Pulse.** Tachycardia may be caused by infection, pain, pulmonary embolus or heart failure.
- **Blood pressure.** This will usually be normal. Check for postural hypotension, which indicates intravascular hypovolaemia.
- **Respiratory rate.** Tachypnoea will usually be present in significant pleural effusions.

Head and neck
- **Trachea.** The trachea may be deviated to the contralateral side in pleural effusion, whereas a collapsed lung causes deviation to the affected side.
- **Lymphadenopathy.** Check for enlarged lymph nodes (infection, malignancy, TB).

Upper limbs
- **Hands.** Check for tar staining, finger clubbing and evidence of rheumatoid arthritis.

Chest
- **Heart.** Search for signs of heart failure, such as a displaced apex beat or a fourth heart sound.
- **Lungs.** There is usually reduced chest expansion on the affected side. Check for stony dull percussion and diminished or absent breath sounds. Localised wheeze or crackles may indicate infection or malignancy. Vocal and tactile fremitus may be reduced.

Abdomen
- **Masses.** Check for any intra-abdominal masses, liver enlargement or ascites if there is a possibility of malignancy.

Lower limbs
- **Peripheral oedema.** This suggests a transudative cause, such as hypoalbuminaemia or heart failure.

Key references and further reading
1. British Thoracic Society Pleural Disease Guideline Group. BTS pleural disease guideline. *Thorax* 2010;65(Suppl. 2):ii32–ii40.
2. Light RW. Pleural effusion. *N Engl J Med* 2002;346:1971–1977.
3. Wong CL, Holroyd-Leduc J, Straus SE. The rational clinical examination: does this patient have a pleural effusion? *JAMA* 2009;301:309–317.

Pulmonary embolism

Key thoughts

Practical points
- **Diagnosis.** Diagnosing pulmonary embolism can be difficult. No symptom or sign is diagnostic, and diagnosis is often made late or missed, particularly if symptoms are mild. It can be particularly difficult to recognise pulmonary embolism in patients with underlying respiratory conditions.
- **Prognosis.** Pulmonary embolism has a high mortality if untreated, and is a common cause of death after elective surgery or childbirth.

Differential diagnosis
- Chest infection.
- Pneumothorax.
- Asthma.
- COPD.
- Myocardial infarction.
- Rare causes such as air embolism, amniotic fluid embolism and fat embolism.

Important risk factors
- Immobilisation for more than 3 days or surgery in the previous 4 weeks.
- Previous deep vein thrombosis or pulmonary embolism.
- Dehydration.
- Abdominal and other major surgery.
- Lower-limb orthopaedic operations.
- Long-distance travel, particularly in people with additional risk factors.
- Thrombophilia and other haematological disorders.
- Pregnancy or birth within the past 6 weeks.
- Malignancy.
- Oestrogens.

RED FLAGS

- Altered level of consciousness
- Haemoptysis
- Systolic blood pressure <90 mmHg
- Heart rate >130 beats per minute
- Respiratory rate >25 breaths per minute
- Oxygen saturation <91%
- Temperature <35 °C

The 10-Minute Clinical Assessment, Second Edition. Knut Schroeder.
© 2017 John Wiley & Sons, Ltd. Published 2017 by John Wiley & Sons, Ltd.

- Presence of risk factors for or signs of thromboembolism
- An alternative diagnosis, such as another respiratory condition (e.g. pneumothorax, pneumonia, acute exacerbation of chronic lung disease), a cardiac cause (e.g. acute coronary syndrome, acute congestive heart failure, dissecting or rupturing aortic aneurysm, pericarditis), musculoskeletal chest pain, gastrooesophageal reflux disease or any cause of collapse.

History

Ideas, concerns and expectations
- **Ideas.** Patients will often not know about the link between deep venous thrombosis and pulmonary embolism.
- **Concerns.** Shortness of breath can be extremely frightening, and the patient may have a feeling of impending doom.
- **Expectations.** Common reasons for consultation include symptom relief and reaching a diagnosis.

History of presenting complaint
- **Context.** Unless patients are very unwell, allow them to tell you about their symptoms in their own words.
- **Quality.** How have symptoms affected day-to-day activities and quality of life?
- **Onset.** Pulmonary embolism often occurs acutely, but it may develop insidiously, with gradually worsening shortness of breath over weeks or months.
- **Respiratory symptoms.** Isolated shortness of breath and rapid breathing are the commonest presenting symptoms. The severity of symptoms depends on the extent to which the pulmonary vascular tree is affected. Pulmonary infarction may present with pleuritic chest pain, haemoptysis and cough. Symptoms of pulmonary embolism usually worsen on exertion and may not be apparent at rest. The absence of dyspnoea makes pulmonary embolism less likely.
- **Circulatory symptoms.** Massive pulmonary embolism may cause acute right heart failure and result in hypotension or circulatory collapse. In elderly patients with pre-existing heart or lung disease, even a small embolus can be serious and life-threatening.
- **Anxiety.** The symptoms of pulmonary embolus can be very frightening and can cause anxiety and resulting hyperventilation. It is easy to dismiss symptoms as related to anxiety when in fact the anxiety is related to the symptoms.
- **Risk factors.** Find out whether any of the risk factors listed at the start of the chapter are present, particularly if there has been unilateral painful leg swelling.

Past and current medical problems
- **Significant past illnesses.** Check for conditions that might affect prognosis, such as respiratory and cardiovascular conditions. Is there a history of a clotting disorder?

- **Operations and trauma.** Surgery and trauma are risk factors for pulmonary embolism.
- **Contraindications to oral anticoagulation.** Consider severe hypertension, peptic ulcers and pregnancy.

Medication
- **Oral contraceptive.** The oral contraceptive pill increases the risk of deep venous thrombosis and pulmonary embolus, particularly in connection with other risk factors, such as smoking and obesity.

Family history
- **Thrombophilia.** Is there a known family history of thrombophilia?

Social history
- **Home.** How has home life been affected by the symptoms?
- **Travel.** Has there been any recent long-distance travel?

Alcohol, smoking and recreational drugs
- **Smoking.** Smoking can contribute to the risk of developing a pulmonary embolus.

Review of previous investigations
- **D-dimer.** A negative test is useful for excluding pulmonary embolism. Near-patient testing kits are available for use outside hospital settings.
- **ECG.** Sinus tachycardia and nonspecific changes are common. Look for atrial fibrillation, right-bundle branch block, right-axis deviation and anterior T-wave inversion. In rare and severe cases, the $S_1Q_3T_3$ pattern may be seen with an S-wave in lead I and a Q-wave and T-wave inversion in lead III.
- **Chest X-ray.** This is often normal, but may show small effusions or linear atelectasis.
- **Leg ultrasound.** The majority of people with pulmonary embolus will have a recent history of deep venous thrombosis.
- **Arterial blood gases.** These can be normal but may show hypoxia and hypocapnia.

Examination

General
- **General condition.** Does the patient look unwell or cyanotic? Is there cardiorespiratory collapse?
- **Breathing.** Is the patient short of breath?

Vital signs
- **Temperature.** There may be a mild fever in pulmonary embolism.

- **Pulse.** Tachycardia with a heart rate >100 beats per minute is an important early sign, and the absence of tachycardia makes pulmonary embolus less likely.
- **Blood pressure.** Blood pressure may be raised due to anxiety or hypertension. Postural hypotension suggests circulatory impairment and impending shock.
- **Respiratory rate.** Tachypnoea >20 breaths per minute is usually present if there is underlying pulmonary embolism, but it may also be the result of anxiety or other causes.

Head and neck
- **JVP.** This may be raised, indicating right ventricular failure due to pulmonary hypertension.

Chest
- **Lungs.** Chest movements may be reduced as a result of pleural pain. Check for localising signs such as a pleural rub. There may be localised wheeze or crackles.
- **Heart.** There may be a loud pulmonary component to the second heart sound and splitting of the second heart sound. Check for atrial fibrillation.

Abdomen
- **Masses.** Check for any intra-abdominal masses, as cancer is a risk factor for thrombosis.

Lower limbs
- **Deep venous thrombosis.** Look for signs of deep venous thrombosis, such as unilateral leg swelling, venous dilation and deep calf tenderness.

Bedside tests
- **Pulse oximetry.** Hypoxia (O_2 saturation <95%) may suggest significant lung involvement, particularly in people with pre-existing lung disease. In young and healthy individuals, oxygen saturation may be normal at rest, but a drop in O_2 saturation on exertion can be a useful marker for pulmonary embolism.
- **Wells score:** If the patient is not severely ill (see Red Flags), assess the two-level PE Wells score to estimate the clinical probability of PE. Wells score >4 = PE likely (admit or arrange immediate CT pulmonary angiogram), Wells score ≤4 points = PE unlikely (arrange D-dimer test). For further management, see NICE (2015).
  - Clinical features of deep venous thrombosis: 1.5 points.
  - Heart rate >100 beats per minute: 1.5 points.
  - Immobilisation >3 days or surgery in previous 4 weeks: 1.5 points.
  - Previous deep venous thrombosis or pulmonary embolism: 1.5 points.
  - Haemoptysis: 1 point.
  - Cancer: 1 point.
  - Alternative diagnosis less likely: 3 points.

Key references and further reading

1. Chunilal SD, Eikelboom JW, Attia J et al. The rational clinical examination: does this patient have pulmonary embolism? *JAMA* 2003;290:2849–2858.

2. National Institute for Health and Care Excellence (NICE). Pulmonary embolism. Clinical Knowledge Summaries. 2015. Available from: http://cks.nice.org.uk/pulmonary-embolism (last accessed 29 April 2016).

3. Robinson G. Pulmonary embolism in hospital practice. *BMJ* 2006;332:156–160.

4. Task Force for the Diagnosis and Management of Acute Pulmonary Embolism of the European Society of Cardiology (ESC). Guidelines on the diagnosis and management of acute pulmonary embolism. *Eur Heart J* 2008:29:2276–2315.

5. Tillie-Leblond I, Marquette C-H, Perez T et al. Pulmonary embolism in patients with unexpected exacerbation of chronic obstructive pulmonary disease: prevalence and risk factors. *Ann Intern Med* 2006;144:390–396.

6. West J, Goodacre S, Sampson F. The value of clinical features in the diagnosis of acute pulmonary embolism: systematic review and meta-analysis. *QJM* 2007;100:763–769.

7. Writing Group for the Christopher Study Investigators. Effectiveness of managing suspected pulmonary embolism using an algorithm combining clinical probability, d-dimer testing, and computed tomography. *JAMA* 2006;295:172–179.

Endocrine and metabolic

Diabetes review

Key thoughts

Practical points
- **Diagnosis.** Symptoms of diabetes are often nonspecific, and a high index of suspicion is required for initial diagnosis. Good control of blood glucose levels reduces the risk of microvascular and macrovascular complications. Regular review is required and a number of issues need to be addressed at the follow-up appointment to ensure optimal care, including problems with glycaemic control, complications, overall health, lifestyle and quality of life.
- **Prognosis.** Long-term prognosis will depend on early identification and management of complications.

Exacerbating factors
- Acute illness.
- Emotional stress.
- Change of diet or activity.
- Medication change or nonadherence.
- Drugs, such as olanzapine, risperidone or steroids.

Important risk factors
- Increasing age, particularly in type 2 diabetes.
- Impaired glucose tolerance or impaired fasting glycaemia.
- Ethnicity (e.g. Afro-Caribbean).
- Family history of diabetes.
- Obesity.
- Polycystic ovary syndrome (PCOS).

RED FLAGS

- Cardiovascular disease (CVD), including cerebrovascular disease, hypertension and peripheral vascular disease
- End-organ damage, such as diabetic retinopathy and nephropathy
- Skin and soft-tissue infections
- Recurrent urinary tract infections
- Peripheral neuropathy
- Foot ulcers
- Diabetic ketoacidosis

The 10-Minute Clinical Assessment, Second Edition. Knut Schroeder.
© 2017 John Wiley & Sons, Ltd. Published 2017 by John Wiley & Sons, Ltd.

History

Ideas, concerns and expectations
- **Ideas.** What does the patient know about diabetes?
- **Concerns.** Lack of confidence about self-management of diabetes is common. Some people with diabetes show little concern about possible complications.
- **Expectations.** Common reasons for consultation are symptom control, reassurance and advice about management.

History of presenting complaint
- **Context.** Allow the patient time to tell you about their symptoms in their own words. How do they feel about being diagnosed with diabetes?
- **Quality of life.** What are the main effects on the quality of life? How is the patient coping with self-management?
- **Onset.** Symptoms of diabetes may be slow to develop and may go unnoticed for a long time. Is the patient aware of any triggers, such as infection or surgery? In people with established diabetes, has there been a change in diet?
- **Symptoms of hyperglycaemia.** Symptoms include thirst, polyuria, malaise, tiredness, recurrent infections, poor wound-healing, weight loss despite good appetite, abdominal pain, headaches, sudden mood changes, wound infections and blurred vision. If symptoms are present, diagnose diabetes if fasting plasma glucose is >7.0 mmol/l or if random plasma glucose is >11.1 mmol/l.
- **Hypoglycaemia.** If diabetes is already established, have there been any episodes of hypoglycaemia? If so, does the patient get any warning symptoms?
- **Diet.** Is the patient aware of dietary measures to improve diabetic control? Does the patient adhere to a healthy diet?
- **Exercise.** Ask about the amount and form of any current exercise routines.
- **Diabetic ketoacidosis.** Features are excessive thirst, nausea, vomiting, abdominal pain, dry skin and mucous membranes, blurred vision, tachypnoea and drowsiness. Patients with type 1 diabetes should be made aware of this medical emergency and should be given test strips for the detection of urinary ketones.
- **Pregnancy.** Is the patient pregnant or planning to have children? Good diabetic control during pregnancy is important in reducing the risk of pregnancy-related complications.

Complications of diabetes
- **Feet.** Ask about infections, ulcers and pain. Does the patient see a podiatrist? Is there any foot pain? Is footwear adequate?
- **Vision.** Ask about any problems with vision and the date of the most recent eye check. Be aware that rapid improvement in glycaemic control can cause short-term deterioration of diabetic eye disease.
- **Neurology.** Ask about numbness, reduced sensation (which may go unnoticed) and features of autonomic neuropathy.
- **Cardiovascular.** Ask about chest pain, shortness of breath and leg swelling.

- **Gastrointestinal tract.** Unexplained diarrhoea, particularly at night, may suggest automic neuropathy affecting the gut.
- **Bladder problems.** In adults with type 1 diabetes who have bladder-emptying problems, consider the possibility of autonomic neuropathy affecting the bladder.
- **Mental health.** All people with diabetes should be screened for depression.
- **Sexual function.** Erectile dysfunction is common and may not be mentioned by male patients unless prompted.

Past and current medical problems
- **Significant past illnesses.** Ask about cardiovascular risk factors such as previous myocardial infarction, hypertension, hyperlipidaemia and a history of transient ischaemic attack or stroke.

Medication
- **Diabetic medication.** Ask about insulin, biguanides, sulphonylureas and thiazolidinediones. Are there problems with injections? How often does the patient forget to take medication? Ask about any side effects. Is the patient coping with taking the medication?
- **CVD.** People with diabetes may need primary or secondary prevention of CVD. Check whether the patient is already taking aspirin, a beta blocker, angeotensin-converting enzyme (ACE) inhibitors, antihypertensives or a statin.
- **Glucogenic medication.** Check whether the patient is taking any medication which may increase blood sugar (e.g. olanzapine, risperidone or steroids).

Alcohol, smoking and recreational drugs
- **Alcohol.** Ask for details about past and present alcohol intake. Alcohol misuse can make good diabetic control much more difficult.
- **Smoking.** Check smoking status. People with diabetes who smoke are at much higher risk of CVD. Has smoking-cessation advice been offered?

Review of previous investigations
- **Haemoglobin A1c (HbA1c).** Check recent values of glycosylated haemoglobin to assess blood glucose control.
- **Urea and electrolytes.** Beware of pseudohyponatraemia in patients with significant hyperglycaemia (glucose >25 mmol/l).
- **Thyroid function.** There is a higher incidence of hypothyroidism in people with diabetes, and thyroid function should be checked annually.
- **Lipid profile.** Diabetic dyslipidaemia is particularly atherogenic, and early statin treatment is recommended.
- **Eye check.** Has there been a recent eye check for diabetic retinopathy?
- **Urine.** Microalbuminuria is currently the earliest marker of renal disease. Improved glycaemic control can reverse the onset of diabetic nephropathy.

Examination

General
- **General condition.** Does the patient look unwell?
- **Dehydration.** If the patient is unwell, then pale skin, lethargy, decreased skin turgor and dry mucosa suggest dehydration.
- **Height and weight.** Check these to estimate the body mass index (BMI) and so allow monitoring of any changes in weight.

Vital signs
- **Blood pressure.** Check for evidence of hypertension. Blood pressure should be maintained at below 130/80 mmHg.

Skin
- **Injection sites.** In patients on insulin, check injection sites for signs of lipoatrophy and lipodystrophy, as well as infection.

Head and neck
- **Eyes.** Look for xanthelasmata (hyperlipidaemia) around the eyes, early cataract formation and ophthalmoplegia. Check visual acuity. Inspect the retina for any diabetic changes (preferably with dilated eyes), unless this has already been done as part of a diabetic retinal-screening programme.
- **Carotids.** Listen for carotid bruits if the history suggests CVD.

Chest
- **Lungs.** Check for signs of infection, if indicated.
- **Heart.** Is there any clinical evidence of cardiomegaly? Check the heart rate and rhythm by auscultation, as atrial fibrillation (AF) may be present.

Abdomen
- **Liver.** Check for hepatomegaly (fatty infiltration).

Lower limbs
- **Pulses.** Check peripheral pulses and look for signs of peripheral vascular disease.
- **Sensation.** Check sensation using a 128 Hz tuning fork and pinprick with special tips or by probing with a 10 g nylon monofilament.
- **Reflexes.** Check ankle and knee reflexes.
- **Feet.** Inspect footwear for suitability. Look for signs of peripheral neuropathy and complications such as deformities, calluses and ulceration.

Bedside tests
- **Blood glucose.** Remember to check blood glucose in people with diabetes or those with unusual illness.

- **Urine dip test.** Check for proteinuria. A test positive for protein, blood and nitrite may suggest urinary tract infection. Microalbuminuria will not be detected by urine dipstick.

Key references and further reading

1. Diabetes UK. www.diabetes.org.uk.
2. Edmonds M, Foster A. ABC of wound healing: diabetic foot ulcers. *BMJ* 2006; 332:407–410.
3. National Institute for Health and Care Excellence (NICE). Type 2 diabetes. NICE guideline [CG66]. May 2008. Available from: http://www.nice.org.uk/guidance/cg66 (last accessed 29 April 2016).
4. National Institute for Health and Care Excellence (NICE). Type 1 diabetes in adults: diagnosis and management. NICE guidelines [NG17]. August 2015. Available from: http://www.nice.org.uk/guidance/ng17 (last accessed 29 April 2016).
5. Scottish Intercollegiate Guidelines Network (SIGN). Management of diabetes. Clinical guideline 116. March 2001. Available from: http://www.sign.ac.uk/pdf/sign116.pdf (last accessed 29 April 2016).

Obesity

Key thoughts

Practical points
- **Diagnosis.** Obesity is common and can lead to a variety of health problems. Identify any underlying causes and complications.
- **Prognosis.** Establish the severity of obesity and assess risk from complications.

Possible causes
- Poor diet.
- Lack of exercise.
- Endocrine (e.g. hypothyroidism, diabetes mellitus, Cushing's disease).
- PCOS.
- Genetic.
- Metabolic syndrome.

Complications
- CVD.
- Type 2 diabetes.
- Hyperlipidaemia.
- Endometrial or breast cancer.
- Fertility problems.
- Osteoarthritis.
- Psychological problems.

RED FLAGS

- Morbid obesity
- Severely reduced mobility
- Suicidal ideation
- Poor self-image
- Diabetes
- Cardiovascular complications

History

Ideas, concerns and expectations
- **Ideas.** In families where all the members are overweight, this may be considered either 'normal' or a 'taboo' subject. How does the patient feel about being overweight?

The 10-Minute Clinical Assessment, Second Edition. Knut Schroeder.
© 2017 John Wiley & Sons, Ltd. Published 2017 by John Wiley & Sons, Ltd.

- **Concerns.** Obese people may worry about having a heart attack or stroke, or that they will develop diabetes. Denial of health risks is common. People aware of the risks may be worried that they will have to make changes in their lifestyle in order to lose weight.
- **Expectations.** Why has the patient come to see you? Common reasons for consultation are a desire to lose weight and the need for help with complications (e.g. high blood pressure, joint problems). Hope for a 'quick fix' and unrealistic expectations about the target weight are common in people who want to lose weight. Many have unsuccessfully tried diets or exercise and request weight-loss medication.

History of presenting complaint

- **Quality of life.** How has being overweight or obese affected the patient's lifestyle and their health (and vice versa)?
- **Onset and duration.** How quickly has the patient gained weight? Has there been a change in diet or activity? How does their family's weight compare? Assuming there are no changes in dietary intake, there is usually a gradual increase in weight through life as activity levels and metabolic requirements fall.
- **Degree of obesity.** Overweight and obesity are commonly assessed by BMI, calculated as weight divided by height (kg/m^2). A BMI of 25.0–29.9 indicates that a patient is overweight (class I obesity: 30.0–34.9; class II: 35.0–39.9; morbid obesity: >40.0). Have there been any recent documented changes in weight? Also look for past values of abdominal girth, which takes account of intra-abdominal fat and is less affected by muscle mass. Higher risks are associated with an abdominal girth of >102 cm in men and >88 cm in women.
- **Concurrent illness.** Does the patient suffer from any associated condition which may lead to weight gain (e.g. hypothyroidism)? Are there any symptoms suggestive of hypothyroidism, such as constipation or cold intolerance? Have complications like type 2 diabetes, CVD, osteoarthritis or certain types of cancer been identified?
- **Menstrual history.** In women, ask about problems with fertility, menorrhagia and irregular vaginal bleeding, which may raise the possibility of endometrial cancer.
- **Motivation.** Although the diagnosis may be obvious, obese people may be poorly motivated to change their lifestyle. They may also be in denial about the problem or the need to do something about it. Without motivation, it is difficult to succeed in helping people to lose weight and reduce health risks.
- **Caloric intake.** Explore details about the patient's dietary habits. What and how much is being eaten? Ask about alcoholic and nonalcoholic drinks, many of which contain a considerable number of calories.
- **Exercise.** Does the patient engage in any physical exercise?
- **Involvement of other health professionals.** Are other team members already involved, such as doctors (e.g. specialists with an interest in obesity), nurses, dieticians or counsellors? Has the patient had any positive or negative experiences with other health professionals in the past?

- **Additional unexplored issues.** Ask the patient if there are any other problems or issues that you have not covered but which might be important. Sleep problems are common and may be caused by obstructive sleep apnoea.

Past and current medical problems
- **Significant past illnesses.** Chronic physical health problems can lead to reduced mobility and excess weight. Consider hypothyroidism, other metabolic and hormonal disorders, osteoarthritis and CVD.
- **Mental health.** Mental health problems are more common in those with weight problems, both as cause and effect.

Medication
- **Medication causing weight gain.** A variety of medications may lead to weight gain, including oral contraception, psychotherapeutics, insulin and oral steroids.
- **Obesity treatments.** Have any obesity treatments been tried, such as orlistat or sibutramine?

Other treatments
- **Surgery.** Has the patient ever had surgical treatment for obesity, such as liposuction or gastric banding?

Family history
- **Obesity.** Does obesity run in the family?
- **Complications and risk factors.** Check for a positive family history of diabetes, CVD or hyperlipidaemia.

Social history
- **Home.** Are there any problems at home that arise directly or indirectly from being overweight or obese? Consider issues around clothing, mobility, sex and relationships.
- **Work.** Moving from a manual to a more sedentary job may contribute to weight gain.
- **Eating habits.** Social and mental health factors (e.g. anxiety, depression) may lead to comfort eating and weight gain, whereas in severe depression, reduced appetite and weight loss are common. What approaches to food and weight do the patient's family and other close people take?

Alcohol, smoking and recreational drugs
- **Alcohol.** Alcohol misuse can contribute to weight gain. Ask for details about previous and current alcohol intake.
- **Smoking.** The risk of cardiovascular complications is substantially increased in obese people who smoke. Has smoking-cessation advice been offered?

Review of previous investigations
- **Full blood count.** A raised mean corpuscular volume (MCV) may occur with alcohol misuse or hypothyroidism.
- **Urea and electrolytes.** Renal problems may occur if the patient is diabetic.
- **Liver function tests.** Abnormalities may arise from fatty infiltration of the liver. Liver function tests need to be monitored if certain drugs are being used for the treatment of obesity.
- **Glucose.** Check results for evidence of diabetes.
- **Lipid profile.** Is cholesterol raised?
- **Thyroid function.** Hypothyroidism may lead to weight gain.
- **Electrocardiogram (ECG).** This may be useful as a baseline and may help detect signs of CVD.

Examination

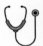

General
- **General condition.** Does the patient look unwell?
- **Hormonal status.** Look for evidence of hypothyroidism, such as thin hair or loss of hair, dry skin, mental slowness and myxoedema. Are there signs of Cushing's disease, such as facial plethora, purpura, puffy face, striae, central obesity and a thick neck (rare)?
- **Body measurements.** Check and record weight, height and abdominal girth to estimate the extent of obesity and as a baseline for weight management. Calculate BMI.

Vital signs
- **Pulse.** Bradycardia may be present in hypothyroidism. Tachycardia may be caused by CVD (e.g. heart failure).
- **Blood pressure.** Hypertension may be associated with obesity and is an important risk factor for CVD.
- **Respiratory rate.** There may be tachypnoea due to heart failure or general lack of fitness.

Skin
- **Striae.** Violaceous striae may occur in Cushing's syndrome or due to treatment with oral steroids. In Cushing's syndrome, skin tends to become thin, fragile and more susceptible to bruises and infections.

Head and neck
- **Neck swelling.** Obesity in Cushing's syndrome or due to steroid use occurs mainly around the trunk, head and neck, with the extremities usually being thin.

Chest
- **Heart.** Examine for signs of CVD, such as cardiomegaly.

Abdomen
- **Palpation.** Abdominal palpation is usually difficult in obese people, and intra-abdominal organs may be impossible to palpate.

Lower limbs
- **Pulses.** Check peripheral pulses and look for signs of peripheral vascular disease.
- **Osteoarthritis.** Check joints for signs of arthritis, which is common in weight-bearing joints such as the hips, knees and ankles.

Bedside tests
- **Glucose.** Check for hyperglycaemia (diabetes).

Key references and further reading

1. National Institute for Health and Care Excellence (NICE). Obesity: identification, assessment and management. NICE guidelines [CG189]. November 2014. Available from: http://www.nice.org.uk/guidance/cg189 (last accessed 29 April 2016).
2. National Institute for Health and Care Excellence (NICE). Obesity. Clinical knowledge summaries. 2015. Available from: http://cks.nice.org.uk/obesity (last accessed 29 April 2016).
3. National Obesity Forum. www.nationalobesityforum.org.uk.
4. World Health Organization (WHO). Obesity. Available from: http://www.who.int/topics/obesity/en/ (last accessed 29 April 2016).

Hirsutism in women

Key thoughts

Practical points
- **Diagnosis.** Hirsutism can be very distressing for patients. PCOS is common, but most cases are idiopathic. In rare cases, consider the possibility of an androgen-secreting tumour.

Differential diagnosis
- Idiopathic hirsutism.
- PCOS.
- Drugs.
- Hypothyroidism.
- Anorexia nervosa.
- Rarely, congenital adrenal hyperplasia, androgen-secreting tumour of the ovary or adrenal glands, Cushing's syndrome, anabolic steroid misuse, hypertrichosis lanuginosa, porphyria.

RED FLAGS

- Systemic symptoms suggestive of malignancy
- Sudden onset and rapid progression of hair growth
- Raised testosterone levels
- Signs of virilisation, such as hair loss from the scalp, voice deepening, increased muscle bulk and clitoromegaly
- Pelvic or abdominal mass
- Features of Cushing's syndrome, such as weight gain (moon face), weight gain in the neck and upper back, stretch marks, easy bruising and proximal muscle weakness

History

Ideas, concerns and expectations
- **Ideas.** What does the patient think is causing excessive hair growth?
- **Concerns.** Excess hair can be very embarrassing and may cause great concern around social interaction. Women might be worried that they are turning into men.
- **Expectations.** Why has the patient come to see you? Common reasons for consultation are advice about cosmetic removal of hair and a desire to identify an underlying cause.

The 10-Minute Clinical Assessment, Second Edition. Knut Schroeder.
© 2017 John Wiley & Sons, Ltd. Published 2017 by John Wiley & Sons, Ltd.

History of presenting complaint

- **Quality of life.** Allow the patient to tell you in their own words how the excessive hair growth is affecting their life.
- **Onset.** Most cases are idiopathic and start gradually. Congenital adrenal hyperplasia usually has a slow onset and may not present until the teenage years or adulthood. Benign androgen-dependent conditions such as PCOS and idiopathic hirsutism usually start during puberty and progress slowly. Consider the possibility of an androgen-secreting tumour of the ovary or adrenal glands if there is late and rapid onset of symptoms.
- **Menstrual problems.** PCOS may cause oligomenorrhoea or amenorrhoea associated with hirsutism. Androgen-secreting tumours may cause sudden menstrual changes, particularly if they are associated with virilisation. The effects of testosterone may be increased in post-menopausal women due to loss of the opposing effects of oestrogen.
- **Features of androgen excess.** Ask about male pattern alopecia, acne, increased muscle mass around the shoulders and loss of breast tissue.
- **Weight change.** Hirsutism or hypertrichosis may occur with anorexia nervosa, which may be concealed. Consider Cushing's syndrome or PCOS if the patient is overweight.
- **Systemic symptoms.** General symptoms, such as weight loss, weight gain, lethargy, general malaise, sweats and loss of appetite may rarely be associated with Cushing's syndrome or tumours.
- **Mental health.** What psychological impact do the symptoms have? Depression and social phobia are relatively common and may not be mentioned by the patient.

Past and current medical problems

- **Endocrine disorders.** Check for any previous endocrine diagnoses, such as Cushing's syndrome, congenital adrenal hyperplasia or hypothyroidism.

Medication and other treatments

- **Treatment for hirsutism.** Cyproterone, the combined oral contraceptive pill or spironolactone may have been tried. Ask about any effects and adverse effects.
- **Hormones.** Drugs containing hormones may contribute to the development of hirsutism. Oral contraceptives containing levonorgestrel, norgestrel or norethisterone may cause androgen-pattern hirsutism. Other hormones, such as prescribed and illicit anabolic steroids, danazole or testosterone, may also be responsible.
- **Drugs causing hypertrichosis.** Minoxidil, phenytoin, ciclosporin and penicillamine may all cause hypertrichosis.
- **Over-the-counter preparations.** Check whether any preparations have been used for the removal of excess hair. This will give you some idea about the severity and progression of the problem. Depilatory creams are commonly used and may lead to skin reactions.

- **Other treatments.** Bleaches, shaving, waxing, plucking, electrolysis and laser therapy may have been used. Ask about any adverse effects, as skin reactions are relatively common. Have any of these been effective?

Family history
- **Inherited disorders.** Idiopathic hirsutism, congenital adrenal hyperplasia and PCOS often run in families.

Social history
- **Home.** Have symptoms affected home life in any way? Are there any relationship problems because of the hair growth?
- **Work.** People in public positions may be embarrassed by their symptoms and find it difficult to go to work.

Review of previous investigations
- **Thyroid function.** Severe hypothyroidism may lead to excessive hair growth.
- **Testosterone.** This may be elevated in PCOS to about three times the level of normal. If levels are higher, consider the possibility of an androgen-secreting tumour.
- **Follicle-stimulating hormone (FSH) and luteinising hormone (LH).** Raised LH occurs in PCOS, and high levels of both LH and FSH may indicate that the patient is menopausal.
- **Cholesterol.** Dyslipidaemia may occur with androgen excess and in hypothyroidism.
- **Endocrine tests.** 17 hydroxyprogesterone may be checked if adrenal hyperplasia is suspected. Two measurements of 24-hour urinary free cortisol help with the diagnosis of Cushing's disease.
- **Pelvic ultrasound.** This is often part of the workup for investigation of amenorrhoea or infertility. Look for evidence of PCOS or tumours.

Examination

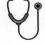

General
- **General condition.** Does the patient look unwell? A deep voice may suggest androgen excess but is a very late sign.
- **Height and weight.** Measure these to calculate BMI. A low BMI can be found in anorexia nervosa. Raised BMI suggests PCOS or Cushing's syndrome.

Hair distribution
- **Pattern.** Identify the pattern of excess hair. Androgen-related hirsutism usually shows a male distribution of hair, with mainly the upper lip, chin, chest and upper back being affected. Generalised growth of hair occurs with hypertrichosis caused by anorexia nervosa, metabolic disorders and some medications.

Skin changes
- **Acanthosis nigricans.** This may be associated with PCOS.
- **Striae.** Deep purple violaceous striae may be found in Cushing's disease.
- **Signs of virilisation.** Look for signs of acne and male pattern baldness, which may suggest high levels of testosterone.

Vital signs
- **Blood pressure.** Hypertension may be present in Cushing's disease.

Abdomen
- **Pelvic examination.** Consider a bimanual pelvic examination if an androgen-secreting tumour is a possibility, although this may only be palpable at a late stage. Clitoromegaly may suggest increased androgens but is also a late sign.

Bedside tests
- **Blood glucose.** This may be raised in Cushing's disease or in other steroid excess.

Key references and further reading
1. Hunter M, Carek P. Evaluation and treatment of women with hirsutism. *Am Fam Physician* 2003;67:2565–2572.
2. National Institute for Health and Care Excellence (NICE). Hirsutism: management. Clinical knowledge summaries. 2014. Available from: http://cks.nice. org.uk/hirsutism (last accessed 29 April 2016).
3. Somani N, Harrison S, Bergfeld WF. The clinical evaluation of hirsutism. *Dermatol Ther* 2008;21:376–391.

Hypothyroidism

Key thoughts

Practical points

- **Diagnosis.** Hypothyroidism is common, with iodine deficiency being the most common cause worldwide. Differentiate between primary hypothyroidism, subclinical hypothyroidism, secondary hypothyroidism and congenital hypothyroidism. Always consider the possibility of hypothyroidism if a patient presents with nonspecific symptoms, as the diagnosis is easily missed.

Possible causes

- **Autoimmune.** Hashimoto's thyroiditis (with a goitre) and atrophic thyroiditis.
- **Iodine deficiency.** Usually presents with a goitre.
- **Iatrogenic.** Surgery, radio-iodine treatment, radiotherapy to the neck.
- **Drugs.** Lithium, amiodarone, contrast media, antithyroid medication, iodides, lithium.
- **Secondary hypothyroidism.** Thyroid-stimulating hormone (TSH) deficiency, hypoparathyroidism, hypothalamic conditions.
- **Infiltration of the thyroid gland (rare).** Amyloidosis, sarcoidosis, haemochromatosis.
- **Congenital.** Absence of the thyroid gland, dyshormonogenesis – will usually have been picked up by newborn screening.

> **RED FLAGS**
>
> - Depression
> - Pregnancy
> - Onset postpartum
> - Treatment with amiodarone or lithium
> - Evidence of pituitary disease (low TSH and T4)
> - Coexisting CVD

History

Ideas, concerns and expectations

- **Ideas.** People with undiagnosed hypothyroidism often have no idea about the possible cause of their symptoms, although they may suspect hypothyroidism if there is a positive family history. Patients may find it difficult to understand that

---

The 10-Minute Clinical Assessment, Second Edition. Knut Schroeder.
© 2017 John Wiley & Sons, Ltd. Published 2017 by John Wiley & Sons, Ltd.

the diagnosis of thyroid disease is not always clear-cut or that individual patients respond differently to treatment.

- **Concerns.** Worries about possible underlying cancer are common in patients presenting with symptoms of hypothyroidism. Alternatively, people may not be too bothered about their symptoms and see them as part of the normal ageing process.
- **Expectations.** Why has the patient come to see you? Common reasons for consultation include symptomatic relief and a search for the underlying diagnosis. Expectations about the success of therapy may be high, and you may need to explain that it can take a while for symptoms to improve once treatment has started (often more than 6 months).

History of presenting complaint

- **Quality of life.** Give the patient time to tell you about their symptoms in their own words. How has day-to-day life been affected? Symptoms of hypothyroidism can reduce quality of life considerably.
- **Onset and duration.** When did symptoms start and how quickly did they develop? Goitre develops slowly, whereas thyroiditis may present more acutely.
- **Symptoms of hypothyroidism.** Ask about typical symptoms, such as tiredness, lethargy, weight gain, decreased appetite, constipation, dry skin, hair loss, general aches, carpal tunnel syndrome, cold intolerance, mental slowing, confusion, depression, deep hoarse voice, reduced libido, menstrual disorders and fertility problems. Which are the most bothersome problems?
- **Goitre.** Development of an anterior neck swelling may be caused by goitre. In areas of iron deficiency (e.g. some mountainous regions), goitre is often endemic.
- **Pregnancy.** If hypothyroidism presents in pregnancy, there is an increased risk of anaemia, pre-eclampsia, low birth weight, stillbirth and postpartum haemorrhage.
- **Diet.** Does the patient follow an unusual diet? Rarely, iodine deficiency may be implicated in the development of hypothyroidism.
- **Mental health.** Ask specifically about any mental health problems, such as depression or confusion. Provide information about self-help groups as appropriate.

Past and current medical problems

- **Thyroid disease.** Ask about previous postnatal thyroiditis or Graves' disease.
- **Surgery and radiotherapy.** Hypothyroidism may occur after thyroid resection or radiotherapy.
- **Pituitary disease.** Pituitary disease is a rare cause of hypothyroidism.
- **Other health problems.** There may be premature CVD due to hypercholesterinaemia. Thyroid replacement therapy will need to be started carefully and with low initial doses if there is a history of angina, particularly in the elderly. Type 1 diabetes is associated with hypothyroidism.

Medication
- **Thyroxine.** If the patient is already taking thyroxine, establish the dosing history and whether there have been any recent changes. Does the current dose control symptoms and keep thyroid function tests within the normal range? Over-replacement with levothyroxine may lead to cardiovascular complications and osteoporosis.
- **Drugs that may affect thyroid function.** Medication such as lithium, carbimazole, amiodarone, interferon alpha, interleukin 2 or iodine may affect thyroid function and cause hypothyroidism.

Family history
- **Hypothyroidism.** There is often a positive family history.
- **Autoimmune disease.** Ask about a family history of autoimmune conditions, which may be associated with hypothyroidism.

Social history
- **Home.** How far have activities of daily living been affected?
- **Work.** Are there any problems with work?

Review of previous investigations
- **Thyroid function.** Raised TSH and low T4 suggest hypothyroidism. Reduced free T4 and total T4 together with a low TSH suggest central hypothyroidism.
- **Full blood count.** A raised MCV occurs in hypothyroidism. There may be anaemia due to vitamin B12 deficiency in pernicious anaemia.
- **Vitamin B12.** Vitamin B12 deficiency is associated with hypothyroidism.
- **Thyroid antibodies.** If these are present, the disease is more likely to progress.

Examination

General
- **General condition.** Does the patient look unwell? Pallor may suggest anaemia. The voice may be husky.
- **Weight.** Check weight as a baseline and compare with any previous measurements.
- **Facial expression.** The typical myxoedema facies may appear in advanced disease. Does the patient look depressed?
- **Mental state.** Consider performing a formal mental state examination if there is a suggestion of reduced cognitive function.

Vital signs
- **Pulse.** Hypothyroidism may cause bradycardia.

Skin
- **Appearance.** The skin may feel dry and thick. Hair loss is common.
- **Vitiligo.** The presence of vitiligo may suggest an autoimmune disorder.

Head and neck

- **Goitre.** Palpate the thyroid gland for evidence of a goitre or tumour. If a goitre is present, does it cause obstructive symptoms? Is there a thyroidectomy scar? An enlarged tender thyroid may indicate subacute thyroiditis.
- **Eyes.** Look for evidence of thyroid ophthalmopathy, such as conjunctival injection and oedema, abnormal eye movements, proptosis, periorbital oedema and keratitis. These signs are commonly associated with Graves' disease but may also occur with autoimmune thyroiditis.

Upper and lower limbs

- **Slow relaxing reflexes.** These are typical for hypothyroidism.
- **Carpal tunnel syndrome.** If suggested by the history, check for evidence of carpal tunnel syndrome.
- **Neurology.** Check for proximal weakness, muscle stiffness and evidence of peripheral neuropathy.

Bedside tests

- **Glucose.** Check blood glucose (possibility of diabetes mellitus).

Key references and further reading

1. Boelaert K, Franklyn JA. Thyroid hormone in health and disease. *J Endocrinol* 2005;187:1–15.
2. Cawood T, Moriarty P, O'Shea D. Recent developments in thyroid eye disease. *BMJ* 2004;329:385–390.
3. Hueston W. Treatment of hypothyroidism. *Am Fam Physician* 2001;64:1717–1724.
4. National Institute for Health and Care Excellence (NICE). Hypothyroidism. Clinical knowledge summaries. 2011. Available from: http://cks.nice.org.uk/hypothyroidism (last accessed 29 April 2016).
5. Negro R, Stagnaro-Green A. Diagnosis and management of subclinical hypothyroidism. *BMJ* 2014;349:g4929.
6. Vaidya B, Pearce HS. Management of hypothyroidism in adults. *BMJ* 2008; 337:a801.

Hyperthyroidism

Key thoughts

Practical points

- **Diagnosis.** Hyperthyroidism can cause a multitude of symptoms. Graves' disease is the most common underlying cause. Rarely, patients may present with a thyrotoxic crisis.

Possible causes

- Graves' disease.
- Toxic nodular goitre.
- Subclinical hyperthyroidism.
- Autoimmune thyroiditis (usually transient hyperthyroidism).
- Drugs such as amiodarone or lithium therapy.

> **RED FLAGS**
>
> - Tracheal compression due to thyroid swelling
> - Solitary nodule increasing in size
> - Unexplained hoarseness or voice symptoms
> - Cervical lymphadenopathy
> - Symptoms in children or older patients (>65 years)
> - Family history of endocrine tumour
> - Thyrotoxic crisis

History

Ideas, concerns and expectations

- **Ideas.** It is rare for people to suspect hyperthyroidism as the cause for their symptoms, which are often nonspecific. A positive family history may give them a clue to the possible underlying cause.
- **Concerns.** Symptoms such as palpitations, unexplained weight loss and anxiety can be very frightening, and people are often worried about a serious underlying illness.
- **Expectations.** Symptomatic relief of symptoms and finding the underlying cause for the symptoms are common reasons for consultation.

The 10-Minute Clinical Assessment, Second Edition. Knut Schroeder.
© 2017 John Wiley & Sons, Ltd. Published 2017 by John Wiley & Sons, Ltd.

History of presenting complaint

- **Quality of life.** Allow patients the time to tell you about their thyroid-related symptoms in their own words. How do they affect day-to-day life?
- **Onset.** Hyperthyroidism may develop at any age and may be transient.
- **Goitre.** Is there a neck swelling, suggesting goitre?
- **Eye symptoms.** Eye symptoms, such as exophthalmos, dry eyes or double vision, suggest the possibility of Graves' disease, particularly if associated with a goitre. Ask about any change in visual acuity or colour vision or an inability to fully close the eye.
- **Thyroid symptoms.** Ask about the typical symptoms of hyperthyroidism, including tiredness, poor short-term memory, muscle weakness, palpitations, tremor, sweating, heat intolerance, bowel frequency or diarrhoea, anxiety, agitation, emotional lability, confusion, skin irritation, menstrual disorders, visual disturbance, neck swelling and disturbed sleep.
- **Pregnancy.** Hyperthyroidism in pregnancy increases the risk of most complications of pregnancy, including pre-eclampsia and miscarriage.
- **Subclinical hyperthyroidism.** This may be present if there is a persistently low TSH level with normal T4 and T3 levels. People with subclinical hyperthyroidism are at higher risk of AF, especially the elderly.
- **Planned surgery.** Thyrotoxicosis can cause problems during anaesthesia.

Past and current medical problems

- **Cardiovascular problems.** Angina, AF, cardiomyopathy and heart failure can result from hyperthyroidism. Refractory arrhythmias in particular increase the chance that the patient has been prescribed amiodarone, which may affect thyroid function.
- **Autoimmune disorders.** Does the patient suffer from associated autoimmune conditions, such as diabetes, vitiligo, pernicious anaemia, Sjögren's syndrome or coeliac disease?
- **Thyroid disease.** Is there a history of postnatal thyroiditis or Graves' disease?

Medication and other treatments

- **Carbimazole.** Is the patient already taking carbimazole? Have there been any adverse drug effects? With the 'block-replace' regime, replacement with levothyroxine is needed to treat hypothyroidism caused by carbimazole.
- **Drugs causing hyperthyroidism.** Check whether the patient is currently being prescribed drugs that may cause hypothyroidism (e.g. amiodarone, lithium).
- **Radioiodine.** This damages the thyroid and is a definitive treatment for hyperthyroidism.
- **Surgery.** Surgery leaves patients euthyroid in most cases, although hypothyroidism may result from surgery. Thyrotoxicosis may also recur. Consider the possibility of recurrent laryngeal nerve problems and parathyroid damage.

Family history
- **Autoimmune disease.** Ask about any relevant family history of any autoimmune conditions.

Social history
- **Home.** How have symptoms affected life at home?
- **Work.** Has work been affected?

Review of previous investigations
- **Thyroid function tests.** Diagnosis is usually confirmed by an elevated T4 and a subnormal TSH.
- **Full blood count.** Look for evidence of neutropenia in any patient taking carbimazole who presents with a sore throat.

Examination

General
- **General condition.** Does the patient look unwell?
- **Weight.** Weight loss due to hyperthyroidism may be considerable. Check and record weight and compare with previous readings.
- **Mental state.** Irritability and anxiety are common.

Vital signs
- **Temperature.** Fever typically accompanies thyrotoxic crisis (rare).
- **Pulse.** Check for tachycardia and arrhythmias, such as AF.
- **Blood pressure.** Hyperthyroidism may contribute to arterial hypertension.

Skin
- **Appearance.** Thinning of skin and hair is common. The skin may feel sweaty and warm.
- **Rash and pruritus.** These may be adverse effects from carbimazole.

Head and neck
- **Eyes.** Look for signs of Graves' disease, such as exophthalmos, corneal opacity, periorbital oedema or papilloedema.
- **Thyroid gland.** The thyroid may be generally enlarged due to goitre, or there may be one or more specific palpable nodules. Check for cervical lymphadenopathy.
- **Throat.** Consider the possibility of agranulocytosis if the patient is taking carbimazole and suffers from sore throat.

Upper limbs
- **Tremor.** Look for a fine tremor in the hands.

Chest
- **Lungs.** Listen for basal crackles as a sign of heart failure.
- **Heart.** Check for evidence of cardiac disease. Check heart rate and rhythm by auscultation to identify AF, which may not always be detected by palpation of the radial pulse alone.

Bedside tests
- **Glucose.** Check blood glucose (diabetes).

Key references and further reading

1. Association for Clinical Biochemistry, British Thyroid Association and British Thyroid Foundation. UK guidelines for the use of thyroid function tests. July 2006. Available from: http://www.british-thyroid-association.org/info-for-patients/Docs/TFT_guideline_final_version_July_2006.pdf (last accessed 29 April 2016).
2. Boelaert K, Franklyn JA. Thyroid hormone in health and disease. *J Endocrinol* 2005;187:1–15.
3. National Institute for Health and Care Excellence (NICE). Hyperthyroidism: management. Clinical knowledge summaries. 2013. Available from: http://cks.nice.org.uk/hyperthyroidism (last accessed 29 April 2016).
4. Reid JR, Wheeler SF. Hyperthyroidism: diagnosis and treatment. *Am Fam Physician* 2005;72:623–630.

Hyponatraemia

Key thoughts

Practical points
- **Diagnosis.** Hyponatraemia is the commonest electrolyte imbalance seen in clinical practice and can have a variety of underlying causes.
- **Prognosis.** Mild hyponatraemia may be self-limiting and asymptomatic, but severe hyponatraemia can lead to severe illness and may be fatal.
- **Volume status.** Try to distinguish between hypovolaemic, euvolaemic and hypervolaemic hyponatraemia.

Differential diagnosis
- Diuretics.
- Fluid depletion due to vomiting or diarrhoea.
- Congestive cardiac failure.
- Liver cirrhosis.
- Hypothyroidism.
- Water overload.
- Renal losses.
- Rarely, Addisonian crisis, pancreatitis, syndrome of inappropriate antidiuretic hormone secretion (SIADH), hypopituitarism, post-transurethral prostatectomy.

> **RED FLAGS**
>
> - Rapid development of hyponatraemia
> - Neurological or other symptoms
> - History of cancer
> - Confusion
> - Deteriorating clinical state and signs of hypovolaemia
> - Suspected SIADH or other endocrine cause
> - Infants
> - Elderly

History

History of presenting complaint
- **Symptoms of hyponatraemia.** Symptoms are usually related to the severity and speed of onset of the fall in plasma sodium concentration. The resulting

---

The 10-Minute Clinical Assessment, Second Edition. Knut Schroeder.
© 2017 John Wiley & Sons, Ltd. Published 2017 by John Wiley & Sons, Ltd.

shift of fluid from the extracellular into the intracellular volume may result in tissue oedema, raised intracranial pressure and neurological symptoms. Mild hyponatraemia (plasma sodium 130–135 mmol/l) does not usually cause any symptoms. Nausea and malaise are common if plasma sodium concentration falls below 125–130 mmol/l. If plasma sodium is between 115 and 120 mmol/l, patients may suffer from lethargy, restlessness, headache, confusion and disorientation. In severe and rapidly developing hyponatraemia, seizures, coma, respiratory arrest or brain-stem herniation may occur, potentially leading to permanent brain damage and death. In chronic hyponatraemia, few symptoms may be present, due to self-regulation of the brain to prevent swelling.

- **Hypovolaemia.** In hypovolaemic hyponatraemia, sodium is lost in larger quantities than water (depletional hyponatraemia). Consider extrarenal losses such as vomiting, diarrhoea, burns, excessive sweating or pancreatitis if urine sodium concentration is <30 mmol/l. Consider renal losses if urine sodium is <30 mmol/l, which may occur as a result of diuretics, cerebral salt wasting, salt-wasting nephropathy or mineralocorticoid deficiency (e.g. Addison's disease).
- **Euvolaemia.** In people with euvolaemic or hypervolaemic hyponatraemia, there is an excess of total body water, causing dilutional hyponatraemia. Consider SIADH, hypothyroidism, adrenocorticotropic hormone (ACTH) deficiency in hypopituitarism or water intoxication, which may all occur in primary polydipsia, excessive administration of parenteral hypotonic fluids or post-transurethral prostatectomy. Urine sodium is usually >30 mmol/l.
- **Hypervolaemia.** If urine sodium is <30 mmol/l, consider liver cirrhosis with ascites, congestive cardiac failure or nephrotic syndrome. If urine sodium is >30 mmol/l, the hyponatraemia is likely caused by chronic renal failure.
- **SIADH.** Consider SIADH if hyponatraemia is associated with high urine osmolality (>100 mOsm/kg) and high urinary sodium (>30 mmol/l) but normal thyroid, renal and adrenal function. Possible causes include lymphoma, small-cell lung cancer, pneumonia, tuberculosis (TB), lung abscess, intracranial disorders (e.g. subarachnoid haemorrhage, infection, tumour) and drugs such as psychotropic medication, carbamazepine and cyclophosphamide.
- **Mental health problems.** There may be an underlying psychiatric problem in people with primary polydipsia.
- **Fainting.** Are there any unexplained episodes of loss of consciousness? Postural hypotension is a sign of volume depletion or, rarely, ACTH deficiency.
- **Fluid balance.** If available, check fluid balance charts for fluid input and output.

Past and current medical problems
- **Autoimmune disease.** Does the patient suffer from autoimmune disease, such as hypothyroidism or Addison's disease?
- **Liver and kidneys.** Is there a history of liver or kidney problems?

Medication
- **Diuretics.** These may cause renal losses of sodium.
- **SIADH.** Look for any drugs that could potentially cause SIADH.

Family history
- **Autoimmune disease.** Ask about any family history of autoimmune disease, such as hypothyroidism or Addison's disease.

Alcohol, smoking and recreational drugs
- **Alcohol.** Ask for details about past and present alcohol consumption (alcoholic liver disease, liver cirrhosis).
- **Smoking.** Heavy smokers are at increased risk of developing lung cancer, which can cause SIADH.

Review of previous investigations
- **Urea and electrolytes.** Check recent results for plasma sodium concentration, to assess the speed with which hyponatraemia has developed.
- **Plasma glucose.** Hyperglycaemia can cause pseudohyponatraemia.
- **Full blood count.** A raised MCV may be caused by hypothyroidism or alcohol misuse. Normocytic anaemia can occur in chronic renal disease.
- **Liver function tests.** Look for evidence of liver disease.
- **Thyroid function.** Hypothyroidism may cause hyponatraemia.
- **Chest X-ray.** This can be useful in establishing a cause for SIADH.
- **Plasma osmolality.** This is rarely discriminant, as it is almost always low in hyponatraemia.

Examination

General
- **Extracellular fluid volume status.** This is the most important aspect of the clinical examination. Assess jugular venous pressure (JVP) and look for oedema in dependant areas. Skin turgor and dry mucous membranes are not particularly useful in establishing fluid status but may provide clues.
- **General condition.** Does the patient look depressed? Are there signs of cognitive impairment (e.g. confusion)? Consider formal mental state examination, if indicated.

Vital signs
- **Temperature.** SIADH may be caused by chest infection.
- **Blood pressure.** Postural hypotension suggests hypovolaemia. Blood pressure may be low in Addison's disease.
- **Respiratory rate.** Tachypnoea may be caused by congestive cardiac failure or respiratory conditions.

Skin
- **Stigmata of chronic liver disease.** If relevant, look for palmar erythema, jaundice, scratch marks and spider naevi.
- **Skin creases.** These may be pigmented in Addison's disease.

Head and neck

- **JVP.** An elevated JVP may suggest hypervolaemia. If indicated, look for signs of superior vena cava obstruction, which may occur in connection with intrathoracic pathology (malignancy).
- **Eyes.** Check pupil reactions, which may be abnormal in central nervous system (CNS) involvement.

Chest

- **Lungs.** Check for any signs of lung or intrathoracic disease, which may cause SIADH. Basal crackles may be heard in congestive cardiac failure.
- **Heart.** Check for a displaced apex beat and a third heart sound, which may occur in congestive cardiac failure.

Abdomen

- **Liver.** Hepatomegaly and ascites may be present in primary liver disease or due to congestive cardiac failure.

Lower limbs

- **Oedema.** Check for signs of peripheral oedema (fluid overload).

Key references and further reading

1. Goh K. Management of hyponatraemia. *Am Fam Physician* 2004;69:2387–2394.
2. National Institute for Health and Care Excellence (NICE). Hyponatraemia. Clinical knowledge summaries. 2015. Available from: http://cks.nice.org.uk/hyponatraemia (last accessed 29 April 2016).
3. Reynolds R, Padfield P, Seckl J. Disorders of sodium balance. *BMJ* 2006;332:702–705.
4. Spasovski G, Vanholder R, Allolio B et al. Clinical practice guideline on diagnosis and treatment of hyponatraemia. *Eur J Endocrinol* 2014;170:G1–G47.

Hypernatraemia

Key thoughts

Practical points
- **Diagnosis.** Hypernatraemia is much less common than hyponatraemia. Try to distinguish between hypovolaemic, euvolaemic and hypervolaemic hypernatraemia. Identifying the underlying cause can be challenging, as there are many potential diagnoses. It is important to assess hydration status in order to narrow down the cause.
- **Prognosis.** Establish the degree of hypernatraemia. Mild hypernatraemia may be self-limiting and asymptomatic, but severe hypernatraemia can lead to severe illness and may be fatal.

Possible causes
- **Hypovolaemia.** Gastrointestinal losses, dermal losses (e.g. burns, sweating), renal failure, diuretics, hyperosmolar nonketotic coma.
- **Hypervolaemia.** Hyperaldosteronism, iatrogenic (saline infusions), excess salt ingestion.
- **Euvolaemia.** Fever, diabetes insipidus, hypodipsia.

> **RED FLAGS**
>
> - Plasma sodium concentrations above 158–160 mmol/l
> - Lack of thirst sensation
> - Altered mental status

History

History of presenting complaint
- **Degree of hypernatraemia.** Hypernatraemia is defined as a plasma sodium concentration of >145 mmol/l. The vast majority of patients have hyperosmolar hypernatraemia, with a reduction in extracellular water rather than a true increase in body sodium.
- **Nonspecific symptoms.** Most people will be asymptomatic, and significant symptoms usually only occur if plasma sodium concentration rises to >160 mmol/l. Patients will be thirsty unless the thalamus is affected, which would suggest probable central diabetes insipidus. Muscle weakness, anorexia, nausea, vomiting and restlessness are relatively early symptoms. Altered mental status, irritability, lethargy, stupor or coma may occur later.

The 10-Minute Clinical Assessment, Second Edition. Knut Schroeder.
© 2017 John Wiley & Sons, Ltd. Published 2017 by John Wiley & Sons, Ltd.

- **Hypovolaemia.** Has the patient suffered from burns or excessive sweating? Ask about any vomiting or diarrhoea. Has body fluid been lost through a fistula? Is the patient taking prescribed diuretics? Are these being taken at the recommended doses?
- **Hypervolaemia.** Does the patient receive additional fluids? Consider causes such as infusion of hypertonic saline, antibiotics containing sodium, tube feeding and hypertonic dialysis. Is there a history of hyperaldosteronism (e.g. Conn's syndrome)? Hypernatraemia in aldosterone excess is usually mild and of little clinical significance.
- **Euvolaemia.** Is there a history of central, nephrogenic or gestational diabetes insipidus? Is there lack of thirst? Ask about any fevers or episodes of hyperventilation. Mechanical ventilation can also lead to hypernatraemia.
- **Diabetes insipidus.** People with diabetes insipidus usually present with polyuria and polydipsia, and hypernatraemia features only if thirst sensation is impaired.
- **Fluid charts.** Review any fluid charts to assess fluid intake and output balance.

Past and current medical problems
- **Renal disease.** Check for a history of acute or chronic renal disease.
- **Adrenal disease.** Is there a history of hyperaldosteronism due to Conn's syndrome?
- **Diabetes.** Hypernatraemia is a feature of hyperosmolar nonketotic coma.
- **Trauma.** Head injury suggests the possibility of a central cause for hypernatraemia.

Medication
- **Loop diuretics.** These may cause fluid depletion, resulting in hypernatraemia.
- **Lithium.** Consider this as a possible cause of nephrogenic diabetes insipidus.
- **Psychotropic medication.** This may lead to altered consciousness, particularly in the elderly, and to subsequent reduction in fluid intake.

Review of previous investigations
- **Creatinine and electrolytes.** Look up recent sodium results for an overview of how quickly the hypernatraemia has developed. Abnormalities may suggest acute or chronic renal disease.
- **Full blood count.** This may show anaemia of chronic disease if there is underlying renal disease.

Examination

General
- **General condition.** Does the patient look unwell?
- **Mental state.** Patients with altered consciousness, confusion or poor thirst sensation are at higher risk of hypernatraemia due to inadequate fluid intake. In these patients, urinary sodium measurement is unlikely to be helpful, as it is

largely reflected by sodium intake. Consider formal mental state examination, if indicated.

- **Extracellular fluid volume status.** This is the most important aspect of the clinical examination. Assess skin turgor and hydration of mucous membranes, although these are weak signs and may only provide clues. Check JVP and look for oedema in relevant areas (feet, sacrum, scrotum).
- **Weight.** Check and record weight regularly to help monitor fluid balance.

Vital signs

- **Temperature.** Check whether there is a possibility of underlying infection.
- **Pulse.** Consider fluid depletion, fluid overload or fever if there is tachycardia.
- **Blood pressure.** Blood pressure may be raised in Conn's syndrome. Check for postural hypotension (fluid depletion).
- **Respiratory rate.** This may be raised in infection or fever. Patients on ventilators may lose fluids and are at increased risk of hypernatraemia.

Chest

- **Lungs.** Basal crackles may suggest fluid overload due to hypertonic infusions, dialysis or salt ingestion.

Upper and lower limbs

- **Tremor.** Look for signs of tremor.
- **Reflexes.** Check for hyperreflexia.
- **Muscle strength.** Muscle strength may be reduced.

Key references and further reading
1. Adrogué HJ, Madias NE. *Hypernatraemia. N Engl J Med* 2000;342:1493–1499.
2. Kugler JP, Hustead T. Hyponatremia and hypernatremia in the elderly. *Am Fam Physician* 2000;61:3623–3630.
3. Reynolds R, Padfield P, Seckl J. Disorders of sodium balance. *BMJ* 2006;332: 702–705.
4. Singer GG, Brenner BM. Fluid and electrolyte disturbances. In: *Harrison's Principles of Internal Medicine* (17th edition). Fauci AS, Braunwald E, Kasper DL et al. (eds). McGraw-Hill, New York; 2008.

Hypokalaemia

Key thoughts

Practical points

- **Diagnosis.** Renal and gastrointestinal losses are common underlying causes.
- **Prognosis.** Hypokalaemia can be life-threatening. Serum potassium <2.5 mmol/l is a medical emergency. Even mild or moderate hypokalaemia may cause problems in patients with underlying CVD.

Possible causes

- Diarrhoea and vomiting.
- Renal conditions.
- Drugs.
- Intestinal fistula.
- Excessive liquorice use.
- Secondary hyperaldosteronism (e.g. liver cirrhosis).
- Rarely, primary hyperaldosteronism (Conn's syndrome), Cushing's syndrome, renal tubular acidosis or hypokalaemic periodic paralysis.

RED FLAGS

- Severe hypokalaemia (<2.5 mmol/l) is associated with life-threatening arrythmias
- Rapidly developing hypokalaemia
- Lack of response to treatment
- Ileus
- History of CVD
- Digoxin toxicity
- ECG changes (flat T-waves, U-waves, ST segment depression)

History

History of presenting complaint

- **Quality of life.** Allow the patient time to tell you about any symptoms that may be caused by hypokalaemia. How far do they affect the quality of life?
- **Symptoms of hypokalaemia.** Mild hypokalaemia is usually asymptomatic. Moderate hypokalaemia can make people feel chronically ill. Serum levels of <3 mmol/l should raise concerns. Tiredness (particularly on exercise), muscle weakness and constipation are common. Muscle necrosis and ascending paralysis can occur with levels <2 mmol/l.

The 10-Minute Clinical Assessment, Second Edition. Knut Schroeder.
© 2017 John Wiley & Sons, Ltd. Published 2017 by John Wiley & Sons, Ltd.

- **Renal problems.** Are there any renal problems that might cause potassium depletion?
- **Gastrointestinal loss.** Consider gastrointestinal losses through diarrhoea, fistulae, nasogastric tubes or laxative abuse. Poor dietary intake, particularly in the elderly, may also play a role.
- **Mineralocorticoid excess.** Conn's and Cushing's syndromes may cause hypokalaemia.
- **Arrhythmias.** Arrhythmias may occur in patients with underlying heart disease, but are uncommon in healthy people.
- **Liquorice.** Excessive liquorice ingestion may cause hypokalaemia.

Past and current medical problems

- **Significant past illnesses.** Is there a personal history of Conn's or Cushing's syndrome?
- **Liver problems.** Liver cirrhosis can cause secondary hyperaldosteronism.
- **CVD.** Consider the possibility of renal artery stenosis as a cause of secondary hyperaldosteronism.
- **Leukaemia.** Hypokalaemia in patients with leukaemia may result from renal potassium wasting.

Medication

- **Diuretics.** Consider loop and thiazide diuretics, particularly in the elderly. Is there a possibility of diuretic misuse?
- **Steroids.** Systemic steroids may lead to hypokalaemia.
- **Laxatives.** Laxative abuse and regular enemas are relatively common causes of hypokalaemia.
- **Antiarrhythmics and digoxin.** If the patient is taking digoxin or antiarrhythmics, hypokalaemia is of particular concern and increases the risk of arrhythmias.
- **Potassium treatment.** If potassium levels have been chronically low, is the patient taking potassium supplements or other potassium-sparing agents?
- **Beta-sympathomimetic drugs.** Check whether the patient is taking decongestants, bronchodilators or inhibitors of uterine contraction, which can all cause hypokalaemia.
- **Antidiarrhoeal agents.** If hypokalaemia is caused by diarrhoea, is the patient taking antidiarrhoeal medication?
- **Mental health.** Laxative or diuretic abuse is common in anorexia nervosa and may be concealed.
- **Other drugs.** Hypokalaemia may also be caused by calcium channel blockers, theophylline or fludrocortisone.

Family history

- **Metabolic conditions.** Ask about a family history of metabolic conditions such as Conn's or Cushing's syndrome.

Alcohol, smoking and recreational drugs
- **Alcohol.** Ask about past and present alcohol intake. Liver cirrhosis can cause secondary hyperaldosteronism and subsequent hypokalaemia.

Review of previous investigations
- **ECG.** This may show the classical appearance of small T-waves and U-waves, ST depression and a prolonged QT interval, but these changes are usually only seen in severe hypokalaemia.
- **Creatinine and electrolytes.** Abnormal values may indicate renal disease. Check for the most recent potassium levels. Have any changes occurred rapidly or slowly?
- **Bicarbonate.** Serum bicarbonate may be high in metabolic alkalosis (causing hypokalaemia).
- **Calcium.** Hypocalcaemia and hypokalaemia may coexist. Correcting hypokalaemia without correcting hypocalcaemia at the same time increases the risk of ventricular arrhythmias.
- **Magnesium.** Magnesium should always be checked if there is hypokalaemia. Magnesium depletion reduces the intracellular potassium concentration and causes renal potassium wasting. It may be impossible to correct hypokalaemia unless hypomagnesaemia is treated simultaneously.
- **Glucose.** Hyperglycaemia may be caused by Cushing's syndrome.
- **Urine.** A 24-hour urine collection for potassium, chloride and calcium may help distinguish between renal and extrarenal causes, but the results may be difficult to interpret (usually done by specialists).
- **Second-line tests.** Check for any results of renin or aldosterone levels. Has the patient ever had urinary free cortisol measured or undergone a dexamethasone suppression test?

Examination

General
- **General condition.** Does the patient look unwell?
- **Signs of liver disease.** Look for stigmata of liver disease, such as jaundice, palmar erythema and spider naevi, as liver cirrhosis may cause secondary hyper-aldosteronism.
- **Hydration.** Assess fluid balance status by looking at a fluid balance chart, if available. Dry mucous membranes and reduced skin turgor suggest dehydration but are weak signs.

Vital signs
- **Pulse.** Tachycardia may occur in fluid depletion or due to fluid overload.
- **Blood pressure.** Blood pressure may be raised due to excess mineralocorticoids in Conn's or Cushing's syndrome – although hypokalaemia may be absent in both these syndromes. Hypokalaemia may also directly increase systolic and dias-tolic blood pressure (likely due to renal sodium retention).

Abdomen

- **Liver.** Check for liver enlargement and ascites, which may be associated with secondary hyperaldosteronism (e.g. alcoholic liver disease).
- **Kidneys.** Listen for the bruit of renal artery stenosis, which may lead to secondary hyperaldosteronism.
- **Bowel sounds.** Reduced bowel sounds may suggest ileus, which is a recognised complication of hypokalaemia.

Limbs

- **Oedema.** Look for pitting oedema in the lower limbs as a sign of fluid overload.
- **Neuromuscular problems.** Paralysis, paraesthesiae and tetany are signs of severe hypokalaemia.

Key references and further reading

1. Gennari FJ. Hypokalemia. *N Engl J Med* 1998;339:451–458.
2. Oram R, McDonaldl J, Vaidya B. Investigating hypokalaemia. *BMJ* 2013;347: f5137.
3. Passare G, Viitanen M, Törring O et al. Sodium and potassium disturbances in the elderly: prevalence and association with drug use. *Clin Drug Investig* 2004;24:535–544.
4. Rastergar A, Soleimani M. Hypokalaemia and hyperkalaemia. *Postgrad Med J* 2001;77:759–764.

Hyperkalaemia

Key thoughts

Practical points
- **Diagnosis.** Renal failure and drugs are the most important causes of hyperkalaemia. Consider spurious hyperkalaemia (due to inadequate sampling procedures) and repeat the sample unless there is another plausible underlying cause.
- **Prognosis.** Severe hyperkalaemia is a medical emergency.

Possible causes
- **Sampling procedure (spurious hyperkalaemia).** Sample deterioration with haemolysis, difficult venepuncture, cold storage.
- **Drugs.** ACE inhibitors, potassium-sparing diuretics.
- **Renal tract.** Renal failure, obstructive uropathy, hyperkalaemic renal tubular acidosis (type IV).
- **Other.** Diabetic ketoacidosis, sickle-cell disease, Addison's disease, hypoaldosteronism, trauma, burns, tumour lysis syndrome.

> **RED FLAGS**
>
> - ECG changes
> - Arrhythmias
> - Bradycardia
> - Myopathy
> - Paralysis
> - Raised serum urea
> - Acute or chronic renal failure
> - Diabetic ketoacidosis

History

History of presenting complaint
- **Symptoms of hyperkalaemia.** Symptoms are usually nonspecific and may not be present. Weakness and lethargy are common. Severe muscle pain may indicate rhabdomyolysis (rare). Shortness of breath may occur due to weakness of the respiratory muscles.
- **Sampling technique and storage.** Difficulties in obtaining a sample or a clenched fist can cause pseudohyperkalaemia. Find out whether a sample was

The 10-Minute Clinical Assessment, Second Edition. Knut Schroeder.
© 2017 John Wiley & Sons, Ltd. Published 2017 by John Wiley & Sons, Ltd.

squirted through the needle or shaken. Contamination with an anticoagulant from another sample (e.g. potassium ethylenediaminetetraacetic acid (EDTA)) may also be responsible. Cooling of the sample or deterioration of the specimen due to the length of storage may contribute to the development of spurious hyperkalaemia.

- **Pre-existing conditions.** Ask about a history of thrombocytosis, severe leucocytosis or red-cell disorders (hereditary or acquired), which can all cause pseudohypokalaemia.
- **Additional unexplored issues.** Ask the patient if there are any other problems or issues that you have not covered but which might be relevant. Urinary symptoms may be present in urinary outflow obstruction.

Past and current medical problems
- **Kidney disease.** Renal failure may present with raised potassium.
- **Urological problems.** Obstructive uropathy may cause hyperkalaemia.

Medication
- **Drugs raising potassium.** Check whether the patient is taking ACE inhibitors, angiotensin receptor blockers, potassium-sparing diuretics or potassium salts.
- **Other drugs.** Corticosteroids, nonsteroidal anti-inflammatory drugs (NSAIDs), trimethoprim or beta blockers may be implicated in the development of hyperkalaemia.

Review of previous investigations
- **Creatinine and electrolytes.** Have parallel measurements of serum and plasma (lithium heparin) potassium been taken? These can help identify spurious hyperkalaemia with intrinsic blood cell-related causes. Look for evidence of kidney disease, such as raised creatinine and reduced estimated glomerular filtration rate <60 ml/min.
- **Full blood count.** This will identify major blood dyscrasias and may point towards red-cell abnormalities. Look in particular for leucocytosis and thrombocytosis, which may both raise potassium levels. A normocytic normochromic anaemia may rarely suggest haemolysis.
- **Bilirubin.** This may be useful if you suspect haemolysis.
- **ECG.** Look for loss of the p-wave, peaked T-waves, prolonged PR interval, widening of the QRS complex, sinus arrest or bradycardia.

Examination

General
- **General condition.** Most patients with hypokalaemia look well, and there will be no specific signs.
- **Muscles.** Check for tender muscles if you suspect rhabdomyolysis (rare).

Vital signs
- **Pulse.** Bradycardia or sinus arrest may occur with severe hyperkalaemia.

Abdomen
- **Bladder.** Check for an enlarged bladder if there is the possibility of obstructive uropathy.
- **Rectal examination.** Check prostate size if obstructive uropathy may be present.

Bedside tests
- **Blood glucose.** Check this if you suspect hyperglycaemia or diabetic ketoacidosis.
- **Urine dipstick.** Check for ketones in diabetic patients (diabetic ketoacidosis).
- **ECG.** ECG monitoring may be required in cases of severe hyperkalaemia or if there are abnormal findings on a resting ECG.

Key references and further reading

1. Clinical Resource Efficiency Support Team (CREST). Guidelines for the treatment of hyperkalaemia in adults. August 2005. Available from: http://www.tdh.org. nz/assets/ED/Misc/Guidelines–Protocols/hyperkalaemia-booklet.pdf?phpMyAd min=VUv7y9CtBOrsmnBFWxFyha%2CKC6d (last accessed 29 April 2016).
2. Hollander-Rodriguez JC, Calvert J. Hyperkalaemia. *Am Fam Physician* 2006;73: 283–290.
3. Johnston JD, Hawthorne SW. How to minimise factitious hyperkalaemia in blood samples from general practice. *BMJ* 1997;314:1200–1201.
4. Smellie WSA. Cases in primary care laboratory medicine: spurious hyperkalaemia. *BMJ* 2007;334:693–695.

Hypocalcaemia

Key thoughts

Practical points

- **Diagnosis.** The most common cause of hypocalcaemia in primary care is vitamin D deficiency. Differentiate between hypocalcaemia with low parathyroid hormone (PTH) levels (hypoparathyroidism) and with high PTH levels (secondary hyperparathyroidism). Phosphate levels can help with the differential diagnosis. Other important causes include hyperventilation and pancreatitis.
- **Prognosis.** Severe hypocalcaemia (<1.9 mmol/l) can potentially be life-threatening and may present as an emergency.

Possible causes

- Vitamin D deficiency.
- Hypoparathyroidism.
- Pseudohypoparathyroidism.
- Hyperventilation.
- Renal failure.
- Acute pancreatitis.
- Overhydration.
- Rarely, PTH resistance, sclerotic metastases, hypomagnesaemia, vitamin D resistance.

RED FLAGS

- Very low calcium levels (<1.9 mmol/l)
- Neurological signs
- Confusion
- Fits
- History of malignancy

History

History of presenting complaint

- **Quality of life.** Allow the patient time to tell you about their symptoms in their own words. How is the quality of life being affected?
- **Severity.** Symptoms usually depend on the speed and magnitude of the fall in serum calcium. Mild hypocalcaemia (2.00–2.12 mmol/l) may be asymptomatic, whereas severe hypocalcaemia (<1.9 mmol/l) may present with neuromuscular irritability.

The 10-Minute Clinical Assessment, Second Edition. Knut Schroeder.
© 2017 John Wiley & Sons, Ltd. Published 2017 by John Wiley & Sons, Ltd.

- **Neurological symptoms.** Symptoms include paraesthesiae around the fingers, toes and mouth. Tetany, muscle cramps and carpal spasm with wrist flexion and fingers drawn together may also occur.
- **Seizures.** Seizures may occur with severe hypocalcaemia.
- **Breathing problems.** Hoarse voice and difficulty in breathing may occur due to laryngospasm or bronchospasm, in which case, there may be associated wheeze. Hyperventilation can also reduce calcium levels.
- **Abdominal pain.** If hypocalcaemia occurs with abdominal pain, consider the possibility of acute pancreatitis.
- **Malabsorption.** Conditions such as coeliac disease may lead to malabsorption of vitamin D, resulting in reduced calcium levels.
- **Malignancy.** Ask if there is a history of malignancy. Osteoblastic metastases from prostate or breast cancer and tumour lysis following chemotherapy may lead to hypocalcaemia.
- **Crush injuries.** Hypocalcaemia may occur in response to rhabdomyolysis after crush injury, although this is rare.

Past and current medical problems
- **Renal disease.** Renal failure is an important cause.
- **Acute pancreatitis.** Is there a history of alcohol misuse or gallstones, which increases the risk of acute pancreatitis?
- **Chronic liver disease.** Vitamin D absorption and activation may be reduced in chronic liver disease and primary biliary cirrhosis.

Medication
- **Bone resorption inhibitors.** Bisphosphonates can cause hypocalcaemia.
- **Drugs affecting vitamin D.** Ketoconazole or phenytoin may affect vitamin D metabolism.
- **Calcium and other supplements.** Have these already been started? Has the patient ever received vitamin D? Has magnesium supplementation been considered, if there is associated hypomagnesaemia?

Review of previous investigations
- **Serum calcium.** Adjustments need to be made for albumin levels, and it is the 'corrected' calcium that is important.
- **PTH.** Levels may be low due to secondary hypoparathyroidism caused by thyroid surgery or autoimmune conditions. There may also be reduced PTH secretion due to gene defects, hypomagnesaemia or other causes. Hypocalcaemia may occur with inappropriately normal or high PTH levels because of secondary hyperparathyroidism. Other causes include vitamin D deficiency, vitamin D resistance and PTH resistance.
- **Creatinine and electrolytes.** Check for evidence of renal failure.
- **Amylase or lipase.** Is there evidence of pancreatitis?
- **Creatinine phosphokinase (CPK).** CPK is likely to be elevated if there is significant muscle damage.

- **Magnesium.** Hypomagnesaemia is associated with hypocalcaemia.
- **25-OH vitamin D.** This may be useful in confirming vitamin D deficiency.
- **ECG.** Look for a prolonged QT interval. Severe hypocalcaemia may lead to ventricular fibrillation or heart block.

Examination

General
- **General condition.** Does the patient look unwell?
- **Mental state.** Dementia and confusion may be present in chronic hypocalcaemia. Consider performing a formal mental state examination, if indicated.

Vital signs
- **Pulse.** Check rate and rhythm. Bradycardia may be caused by heart block.
- **Respiratory rate.** Tachypnoea may indicate hyperventilation, which is an important cause of hypocalcaemia.

Head and neck
- **Chvostek's sign.** Tapping over the facial nerve with the mouth slightly open may cause the facial muscles to twitch, but this can also happen in people with normal calcium levels.
- **Eyes.** Look for any obvious cataract, which may occur with prolonged hypocalcaemia.
- **Papilloedema.** Raised intracranial pressure may occur with hypocalcaemia.

Upper limbs
- **Trousseau's sign.** Inflating a blood pressure cuff on the upper arm for 3 minutes may cause carpal spasm with metacarpophalangeal flexion, hyperextended fingers and flexion of the thumb on to the palm.

Chest
- **Lungs.** Search for evidence of bronchospasm causing hyperventilation.

Abdomen
- **Liver.** Check for hepatomegaly if liver problems are suspected.
- **Tenderness.** Consider the possibility of acute pancreatitis if there is abdominal tenderness.

Key references and further reading
1. Bushinsky DA, Monk RD. Electrolyte quintet: calcium. *Lancet* 1998;352:305–311.
2. Cooper MS, Gittoes NJL. Diagnosis and management of hypocalcaemia. *BMJ* 2008;336:1298–1302.
3. Fong J, Khan A. Hypocalcaemia: updates in diagnosis and management for primary care. *Can Fam Physician* 2012;58:158–162.

Hypercalcaemia

Key thoughts

Practical points
- **Diagnosis.** The normal range for serum calcium is usually between 2.25 and 2.50 mmol/l and depends on protein levels, so laboratories usually give the 'corrected' calcium level. Primary hyperparathyroidism and malignancy are important causes. Investigation of renal impairment is a common reason for measuring calcium levels.

Possible causes
- Primary hyperparathyroidism.
- Malignancy.
- Drugs such as vitamin D or A supplements.
- Renal problems, including chronic renal failure, renal dialysis, post-kidney transplant.
- Tuberculosis.
- Milk–alkali syndrome.
- Acquired immunodeficiency syndrome (AIDS).
- Rarely, sarcoidosis, thyrotoxicosis, familial hypocalciuric hypercalcaemia.

> **RED FLAGS**
>
> - Serum calcium >3.5 mmol/l
> - Pancreatitis
> - Vomiting
> - Dehydration
> - Kidney stones
> - Renal impairment
> - Back pain
> - Breast lump
> - Change in bowel habit
> - Haematuria
> - Systemic features suggesting malignancy (e.g. weight loss, malaise, fatigue, sweats, fever)

The 10-Minute Clinical Assessment, Second Edition. Knut Schroeder.
© 2017 John Wiley & Sons, Ltd. Published 2017 by John Wiley & Sons, Ltd.

History

History of presenting complaint

- **Quality of life.** What are the main problems? How far have they affected the quality of life?
- **Onset of symptoms.** Hypercalcaemia due to cancer is usually accompanied by symptoms of the cancer itself and often develops over a few weeks.
- **General symptoms.** Ask about weakness, fatigue and lethargy. Patients often complain of polyuria and polydipsia. Visual problems may occur if there are corneal deposits in chronic hypercalcaemia.
- **Pain.** Ask about any muscle or bone pain. Abdominal pain and pain due to stone formation are important presenting features.
- **Mental health.** Depression and confusion may be the only presenting features of hypercalcaemia.
- **Abdominal symptoms.** In addition to abdominal pain, nausea and vomiting are common. Ask about problems with constipation. Consider milk–alkali syndrome if the patient has a high intake of over-the-counter indigestion medicines.
- **Calcium levels <2.8 mmol/l.** Patients usually feel just generally unwell, but may also complain of polyuria, nocturia and polydipsia. Dyspepsia, mild cognitive impairment and the symptoms of depression may also be present.
- **Calcium levels 2.8–3.5 mmol/l.** Ask about muscle weakness and constipation. Anorexia, nausea and fatigue may also be present. Is there any bone pain?
- **Calcium levels >3.5 mmol/l.** Patients are usually unwell at this level. Features may include vomiting, abdominal pain, constipation, lethargy and dehydration. There may be associated pancreatitis or coma.
- **Symptoms of cancer.** Check for symptoms of malignancy, particularly myeloma (e.g. back pain) and cancers of the breast (breast lump), lung (cough, smoking), prostate (urinary symptoms), colon (change in bowel habit, rectal bleeding), kidney (haematuria), thyroid (neck swelling) and ovary (abdominal pain and swelling).
- **Calcium deposits.** In chronic hypercalcaemia, calcium may lead to renal stone disease, nephrocalcinosis or chondrocalcinosis.
- **Exogenous calcium.** Does the patient receive intravenous fluids or parenteral nutrition containing calcium?
- **Immunodeficiency and infections.** Hypercalcaemia may occur in AIDS or tuberculosis.

Past and current medical problems

- **Renal disease.** Ask about a history of kidney problems, including renal failure. Hypercalcaemia may occur after kidney transplant or in chronic dialysis.

Medication

- **Diuretics.** Thiazide diuretics may rarely increase calcium levels.
- **Vitamins.** Ask about any vitamin D or A supplements.

- **Digoxin.** Check whether the patient is taking digoxin (digoxin toxicity is increased in hypercalcaemia).
- **Lithium.** Lithium may also cause hypercalcaemia.

Family history
- **Disorders of calcium metabolism.** Ask about a family history of familial hypocalciuric hypercalcaemia.

Review of previous investigations
- **Serum calcium.** Adjustments need to be made for albumin levels – it is the 'corrected' calcium that is important (this is what is usually reported by laboratories).
- **Liver function tests.** A normal alkaline phosphatase may occur in milk–alkali syndrome, myeloma, thyrotoxicosis or sarcoidosis. If the alkaline phosphatase is raised, suspect bony metastases, thyrotoxicosis or sarcoidosis.
- **Calcitonin.** A raised calcitonin level may occur with B-cell lymphoma.
- **PTH.** Raised PTH levels may be caused by primary or secondary hyperparathyroidism, as well as familial hypercalciuric hypercalcaemia (rare). Levels are usually low with iatrogenic causes, such as renal dialysis, granulomatous disease, thyrotoxicosis, adrenal insufficiency and vitamin D intoxication. In malignancy, levels tend to be normal or low.
- **Prostate-specific antigen (PSA).** This should be tested if prostate cancer is suspected.
- **X-rays.** These may show demineralisation, pathological fractures, bone cysts or bony metastases.
- **Ultrasound, computerised tomography (CT) and intravenous urogram.** These may help identify abnormalities in the urinary tract, such as stones or calcification.

Examination

General
- **General condition.** Does the patient look unwell or depressed? Cachexia may suggest malignancy.
- **Dehydration.** Dry mucus membranes and reduced skin turgor may suggest dehydration, but these are weak signs.
- **Mental state.** Is the patient confused or restless? Consider formal mental state examination, if appropriate.

Vital signs
- **Pulse.** Tachycardia may be caused by dehydration.
- **Blood pressure.** Check for postural hypotension (dehydration).

Neck
- **JVP.** A low JVP is a sign of hypotension, but it may be difficult or impossible to elicit.
- **Lumps.** Check for lymphadenopathy and evidence of thyroid cancer.

Chest
- **Lungs.** Is there any clinical evidence of tuberculosis, sarcoidosis or lung cancer?
- **Breast.** Check the breasts for any lumps if breast cancer is a possibility.

Abdomen
- **Distension.** Abdominal distension may occur with hypercalcaemia.
- **Masses.** Check for any masses. Renal and ovarian masses may, in rare cases, be palpable in advanced cancer of the kidney or ovary.
- **Bowel sounds.** These may be decreased in hypercalcaemia.
- **Rectal examination.** Consider digital rectal examination if there is a possibility of prostate or bowel cancer.

Limbs
- **Muscles.** Assess muscular tone and strength.
- **Reflexes.** Deep-tendon reflexes may be depressed.

Bedside tests
- **Urine glucose.** Glucosuria may be associated with hypercalcaemia.

Key references and further reading

1. Bajorunas DR. Clinical manifestations of cancer-related hypercalcaemia. *Semin Oncol* 1990;17:16–25.
2. Mahon SM. Signs and symptoms associated with malignancy-induced hypercalcaemia. *Cancer Nurs* 1989;12:153–160.
3. National Institute for Health and Care Excellence (NICE). Hypercalcaemia. Clinical knowledge summaries. 2014. Available from: http://cks.nice.org.uk/hypercalcaemia (last accessed 29 April 2016).
4. Pecherstorfer M, Brenner K, Zojer N. Current management strategies for hypercalcemia. *Treat Endocrinol* 2003;2:273–292.

Gastrointestinal

Nausea and vomiting

Key thoughts

Practical points
- **Diagnosis.** Nausea and vomiting are common symptoms and often occur as a result of acute viral infections or adverse drug effects. A number of nongastrointestinal conditions may need to be considered if vomiting is severe, persistent or otherwise unexplained. Rarely, serious underlying causes (e.g. raised intracranial pressure) will need urgent action. Investigations are not usually necessary unless symptoms suggest serious disease or are prolonged.

Possible causes
- Acute viral infection.
- Drug adverse effect (e.g. opioids, nonsteroidal anti-inflammatory drugs (NSAIDs), chemotherapy).
- Psychological (anxiety).
- Food poisoning.
- Alcoholic gastritis.
- Pregnancy.
- Migraine.
- Vestibular conditions.
- Myocardial infarction.
- Head injury.
- Peptic ulcer and *Helicobacter pylori* infection.
- Rarely hypercalcaemia, central nervous system (CNS) causes (e.g. meningitis, raised intracranial pressure), bulimia, postoperative exogenous toxins.

RED FLAGS

- Prolonged or severe vomiting
- Haematemesis
- Head injury
- Papilloedema
- Rash and fever (meningitis)
- Dehydration
- Systemic symptoms (e.g. weight loss, malaise, fatigue, sweats, fever)
- Eating disorder

The 10-Minute Clinical Assessment, Second Edition. Knut Schroeder.
© 2017 John Wiley & Sons, Ltd. Published 2017 by John Wiley & Sons, Ltd.

History

Ideas, concerns and expectations
- **Ideas.** Can the patient give any clues as to what might be the underlying cause?
- **Concerns.** Patients often worry that they may have cancer if symptoms persist.
- **Expectations.** The most common reason for consultation is for symptom relief. Many patients will expect further investigation or specialist referral.

History of presenting complaint
- **Quality of life.** Allow the patient to tell you their story in their own words. How do symptoms affect their quality of life? Mood is commonly affected, and persistent symptoms of nausea and vomiting can be very distressing and disabling.
- **Onset and progression.** How long have the symptoms been present? Acute onset occurs in gastroenteritis and with food poisoning. Many drugs can cause chronic nausea. Consider the possibility of pregnancy in women of childbearing age who present with unexplained nausea. Has there been a recent head injury?
- **Severity.** How severe are the symptoms? Severe vomiting can lead to dehydration and electrolyte imbalances.
- **Gastrointestinal symptoms.** Is the patient able to eat and drink? Diarrhoea is common and suggests gastroenteritis. Rarely, consider bowel obstruction or ileus if there is absolute constipation with abdominal distension. Consider peptic ulcer disease, gastrooesophageal reflux or, rarely, pancreatitis if there is epigastric pain or symptoms of heartburn. Associated right iliac fossa pain may indicate appendicitis. If there is right upper quadrant pain, consider biliary colic or cholecystitis. Has there been haematemesis?
- **Other associated symptoms.** If there is fever, consider infectious causes such as acute viral illness, gastroenteritis, urinary tract infection or, rarely, meningitis, hepatitis or septicaemia. Consider vestibular causes if nausea and vomiting occur on movement and are associated with vertigo. Ask about any CNS symptoms, such as headache, visual problems and reduced consciousness, which may indicate migraine or, in rare cases, intracranial causes such as tumour, haemorrhage or meningitis. Cerebral causes may lead to vomiting on lying flat due to meningeal irritation or raised intracranial pressure.
- **Systemic symptoms.** Consider the possibility of underlying cancer if nausea is chronic and there are systemic symptoms such as fever, night sweats, weight loss, anorexia or bone pain.
- **Mental health.** Nausea and vomiting may occur with anxiety, depression or eating disorders such as anorexia nervosa and bulimia.
- **Alcohol.** Alcohol misuse commonly leads to nausea and vomiting.

Review of previous investigations
- **Full blood count.** Look for evidence of infection and anaemia.
- **Renal function.** Consider renal failure and look for raised creatinine and/or urea.

- **Liver function test.** Look for a raised gamma-glutamyl transpeptidase (GGT) and alkaline phosphatase (bile duct obstruction).
- **Calcium.** Hypercalcaemia may present with nausea and vomiting.
- **Lipase and amylase.** These are helpful in the diagnosis of pancreatitis.
- **Bone profile.** Is there any evidence of hypercalcaemia?
- **Endoscopy.** This is helpful in the diagnosis of persistent vomiting.

Past and current medical problems
- **Gastrointestinal problems.** Is there a history of bowel problems?
- **Trauma.** Consider raised intracranial pressure if there is a history of recent head injury.
- **Operations.** Postoperative vomiting is common, particularly after bowel, gynaecological or ear, nose and throat (ENT) surgery.

Medication and other treatments
- **Antiemetics.** Ask whether any antiemetics have been used. Extrapyramidal adverse effects are rare, but they tend to be more common in young and old people.
- **Drugs causing nausea or vomiting.** Many drugs can cause nausea and vomiting, particularly opioid analgesics, NSAIDs, drugs used in chemotherapy, antibiotics and aminoglycosides. Also ask about over-the-counter and herbal medicines.
- **Cancer treatments.** Radiation and chemotherapy commonly cause nausea and vomiting.

Social history
- **Home.** How has home life been affected? Is the patient able to look after dependants at home?
- **Work.** Has work been affected? Is a sick note needed?

Alcohol, smoking and recreational drugs
- **Alcohol.** Ask for details about usual alcohol consumption. Vomiting is common in alcohol misuse and a serious symptom in alcohol withdrawal.
- **Drugs.** Nausea and vomiting are common symptoms of drug misuse or withdrawal.

Examination

General
- **General condition.** Does the patient look unwell?
- **Dehydration.** Look for any clues suggesting dehydration, such as dry mucous membranes and reduced skin turgor (weak signs).

Vital signs
- **Temperature.** Raised temperature suggests infection.

- **Pulse.** Tachycardia may occur with serious underlying illness, dehydration or fever. If there is bradycardia, consider an intracranial cause.
- **Blood pressure.** Check lying and standing blood pressure for postural hypotension (hypovolaemia).
- **Respiratory rate.** Tachypnoea suggests possible chest infection.

Head and neck

- **Sclerae.** Look for evidence of jaundice.
- **Conjunctivae and mucous membranes.** Is the patient clinically anaemic?
- **Neck stiffness.** Check for neck stiffness if meningitis is a possibility (rare).
- **Optic fundi.** Look for papilloedema, indicating raised intracranial pressure in rare cases.

Abdomen

- **Distension.** Consider pregnancy, constipation, ascites, cancer or bowel obstruction if the abdomen is distended.
- **Tenderness.** Epigastric tenderness may suggest gastritis, peptic ulcer or, rarely, pancreatitis. Right upper quadrant tenderness occurs as a result of biliary colic or cholecystitis. Consider appendicitis if there is right iliac fossa tenderness. Loin tenderness suggests the possibility of pyelonephritis.
- **Masses.** Any masses may rarely suggest malignancy. Check the groins for evidence of inguinal hernia.

Bedside tests

- **Pregnancy test.** This is essential in women of childbearing age if pregnancy is a possibility and there is no convincing alternative diagnosis.
- **Urine dipstick.** Proteinuria may suggest renal problems. Consider urinary tract infection if the dipstick test is positive for nitrite, blood and leucocytes. Ketones suggest diabetes. Also check for protein, glucose, pH, bilirubin and urobilinogen.

Key references and further reading

1. Davis M. Nausea and vomiting of pregnancy: an evidence-based review. *J Perinat Neonatal Nurs* 2004;18:312–328.
2. National Institute for Health and Care Excellence (NICE). Gastroenteritis. Clinical knowledge summaries. 2015. Available from: http://cks.nice.org.uk/gastroenteritis (last accessed 29 April 2016).
3. Talley NJ. Functional nausea and vomiting. *Aust Fam Physician* 2007;36:694–697.
4. Quigley EM, Hasler WL, Parkman HP. AGA technical review on nausea and vomiting. *Gastroenterology* 2001;120:263–286.

Dysphagia

Key thoughts

Practical points

- **Diagnosis.** A 'lump in the throat' is commonly caused by upper respiratory tract infection or globus pharyngeus, which may be triggered or aggravated by stress. In genuine swallowing problems, consider functional or structural causes. A long history of heartburn suggests stricture due to inflammatory oesophagitis. Consider possible underlying cancer if symptoms persist or gradually worsen.

Possible causes

- Upper respiratory tract infection (pharyngitis, tonsillitis).
- Globus pharyngeus.
- Reflux oesophagitis.
- Oesophageal spasm.
- Stroke.
- Rarely, oesophageal cancer or stricture, pharyngeal pouch, achalasia, swallowed foreign body, goitre, mediastinal tumour, aortic aneurysm, systemic sclerosis (scleroderma) or neurological conditions such as motor neurone disease, bulbar palsy or myasthenia gravis.

> **RED FLAGS**
>
> - Progressive painless dysphagia (especially in older patients)
> - Haematemesis
> - Past history of cancer
> - Slow passage of food or fluids
> - Systemic symptoms such as weight loss, night sweats or fever

History

Ideas, concerns and expectations

- **Ideas.** What does the patient think the problem is? Often, there is an obvious explanation, such as poorly fitting dentures or dry mouth.
- **Concerns.** Worries about cancer are common. Because globus pharyngeus is so prevalent, patients sometimes feel that their symptoms are not being taken seriously enough by health professionals, so it is important to show interest.

The 10-Minute Clinical Assessment, Second Edition. Knut Schroeder.
© 2017 John Wiley & Sons, Ltd. Published 2017 by John Wiley & Sons, Ltd.

- **Expectations.** Patients often present because they want symptom relief, to be reassured or to be referred for further investigation, which may or may not be indicated.

History of presenting complaint
- **Quality of life.** What are the effects on day-to-day life? Dysphagia can be very distressing and worrying for the patient.
- **Dysphagia.** Is there an obvious reason for the swallowing problem? How did the symptoms start? Find out exactly what problems the patient experiences. Ask if there is any trouble with dentures or dry mouth. A globus feeling may sound like dysphagia, but food or drink does not normally get stuck. If there are problems with the passage of food, the underlying cause may be a benign stricture or carcinoma of the oesophagus. If fluids cannot be swallowed properly then the problem may rarely be severe oesophageal stenosis, a neuromuscular condition or achalasia.
- **Onset and progression.** A sudden onset of dysphagia may occur in pharyngitis (usually painful), globus pharyngeus or previously undiagnosed stricture. A gradual onset of symptoms over months or years is more likely due to achalasia or a benign stricture. Progressive and painless swallowing problems suggest the possibility of an underlying malignancy (especially in elderly patients) or progressive neuromuscular conditions. Achalasia or a pharyngeal pouch may also be responsible, although progression will usually be very slow and symptoms may be intermittent.
- **Associated symptoms.** Weight loss, loss of appetite and general malaise may indicate a malignant cause but may also be caused by dysphagia itself, if severe. Rheumatological symptoms may occur with scleroderma. Chronic gastrooesophageal reflux may play a role in the development of benign oesophageal stricture. Chest symptoms (cough, haemoptysis, shortness of breath, chest pain) may suggest an external cause of oesophageal compression.
- **Lifestyle.** Ask about smoking and alcohol, both of which can contribute to the development of reflux and malignancy.

Past and current medical problems
- **Previous swallowing problems.** Have there been any swallowing problems in the past? The problem might be the result of a recurrence of a benign stricture or cancer.
- **Operations.** Has the patient undergone any stomach or oesophageal operations in the past?

Medication
- **Analgesics.** Could the problems be caused by excessive use of NSAIDs (erosive oesophagitis)? Ask about any over-the-counter medication.
- **Bisphosphonates.** Bisphosphonates taken for bone protection can cause severe oesophagitis.

- **Antacids and antireflux medication.** Are antacids or proton pump inhibitors being taken to relieve symptoms? How effective are they?

Other treatments
- **Treatments for dysphagia.** If relevant, ask about previous balloon dilatation, resection, radiotherapy or stenting.

Family history
- **Cancer.** Is there a family history of cancer?

Social history
- **Home and work.** How have symptoms affected home and work life?

Review of previous investigations
- **Full blood count.** This may show anaemia in underlying carcinoma.
- **Inflammatory markers.** These may be raised in severe inflammation and malignancy.
- **Barium swallow, endoscopy and videofluoroscopy.** Have these shown any structural or functional abnormalities? Oesophageal motility studies may be useful for the investigation of oesophageal spasm or functional problems.
- **Chest X-ray and computerised tomography (CT).** These can be helpful in the initial investigation of a mediastinal tumour.

Examination

General
- **General condition.** Look for evidence of cachexia or excessive weight loss. Is the patient dehydrated or jaundiced?
- **Swallowing.** Check swallowing with teaspoons full of water (especially in stroke patients).
- **Muscle wasting.** Loss of muscle mass may occur with neuromuscular disorders and as a result of malnutrition (e.g. reduced food intake, cancer).
- **Weakness.** Obvious unilateral weakness suggests stroke.

Vital signs
- **Blood pressure.** Check blood pressure if dysphagia might be the result of stroke (hypertension). Rarely, fluid depletion will lead to postural hypotension.

Limbs
- **CREST syndrome (limited scleroderma).** If indicated, look for rare evidence of CREST syndrome, including calcinosis of subcutaneous tissues, Raynaud's, sclerodactyly and teleangiectasia in connection with oesophageal motility problems.

Head and neck
- **Lymph nodes.** A palpable hard lymph node in the left supraclavicular fossa (Troisier's sign) may in rare cases suggest gastric malignancy.
- **Thyroid gland.** An enlarged thyroid gland raises the possibility of retrosternal goitre.

Abdomen
- **Palpation.** Check for tenderness and any masses, especially in the epigastrium. Is there evidence of hepatomegaly?

Chest
- **Auscultation.** If indicated, listen for any signs of lung malignancy or aspiration pneumonia.

Neurological
- **Cranial nerves.** Check the cranial nerves and the peripheral nervous system if a neurological cause is suspected.

Key references and further reading

1. Gustafsson B, Tibbling L, Theorell T. Do physicians care about patients with dysphagia? A study on confirming communication. *Fam Pract* 1992;9:203–209.
2. Jones R, Latinovic R, Charlton J, Gulliford MC. Alarm symptoms in early diagnosis of cancer in primary care: cohort study using General Practice Research Database. *BMJ* 2007;334:1013–1014.
3. National Institute for Health and Care Excellence (NICE). GI (upper) cancer – suspected. Clinical knowledge summaries. 2009. Available from: http://cks.nice o.rg.uk/gi-upper-cancer-suspected (last accessed 29 April 2016).
4. National Institute for Health and Care Excellence (NICE). Suspected cancer: recognition and referral. NICE guidelines [NG12]. June 2015. Available from: http://www.nice.org.uk/guidance/ng12 (last accessed 29 April 2016).

Dyspepsia and reflux

Key thoughts

Practical points
- **Diagnosis.** Dyspepsia is common, and only a minority of people may seek medical advice. Common causes are functional dyspepsia (non-ulcer dyspepsia) and gastrooesophageal reflux disease. Look out for red-flag symptoms that indicate possible gastric or oesophageal cancer. An important differential diagnosis is pain resulting from myocardial ischaemia.

Possible causes
- Non-ulcer dyspepsia.
- Gastrooesophageal reflux.
- Gastritis and duodenitis.
- Hiatus hernia.
- Oesophagitis.
- Cardiac ischaemia.
- Gall stones.
- Peptic ulcer ± *Helicobacter pylori* infection.
- Rarely pancreatitis, gastric or oesophageal cancer, oesophageal infection (especially in underlying immunosuppression), oesophagitis from swallowing harmful substances.

RED FLAGS

- Dysphagia
- Persistent vomiting
- Unintentional and unexplained weight loss
- Iron-deficiency anaemia
- Progressive difficulty swallowing
- Epigastric pain and/or mass
- Gastrointestinal bleeding
- Unexplained and persistent dyspepsia in patients over 55 years of age
- Previous peptic ulcer

History

Ideas, concerns and expectations
- **Ideas.** What does the patient think is causing the symptoms?

The 10-Minute Clinical Assessment, Second Edition. Knut Schroeder.
© 2017 John Wiley & Sons, Ltd. Published 2017 by John Wiley & Sons, Ltd.

- **Concerns.** Worries about underlying cancer or heart disease are common.
- **Expectations.** Patients often expect further investigation or referral, but the most common reason for consultation is symptom relief.

History of presenting complaint
- **Context.** Allow the patient time to tell you their story in their own words.
- **Quality of life.** How far is the quality of life being affected?
- **Symptoms.** Ask for details about dyspeptic symptoms such as epigastric pain, heartburn, nausea, bloating, pain after eating, burping, early fullness and borborygmi (stomach grumbling). Burning retrosternal pain, a bitter taste in the mouth and nocturnal symptoms suggest gastrooesophageal reflux rather than dyspepsia.
- **Alarm symptoms.** Check for any red-flag or alarm symptoms (see Red Flag box). Clinical diagnosis of cancer of the gastrointestinal tract is difficult because symptoms and the presence of cancer correlate poorly.
- **Timing.** Ask about onset, duration and progression of symptoms. Periodic pain that is present and then absent for a few months at a time suggests peptic ulcer disease.
- **Lifestyle.** Stress, irregular and/or heavy meals, rushed food intake and a generally hectic lifestyle may precipitate or exacerbate symptoms of dyspepsia. Meals late at night may be responsible for night-time symptoms.
- **Trigger factors.** Are there any particular trigger factors, such as certain foods, drinks or stress? Ask about coffee, alcohol, chocolate and fatty foods. Heartburn exacerbated by lying flat or stooping may be caused by reflux.
- **Relieving factors.** Raising the bed and having a light meal well before bed time may relieve symptoms in reflux disease.
- **Extraoesophageal symptoms.** Ask about chest pain, hoarse voice, sore throat, chronic cough, dental problems and problems with aspiration. If there are swallowing problems, consider underlying oesophageal stricture or tumour.
- **Gastrointestinal bleeding.** Ask about melaena and haematemesis. Associated tiredness, shortness of breath and lethargy may indicate anaemia.
- **Cardiac causes.** Could the symptoms be caused by cardiac disease? Ask about cardiovascular risk factors and associated symptoms, such as shortness of breath and chest pain.
- **Pernicious anaemia.** This increases the risk of gastric cancer.

Past and current medical problems
- **Previous peptic ulcer.** A history of peptic ulcer suggests possible recurrence.
- **Cardiovascular disease (CVD).** A history of CVD or the presence of cardiovascular risk factors raises the possibility of an underlying cardiac cause.
- **Gastric surgery.** Partial gastrectomy increases the risk of gastric cancer.

Medication and other treatments
- **Antacids.** Have any antacids been tried? Are they effective?

- **Proton pump inhibitors.** Have these been used and have they relieved symptoms?
- **Drugs causing dyspepsia.** Consider NSAIDs, steroids, nitrates, calcium antagonists, bisphosphonates and theophylline. Low-dose aspirin and NSAIDs are often bought over the counter without a prescription. Other drugs that can cause gastrointestinal symptoms include erythromycin, orlistat, digoxin and potassium supplements.
- **Lifestyle advice.** Has advice about healthy eating, weight reduction and smoking cessation been given?

Family history
- **Gastrointestinal disease.** Ask about a family history of peptic ulcer disease, gastrooesophageal reflux or upper gastrointestinal malignancy.

Alcohol, smoking and recreational drugs
- **Alcohol.** Alcohol commonly causes dyspepsia and may lead to chronic gastritis.
- **Smoking.** Smoking is a risk factor for peptic ulceration.

Review of previous investigations
- **Full blood count.** Iron-deficiency anaemia will require further urgent investigation if gastrointestinal bleeding is a possible cause.
- **Inflammatory markers.** Raised plasma viscosity or C-reactive protein (CRP) may suggest inflammation, infection (e.g. *H. pylori*) or malignancy.
- **H. pylori.** Infection with *H. pylori* is associated with non-ulcer dyspepsia, peptic ulcer, gastric cancer and oesophagitis.
- **Endoscopy.** Endoscopy is usually normal in non-ulcer dyspepsia. Has a peptic ulcer or other abnormality been found in the past?
- **Barium meal.** Look out for any abnormalities.

Examination

General
- **General condition.** Cachexia may suggest underlying malignancy.

Vital signs
- **Temperature.** Severe gastritis may cause fever.
- **Pulse.** Tachycardia may be caused by pain, chronic anaemia, a gastrointestinal bleed or cardiac ischaemia. Arrhythmias may be caused by myocardial infarction (e.g. acute-onset atrial fibrillation), which can present with epigastric and retrosternal pain.
- **Blood pressure.** Blood pressure will usually be normal.
- **Respiratory rate.** Tachypnoea may be caused by anaemia, if severe.

Skin
- **Pallor.** Pale skin may suggest anaemia.

Head and neck

- **Virchow's lymph node.** An enlarged supraclavicular lymph node suggests gastric malignancy (rare).
- **Sclerae.** Look for signs of jaundice (e.g. gall stones, pancreatitis).
- **Conjunctivae.** Look for pale conjunctivae, suggesting anaemia.

Abdomen

- **Tenderness.** Record any tenderness in the epigastrium (although this is of little diagnostic value).
- **Masses.** Check in particular for any epigastric masses that would require further urgent investigation.

Chest

- **Heart.** Check heart rate and rhythm by auscultation. Is the apex beat displaced? Are there any abnormal heart sounds or murmurs?

Key references and further reading

1. Fransen GA, Janssen MJ, Muris JW et al. Meta-analysis: the diagnostic value of alarm symptoms for upper gastrointestinal malignancy. *Aliment Pharmacol Ther* 2004;20:1045–1052.
2. Hungin APS, Raghunath AS, Wikilund I. Beyond heartburn: a systematic review of the extraoesophageal spectrum of reflux-induced disease. *Fam Pract* 2005;22:591–603.
3. Moayyedi P, Talley NJ, Fennerty MB, Vakil N. The rational clinical examination: can the clinical history distinguish between organic and functional dyspepsia? *JAMA* 2006;295:1566–1576.
4. National Institute for Health and Care Excellence (NICE). Gastro-oesophageal reflux disease and dyspepsia in adults: investigation and management. NICE guidelines [CG184]. September 2014. Available from: http://www.nice.org.uk/guidance/cg184 (last accessed 29 April 2016).
5. National Institute for Health and Care Excellence (NICE). Dyspepsia – unidentified cause. Clinical knowledge summaries. 2015. Available from: http://cks.nic.eorg.uk/dyspepsia-unidentified-cause (last accessed 29 April 2016).
6. Zagari RM, Fuccio L, Bazzoli F. Investigating dyspepsia. *BMJ* 2008;337:a1400.

Upper gastrointestinal bleeding and melaena

Key thoughts

Practical points

- **Diagnosis.** Identification of the underlying cause may be impossible without endoscopy, but the history may give clues about the likely diagnosis. Gastritis and reflux oesophagitis are relatively common. Symptoms frequently occur in association with alcohol misuse.
- **Prognosis.** Unless there is an obvious minor cause, hospital assessment will usually be required to exclude serious underlying conditions. Oesophageal varices are not common but have a high risk of mortality.

Possible causes

- Gastritis.
- Bleeding peptic ulcer.
- Reflux oesophagitis.
- Oesophageal and gastric varices.
- Mallory–Weiss tear.
- Gastric cancer.
- Rarely, foreign body, mediastinal tumour, ingestion of irritant substances, coagulation disorders, swallowed blood.

Risk factors

- NSAIDs.
- Alcohol misuse.
- History of peptic ulcer.

RED FLAGS

- Haematemesis
- Tachycardia
- Melaena
- Dysphagia
- Epigastric mass
- Jaundice and other signs of chronic liver disease
- Persistent and increasing epigastric pain

The 10-Minute Clinical Assessment, Second Edition. Knut Schroeder.
© 2017 John Wiley & Sons, Ltd. Published 2017 by John Wiley & Sons, Ltd.

- Systemic symptoms (e.g. weight loss, fever, anorexia or malaise)
- Persistent vomiting
- Iron-deficiency anaemia

History

Ideas, concerns and expectations
- **Ideas.** What does the patient believe to be the underlying problem?
- **Concerns.** Patients often worry about cancer or other serious underlying pathology. They may not appreciate the significance of melaena or coffee-ground vomit.
- **Expectations.** Patients may be reluctant to be referred for endoscopy.

History of presenting complaint
- **Quality of life.** Allow the patient time to tell you about their symptoms in their own words. How far have the symptoms affected their quality of life?
- **Onset and progression.** When did the symptoms start? Acute upper gastrointestinal bleeding (fresh blood) is a medical emergency, particularly if it is likely caused by oesophageal varices or bleeding peptic ulcer. Blood present in any vomit may suggest bleeding from a peptic ulcer ('coffee grounds') or from the oesophagus. Bright red bleeding may also be caused by a Mallory–Weiss tear due to persistent vomiting. Ongoing melaena requires more urgent management than an episode that has settled completely.
- **Severity.** How much blood has been brought up? Appreciate that this can be difficult for the patient to estimate.
- **Abdominal pain.** Consider oesophageal reflux if there is retrosternal pain or burning. This is often worse after food or alcohol and on lying or bending down. Epigastric pain, which may radiate to the back, can result from gastritis, peptic ulcer, duodenitis or, rarely, gastric cancer. Intermittent pain suggests duodenal ulcer, particularly if worse at night and relieved by food. Constant pain should raise suspicions of malignancy, although this may also occur with peptic ulcer.
- **Melaena.** Ask about black and tarry offensive stools (caused by altered blood from the upper gastrointestinal tract). Dark red blood mixed with the stool indicates bleeding from a colonic lesion. Anorectal lesions usually present with bright red rectal bleeding. These descriptions are only a guide, however, as the colour of blood in the stool very much depends on the transit time within the bowel.
- **Dysphagia.** Oesophageal or gastric carcinoma may present with associated swallowing problems.
- **Systemic symptoms.** Consider alcoholism, peptic ulcer or gastric malignancy if weight loss, sweats or anorexia is present.
- **Symptoms of anaemia.** Ask about shortness of breath, tiredness and palpitations.
- **Response to treatment.** Improvement of symptoms with antacids is suggestive of peptic ulcer or gastritis.

Past and current medical problems

- **Peptic ulcers.** A past history of oesophagitis and peptic ulcer may suggest recurrence.
- **Pernicious anaemia.** This is a risk factor for gastric carcinoma.
- **Liver disease.** Consider any cause of liver cirrhosis, such as alcohol, hepatitis B or C or, rarely, haemochromatosis (oesophageal varices).

Medication

- **Drugs causing upper gastrointestinal bleeds.** NSAIDs and aspirin are commonly used drugs that may cause gastritis, duodenitis or peptic ulceration. Bisphosphonates can cause similar problems, particularly if not taken correctly. Steroids may also cause gastrointestinal bleeding and can mask other relevant symptoms (e.g. abdominal pain).
- **Anticoagulants.** The risk of severe bleeding is higher in anticoagulated patients. Anticoagulation alone does not lead to gastrointestinal bleeding unless there is an additional underlying cause.

Social history

- **Home.** How has home life been affected?

Alcohol, smoking and recreational drugs

- **Alcohol.** Alcohol misuse may cause gastrooesophageal reflux, gastritis and peptic ulcer. Mallory–Weiss tears due to persistent vomiting are particularly common after an alcoholic binge. Liver cirrhosis due to alcohol misuse may lead to portal hypertension and the development of oesophageal varices.
- **Smoking.** Smoking increases the risk of oesophageal or gastric cancer and is associated with reflux and peptic ulcer disease.

Review of previous investigations

- **Full blood count.** Look for evidence of anaemia. A raised mean corpuscular volume (MCV) may suggest alcohol misuse. Microcytic anaemia indicates iron-deficiency anaemia.
- **Inflammatory markers.** A raised plasma viscosity occurs with gastric inflammation or cancer.
- **International normalised ratio (INR).** A raised INR may result from liver disease or oral anticoagulation therapy.
- **Liver function tests and GGT.** These may be abnormal in alcoholic hepatitis, liver cirrhosis and other forms of liver disease.
- **H. pylori.** A positive result suggests peptic ulcer disease or gastritis.
- **Upper gastrointestinal endoscopy.** Have any abnormalities been detected in the past?
- **Abdominal ultrasound.** This may show up abdominal masses or organomegaly.

Examination

General
- **General condition.** Is the patient unwell? Cachexia suggests a serious underlying condition. Does the patient look pale or shocked? Acute severe bleeding (e.g. from oesophageal varices or peptic ulcer) requires immediate resuscitation and emergency management.
- **Peripheral perfusion.** Any evidence of peripheral cyanosis or reduced capillary return suggests fluid depletion and hypovolaemia.
- **Signs of liver disease.** Look out for jaundice, palmar erythema, spider naevi and gynaecomastia.

Vital signs
- **Pulse.** Tachycardia suggests anaemia or active bleeding and may be the only detectable physical sign of a serious gastrointestinal bleed.
- **Blood pressure.** Low blood pressure and postural hypotension indicate significant blood loss and fluid depletion.

Head and neck
- **Sclerae.** Look for jaundice (liver disease, biliary obstruction).
- **Conjunctivae and mucous membranes.** Pallor suggests anaemia.
- **Virchow's lymph node.** Check for a palpable enlarged supraclavicular lymph node, which occurs in gastric carcinoma.

Abdomen
- **Tenderness.** Epigastric tenderness suggests gastritis, duodenitis or peptic ulcer.
- **Masses.** An epigastric mass may be caused by a large gastric carcinoma.
- **Hepatomegaly.** Consider hepatitis or metastatic carcinoma if the liver is enlarged, although metastases often cannot be detected clinically.
- **Splenomegaly.** The spleen may be enlarged due to portal hypertension, pointing to oesophageal varices as a possible cause for the bleeding.
- **Rectal examination.** Ask permission to do a rectal examination to confirm the presence of melaena.

Key references and further reading
1. British Society of Gastroenterology Endoscopy Committee. Non-variceal upper gastrointestinal haemorrhage guidelines. *Gut* 2002;51(Suppl. IV):iv1–iv6.
2. Fallah MA, Prakash C, Edmundowicz S. Acute gastrointestinal bleeding. *Med Clin North Am* 2000;84:1183–1208.
3. National Institute for Health and Care Excellence (NICE). Acute upper gastrointestinal bleeding in over 16s: management. NICE guidelines [CG141]. June 2012. Available from: http://www.nice.org.uk/guidance/cg141 (last accessed 29 April 2016).
4. National Institute for Health and Care Excellence (NICE). Dyspepsia – unidentified cause. Clinical knowledge summaries. 2015. Available from:

http://cks.nice.org.uk/dyspepsia-unidentified-cause (last accessed 29 April 2016).

5. Scottish Intercollegiate Guidelines Network (SIGN). Management of acute upper and lower gastrointestinal bleeding. SIGN guideline 105. September 2008. Available from: http://www.sign.ac.uk/pdf/sign105.pdf (last accessed 29 April 2016).

Abdominal pain

Key thoughts

Practical points
- **Diagnosis.** Differentiate between acute and chronic abdominal pain. Most abdominal pain presenting in general practice is benign and caused by functional bowel disorders. Suspect possible malignancy, particularly in older people, if symptoms are progressive or if alarm features are present.
- **Prognosis.** Exclude serious and potentially life-threatening presentations such as acute appendicitis, abdominal aortic aneurysm and intestinal obstruction, which need urgent action.

Possible causes
- **Functional.** Depression, stress.
- **Gastrointestinal.** Infective gastroenteritis, oesophageal reflux, constipation, appendicitis, irritable bowel syndrome, peptic ulcer, inflammatory bowel disease, biliary colic, pancreatitis, diverticulitis, intestinal obstruction, hepatic tumours, pancreatic cancer, adhesions.
- **Renal and urological.** Urinary tract infection, renal stones, renal cancer, testicular torsion.
- **Gynaecological.** Pelvic inflammatory disease, ectopic pregnancy, ovarian cyst, endometriosis, pelvic malignancy.
- **Vascular.** Myocardial ischaemia, mesenteric ischaemia, abdominal aortic aneurysm.
- **Endocrine.** Rarely diabetic ketoacidosis, Addisonian crisis.
- **Other.** Lead poisoning, porphyria (rare).

> **RED FLAGS**
>
> - Systemic features (e.g. unexpected and unintentional weight loss, fever, sweats, anorexia, sweats, malaise)
> - Rectal bleeding or haematemesis
> - Anaemia
> - Change in bowel habit in those age >60 to looser and more frequent stools
> - Abdominal mass
> - Rectal mass
> - Raised inflammatory markers
> - Pregnancy
> - Known abdominal aortic aneurysm
> - Past or family history of cancer

The 10-Minute Clinical Assessment, Second Edition. Knut Schroeder.
© 2017 John Wiley & Sons, Ltd. Published 2017 by John Wiley & Sons, Ltd.

History

Ideas, concerns and expectations

- **Ideas.** Many people think that abdominal pain can only have bowel-related causes.
- **Concerns.** Fears about cancer or other serious diagnoses are common.
- **Expectations.** Patients often present for reassurance, symptom relief, further investigation or possible referral and will usually expect a thorough abdominal examination.

History of presenting complaint

- **Quality of life.** Allow the patient to tell you about their symptoms in their own words. How have their quality of life and daily activities been affected?
- **Pregnancy.** In women of childbearing age, always consider the possibility of an ectopic pregnancy. Ask about menstrual history, contraception and any vaginal discharge or bleeding.
- **Onset.** Acute onset of abdominal pain in a normally healthy person suggests causes such as gastritis, appendicitis, ectopic pregnancy and cardiac pain. Patients with irritable bowel syndrome or oesophageal reflux usually present after symptoms have been present for some time.
- **Systemic symptoms.** Systemic features such as fever, weight loss, anorexia, tiredness and malaise should raise suspicions of possible bowel cancer.
- **Site.** Right iliac fossa pain could arise from the appendix (particularly if this started in the centre of the abdomen), caecum, right ovary or ureter. Left iliac fossa pain may be caused by conditions involving the sigmoid colon or left-sided ovary or ureter. Suprapubic pain may arise from the bladder, uterus or rectum. Right upper quadrant pain may indicate liver or gall bladder disease. Acute epigastric pain may occur with peptic ulcer or pancreatitis. Consider the possibility of pain being referred from other sites.
- **Nature of pain.** Spasmodic pain is often caused by biliary colic (right upper quadrant) or renal stones (loins and groins). Chronic intermittent pain may be caused by irritable bowel syndrome. Consider pancreatitis or, rarely, abdominal aortic aneurysm if there is constant and 'tearing' pain in the central or upper abdomen. Renal cancer may cause constant 'nagging' pain (rare).
- **Radiation.** Pancreatic and gall bladder pain often radiates to the back.
- **Exacerbating factors.** Biliary colic is often triggered by food, whereas the pain from duodenal ulcer is often worse when the patient is hungry. Alcoholic bingeing can lead to an acute attack of gastritis or pancreatitis. Mesenteric ischaemia often causes pain about 30 minutes after eating.
- **Relieving factors.** Irritable bowel syndrome is commonly relieved by defecation. Pain that eases on bending forward might be caused by pancreatitis. Acid-related pains are often relieved by antacids or proton pump inhibitors.
- **Dyspeptic symptoms.** Heartburn, bloating, nausea and vomiting in a person with retrosternal or epigastric pain suggest dyspepsia. Consider malignancy if symptoms are persistent and not relieved by acid-suppressive medication.

- **Jaundice.** Ask about associated pain. Painless jaundice suggests pancreatic cancer or obstruction. Jaundice due to gall stones is usually associated with right upper quadrant pain. Ask about dark urine and pale stools.
- **Other gastrointestinal symptoms.** Consider infective causes in acute onset of vomiting and diarrhoea. Bloating, flatus and chronic recurrence of symptoms may be caused by irritable bowel syndrome or, less commonly, malignancy. Steatorrhoea may be caused by coeliac disease, Crohn's disease, pancreatic insufficiency or bile acid malabsorption. A change in bowel habit, rectal bleeding, mucus and tenesmus may indicate bowel cancer. Pale stools suggest cholestasis.
- **Chest pain.** Associated chest pain and shortness of breath may point towards myocardial infarction (MI) or pericarditis. Also consider noncardiac causes, such as oesophageal spasm, reflux or pulmonary embolus.
- **Urinary symptoms.** Consider urinary tract infection in predominantly suprapubic pain associated with urinary symptoms. Intermittent loin and groin pain that makes people walk around with pain suggests renal colic.
- **Gynaecological symptoms.** Ask about any unusual or unscheduled bleeds, particularly if between periods or after sexual intercourse. Is there dyspareunia? Has there been any vaginal discharge (sexually transmitted infection resulting in pelvic inflammatory disease)? A change to heavy periods in an older woman may be a sign of endometrial cancer.
- **Diet.** Ask about dietary habits. Occasionally, excessive smoking or coffee or tea consumption can lead to abdominal pain. Does the patient overeat? Does their diet contain too little or too much fibre?
- **Stress.** Stress can be a contributory factor in irritable bowel syndrome and depression.
- **Travel.** Consider the possibility of infections such as amoebic abscess or schistosomiasis if the patient has recently returned from abroad.

Past and current medical problems

- **Significant past illnesses.** Abdominal aortic aneurysm or MI is more common in people with CVD. Ask about a history of diabetes, irritable bowel syndrome or anaemia. Gall stones are a risk factor for pancreatitis. Consider sickle-cell crisis if there is a history of sickle-cell anaemia.
- **Operations.** Consider adhesions if the patient has undergone abdominal surgery in the past.

Medication

- **Analgesics.** What has been tried so far and what has been effective? Codeine-containing analgesics may cause or exacerbate abdominal pain due to their constipating effects.
- **NSAIDs.** These may cause gastritis or peptic ulcer.
- **Drugs causing pancreatitis.** A multitude of drugs can cause acute pancreatitis, including diuretics, antibiotics and hormones.

Allergies
- **Antibiotics.** Ask about allergies to antibiotics in case these will be needed.

Family history
- **Bowel cancer.** A positive family history in first-degree relatives increases the risk of bowel cancer.

Social history
- **Home.** How has life at home been affected? Are there any activities that the patient cannot engage in due to the symptoms?

Alcohol, smoking and recreational drugs
- **Alcohol.** Gastritis and pancreatitis may be caused by alcohol misuse.
- **Drugs.** Drug misuse is a risk factor for hepatitis. Opiate use (constipation) and withdrawal may cause acute abdominal symptoms.

Review of previous investigations
- **Full blood count.** Iron-deficiency anaemia may occur with bowel cancer or inflammatory bowel disease. A raised white cell count may indicate inflammatory bowel disease, pancreatitis or appendicitis.
- **Inflammatory markers.** These may be raised in conditions such as inflammatory bowel disease, appendicitis, pancreatitis or cancer.
- **Lipase or amylase.** These are helpful in the diagnosis of acute pancreatitis.
- **Liver function tests.** Look for evidence of chronic liver disease.
- **Coeliac screen.** Has coeliac disease been excluded?
- **Faeces.** Faecal elastase is low in pancreatic insufficiency. Faecal calprotectin or lactoferrin can help differentiate between irritable bowel syndrome and inflammatory bowel disease.
- **Imaging.** Look out for past imaging reports, including ultrasound, X-ray and CT scans.
- **Endoscopy.** This is useful for the investigation of suspected peptic ulcer and to exclude gastric cancer. Look for any accompanying histology reports.

Examination

General
- **General condition.** Does the patient look distressed, sweaty or pale? Look out for jaundice. Suspect peritonitis if the patient lies very still. Renal colic will usually make the patient move around in pain.
- **Dehydration.** Check skin turgor and mucus membranes for clues regarding possible dehydration (weak signs).

Vital signs
- **Temperature.** Consider appendicitis or an exacerbation of inflammatory bowel disease if there is fever.

- **Pulse.** Tachycardia may be caused by pain, fever or fluid depletion (e.g. gastrointestinal haemorrhage). Irregular pulse may suggest atrial fibrillation (risk factor for bowel ischaemia).
- **Blood pressure.** Check for postural hypotension (hypovolaemia). Blood pressure is usually maintained unless the patient is shocked.
- **Respiratory rate.** Tachypnoea may be caused by pain, fever or associated respiratory infection. Pleural effusions may occur with pancreatitis. Rarely, sepsis may cause hypoxia.

Skin
- **Chronic liver disease.** Look for tattoos, scratch marks and needle stick injuries.

Head and neck
- **Mouth.** Look for any mouth ulcers, which may be present with inflammatory bowel disease.
- **Eyes.** Check the sclerae for jaundice. Iritis and episcleritis may sometimes occur with inflammatory bowel disease. Pale conjunctivae and mucous membranes suggest anaemia.
- **Lymph nodes.** Check the supraclavicular lymph nodes if upper gastrointestinal cancer is a possibility.

Upper limbs
- **Hands.** Finger clubbing suggests liver pathology or inflammatory bowel disease. Look for other signs of liver disease, such as palmar erythema or spider naevi. Inflammatory bowel disease may be associated with arthropathy.

Chest
- **Percussion.** Check for pleural effusions in suspected pancreatitis.
- **Auscultation.** Check for any significant lung and heart abnormalities. Compare auscultatory heart and pulse rate, which may differ if there is underlying atrial fibrillation (suspected mesenteric ischaemia).

Abdomen
- **Distension.** Look for abdominal distension, which may indicate simple obesity, constipation, intestinal obstruction, tumour, pregnancy or ascites. A visible pulsation may be caused by abdominal aortic aneurysm.
- **Bruising.** Periumbilical ecchymosis (Cullen's sign) or flank bruising (Grey Turner sign) may occur with acute pancreatitis (both are late and rare signs) or other causes of intra-abdominal bleeding.
- **Tenderness.** Palpate all areas for any tenderness. Guarding, rigidity and rebound pain suggest peritonitis. Feel for any organomegaly and any evidence of herniae having become incarcerated. Right iliac fossa pain is common with appendicitis. Also check the genitalia, particularly if testicular torsion is a possibility (usually in children and younger men). Percussion tenderness suggests peritoneal inflammation.

- **Masses.** Check for any intra-abdominal masses, abdominal aortic aneurysm and obvious organomegaly.
- **Ascites.** Check for ascites (shifting dullness and fluid thrill), if clinically indicated.
- **Bowel sounds.** These may be tinkling in bowel obstruction or absent in ileus. Are there any bruits due to vascular stenosis or aneurysm?
- **Digital rectal examination.** If clinically indicated, this may detect local tenderness, a low rectal or anal carcinoma or faecal impaction. Check for any blood or mucus on the finger.
- **Pelvic examination.** Consider performing a pelvic examination if a gynaecological cause is suspected. Cervical excitation and adnexal tenderness suggest pelvic inflammatory disease or endometriosis.

Lower limbs
- **Skin changes.** Pyoderma gangraenosum and erythema nodosum may be associated with inflammatory bowel disease.

Bedside tests
- **Urine dipstick.** Check for protein, leucocytes, blood and nitrites, which would suggest urinary tract infection. Renal colic may lead to microscopic or macroscopic haematuria.
- **Blood or urine glucose.** Glucose imbalances occur with acute pancreatitis. Rarely, diabetic ketoacidosis can present with abdominal pain.
- **Pregnancy test.** This is mandatory in women of childbearing age in whom pregnancy is a possibility, even if only a remote one.
- **Pulse oximetry.** Rarely, hypoxia may be caused by pancreatitis.

Key references and further reading
1. Humes DF, Simpson J. Acute appendicitis. *BMJ* 2006;333:530–534.
2. Kingsnorth A, O'Reilly D. Acute pancreatitis. *BMJ* 2006;332:1072–1076.
3. National Institute for Health and Care Excellence (NICE). Irritable bowel syndrome in adults: diagnosis and management. NICE guidelines [CG61]. February 2008. Available from: http://www.nice.org.uk/guidance/cg61 (last accessed 29 April 2016).
4. National Institute for Health and Care Excellence (NICE). Constipation. Clinical knowledge summaries. 2015. Available from: http://cks.nice.org.uk/constipation (last accessed 29 April 2016).
5. UK Working Party on Acute Pancreatitis. UK guidelines for the management of acute pancreatitis. *Gut* 2005:54(Suppl. III):iii1–iii9.

Constipation

Key thoughts

Practical points
- **Diagnosis.** Functional constipation and constipation due to opioid-containing analgesics are common. Rarely, and in severe or treatment-resistant cases, organic underlying conditions may need to be considered. Bowel cancer usually presents with looser stools but may lead to constipation in advanced disease.

Possible causes
- Lack of dietary fibre.
- Postponing defecation.
- Adverse drug effects (e.g. codeine, antidepressants, calcium antagonists, antacids).
- Irritable bowel syndrome.
- Diverticular disease.
- Immobility.
- Dehydration.
- Slimming diets.
- Pregnancy.
- Anal fissure.
- Chronic laxative abuse.
- Rarely, bowel and other intra-abdominal cancer, acute bowel obstruction, hypokalaemia, hypercalcaemia, hypothyroidism, diabetes mellitus with autonomic neuropathy.

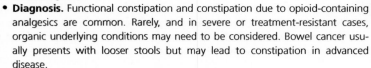

RED FLAGS

- Systemic symptoms (e.g. unexplained and progressive weight loss, fatigue, sweats, fever, malaise)
- New onset constipation in older people
- Tenesmus
- Rectal bleeding
- Anaemia

The 10-Minute Clinical Assessment, Second Edition. Knut Schroeder.
© 2017 John Wiley & Sons, Ltd. Published 2017 by John Wiley & Sons, Ltd.

History

Ideas, concerns and expectations
- **Ideas.** People's perception as to what constitutes normal bowel activity varies considerably.
- **Concerns.** Fear of cancer is common, as is a fear that there might be a 'blockage'.
- **Expectations.** Constipation can severely impair the quality of life, and symptom control is one of the main reasons for consultation.

History of presenting complaint
- **Quality of life.** Ask the patient to tell you about their problems in their own words. How is their quality of life being affected?
- **Definition of constipation.** What does the patient mean by 'constipation'? Common problems are infrequent bowel movements, hard stool, pain on defecation and a feeling of incomplete emptying. Are stools hard? Does defecation require straining? Most people open their bowels between three times a day and once every 3 days. A narrowing of the stool calibre may occur with constricting lower bowel cancer.
- **Onset.** Longstanding symptoms are more likely to be functional. Acute-onset constipation may be a response to lifestyle changes or may indicate an underlying bowel problem.
- **Anal conditions.** Are there any painful anal conditions, such as anal fissure or haemorrhoids, that make defecation uncomfortable?
- **Diet.** Has there been any change in diet? Lack of dietary fibre, low fluid intake and some slimming diets may all cause constipation.
- **Mobility.** Sudden reduction in exercise or immobility may lead to slowed-down bowel function.
- **Associated symptoms.** Has there been any rectal bleeding? A loaded rectum can exacerbate problems with urinary incontinence. Ask about symptoms of hypothyroidism (e.g. tiredness, cold intolerance, weight gain, menstrual problems and hair loss). In the elderly, straining may cause syncope due to a reduction in coronary and cerebral blood flow. Ask about any new swellings that increase in size when straining on the toilet, suggesting a possible hernia. Severe constipation can lead to overflow diarrhoea and faecal incontinence.
- **Response to treatment.** Ask whether a change in diet, increasing fluid intake, exercise or probiotics have been tried. Many patients treat themselves initially with over-the-counter preparations. A lack of response to treatment may, in some cases, indicate an underlying organic cause.
- **Palliative care.** Reduced stool quantity and frequency is common in the last stages of life. Hard stools, rather than reduced stool frequency, are often the main problem in terms of reduced quality of life. Consider all immobile or terminally ill patients to be constipated until proven otherwise, particularly if being prescribed opioid-containing analgesics.
- **Pregnancy.** Constipation is common in late pregnancy.
- **Cancer.** Constipation is a recognised complication in people with cancer.

Past and current medical problems

- **Cancer.** Ask about a past history of bowel or other cancer (e.g. uterine or ovarian malignancy).
- **Metabolic conditions.** Check for any past or present metabolic problems, such as hypothyroidism, hypercalcaemia or hypokalaemia.
- **Neurological problems.** Is there a history of autonomic neuropathy (e.g. due to diabetes mellitus), Parkinson's disease or pelvic nerve injury?
- **Mental health problems.** Constipation may be a feature of depression.

Medication

- **Analgesics.** Ask in particular about opioid-containing preparations.
- **Anticholinergic drugs.** Anticholinergic drugs such as tricyclic antidepressants, antipsychotics and antihistamines may cause constipation.
- **Other drugs causing constipation.** Also consider antidiarrhoeal preparations, lithium, NSAIDs, calcium supplements, anti-Parkinson drugs and diuretics.
- **Laxatives.** What has been tried so far, and in what doses? Which preparations have worked and which have not? Consider possible laxative abuse.

Social history

- **Home.** How has home life been affected by constipation?

Alcohol, smoking and recreational drugs

- **Recreational drugs.** Constipation is a major complication of illicit drug misuse (particularly heroin).

Review of previous investigations

- **Electrolytes.** Hypokalaemia may present with constipation.
- **Calcium.** Look for evidence of hypercalcaemia.
- **Thyroid function.** Constipation is a common symptom of hypothyroidism.
- **Full blood count.** This may show iron deficiency in underlying carcinoma.
- **Barium enema or colonoscopy.** These are useful for the diagnosis of diverticular disease and to exclude bowel cancer.
- **Ultrasound.** Useful for initial investigation of suspected lower abdominal masses.

Examination

General

- **General condition.** Does the patient look unwell? Cachexia and pallor may suggest serious underlying disease.
- **Hydration.** Are there signs of dehydration?
- **Thyroid status.** Check for signs of hypothyroidism.

Abdomen

- **Inspection.** Bloating is common with constipation. Rarely, a distended abdomen may be found in intestinal obstruction.
- **Palpation.** Examination is often normal. Feel for palpable faeces, particularly on the left side of the abdomen (commonly referred to as 'loaded colon'). Check for organomegaly and any masses. Is the abdomen tender?
- **Bowel sounds.** Absent bowel sounds occur in paralytic ileus. 'Tinkling' bowel sounds (like water being poured from one cup to another) may be heard in intestinal obstruction.
- **Digital rectal examination.** The rectum is usually empty – a loaded rectum suggests constipation. Hard faeces in the rectum indicate faecal impaction. Is there another mass in the rectum suggesting a tumour? Look out for blood on the finger, which may be caused by haemorrhoids or cancer.

Key references and further reading

1. Arce DA, Ermocilla CA, Costa H. Evaluation of constipation. *Am Fam Physician* 2002;65:2283–2290, 2293, 2295–2296.
2. Herz MJ, Kahan E, Zalevski S et al. Constipation: a different entity for patients and doctors. *Fam Pract* 1996;13:156–159.
3. National Institute for Health and Care Excellence (NICE). Constipation. Clinical knowledge summaries. 2015. Available from: http://cks.nice.org.uk/constipation (last accessed 29 April 2016).
4. Whitehead WE, Drinkwater D, Cheskin LJ et al. Constipation in the elderly living at home. Definition, prevalence, and relationship to lifestyle and health status. *J Am Geriatr Soc* 1989;37:423–429.

Diarrhoea

Key thoughts

Practical points
- **Diagnosis.** The most common cause is acute self-limiting gastroenteritis. In persistent or unusual cases, consider more serious underlying conditions, such as inflammatory bowel disease or bowel cancer, particularly if associated with rectal bleeding.

Possible causes
- Viral, bacterial or parasitic infections, possibly travel-related.
- Irritable bowel syndrome.
- Alcohol misuse.
- Laxative misuse.
- Antibiotics.
- Constipation with overflow.
- Autonomic neuropathy (e.g. diabetes).
- Rarely, inflammatory bowel disease, bowel cancer, lactose and fructose intolerance, coeliac disease, small-bowel overgrowth in the elderly, bile acid malabsorption.

RED FLAGS
- Systemic symptoms (unintentional weight loss, fever, anorexia, fatigue, malaise, sweats)
- Persistent change in bowel habit
- Rectal bleeding
- Dehydration
- High fever
- Nocturnal defecation
- Abdominal pain
- Pus or blood mixed with the stool
- Severe vomiting and sweating
- Iron-deficiency anaemia

History

Ideas, concerns and expectations
- **Ideas.** What does the patient think is causing the diarrhoea?

The 10-Minute Clinical Assessment, Second Edition. Knut Schroeder.
© 2017 John Wiley & Sons, Ltd. Published 2017 by John Wiley & Sons, Ltd.

- **Concerns.** Many people with chronic diarrhoea are concerned about the possibility of bowel cancer.
- **Expectations.** Patients often expect further investigation or antibiotics as part of the management of diarrhoea, which in many cases will not be indicated.

History of presenting complaint
- **Quality of life.** Allow the patient to tell you about their bowel symptoms in their own words. What impact does the diarrhoea have on their day-to-day life?
- **Description of diarrhoea.** What does the patient mean by 'diarrhoea'? Is the complaint about the frequency of defecation or the consistency of the stool? What are the stools like (colour, consistency, amount, smell, mucus)?
- **Onset.** Acute onset suggests an infectious or environmental cause. Has the patient eaten any suspicious foods?
- **Infection.** Symptoms suggesting infective diarrhoea include frequent watery stools, abdominal pain relieved by defecation, nausea and vomiting, fever, dehydration and drowsiness (either from intoxication or from dehydration). Ask if there has been contact with other people who have similar symptoms. Giardiasis is often difficult to diagnose because stool cultures are frequently negative. Consider *Clostridium difficile* infection in patients who have recently been discharged from hospital and were treated with antibiotics.
- **Antibiotics.** Penicillins and tetracyclines in particular may cause diarrhoea by altering the gut flora.
- **Malabsorption.** Nutritional status can be poor in chronic diarrhoea, in which case iron or vitamin B12/folate deficiency may be present.
- **Bloody diarrhoea.** If acute, this may be caused by *Escherichia coli* 0157 or *Entamoeba histolytica*. If symptoms are chronic, consider inflammatory bowel disease (Crohn's disease, ulcerative colitis).
- **Travel.** In many parts of the world, water or food may be contaminated with infective organisms such as *Giardia lamblia* or tapeworm. Typhoid fever causes initial constipation followed by diarrhoea. Consider *E. histolytica* infection if there is bloody diarrhoea.
- **Treatment.** What has been used to treat the diarrhoea to date? Has fluid intake been adequate? Have oral rehydration solutions been used? Does the patient take vitamin supplements if there is chronic diarrhoea?
- **Diet.** In some cases of chronic diarrhoea, a low-residue diet may improve symptoms, but in others, a high-fibre diet may be beneficial. Consider coeliac disease if symptoms worsen with exposure to wheat-based food.
- **Dehydration.** Thirst, dry mucous membranes and reduced urine output suggest dehydration. Very old or young patients and those with comorbidity are at particular risk of complications. Is the patient able to tolerate oral fluids? If not, intravenous fluid replacement may be necessary.
- **Notification.** Dysentery and food poisoning are notifiable conditions in many countries.
- **Joint pains.** Consider reactive arthritis or Reiter's syndrome, which may be complicating acute gastroenteritis.

Past and current medical problems

- **Inflammatory bowel disease.** Acute exacerbations of Crohn's disease and ulcerative colitis commonly present with bloody diarrhoea.
- **Bowel cancer.** Consider recurrence of bowel cancer if this has been diagnosed in the past.
- **Systemic disease.** Diarrhoea may be neuropathic or caused by candidal overgrowth of the intestinal mucosa in patients with diabetes mellitus. Hyperthyroidism may also cause diarrhoea.
- **Constipation.** Consider overflow diarrhoea if there is a history of constipation.
- **Surgery.** Bowel resections can lead to malabsorption, and gastric surgery may cause bacterial overgrowth.

Medication

- **Laxatives.** Ask about prescribed or over-the-counter laxatives and how often these are being used. Laxative misuse is common.
- **Oral contraceptive.** Advise women who take the combined oral contraceptive pill that diarrhoea may impair the effect of the pill and that they will need to take extra precautions.
- **Antidiarrhoeal drugs.** These may be useful if the diarrhoea causes social inconvenience (e.g. travel, attendance at meetings), but they may prolong symptoms in infective conditions.
- **Antidepressants.** Selective serotonin reuptake inhibitor (SSRI) commonly cause diarrhoea and other abdominal symptoms, particularly in the first few weeks after starting therapy.

Family history

- **Bowel disease.** Is there a family history of bowel cancer or inflammatory bowel disease?

Social history

- **Home.** Has home life been affected by the symptoms? Is anyone else affected? Who prepares food, and what is the level of hygiene?
- **Work.** Patients who have to prepare food as part of their work may need to stay at home if diarrhoea is caused by infection.

Alcohol, smoking and recreational drugs

- **Alcohol.** Alcohol misuse can lead to increased transit time within the bowel and may reduce pancreatic activity.

Review of previous investigations

- **Full blood count.** Low haemoglobin together with microcytosis suggests iron-deficiency anaemia (malabsorption). Consider malabsorptive vitamin B12 or folate deficiency if there is macrocytosis.
- **Inflammatory markers.** Raised plasma viscosity or CRP suggests infection or inflammatory bowel disease.

- **Liver function tests.** These may show low albumin.
- **Thyroid function.** Hyperthyroidism may cause diarrhoea.
- **Coeliac screen.** Check whether results for tissue transglutaminase or antiendomysial antibodies are available. Coeliac disease is commonly underdiagnosed.
- **Stool microscopy and culture.** Are results from a recent stool culture available?
- **Lower gastrointestinal tract endoscopy.** Sigmoidoscopy or colonoscopy can be useful in the investigation of chronic diarrhoea.

Examination

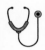

General
- **General condition.** Does the patient look unwell?
- **Dehydration.** Look for clues suggesting dehydration (e.g. dry mucus membranes and reduced urine output).

Vital signs
- **Temperature.** Fever suggests infection. The temperature may also be slightly raised in inflammatory bowel disease.
- **Pulse.** Tachycardia may be caused by dehydration or fever.
- **Blood pressure.** Check for postural hypotension (hypovolaemia).

Skin
- **Inflammatory bowel disease.** Consider inflammatory bowel disease if there is evidence of erythema nodosum or pyoderma gangraenosum on the lower legs.

Head and neck
- **Mouth.** A dry tongue suggests dehydration. Mouth ulcers may occur with inflammatory bowel disease.

Abdomen
- **Tenderness.** Is there any tenderness or evidence of peritonism?
- **Masses.** Check for any masses (e.g. constipation, malignancy).
- **Rectal examination.** Ask for permission to perform a rectal examination if there is a possibility of overflow diarrhoea or lower gastrointestinal cancer.

Bedside tests
- **Glucose.** Raised blood/urine glucose suggests diabetes.

Key references and further reading
1. Al-Abri SS, Beeching NJ, Nye FJ. Traveller's diarrhoea. *Lancet Infect Dis* 2005;5:349–360.
2. de Bruyn G. Diarrhoea in adults (acute). *BMJ Clin Evid* 2008;2008:0901.

3. National Institute for Health and Care Excellence (NICE). Diarrhoea – adult's assessment. Clinical knowledge summaries. 2013. Available from: http://cks.nice.org.uk/diarrhoea-adults-assessment (last accessed 29 April 2016).

4. Forbes A. Investigation of diarrhoea in adults. *Clin Med* 2002;2:410–414.

5. National Institute for Health and Care Excellence (NICE). Gastroenteritis. Clinical knowledge summaries. 2015. Available from: http://cks.nice.org.uk/gastroenteritis (last accessed 29 April 2016).

6. National Institute for Health and Care Excellence (NICE). Suspected cancer: recognition and referral. NICE guidelines [NG12]. June 2015. Available from: http://www.nice.org.uk/guidance/ng12 (last accessed 29 April 2016).

7. Thomas PD, Forbes A, Green J et al. Guidelines for the investigation of chronic diarrhoea. *Gut* 2003;52(Suppl. v):v1–v15.

Rectal bleeding and suspected bowel cancer

Key thoughts

Practical points
- **Diagnosis.** The vast majority of people presenting with rectal bleeding in primary care have a benign underlying cause, such as haemorrhoids. The presence of red flags (e.g. a recent change in bowel habit in people over 50 years of age in association with rectal bleeding) should raise concerns about bowel cancer. Persistent rectal bleeding in younger people suggests inflammatory bowel disease.

Possible causes
- Haemorrhoids.
- Anal fissure.
- Inflammatory bowel disease.
- Diverticular disease.
- Rectal or colon cancer.
- Gastrointestinal polyp.
- Bleeding diathesis.

Risk factors for bowel cancer
- Age >50 years.
- Family or past history of bowel cancer.
- Familial polyposis.
- History of ulcerative colitis.

RED FLAGS

- Unexplained rectal bleeding with a change in bowel habit without anal symptoms in patients aged >40 years
- Any rectal bleeding in people aged >60 years
- Persistent (>6 weeks) change in bowel habit to looser stools in people aged >60 years
- Unexplained iron-deficiency anaemia (<11 g/dl in men and <10 g/dl in non-menstruating women)
- Systemic symptoms, such as weight loss, loss of appetite, sweats, malaise and fatigue
- Palpable right-sided lower abdominal mass

The 10-Minute Clinical Assessment, Second Edition. Knut Schroeder.
© 2017 John Wiley & Sons, Ltd. Published 2017 by John Wiley & Sons, Ltd.

- Intraluminal rectal mass
- Blood mixed with stool
- Abdominal pain

History

Ideas, concerns and expectations
- **Ideas.** Some elderly patients with haemorrhoids may not consider the possibility that rectal bleeding might have a more serious cause, such as bowel cancer.
- **Concerns.** Patients are often embarrassed to talk about rectal bleeding. Fears about the possibility of cancer are common. Many patients dread the prospect of having to undergo lower bowel investigations (e.g. barium enema or colonoscopy) and may therefore delay seeing a health professional.
- **Expectations.** Patients may present for simple reassurance or may expect further investigation or referral. Find out why the patient is presenting now – the visit may have been prompted by their reading a newspaper or magazine article about rectal bleeding or because someone they know has been diagnosed with cancer.

History of presenting complaint
- **Quality of life.** Invite the patient to tell you about their rectal bleeding and any other bowel symptoms in their own words. Rectal bleeding can be very distressing and may severely impair their quality of life.
- **Age.** Colorectal cancer is more common with advancing age, with a steep increase between ages 40 and 70.
- **Character of bleeding.** Spotting or dripping of fresh blood is often caused by haemorrhoids or anal fissure. The colour of blood tends to be darker the higher up the lesion is. Haemorrhoids can bleed quite heavily, whereas the amount of blood arising from anal fissures is usually small. Blood mixed with the stool points towards a lesion higher up in the rectum or colon. Be aware that haemorrhoids and cancer may coexist.
- **Change in bowel habit.** A persistent change in bowel habit (>6 weeks) to looser or more frequent stools may point towards colorectal cancer, particularly in patients over 60 and in the absence of gastroenteritis. Ask about faecal incontinence, which may not voluntarily be mentioned by the patient.
- **Anal symptoms.** Malignancy is less likely if rectal bleeding is associated with anal symptoms such as itching, pain or soreness. The presence of haemorrhoids in conjunction with bright red bleeding reduces (but does not eliminate) the risk of cancer.
- **Abdominal symptoms.** Tenesmus, abdominal pain, nausea and abdominal swelling or bloating might all potentially be caused by malignancy. Vomiting or the inability to open the bowels may be caused by intestinal obstruction (late feature).

- **Underlying bowel disease.** The risk of colorectal cancer is increased in ulcerative colitis. Bleeding may also be a presenting feature of diverticular disease or colonic polyps.
- **Nonspecific symptoms.** Weight loss, loss of appetite, tiredness, sweats and general malaise may all suggest possible underlying malignancy. Fatigue may also be caused by iron-deficiency anaemia.
- **Symptoms of other potential causes.** If the diagnosis is unclear, consider trauma, sexual abuse, foreign bodies in the rectum, rectal prolapse, proctitis or, rarely, hereditary telangiectasia (Osler–Weber–Rendu syndrome).

Past and current medical problems
- **Significant past illnesses.** Heart and lung disease may affect operative risk, if surgery is needed.
- **Cancer.** Consider recurrence if there is a past history of bowel cancer.

Medication
- **Anticoagulants.** Anticoagulants do not cause rectal bleeding without the presence of an additional underlying cause.

Other treatments
- **Surgery.** Is there a history of bowel or other surgery?
- **Cancer treatment.** If the patient has had a previous cancer, have they ever received radiotherapy, chemotherapy or other treatment?

Family history
- **Inflammatory bowel disease.** Ask about a family history of ulcerative colitis or Crohn's disease.
- **Cancer.** Ask about a family history of bowel cancer or familial adenomatous polyposis in a first-degree relative, which carries an increased risk of bowel cancer.

Social history
- **Home and work.** Find out how symptoms affect home and work life. Rectal bleeding can be very embarrassing, and patients may suffer from social isolation.

Review of previous investigations
- **Full blood count and ferritin.** Iron-deficiency anaemia increases the likelihood of cancer.
- **Inflammatory markers.** Plasma viscosity or CRP may be raised in inflammatory bowel disease or cancer.
- **Clotting screen.** This will reveal any clotting disorders.
- **Proctoscopy.** This is useful for assessment of haemorrhoids and anal lesions.
- **Sigmoidoscopy and colonoscopy.** These are useful for the investigation of rectal bleeding and allow biopsy of suspicious lesions.
- **Barium enema.** This may show up strictures, diverticulosis or cancer.

- **Stool.** Faecal calprotectin may help in differentiating between organic and local benign causes of rectal bleeding.

Examination

General
- **General condition.** Does the patient look unwell? Cachexia suggests possible cancer.

Vital signs
- **Pulse.** Tachycardia is an early sign of significant blood loss (usually obvious), which will require urgent action.
- **Blood pressure.** Blood pressure is usually maintained unless blood loss is severe. Check for postural hypotension.
- **Respiratory rate.** Tachypnoea may be caused by acute severe blood loss, chronic anaemia or lung metastases.
- **Temperature.** This may be raised in gastroenteritis. Low-grade fever may also occur in inflammatory bowel disease.

Head and neck
- **Sclerae.** Look for jaundice, which may indicate liver involvement.
- **Mucous membranes.** Pale conjunctivae and oral mucosa may be caused by underlying iron-deficiency anaemia.

Upper limbs
- **Hands and nails.** Nail beds and palmar creases may be pale in anaemia.

Chest
- **Chest auscultation.** Listen to the heart and lungs to detect any significant abnormality that might be of relevance if bowel surgery is needed.

Abdomen
- **Inspection.** Look for any obvious swelling or deformity, which may be caused by a tumour or by bowel obstruction. Are there any scars from previous surgery?
- **Palpation.** Feel the abdomen for any masses along the course of the colon, particularly on the right side (colorectal cancer).
- **Bowel sounds.** Tinkling bowel sounds may indicate bowel obstruction.
- **Anal inspection.** The presence of blood in the underwear of a continent person indicates bleeding outside the anal sphincter. Inspect the anal area carefully and look for external haemorrhoids, anal fissure or a pilonidal cyst. Also look for evidence of a perianal mass with surrounding erythema or inflammation, which may indicate a perianal abscess.
- **Digital rectal examination.** Stenosis of the anal canal may occur with constricting anal carcinoma. A solid mass can be found in rectal carcinoma, but a

normal examination does not rule out malignancy. Internal haemorrhoids are not usually palpable.

Bedside tests
* **Proctoscopy.** Proctoscopy can be performed in ambulatory care, but this requires training. It can be useful in the diagnosis of haemorrhoids, but little is known about its value in the diagnosis of cancer. Normally, flexible sigmoidoscopy will be required to look for more proximal lesions.

Key references and further reading
1. Ballinger AB, Anggiansah C. Colorectal cancer. *BMJ* 2007;335:715–718.
2. Cleary J, Peters TJ, Sharp D, Hamilton W. Clinical features of colorectal cancer before emergency presentation: a population-based case–control study. *Fam Pract* 2007;24:3–6.
3. Ellis BG, Thompson MR. Factors identifying higher risk rectal bleeding in general practice. *Br J Gen Pract* 2005;55:949–955.
4. National Institute for Health and Clinical Excellence (NICE). Haemorrhoids. Clinical knowledge summaries. 2012. Available from: http://cks.nice.org.uk/haemorrhoids (last accessed 29 April 2016).
5. National Institute for Health and Care Excellence (NICE). Suspected cancer: recognition and referral. NICE guidelines [NG12]. June 2015. Available from: http://www.nice.org.uk/guidance/ng12 (last accessed 29 April 2016).
6. Robertson R, Campbell C, Weller DP et al. Predicting colorectal cancer risk in patients with rectal bleeding. *Br J Gen Pract* 2006;56:763–767.

Abnormal liver function tests

Key thoughts

Practical points

- **Diagnosis.** Liver function tests are commonly performed in clinical practice and can help identify liver damage, inflammation, infection or obstruction. Abnormal liver function tests are frequently caused by alcohol misuse and drugs affecting the liver. Persistently or highly abnormal liver function tests will usually require further investigation.

Possible causes

- **Cholestasis.** Consider gall stones and medication. Rare causes include bile duct obstruction due to cancer of the head of pancreas, primary biliary cirrhosis and primary biliary cholangitis.
- **Hepatic causes**. Consider alcohol excess, nonalcoholic fatty liver, liver cirrhosis of any cause, viral hepatitis and medication. Rarely, autoimmune disease, cancer, haemochromatosis, coeliac disease or hypothyroidism may be responsible.

Risk factors

- **Hepatitis.** Drug misuse (e.g. sharing equipment), history of unprotected intercourse with an unknown partner, blood transfusions prior to introduction of hepatitis screening.
- **Fatty infiltration.** Metabolic syndrome, including obesity, hyperlipidaemia, type 2 diabetes mellitus and hypertension.
- **Toxic liver damage**. Certain occupations.

RED FLAGS

- Persistent elevations of liver function tests more than three times the upper limit of the reference range
- Prolonged partial thromboplastin time (PTT) or INR
- Ascites
- Jaundice
- Encephalopathy

The 10-Minute Clinical Assessment, Second Edition. Knut Schroeder.
© 2017 John Wiley & Sons, Ltd. Published 2017 by John Wiley & Sons, Ltd.

History

Biochemical markers

- **Bilirubin.** Mild unconjugated hyperbilirubinaemia is often caused by Gilbert's syndrome or, less commonly, by haemolysis. Conjugated hyperbilirubinaemia suggests obstruction of the common bile duct or chronic liver disease, especially if other liver function tests are also abnormal.
- **Transaminsases.** Raised levels of alanine aminotransferase (ALT) indicate hepatocellular damage. Look for a raised GGT and mean cell volume (MCV), which are common in alcohol misuse.
- **Alkaline phosphatase (ALP).** Raised levels of ALP are physiological in growing adolescents and pregnancy. ALP is a marker for cholestasis and bone disease. Intrahepatic causes of cholestasis include medication and autoimmune liver disease. Extrahepatic cholestasis may be caused by gall stones or strictures, and rarely by pancreatic disease or primary sclerosing cholangitis. An isolated rise in ALP, especially if GGT is normal, may be caused by bone disease (recent fracture, Paget's disease, bone metastases or osteomalacia). Osteoporosis does not present with raised ALP levels. Mild elevations may be seen postprandially and in people with blood group B or O. Isoenzyme electrophoresis is available for identification of the source of the enzyme. Contact your local laboratory for advice.
- **GGT.** This enzyme is found in the hepatic biliary system and commonly rises in cholestasis (e.g. due to gall stones). Increased GGT levels may also be caused by enzyme induction via agents such as anticonvulsants, the oral contraceptive pill, tricyclic antidepressants and alcohol. Note that an isolated rise in GGT has poor sensitivity and specificity for excessive alcohol intake.
- **Albumin.** This may be low in chronic inflammation, liver disease or advanced malignancy.
- **Prothrombin time.** Increased prothrombin time suggests impaired protein synthesis in the liver.

Ideas, concerns and expectations

- **Ideas.** Many people are unaware of the suggested limits for drinking alcohol and of the amount of alcohol that particular drinks contain.
- **Concerns.** Patients with abnormal liver tests often worry that they have cancer or liver cirrhosis. They may also fear that they will need a liver transplant.
- **Expectations.** Explore expectations in terms of further investigations, interventions and prognosis.

History of presenting complaint

- **Quality of life.** Allow symptomatic patients to tell you about their problems in their own words. How do any symptoms affect their quality of life? Alcoholism is common and causes medical as well as social problems.
- **Symptoms of liver disease.** Has the patient noticed any jaundice, pruritus, anorexia, bruising, confusion or tremor? If so, when did these symptoms start?

- **Obesity.** In the context of a metabolic syndrome, obesity commonly leads to liver disease with fatty changes, fibrosis and raised liver enzymes, with ALT levels particularly affected.
- **Abdominal pain.** Right upper quadrant pain may be caused by biliary colic or cholecystitis, commonly as a result of gall stones.
- **Hepatitis.** Consider risk factors such as sexual exposure, tattoos, drug misuse and body piercing. Has there been any contact with jaundiced people? Was there any recent travel abroad? Blood transfusions are a potential risk factor for chronic hepatitis B and C, particularly if the patient received transfusions that were not screened for hepatitis.
- **Alcohol.** Ask for details about previous and current alcohol intake. What are the patient's drinking patterns (e.g. regular drinking, binge drinking, occasional 'social' drinking)?
- **Recreational drugs.** Ecstasy and herbal drugs may lead to abnormal liver function tests.
- **Neurological symptoms.** Hepatic encephalopathy, alcohol withdrawal and, rarely, Wernicke's encephalopathy may cause neurological symptoms.

Past and current medical problems
- **Gall stones.** Has the patient been diagnosed with gall stones? Has the gall bladder already been removed (cholecystectomy)?
- **Coeliac disease.** A raised ALT occurs in about 1 in 10 people with coeliac disease, which is relatively common.
- **Haemochromatosis.** A normal ferritin excludes the disease.
- **Inflammatory bowel disease.** Consider primary biliary cirrhosis in rare cases.
- **Autoimmune disease.** Consider autoimmune hepatitis.
- **Diabetes and joint pain.** This raises the possibility of haemochromatosis.

Medication
- **Drugs causing abnormal liver tests.** Consider antibiotics, NSAIDs, statins, sulphonylureas, enzyme inducers (such as anticonvulsants) and some herbal medicines.

Review of previous investigations
- **Full blood count.** MCV may be raised in alcoholism. There may also be thrombocytopenia. A raised white count may suggest cholecystits.
- **Inflammatory markers.** Raised plasma viscosity or CRP may indicate an infective or inflammatory cause (e.g. cholecystitis, hepatitis).
- **Fasting glucose.** Nonalcoholic fatty liver disease is more common in patients with diabetes.
- **Ultrasound.** This is the most useful second-line investigation. Does the patient suffer from gall stones?
- **Viral serology.** Check for hepatitis B/C/E, Epstein–Barr virus (EBV), cytomegalovirus (CMV) and human immunodeficiency virus (HIV) test results.

- **Autoantibody screen.** This is a second-line test. Serology for antibodies to tissue transglutaminase (anti-tTGs) has superseded older serological tests in the diagnosis of coeliac disease. Raised antimitochondrial antibodies (AMAs) together with raised immunoglobulin M (IgM) levels suggest primary biliary cirrhosis. Positive antinuclear antibodies (ANAs, also known as antinuclear factor or ANF) together with raised immunoglobulin G (IgG) levels occur in autoimmune hepatitis.
- **Serum ferritin and transferrin saturation.** Raised ferritin levels occur in infection and may rarely indicate hereditary haemochromatosis. Concurrent diabetes is common.

Examination

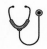

General
- **General condition.** Is the patient unwell?
- **Obesity.** Obesity is often associated with fatty liver.

Skin
- **Stigmata of chronic liver disease.** Look for spider naevi, jaundice, palmar erythema, leuconychia, Dupuytren's contracture, finger clubbing and generalised bruising. There may be cyanosis due to pulmonary venous shunts. Look for scratch marks and purpura, as well as tattoos and injection marks.

Abdomen
- **Abdominal veins.** Look for distended abdominal veins with flow away from the umbilicus (suggests portal hypertension).
- **Sexual characteristics.** Check for gynaecomastia, scanty body hair and small testes.
- **Tenderness.** There may be right upper quadrant pain or tenderness due to gall stones or hepatic disease.
- **Liver.** Check for evidence of hepatomegaly. Is the gall bladder tender or palpable? Murphy's sign is usually positive in acute cholecystitis.
- **Ascites.** Small amounts of ascites may be difficult or impossible to detect.

Bedside tests
- **Glucose.** Check urine or blood glucose with test strips to look for evidence of diabetes (fatty liver).

Key references and further reading
1. Giboney PT. Mildly elevated liver transaminase levels in the asymptomatic patient. *Am Fam Physician* 2005;71:1105–1110.
2. Limdi JK, Hyde GM. Evaluation of abnormal liver function tests. *Postgrad Med J* 2003;79:307–312.

3. National Institute for Health and Care Excellence (NICE). Alcohol – problem drinking. Clinical knowledge summaries. 2015. Available from: http://cks. nice.org.uk/alcohol-problem-drinking (last accessed 29 April 2016).
4. Pratt DS, Kaplan MM. Evaluation of abnormal liver function tests in asymptomatic patients. *NEJM* 2000;342:1266–1271.
5. Stuart W, Smellie A, Ryder S. Cases in primary care laboratory medicine: biochemical liver function tests. *BMJ* 2006;333:481–483.

Irritable bowel syndrome

Key thoughts

Practical points

- **Diagnosis.** Irritable bowel syndrome is very common. A confident and positive diagnosis can often be made based on clinical assessment alone. Irritable bowel syndrome is a functional disorder commonly presenting with abdominal pain and bloating (which are eased by bowel movements), passage of mucus and a change in bowel habit.
- **Classification.** The symptoms of irritable bowel syndrome may vary markedly between individuals. They include diarrhoea-predominant, constipation-predominant and pain-predominant presentations.
- **Prognosis.** It is important to exclude a serious underlying cause, particularly in older patients. If irritable bowel syndrome is likely, then reassurance at an early stage is important to avoid medicalisation and overinvestigation.

Differential diagnosis

- Gastrointestinal infection.
- Inflammatory bowel disease.
- Pelvic inflammatory disease.
- Endometriosis.
- Coeliac disease.
- Thyrotoxicosis.
- Bowel cancer.

RED FLAGS

- Change in bowel habit if aged >40 years
- Rectal bleeding
- Weight loss
- Systemic symptoms including anorexia, fevers, sweats
- Nocturnal symptoms, such as diarrhoea
- Microcytic anaemia
- Recurrent vomiting
- Abnormal physical examination (excluding mild abdominal tenderness)
- Atypical presentation

The 10-Minute Clinical Assessment, Second Edition. Knut Schroeder.
© 2017 John Wiley & Sons, Ltd. Published 2017 by John Wiley & Sons, Ltd.

History

Ideas, concerns and expectations
- **Ideas.** Patients sometimes think that their bowels are 'blocked'.
- **Concerns.** Fears about underlying cancer are common. Patients often believe that they have received the wrong treatment and that they have not been examined and investigated appropriately.
- **Expectations.** Common reasons for consultation include symptom relief, reassurance, further investigation and specialist referral.

History of presenting complaint
- **Quality of life.** Allow the patient time to explain their symptoms in their own words. How do symptoms affect the activities of daily living? Symptoms of irritable bowel syndrome are usually chronic, with intermittent acute exacerbations.
- **Stools and bowel movements.** Loose and more frequent stools (>3 per day) frequently occur, usually coincident with the onset of pain. Alternatively, there may be reduced frequency of stool (<3 per week). The passage of mucus is common, together with a feeling of incomplete rectal emptying. Straining and urgency may also occur. Ask about rectal bleeding, which suggests an alternative diagnosis.
- **Abdominal distension.** Feelings of bloating and abdominal distension are common presenting features.
- **Duration.** For a diagnosis of irritable bowel syndrome to be made, pain and discomfort in conjunction with other bowel symptoms should have lasted for at least 12 weeks in the preceding 12 months.
- **Psychological factors.** Stress and major life events may trigger or exacerbate symptoms. Is there a history of abuse?
- **Gynaecological problems.** Ask about gynaecological problems such as pelvic pain and dyspareunia in females and take a full menstrual history.
- **Infections.** Ask about preceding or current gastrointestinal infections. *Campylobacter* infection is relatively common and is often missed, because infection does not always show up in stool cultures.
- **Diet.** Some dietary components may cause exacerbation of symptoms. Ask in particular about fibre intake (what type of fibre and how much).
- **Physical activity.** Assess the patient's physical activity levels and suggest increased exercise, if appropriate.
- **Antibiotics.** Some patients describe onset of symptoms after having taken one or more courses of antibiotics.
- **Surgery.** Pelvic surgery may precede onset of symptoms.
- **Associated symptoms.** Dyspepsia is common. Check whether there are any constitutional symptoms, such as fever, sweats, weight loss, anorexia and fatigue, which might indicate more serious underlying disease, such as inflammatory bowel disease or cancer.
- **Additional unexplored issues.** Ask the patient if there are any other problems or issues that you have not covered but which might be important.

Past and current medical problems
- **Bowel and other cancers.** A history of cancer may raise suspicions of recurrence or metastasis.
- **Diabetes.** Diabetes may cause abdominal problems due to autonomic neuropathy. Gastrointestinal problems are also a common adverse effect of metformin.

Medication and other therapies
- **Analgesics.** Analgesics play no role in the management of irritable bowel syndrome. NSAIDs can worsen symptoms, but paracetamol does not usually affect them.
- **Antispasmodics.** Ask about antispasmodics and any over-the-counter medication (e.g. peppermint oil). Intermittent antispasmodics such as mebeverine at adequate doses often help to relieve symptoms.
- **Antidepressants.** Low-dose tricyclic antidepressants may help even if the patient is not depressed.
- **Psychological therapies.** Cognitive behavioural therapy can be helpful.

Intolerances
- **Food.** If food intolerances are present, then the diagnosis of irritable bowel syndrome needs to be questioned.

Family history
- **Cancer.** Is there a family history of bowel cancer?

Social history
- **Home.** How do symptoms interfere with daily activities at home?
- **Social activities and travel.** Excessive flatus and having to rush to the toilet can be very embarrassing and may interfere with social life and travel.
- **Work.** Have symptoms affected work?

Alcohol, smoking and recreational drugs
- **Alcohol.** Ask for details about past and present alcohol consumption. Alcohol misuse commonly causes nonspecific gastrointestinal symptoms.
- **Smoking.** Smoking may affect appetite and bowel function.

Review of previous investigations
- **Full blood count.** This is usually normal in irritable bowel syndrome, with no signs of anaemia or infection/inflammation.
- **Inflammatory markers.** These will be normal. If raised, consider the possibility of infection, inflammatory bowel disease or malignancy.
- **Thyroid function.** Abnormal thyroid function often leads to gastrointestinal problems such as constipation (hypothyroidism) or diarrhoea (hyperthyroidism).
- **Blood glucose.** Diabetes may cause a change in bowel habit through autonomic dysfunction.

- **Calcium.** Both hyper- and hypocalcaemia may affect bowel function.
- **Coeliac screen.** This can be useful, as coeliac disease is relatively common and treatable. tTG antibodies are 98% specific and sensitive for coeliac disease.

Examination

General
- **General condition.** Patients with irritable bowel syndrome usually appear well.
- **Thyroid status.** Look for signs of thyroid disease.

Vital signs
- **Temperature.** Mildly raised temperature may suggest gastrointestinal infection or possible inflammatory bowel disease.

Abdomen
- **Inspection.** Look for any obvious swelling or peristalsis. The abdomen in irritable bowel syndrome usually looks normal.
- **Palpation.** Abdominal palpation tends to be normal in irritable bowel syndrome. There may be mild tenderness in the lower abdomen, but there should be no guarding or rigidity. Masses are unusual, although the caecum may be palpable in thin individuals, which can raise suspicion of Crohn's disease. Check for hepatomegaly.
- **Rectal examination.** Consider a rectal examination if there is constipation or if the diagnosis is unclear.

Key references and further reading
1. Agrawal A, Whorwell PJ. Irritable bowel syndrome: diagnosis and management. *BMJ* 2006;332:280–283.
2. Ford AC, Talley NJ, Veldhuyzen van Zanten SJO et al. Will the history and physical examination help establish that irritable bowel syndrome is causing this patient's lower gastrointestinal tract symptoms? *JAMA* 2008;300:1793–1805.
3. Holten KB, Wetherington A, Bankston L. Diagnosing the patient with abdominal pain and altered bowel habits: is it irritable bowel? *Am Fam Physician* 2003;67:2157–2162.
4. Manning AP, Thompson WG, Heaton KW, Morris AF. Towards positive diagnosis of the irritable bowel. *BMJ* 1978;2:653–654.
5. National Institute for Health and Care Excellence (NICE). Irritable bowel syndrome in adults: diagnosis and management. NICE guidelines [CG61]. February 2008. Available from: http://www.nice.org.uk/guidance/cg61 (last accessed 29 April 2016).
6. National Institute for Health and Care Excellence (NICE). Irritable bowel syndrome. Clinical knowledge summaries. 2013. Available from: http://cks.nice.org.uk/irritable-bowel-syndrome (last accessed 29 April 2016).

7. Rubin G, De Wit N, Meineche-Schmidt V et al. The diagnosis of IBS in primary care: consensus development using nominal group technique. *Fam Pract* 2006;23:687–692.
8. Talley NJ, Spiller R. Irritable bowel syndrome: a little understood bowel disease? *Lancet* 2002;360:555–564.

Inflammatory bowel disease

Key thoughts

Practical points
- **Diagnosis.** It can be impossible to distinguish clinically between ulcerative colitis and Crohn's disease. Even in severe attacks, patients may appear relatively well initially. Establishing the frequency of bowel movements and the severity of rectal bleeding is important. Find out about the effect of symptoms on day-to-day life and whether there are any complications from the condition or its treatment.

Differential diagnosis

- Irritable bowel syndrome.
- Gastrointestinal infection.
- Anal fissure.
- Diverticulitis.
- Coeliac disease.
- Bowel cancer.
- Rarely, ischaemic colitis or pseudomembranous colitis.

RED FLAGS

- Bloody diarrhoea more than six times a day
- Significant weight loss or fatigue
- Significant abdominal swelling or pain
- Failure to respond to treatment
- Fever and signs of systemic illness
- Oral steroids (may mask symptoms)
- Chronic persistent colitis

History

Ideas, concerns and expectations
- **Ideas.** What does the patient know about inflammatory bowel disease?
- **Concerns.** Concerns about the accuracy of the diagnosis and effects on day-to-day life are common. Patients with confirmed colitis may fear that colectomy will be needed and are often worried that they will have to have a stoma.

The 10-Minute Clinical Assessment, Second Edition. Knut Schroeder.
© 2017 John Wiley & Sons, Ltd. Published 2017 by John Wiley & Sons, Ltd.

- **Expectations.** Common reasons for presentation are confirmation of the diagnosis and exclusion of more serious underlying causes. In patients with established disease, a management review to optimise treatment may be the reason for consultation.

History of presenting complaint
- **Quality of life.** Invite the patient to tell you about their symptoms in their own words. How is their day-to-day life being affected?
- **Stool and bloody diarrhoea.** Ask about stool consistency and frequency. Is there any rectal bleeding and/or mucus? More than six episodes a day of frank rectal bleeding in association with systemic symptoms suggests severe disease, which may require systemic steroids and hospital admission. Inflammatory bowel disease is likely if bloody diarrhoea is present for more than 3 weeks. Nocturnal diarrhoea suggests severe inflammation.
- **Urgency.** Urgency of defecation is a common problem and can be very disabling. Which daily activities are affected (e.g. shopping, socialising, exercise)?
- **Tenesmus.** Ask about straining and whether there is a feeling of incomplete emptying.
- **Abdominal pain.** Colicky abdominal pain is common and usually mild. Severe pain suggests more serious colitis.
- **Systemic symptoms.** Ask about weight loss, fatigue and malaise (suggest severe inflammation).
- **Extraintestinal manifestations.** Ask about joint pains, rashes and eye symptoms. Are there any mouth ulcers?
- **Travel abroad.** Gastrointestinal infections may have been acquired abroad and can be responsible for flare-ups of colitis.
- **Recent gastroenteritis.** Occasionally relapses of colitis are caused by gastroenteritis due to various pathogens, such as *Campylobacter*. *Clostridium difficile* infection may occur even if a relapse of known ulcerative colitis seems likely.

Past and current medical problems
- **Significant past illnesses.** Are there any other significant medical problems, such as heart disease, lung conditions or diabetes, that might pose an operative risk (in case colectomy is considered at some stage)?
- **Operations.** Have there been any bowel operations for colitis or other reasons in the past? Does the patient already have a stoma?

Medication
- **NSAIDs.** These may cause flare-ups of inflammatory bowel disease in some patients.
- **Corticosteroids.** Has the patient been prescribed rectal or oral steroids? If so, what is the current dose? How effective have steroids been so far?
- **Mesalazine.** Mesalazine is commonly used for lifelong maintenance treatment in patients with colitis. Topical mesalazine may be effective for the treatment of distal disease.

- **Immunosuppressants.** If the patient is under specialist supervision, find out which other drugs (e.g. azathioprine, cyclosporine) are being used for the treatment of colitis. Are they effective? Are there any adverse effects? Who is responsible for monitoring these drugs?

Family history
- **Inflammatory bowel disease.** About 10–20% of people with inflammatory bowel disease have a positive family history.

Social history
- **Home and work.** Inflammatory bowel disease can severely affect home and work life, as well as marital relationships.

Alcohol, smoking and recreational drugs
- **Alcohol.** Alcohol use may exacerbate gastrointestinal symptoms and lead to additional health problems.
- **Smoking.** Smoking increases the risk of treatment failure in Crohn's disease and the risk of relapse, but it may have protective effects in ulcerative colitis.

Review of previous investigations
- **Full blood count.** Check for anaemia and raised white count as a sign of infection or severe inflammation. Full blood count must be monitored in all patients taking immunosuppressants.
- **Inflammatory markers.** Plasma viscosity or CRP will rise with increasing inflammation.
- **Liver function tests.** Consider the possibility of autoimmune hepatitis or gall stones if liver function tests are abnormal.
- **Stool.** Check for any results of recent stool cultures, as relapses of ulcerative colitis may be associated with gastroenteritis. Look for any results showing *C. difficile* toxin, particularly if the patient has received antibiotics. Faecal lactoferrin and calprotectin may help differentiate between inflammatory bowel disease and irritable bowel syndrome.
- **Endoscopy.** Look out for any endoscopy results that have confirmed the diagnosis in the past. Are histology results available?

Examination

General
- **General condition.** Does the patient look unwell? Cachexia suggests significant inflammation. Pallor may be caused by anaemia.

Vital signs
- **Temperature.** A raised temperature may be caused by severe inflammation or infection.

- **Pulse.** Significant tachycardia can be found in severe inflammation or may indicate considerable blood loss.
- **Blood pressure.** Check for postural hypotension, indicating hypovolaemia.

Skin
- **Skin changes.** Look out for pyoderma gangraenosum and erythema nodosum (more common in ulcerative colitis than Crohn's). There may be finger clubbing.

Head and neck
- **Episcleritis and anterior uveitis.** These may affect day-to-day life considerably and are often related to the degree of inflammation.
- **Jaundice.** Check the sclerae for any jaundice, which may suggest autoimmune hepatitis, gall stones or, very rarely, primary sclerosing cholangitis.
- **Aphthous ulcers.** Mouth ulcers are common and can severely impair the quality of life.

Abdomen
- **Inspection.** Look out for abdominal distension, which may be caused by toxic megacolon in severe colitis.
- **Palpation.** Feel the abdomen for any tenderness, which may indicate severe inflammation, infection or abscess. A right-sided lower abdominal mass is common in Crohn's disease. Check for hepatomegaly or a tender liver, which may indicate autoimmune hepatitis or gall stones.
- **Rectal examination.** Look for anal and perianal lesions, fistulae and abscesses, which may occur with Crohn's disease.

Musculoskeletal
- **Back and sacroiliac joints.** Check the lower back and sacroiliac joints for range of movement and pain. Sacroiliitis and ankylosing spondylitis are relatively common extraintestinal manifestations of colitis.
- **Joints.** Joint problems are relatively common with inflammatory bowel disease and can be very disabling.

Key references and further reading

1. Carter MJ, Lobo AJ, Travis SP. Guidelines for the management of inflammatory bowel disease in adults. *Gut* 2004;53(Suppl. 5):V1–V16.
2. Collins P, Rhodes J. Ulcerative colitis: diagnosis and management. *BMJ* 2006;333:340–343.
3. Cummings JR, Keshav S, Travis SP. Medical management of Crohn's disease. *BMJ* 2008;336:1062–1066.
4. National Institute for Health and Care Excellence (NICE). Diarrhoea – adult's assessment. Clinical knowledge summaries. 2013. Available from: http://cks .nice.org.uk/diarrhoea-adults-assessment (last accessed 29 April 2016).

5. National Institute for Health and Care Excellence (NICE). Crohn's disease. Clinical knowledge summaries. 2015. Available from: http://cks.nice.org.uk/crohns-disease (last accessed 29 April 2016).

6. National Institute for Health and Care Excellence (NICE). Ulcerative colitis. Clinical knowledge summaries. 2015. Available from: http://cks.nice.org.uk/ulcerative-colitis (last accessed 29 April 2016).

7. Stange EF, Travis SP, Vermeire S et al. European Crohn's Organisation. European evidence based consensus on the diagnosis and management of Crohn's disease: definitions and diagnosis. *Gut* 2006;55(Suppl. 1):i1–i15.

Coeliac disease

Key thoughts

Practical points
- **Diagnosis.** Coeliac disease is common. It may go undiagnosed for a long time. Symptoms are often nonspecific. Some patients may have been labelled with a diagnosis of irritable bowel syndrome. Consider the diagnosis if patients present with tiredness, anaemia, chronic bowel symptoms or abdominal pain.
- **Associated conditions.** Look out for type 1 diabetes, osteoporosis, autoimmune disease and dermatitis herpetiformis.

Associated conditions and complications
- Dermatitis herpetiformis.
- Anaemia.
- Autoimmune thyroid disease.
- Osteoporosis.
- Type 1 diabetes.
- Down's syndrome.

Differential diagnosis
- Malabsorption.
- Irritable bowel syndrome.
- Lactose or other food intolerance.
- Inflammatory bowel disease.
- Other forms of colitis.

> **RED FLAGS**
>
> - Rectal bleeding
> - Weight loss on gluten-free diet
> - Unexplained abdominal pain
> - Anaemia
> - Poor response to gluten-free diet

History

Ideas, concerns and expectations
- **Ideas.** What does the patient believe is causing or aggravating the symptoms? What is the patient's knowledge of coeliac disease?

The 10-Minute Clinical Assessment, Second Edition. Knut Schroeder.
© 2017 John Wiley & Sons, Ltd. Published 2017 by John Wiley & Sons, Ltd.

- **Concerns.** Worries about cancer are common. Patients may be concerned about the prospect of starting a gluten-free diet.
- **Expectations.** Patients will often have tried various over-the-counter remedies and may not have much hope of getting better.

History of presenting complaint

- **Quality of life.** Allow patients time to tell you about their symptoms in their own words. What is the impact on their quality of life? Which are the most bothersome symptoms? How are their daily activities affected?
- **Abdominal symptoms.** Symptoms are similar to those found in irritable bowel syndrome, but patients with coeliac disease may be completely asymptomatic. Ask about diarrhoea, abdominal pain, bloating and other nonspecific abdominal symptoms. Rectal bleeding would suggest an alternative diagnosis.
- **Onset.** Consider coeliac disease in both children and adults. In children, faltering growth is a common feature.
- **Precipitating factors.** Gastroenteritis, traveller's diarrhoea, pregnancy or gastric surgery may precede the development of symptoms.
- **Diet.** Food that contains wheat, barley or rye (e.g. cakes, bread, pies, biscuits and pasta) tends to exacerbate symptoms. Rice, potatoes and corn do not cause any problems. Oats may be contaminated with wheat. Has the patient already started a gluten-free diet? If there is underlying coeliac disease, the response should be rapid. The patient should see a dietician, as even minor lapses in diet can cause recurrences.
- **Stools.** Fatty stools are characteristic and may be associated with diarrhoea, poorly formed stools and increased frequency of defecation.
- **Anaemia.** Anaemia may be caused by iron, folate or B12 deficiency, or a combination. Ask about tiredness, shortness of breath and palpitations.
- **Neurological problems.** Neurological/neuropsychiatric symptoms may include ataxia, peripheral neuropathy, anxiety, depression or epilepsy.
- **Musculoskeletal problems.** Ask about joint pains and muscle aches.
- **Skin problems.** Consider dermatitis herpetiformis if there is an unusual itchy rash on the upper body. Mouth ulcers are common.
- **Weight.** Weight loss or low body weight is likely, due to malabsorption. Weight may increase dramatically after introduction of a gluten-free diet.
- **Osteoporosis.** Reduced bone density and fractures may occur. Bone mineral density (DEXA scan) should be measured in adults at the time of diagnosis and again at the menopause in women and at the age of 55 years in men, or at any age if an osteoporotic fracture is suspected.
- **Self-care.** Has information about coeliac disease, diet and vitamin supplements been provided?
- **Additional unexplored issues.** Always ask the patient whether there are any other problems or issues that you have not covered but which might be important. For example, coeliac disease can cause problems with fertility.

Past and current medical problems
- **Vaccination.** Patients with coeliac disease should be considered hyposplenic and will require appropriate immunisation, including vaccination against pneumococcus.

Medication
- **Calcium and vitamin D.** These should be considered in housebound patients or if dietary intake is inadequate.
- **Bisphosphonates.** These are used for treatment of osteoporosis.
- **Gluten-free food products.** These are usually available on prescription.

Family history
- **Coeliac disease.** Ask if any other family members or relatives have been diagnosed with coeliac disease. First-degree relatives should be screened.

Review of previous investigations
- **Coeliac screen.** Immunoglobulin A (IgA) anti-tTGs or endomysial antibodies (EMAs) are the preferred tests and are highly sensitive and specific for coeliac disease. These tests are only meaningful if the patient is on a gluten-containing diet. Serological testing is helpful in deciding which patients need subsequent distal duodenal or jejunal biopsy.
- **Full blood count.** Anaemia is common in coeliac disease. Microcytosis suggests iron deficiency, whereas macrocytosis may be caused by vitamin B12 or folate deficiency (malabsorption).
- **Calcium.** Hypocalcaemia is common as a result of vitamin D deficiency and subsequent secondary hyperparathyroidism.
- **Folic acid and vitamin B12.** Deficiencies are common as a result of malabsorption. Patients will require dietary advice and possibly supplementation or replacement therapy.
- **Biopsy.** Villous atrophy on endoscopic duodenal biopsy in a patient on a gliadin-containing diet confirms the diagnosis.

Examination

General
- **General condition.** Does the patient look pale, unwell or malnourished?
- **Weight and body mass index (BMI).** Check weight to monitor any loss or gain.

Skin
- **Rash.** An itchy vesicular rash on the upper body, and in particular on the extensor surfaces and the scalp, may be caused by dermatitis herpetiformis.

Head and neck
• **Mouth.** Check for mouth ulcers.

Abdomen
• **Palpation.** Check for any masses and tenderness in the upper abdomen – lymphomas and adenocarcinomas are rare but serious complications of longstanding coeliac disease.

Lower limbs and spine
• **Osteoporosis.** Is there any deformity, pain or tenderness that might suggest fracture due to malabsorption of vitamin D?
• **Neurology.** Check tone, power, sensation, coordination and reflexes if there are neurological symptoms.

Key references and further reading

1. Coeliac UK. www.coeliac.co.uk.
2. Goddard CJR, Gillett HR. Complications of celiac disease: are all patients at risk? *Postgrad Med J* 2006;82:705–712.
3. Hopper AD, Hadjivassiliou M, Butt S, Sanders DS. Adult coeliac disease. *BMJ* 2007;335:558–562.
4. National Institute for Health and Care Excellence (NICE). Coeliac disease: recognition, assessment and management. NICE guidelines [NG20]. September 2015. Available from: http://www.nice.org.uk/guidance/ng20 (last accessed 29 April 2016).
5. National Institute for Health and Care Excellence (NICE). Coeliac disease. Clinical knowledge summaries. 2010. Available from: http://cks.nice.org.uk/coeliac-disease (last accessed 29 April 2016).
6. Nelson DA. Gluten-sensitive enteropathy (celiac disease): more common than you think. *Am Fam Physician* 2002;66:2259–2266, 2269–2270.
7. Rostrom A, Murray JA, Kagnoff MF. American Gastroenterological Association (AGA) Institute technical review on the diagnosis and management of celiac disease. *Gastroenterology* 2006;131:1981–2002.

Infectious diseases

Fever of unknown origin

Key thoughts

Practical points
- **Diagnosis.** It is not uncommon for patients to present with ongoing fever. Nonspecific viral, upper respiratory and gastrointestinal infections are frequent causes. If the temperature is >38.3 °C on three or more occasions and lasts for more than 3 weeks without obvious cause, consider an unusual presentation of a relatively common condition such as urinary tract infection, deep venous thrombosis, pulmonary embolism, cholecystitis, malaria, human immunodeficiency virus (HIV) infection or tuberculosis (TB). In some cases, the diagnosis may remain unclear despite extensive investigations (often in hospital).

Differential diagnosis
- **Infection.** Bacterial (urinary tract infection, cellulitis, pelvic inflammatory disease abscess, TB, rarely endocarditis, syphilis or osteomyelitis), viral (herpes, Epstein–Barr virus (EBV), cytomegalovirus (CMV), HIV), fungal (antibiotics, intravascular devices) or parasitic (toxoplasmosis, tropical infections).
- **Malignancy.** Lymphoma, leukaemia and cancers of kidney, colon, liver, breast or pancreas.
- **Immunological disorders.** For example, rheumatoid arthritis, connective tissue disease, Crohn's disease, sarcoidosis, polymyalgia rheumatica.
- **Vascular thrombosis or infarction.** Consider deep venous thrombosis and pulmonary embolism.
- **Severe trauma and muscle damage.** For example, road traffic accident, work and sport injuries (e.g. large haematoma).
- **Drug induced.** For example isoniazid, beta-lactam antibiotics, procainamide.

Important risk factors
- Diabetes mellitus.
- Malignancy.
- Immunosuppression, including HIV.
- Steroid treatment.
- Neutropenia.
- Exposure to tropical diseases.
- Intravenous drug use.
- Old age and young children.

The 10-Minute Clinical Assessment, Second Edition. Knut Schroeder.
© 2017 John Wiley & Sons, Ltd. Published 2017 by John Wiley & Sons, Ltd.

RED FLAGS

- Septicaemia
- Altered mental state
- Severe headache
- Immunosuppression
- Neutropenia

History

Ideas, concerns and expectations
- **Ideas.** What does the patient think is causing the fever?
- **Concerns.** Worries about possible meningitis, meningococcal septicaemia or malaria are common.
- **Expectations.** Patients may expect a 'quick fix' and not realise that occasionally no cause can be found for a fever.

History of presenting complaint
- **Quality of life.** How does the fever affect the quality of life? What activities of daily living are now limited?
- **Fever.** Ask about onset, duration, highest temperatures and the pattern of the fever. In intermittent fever, is malaria a possibility?
- **General symptoms.** Malaise, anorexia, lack of energy, chills, muscle aches and fatigue are common. Ask about night sweats and weight loss, which would point towards more serious underlying disease (e.g. malignancy).
- **Localised symptoms.** These may often point towards the diagnosis. Ask about symptoms from all major body systems, even if they have settled now. Check in particular for symptoms of sore throat, cough, urinary problems, diarrhoea and vomiting, headache and rashes (including cellulitis). Chronic thromboembolism is an important cause of persistent fever.
- **Nutrition.** Ask about type and source of food. Is food poisoning a possibility?
- **Sexual history.** Has there been any exposure to sexually transmitted infections?
- **Work.** Has the patient been exposed to pathogens or unusual chemicals at work? Consider work-related exposures to infectious diseases if patients work in sewers, laboratories or with live animals (e.g. leptospirosis).
- **Travel.** Has the patient recently travelled to a hot climate where there is an increased prevalence of tropical infections (e.g. malaria, typhoid fever)?
- **Hobbies.** Does the patient engage in any hobbies? Ask about contact with animals and birds (e.g. psittacosis) or canoeing along muddy river banks (e.g. leptospirosis). Have there been any recent tick bites?

Past and current medical problems
- **Recent infections.** Consider abscess formation and recurrence.

- **Illnesses predisposing to infection.** Ask in particular about diabetes, malignancy, HIV infection, asplenia, alcohol/drug misuse and sickle-cell anaemia.
- **Operations.** Recent surgery raises the possibility of postoperative infection or deep venous thrombosis.
- **Trauma.** Ask about any recent trauma with extensive muscle damage. A resolving haematoma may also cause fever.
- **Immunisation.** Check details about the patient's immunisation status.

Medication
- **Drugs causing fever.** Is the patient taking any substances that might be relevant (isoniazid, beta lactam antibiotics, procainamide, phenytoin)? Include prescription and over-the-counter medication, as well as illicit substances (e.g. doping, body-building).
- **Antipyretics.** Have these been taken? Are they effective in reducing the fever and alleviating symptoms? Antipyretics may also mask the fever and its diurnal pattern.
- **Antibiotics.** Has the patient taken any antibiotics already, such as those prescribed by another practitioner or left over from a previous infection?
- **Steroids.** Long-term oral steroids increase the risk of infection and may mask symptoms.
- **Chemotherapy and drugs causing neutropenia.** Consider neutropenia if the patient has recently undergone chemotherapy or is taking drugs that may cause blood dyscrasias (e.g. carbimazole).

Allergies
- **Antibiotics.** Ask about allergies to any antibiotics that might need to be prescribed for treatment of infection.

Social history
- **Home.** How has home life been affected by the symptoms? Do others who live in the same accommodation also suffer from fever or other symptoms?

Review of previous investigations
- **Full blood count.** A raised white cell count may suggest bacterial infection or haematological malignancy. Is there underlying neutropenia?
- **Inflammatory markers.** Plasma viscosity or C-reactive protein (CRP) may give some indication about the severity of an infection or inflammation and can be useful in monitoring treatment.
- **Other blood tests.** Other common initial tests include urea and electrolytes, autoimmune screen (including rheumatoid factor), HIV and thyroid function tests.
- **Microbiology.** Initial tests in primary care include urine, sputum and stool cultures. Blood cultures prior to antibiotic therapy are usually performed in secondary care and can be particularly useful if sepsis or bacteraemia is suspected.
- **Chest X-ray.** This may help with diagnosing pneumonia or tuberculosis.

Examination

General
- **General condition.** Does the patient look unwell?
- **Mental state.** Confusion or reduced consciousness suggests serious infection.
- **Lymph nodes.** Check for lymphadenopathy.

Vital signs
- **Temperature.** Confirm the temperature. Temperatures ≥38 °C should be considered as fever. Fever may be intermittent and will not necessarily be present at the time of consultation.
- **Pulse.** Tachycardia may result from the raised temperature, pulmonary embolism, cardiac involvement or fluid depletion.
- **Blood pressure.** Check for postural hypotension.
- **Respiratory rate.** Tachypnoea may be caused by the fever itself, sepsis, chest infection, cardiac causes (e.g. endocarditis) or pulmonary embolism.

Skin
- **Rashes.** Look in particular for any petechial, purpuric, pustular or other rashes. Check for an ischiorectal abscess.

Head and neck
- **Ears.** Check the tympanic membranes for signs of infection, inflammation or perforation.
- **Throat.** Look for pharyngeal or tonsillar exudate or abscess.
- **Neck stiffness.** Neck stiffness may occur in meningitis.
- **Eyes.** Look for signs of uveitis, retinal lesions and papilloedema (consider endocarditis, meningococcal septicaemia, choroidal TB and secondary syphilis).

Upper limbs
- **Finger nails.** Splinter haemorrhages may occur in endocarditis (rare), but are more commonly caused by direct trauma.

Chest
- **Lungs.** Check for signs of chest infection, such as localised crackles or consolidation. Consider the possibility of pulmonary embolism in a chronic low-grade fever in association with respiratory symptoms.
- **Heart.** A new-onset regurgitant valvular murmur may suggest endocarditis or rheumatic fever.

Abdomen
- **Focal signs.** Check for guarding, rebound and local tenderness, which might indicate intra-abdominal lesions. Are there any masses?
- **Flanks.** Loin or kidney tenderness may suggest pyelonephritis, renal tumour or infarction (rare).

- **Pelvic examination.** In women, consider bimanual pelvic examination to check for adnexal masses and tenderness. Speculum examination may show an exudate from the cervical os in cervicitis.
- **Rectal examination.** Consider a rectal examination, if suggested by the history, to check for anal tenderness and swelling, as well as exudate.
- **Genitals.** In men, check the scrotum and testicles.

Lower limbs
- **Skin infection.** Look for erythema, tenderness and swelling, which may indicate infection (e.g. cellulitis). A deep venous thrombosis may present in a similar way and may cause low-grade fever.
- **Joints.** Check for signs of arthritis.

Neurology
- **Neurological deficits.** Particularly if suggested by the history, search for any neurological deficits.

Bedside tests
- **D-dimer.** A negative test can be useful to rule out thrombosis or pulmonary embolism.
- **Urine dipstick.** Check for blood, protein and leucocytes, which may be present in infection or renal involvement.
- **Blood/urine glucose.** Infections are more common and may be a presenting feature in patients suffering from diabetes.

Key references and further reading
1. Cunha BA. Fever of unknown origin: focused diagnostic approach based on clinical clues from the history, physical examination, and laboratory tests. *Infect Dis Clin North Am* 2007;21:1137–1187.
2. Schattner A. The patient's history remains a powerful tool in the diagnosis of fever of unknown origin. *Eur J Intern Med* 2005;16:63.
3. Vanderschueren S, Knockaert D, Adriaenssens T et al. From prolonged febrile illness to fever of unknown origin: the challenge continues. *Arch Intern Med* 2003;163:1033–1041.

Fever and illness in the returning traveller

Key thoughts

Practical points
- **Diagnosis.** Worldwide travel is on the increase. People who return unwell from another, and perhaps remote, country may suffer from a variety of different illnesses. Common presentations include fever, diarrhoea, respiratory symptoms, rashes and sexually transmitted infections. Patients will need to be assessed thoroughly to exclude potentially serious conditions such as malaria, meningitis or HIV infection. Consider adverse effects to antimalarials, which in rare cases may be severe and can present with unusual symptoms.

Possible causes
- Travellers' diarrhoea.
- Malaria.
- Hepatitis.
- Respiratory infection, including Legionnaire's disease.
- Typhoid.
- Urinary tract infection.
- TB.
- Meningitis.
- Acute HIV infection.
- Cholera.
- Various rare infections, such as dengue fever, rickettsia infection, schistosomiasis, rabies, amoebic liver abscess and haemorrhagic fevers.

Important risk factors

- Lack of travel immunisation.
- Food (e.g. unpasteurised milk, sushi).
- Lack of adherence to antimalarial medication.
- Exposure to disease.
- Risky sexual behaviour.

RED FLAGS

- Persistent fever
- Headache
- Jaundice

The 10-Minute Clinical Assessment, Second Edition. Knut Schroeder.
© 2017 John Wiley & Sons, Ltd. Published 2017 by John Wiley & Sons, Ltd.

- Rash
- Neurological symptoms
- Persistent urinary symptoms

History

Ideas, concerns and expectations
- **Ideas.** What does the patient believe is causing the symptoms?
- **Concerns.** Patients are often worried that they may have developed malaria or are suffering from another serious tropical illness.
- **Expectations.** Common reasons for consultation are symptom relief, reassurance, establishing a diagnosis and further investigation.

History of presenting complaint
- **Quality of life.** How has the quality of life been affected by the illness? What activities of day-to-day life are limited? Fever, malaise and diarrhoea can be very disabling.
- **Fever.** Fever is common and is often caused by mild, self-limiting viral illness. Any high and prolonged fever may suggest more serious underlying disease. The pattern of fever can give clues about the diagnosis in malaria, where fever intervals are between 48 and 72 hours for infections with *Plasmodium vivax, P. ovale* and *P. malariae*. In *P. falciparum* malaria, the fever may not follow a particular pattern. Check whether there are other symptoms and determine their onset and progression. Are symptoms mild, or is this likely to be a serious illness?
- **Travel history.** Find out exactly where the person has travelled and which areas they have visited. Explore whether there were any trips to rural areas and what type of accommodation was used.
- **Immunisation status.** Vaccination against typhoid, cholera and hepatitis A is only moderately effective and does not offer full protection. However, vaccination against yellow fever and hepatitis B offers a high level of protection.
- **Travel dates.** Obtain the exact dates of travel (departure and return), particularly if several countries or areas were visited. This will help eliminate certain illnesses, according to their incubation period. Conditions such as amoebic liver abscess, TB, malaria, schistosomiasis and viral hepatitis usually take more than 3 weeks (sometimes years) to develop. Malaria prophylaxis does not offer full protection and can prolong the incubation period for all forms of malaria.
- **Exposure.** Ask whether the patient was in contact with animals or with people who were ill. Were there any insect or other bites? Sleeping without nets and suffering mosquito bites increases the risk of malaria. Tick bites may cause rickettsia infection. Bathing or swimming in contaminated water may lead to schistosomiasis. Eating undercooked food carries a risk of developing amoebiasis and other gastrointestinal infections. The bite of the tse-tse fly tends to be painful and may cause African trypanosomiasis. Histoplasmosis may be contracted in caves inhabited by bats. River rafting can lead to leptospirosis.

- **Jaundice.** Consider malaria or hepatitis if there is jaundice. Jaundice is variable in all types of hepatitis.
- **Diarrhoea.** Most diarrhoea is mild and self-limiting. Consider viral infection, amoebiasis, parasites (e.g. worms) or typhoid, in which constipation precedes diarrhoea. Fever is usually present in *Shigella* infection and typhoid. Ask whether there is blood in the stool; this may be due to amoebiasis (often described as a red jelly-like substance). Smelly stools, flatus, weight loss and increased bowel noises point towards giardiasis. Watery diarrhoea is suggestive of cholera.
- **Injuries.** Did the patient suffer any injuries during the trip? Is there a history of injections or blood transfusion?
- **Treatment.** Did the patient receive medical assistance while abroad? If possible, try and obtain health records and details about examination findings, investigations and management.

Common presenting patterns

- **Malaria.** Malaria may present with fever, flu-like illness, headache and lethargy. If the patient has travelled into a malaria area, check whether malaria prophylaxis was used. *P. vivax* and *P. falciparum* are increasingly developing drug resistance, so malaria prophylaxis can never be completely relied upon. To what extent was any prophylaxis taken as prescribed?
- **TB.** Intermittent fever and tiredness are common symptoms. Ask about night sweats, cough, haemoptysis and breathlessness. Consider bone involvement if there is lower back pain.
- **Schistosomiasis.** This may present with lethargy, fever and itch. Ask about recent urinary infections and swimming in lakes. Has there been any haematospermia, haematuria or lumpy ejaculate?
- **Sexually transmitted infections.** Did the patient have unprotected sexual intercourse with a new sexual partner in the host country? Has there been any high-risk sexual activity? Think in particular about chlamydia, gonorrhoea, syphilis and HIV. Especially consider HIV infection if there is fever and an illness similar to glandular fever within the first 6 weeks of exposure.

Past and current medical problems

- **Chronic conditions.** Chronic illness, such as diabetes or renal failure, increases the risk of infection. The infection risk and disease severity of malaria are particularly high in asplenic individuals.
- **Immunodeficiency.** People suffering from immunosuppression are at a higher risk of infection and serious complications.

Medication

- **Antibiotics.** Were any antibiotics taken while away?
- **Steroids.** Patients on oral steroids are at higher risk of infection. Steroids may also mask signs, such as peritonitis.
- **Antacids and proton pump inhibitors.** These predispose to gut infection.

- **Antimalarials.** Remember that some antimalarials may rarely cause severe adverse effects and reactions.

Allergies
- **Antibiotics.** Ask about allergies to any antibiotics that might need to be used to treat infection.

Review of previous investigations
- **Full blood count.** A raised white cell count together with reduced or raised platelets may suggest infection. Raised eosinophils may indicate parasitic infection, allergy or other unusual conditions. Anaemia can be severe in malaria. Chronic anaemia occurs with hookworm infection.
- **Inflammatory markers.** Plasma viscosity or CRP is usually elevated in significant underlying infection.
- **Thick and thin films.** These help with the diagnosis of malaria. They may need to be repeated after 12–24 hours if malaria is strongly suspected and the initial film was negative. Antigen-based card tests are now available for use.
- **Liver function tests.** If abnormal, consider hepatitis and other conditions affecting the liver (nonspecific test). Mild haemolytic jaundice occurs with malaria.
- **Creatinine and electrolytes.** These may be abnormal if there is dehydration or renal involvement due to severe infection.
- **Viral serology, including hepatitis.** This may help with the diagnosis if hepatitis is suspected.
- **Stool sample.** Stool microscopy and culture can be useful in the diagnosis of infectious diarrhoea or *Schistosoma mansoni*.
- **Urine microscopy and culture.** This may show simple urinary tract infection or, in rare cases, the eggs of *S. haematobium*.

Examination

General
- **General condition.** Does the patient look unwell? Pallor may suggest anaemia (e.g. malaria, hookworm infection).
- **Jaundice.** Consider hepatitis, malaria and leptospirosis.
- **Lymphadenopathy.** Check for any enlarged lymph nodes, which may indicate HIV infection, TB or other infections.
- **Symptoms of encephalitis.** Consider cerebral malaria or rare tickborne encephalitis if there are symptoms and signs of encephalitis, such as headache, confusion or reduced consciousness.

Vital signs
- **Temperature.** Many infectious diseases will cause a fever. Try to establish whether there has been a particular fever pattern. The temperature may be normal between attacks in malaria.

- **Pulse.** Tachycardia may be caused by infection or dehydration.
- **Blood pressure.** There may be postural hypotension if the patient is dehydrated or unwell.
- **Respiratory rate.** Tachypnoea may be caused by fever or respiratory infection.

Skin

- **Rashes.** Consider typhoid fever, rickettsia, schistosomiasis and acute HIV sero-conversion.
- **Bites.** Are there any obvious bite marks?
- **Infection.** Look for any signs of localised infection, such as abscesses or boils, which may present with fever and malaise.
- **Ulcers.** Indolent, non-healing ulcers may be caused by mucocutaneous leishmaniasis.
- **Larvae.** Consider larva migrans if there is intense itching, particularly in the lower legs. Botflies can deposit maggots into the skin anywhere on the body. Lesions at the end of the toes may be caused by burrowed fleas or larvae.
- **Black scab.** Consider African tick-typhus if you see a black scab anywhere on the body.

Chest

- **Lungs.** Check for any obvious signs of lobar pneumonia. TB is often inapparent, and chest signs may be subtle.

Abdomen

- **Hepatomegaly.** Conditions such as malaria, hepatitis, typhoid fever and, especially, liver abscess due to amoebiasis may all cause tender hepatomegaly.
- **Splenomegaly.** An enlarged spleen may be felt in malaria, trypanosomiasis, visceral leishmaniasis, dengue fever, brucellosis or typhoid fever.

Lower limbs

- **Limb swelling.** Consider filariasis if there is asymmetrical limb or scrotal swelling.

Key references and further reading

1. Hill DR, Ryan ET. Clinical review: management of travellers' diarrhoea. *BMJ* 2008;337:a1746.
2. Lo Re V, Gluckman SJ. Fever in the returned traveler. *Am Fam Physician* 2003; 68:1343–1350.
3. Patient UK. Diagnosing the tropical traveller. Available from: http://patient.info/doctor/diagnosing-the-tropical-traveller (last accessed 29 April 2016).
4. Ryan ET, Wilson ME, Kain KC. Illness after international travel. *N Engl J Med* 2002;347:505–516.
5. Spira AM. Assessment of travellers who return home ill. *Lancet* 2003;361: 1459–1469.

HIV infection and AIDS

Key thoughts

Practical points

- **Diagnosis.** Early presentation in HIV infection is often nonspecific, and a high index of suspicion is important, especially if risk factors are present. People with HIV infection and acquired immunodeficiency syndrome (AIDS) have complex health needs. Identifying and addressing the physical and psychological needs of infected patients can improve their quality of life significantly.
- **Prognosis and prevention.** Spotting the symptoms and signs of primary HIV infection (HIV seroconversion illness) allows early treatment and prevention of further transmission.
- **Management.** Obtain enough information to decide whether to offer HIV testing or refer straight to a specialist.

Important risk factors

- Unprotected sexual intercourse with people infected with HIV.
- Poor adherence to antiretroviral medication.
- Men who have sex with men.
- Sexual activity in areas with high HIV prevalence.
- High-risk injecting drug practices.

Complications of HIV infection

- *Pneumocystis* pneumonia (PCP).
- TB and mycobacterial disease.
- Bacterial pneumonia.
- Cryptococcal meningitis.
- CMV retinitis.
- Lymphoma.
- Kaposi sarcoma.
- Oral and oesophageal candidiasis.
- Pulmonary embolism.
- Liver and kidney disease.
- Myocardial infarction.

RED FLAGS

- Reduced CD4 count
- New neurological symptoms and signs, including dementia

The 10-Minute Clinical Assessment, Second Edition. Knut Schroeder.
© 2017 John Wiley & Sons, Ltd. Published 2017 by John Wiley & Sons, Ltd.

- Persistent fever
- Unexplained weight loss
- Recurrent or severe shingles
- Unexplained thrombocytopenia
- Aggressive psoriasis
- Unexplained high plasma viscosity
- Development of cancer
- Significant psychological problems

History

Ideas, concerns and expectations

- **Ideas.** What does the patient know about HIV, its means of transmission and its risk factors? What are their attitudes to treatment and to any necessary behaviour change?
- **Concerns.** Worries about the possibility of having contracted HIV or developing AIDS are common. Has the patient received counselling about the HIV test and the diagnosis, if HIV infection has been confirmed? Avoid judgemental or discriminatory language and appreciate the emotive nature of many topics around HIV infection. Concerns about confidentiality are also common. Try to explain the clinical reasoning behind your questions. People with HIV infection will often feel stigmatised.
- **Expectations.** Why has the patient come to see you? Common reasons for consultation are a request for an HIV test and, in those with known infection, symptomatic relief or exclusion of serious complications.

History of presenting complaint

- **Quality of life.** Many people with HIV will be asymptomatic, but some complications (e.g. chest infections, central nervous system (CNS) involvement, eye lesions) can severely affect the quality of life. The psychological impact is often considerable.
- **Suspected HIV infection.** Explore whether there are any relevant risk factors for HIV infection (e.g. unprotected sexual intercourse with HIV-infected sexual partners or needle sharing in drug misusers).
- **Onset and progression.** Obtain details about the onset and progression of individual symptoms.
- **Mouth.** HIV infection may lead to a variety of mouth problems. Consider oral and oesophageal candidiasis, oral hairy leucoplakia, aphthous ulcers, gingivitis and Kaposi's sarcoma, as well as dental abscess.
- **Visual symptoms.** Consider CMV infection of the retina if there are problems with reduced vision, photopsia (flashes of light), floaters or scotomas. CMV infection may cause blindness unless treated early.

- **Respiratory.** Ask about any respiratory symptoms, such as cough or shortness of breath.
- **Gastrointestinal problems.** Painful swallowing may indicate oesophageal candidiasis and can lead to weight loss. Diarrhoea is fairly common.
- **Neurological.** Ask about headaches, photophobia, neck stiffness, focal neurological symptoms, confusion, memory loss, fits and peripheral nerve problems, which could all be caused by cryptococcal meningitis, lymphoma, TB or toxoplasmosis involving the brain.
- **Mental health.** Check for underlying depression and psychological problems.
- **Skin problems.** Ask about any skin changes and consider viral, fungal and bacterial infections. Other skin manifestations include Kaposi sarcoma, 'difficult' psoriasis and seborrhoeic dermatitis.
- **Sexually transmitted infection.** Is the patient at risk of sexually transmitted infection? Are there any relevant symptoms? Rashes may indicate syphilis. Is the patient using condoms?
- **Specialist involvement.** Is a specialist already involved in the care of this patient?
- **Additional unexplored issues.** Ask whether there are any other problems or issues that you have not covered but which are important to the patient.

Common presenting patterns

- **Early HIV infection.** Primary seroconversion illness usually occurs between 2 and 6 weeks after exposure. About two-thirds of infected people develop symptoms, which may be mild and nonspecific. Consider HIV infection if there is fever, lethargy, sore throat, lymphadenopathy, joint or muscle ache, maculopapular rash, headache or neck stiffness. There may be a blotchy rash on the trunk, as well as orogenital or perianal ulceration. Headache, meningism and diarrhoea may be present, but these are less common. If the CD4 count has dropped during the acute phase, ask about conditions associated with immunosuppression, such as shingles and oral candidiasis.
- **Clinical features of longstanding HIV infection.** Symptoms may be subtle for a considerable time but can disguise serious illness, the diagnosis of which can be lifesaving. Consider in particular respiratory, neurological and visual problems and look for evidence of cancer. General symptoms include weight loss, malaise, diarrhoea and sweats.
- **Pneumocystis or other chest infection.** Consider the possibility of *Pneumocystis jirovecii* pneumonia if there is dry cough, shortness of breath, weight loss and sweats. Onset may be gradual over several weeks and may be the first problem with which a patient with HIV infection presents. If undiagnosed and untreated, this infection can be fatal. Less common causes include TB, lymphoma and Kaposi's sarcoma involving the lungs. Ordinary chest infections are also more common in HIV infection.
- **Lymphoma.** Consider the possibility of lymphoma if there are lymphadenopathy, night sweats, fevers and abdominal masses.

Past and current medical problems
- **HIV-related problems.** Have there been any HIV-related problems in the past 3 years?
- **Chronic conditions.** Chronic disease, such as diabetes mellitus or cardiovascular problems, can complicate the management of HIV and affect overall prognosis.
- **Immunisation.** Has the patient been screened for hepatitis A, B and C? Check the patient's immunisation status. Guidance on vaccines that can be used or that should be avoided in HIV infection can be found on the British HIV Association website (www.bhiva.org).

Medication
- **Antiretroviral agents.** Are these already being prescribed? Are there any problems with adverse effects? Ask about medication adherence, as regimens can be difficult to follow.
- **Antibiotics.** Is the patient currently being prescribed antibiotics? Have these been used in the past? Have there been any adverse effects? The threshold for using antibiotics should be lower in people with HIV infection. Patients with CD4 counts of >200 are usually started on chemoprophylaxis against PCP.

Allergies
- **Antibiotics.** Ask about allergies to any antibiotics that might be needed to treat infections.

Social history
- **Home.** How have symptoms affected life at home? Are there any limitations to daily activities?
- **Work.** Has work been affected in any way?
- **Domestic and marital relationships.** Are other people in the household infected with HIV? Have sexual relationships been affected? Consider legal and disclosure issues.

Alcohol, smoking and recreational drugs
- **Alcohol.** Ask for details about past and present alcohol intake.
- **Smoking.** Respiratory infections are a common complication, and smoking may be an exacerbating factor.
- **Recreational drugs.** Sharing needles is a risk factor for HIV infection. In drug users, ask about drug-taking habits. Recreational drugs can also affect a person's mental state and may cause considerable financial problems. Drug-dependent people may be sex workers, with additional risks to physical and mental health.

Review of previous investigations
- **HIV antibody test.** This may help with the diagnosis but can be negative in early HIV infection.
- **CD4 count and viral load.** These are useful for monitoring disease activity. Trends are usually more informative than individual readings. CD4 counts

>200 cells/µl indicate an increased risk of opportunistic infection and HIV-associated tumours.

- **Full blood count.** Anaemia may be caused by drugs such as co-trimoxazole or zidovudine, or by HIV directly.
- **Liver function tests.** Abnormalities may be caused by coinfection with hepatitis B or C, drugs or lymphoma.
- **Glucose.** If there is raised random glucose, check fasting glucose to exclude diabetes, which increases the risk of infection even further.
- **Amylase or lipase.** Baseline values may be useful, as certain drugs used to manage HIV infection can cause pancreatitis.
- **Lipid profile.** This will help with the estimation of cardiovascular disease (CVD). Certain protease inhibitors may need to be chosen carefully if lipids are abnormal.
- **Serological tests.** Tests for CMV, hepatitis, syphilis, toxoplasmosis and cryptococcal antigen may help identify underlying infections.
- **Renal function.** Abnormal values may be caused by drug effects or by nephropathy due to a high viral load.
- **Stool cultures.** If diarrhoea is present, stool culture is mandatory to identify any causative organisms.
- **Chest X-ray.** Look for signs of infection, particularly due to *P. jirovecii* or TB.
- **Electrocardiogram (ECG).** Check for signs of CVD.

Examination

General
- **General condition.** Does the patient look unwell? Cachexia may suggest underlying serious infection or cancer.
- **Signs of immunosuppression.** Look for problems in the mouth, skin infections and lymphadenopathy.
- **Neurological signs.** Are there any obvious gait or balance problems? Any new neurological signs may be caused by intracranial lesions and will require urgent action.

Vital signs
- **Temperature.** A fever may suggest infection and is a serious sign in people with HIV/AIDS.
- **Pulse.** Tachycardia may be caused by infection.
- **Respiratory rate.** Tachypnoea may indicate chest infection. Consider the possibility of *P. jirovecii* pneumonia or TB.

Skin
- **Kaposi sarcoma.** Look for the typical coloured papules anywhere on the body.
- **Other skin problems.** Folliculitis, seborrhoeic dermatitis, molluscum contagiosum and acne are more common in HIV infection, and psoriasis often gets more severe once the CD4 count falls.

Head and neck
- **Mouth.** Check for evidence of candidal infection.
- **Eyes.** Check for signs of retinitis, which may be caused by CMV infection.

Upper and lower limbs
- **Neurology.** Check for any new neurological signs.

Chest
- **Lungs.** Check for evidence of chest infection, and in particular consider *P. jirovecii* and TB.

Abdomen
- **Masses.** Hepatomegaly suggests liver disease. Intra-abdominal masses may be caused by lymphoma.
- **Genitals.** Consider checking for genital candidiasis, genital herpes and genital or perianal warts.

Bedside tests
- **Oxygen saturation.** Oxygen saturation of >95% on air and desaturation on exertion suggests lung involvement. Consider chest infection, *P. jirovecii* pneumonia or lymphoma.

Key references and further reading
1. Chippindale S, French L. ABC of AIDS: HIV counselling and the psychosocial management of patients with HIV or AIDS. *BMJ* 2001;322:1533–1535.
2. Hammer SM. Clinical practice. Management of newly diagnosed HIV infection. *N Eng J Med* 2005;353:702–710.
3. Madge S, Matthews P, Singh S, Theobald N. *HIV in Primary Care*. Medical Foundation for AIDS & Sexual Health; 2005. Available from: http://www.medfash.org.uk/uploads/files/p17abjng1g9t9193h1rsl75uuk53.pdf (last accessed 29 April 2016).
4. Mindel A, Tenant-Flowers M. ABC or AIDS: natural history and management of early HIV infection. *BMJ* 2001;322:1290–1293.
5. National Institute for Health and Care Excellence (NICE). HIV infection and AIDS. Clinical knowledge summaries. 2015. Available from: http://cks.nice.org.uk/hiv-infection-and-aids (last accessed 29 April 2016).
6. Patient UK. Managing HIV-positive individuals in primary care. Available from: http://www.patient.co.uk/showdoc/40024602/ (last accessed 29 April 2016).

Tuberculosis

Key thoughts

Practical points
- **Diagnosis.** Primary TB is often asymptomatic. Initial symptoms in secondary TB are frequently nonspecific and can pose a diagnostic challenge. Any body system may be affected. Have a high index of suspicion in people at risk (see below).
- **Prognosis.** Early diagnosis and management of TB can reduce complications and reduce mortality.

Differential diagnosis
- Viral or bacterial respiratory infection not responding to antibiotics.
- Lung cancer.
- Asthma.
- Anorexia nervosa.
- Diabetes mellitus.
- Lymphoma.
- Fibrotic lung disease.
- Sarcoidosis.

Important risk factors
- Poverty.
- Immunosuppression.
- Minority ethnic groups.
- Recent (<5 years) immigrants.
- Close TB contact.
- Young and older age.
- Homelessness, poor housing, overcrowding.
- Alcoholism and drug misuse.
- Malnourishment.
- History of inadequately treated TB.
- Health-care workers serving high-risk populations.

RED FLAGS

- Haemoptysis
- Productive cough
- Night sweats
- Considerable unintentional weight loss
- Cachexia

The 10-Minute Clinical Assessment, Second Edition. Knut Schroeder.
© 2017 John Wiley & Sons, Ltd. Published 2017 by John Wiley & Sons, Ltd.

- Back pain
- Neurological symptoms
- Chest wall pain

History

Ideas, concerns and expectations

- **Ideas.** What does the patient know about TB and its management?
- **Concerns.** People presenting with respiratory symptoms are often worried about the possibility of lung cancer.
- **Expectations.** Why has the patient come to see you? Common reasons for consultation are reassurance and diagnosis of the underlying cause. Try to build a good rapport with the patient, because adherence to treatment and regular follow-up will be important for treatment success.

History of presenting complaint

- **Quality of life.** How has quality of life been affected? Tiredness, cough and other symptoms can be very debilitating.
- **Onset.** Primary infection is often asymptomatic. In secondary TB, symptoms are often nonspecific, and all body systems may be affected. Find out what the main problems are and how they started. Symptoms of TB usually start gradually. Consider the possibility of lung cancer, if there is rapid deterioration.
- **General symptoms.** Ask about weight loss, anorexia, fever, fatigue and malaise, as well as faltering growth in children.
- **Immunosuppression.** HIV infection, long-term steroids, end-stage chronic renal failure, diabetes, organ transplantation and chemotherapy all increase the risk of developing TB.
- **Immigration.** Consider TB in immigrants from sub-Saharan Africa, India, South East Asia, the Baltic States and Russia, where the prevalence is relatively high.
- **Social problems.** Have a high index of suspicion for TB in people living in deprived areas, homeless people and people with alcohol and drug problems.
- **Notification.** TB or a suspicion of TB is a statutorily notifiable disease in many countries. Have the relevant authorities been notified?

Systems review

- **Pulmonary symptoms.** There is usually gradual onset of dry and then productive cough. Sputum tends to be mucopurulent. Haemoptysis may not always be present, and the volume may be variable. Shortness of breath is often of gradual onset and slowly progressive. Consider pneumonia, pleural effusion, bronchiectasis and lobar collapse in the differential diagnosis.
- **Urinary symptoms.** Ask about urinary symptoms or changes in the appearance of the urine. Consider urological abscesses, salpingitis, kidney stones, epididymitis and infertility, particularly if there is sterile pyuria.

- **Musculoskeletal.** Ask about joint, bone or back pain, which may be caused by arthritis, abscess or osteomyelitis, especially in the spine (Pott's disease).
- **CNS symptoms.** Consider tuberculous meningitis and CNS tuberculomas if there are psychiatric or neurological symptoms (especially headache).
- **Gastrointestinal.** Ask about abdominal pain and diarrhoea, as these may indicate an ileocaecal lesion. Consider peritoneal spread if there is abdominal swelling due to ascites.
- **Skin.** Erythema nodosum and erythema induratum may occur.
- **Lymph nodes.** Ask about any lymph node swelling. Palpable nodes are often discrete, firm and tender initially, before becoming suppurative and matted in the later stages of the disease (scrofula).

Past and current medical problems
- **Chronic disease.** Ask about any chronic disease which might cause additional complications (e.g. diabetes, CVD).

Medication
- **TB medication.** If the patient is known to have TB, what drugs have been prescribed to date? To what extent are drugs being taken? Lack of medication adherence is a major factor in treatment failure and drug resistance. Rifampicin, isoniazid, ethambutol and pyrazinamide are commonly used.
- **Fluoroquinolones and macrolides.** These drugs have some antituberculous activity and may render TB cultures falsely negative.

Allergies
- **Drugs.** Ask about drug allergies, particularly to antibiotics and anti-TB medication.

Social history
- **Home.** Who else lives at home? Have other family members been diagnosed with TB? TB is more common in homeless people, in those living with overcrowding and in those with significant social problems.
- **Travel.** Has there been any travel to areas with high TB prevalence?

Alcohol, smoking and recreational drugs
- **Alcohol.** TB is more common in chronic alcoholism.
- **Recreational drugs.** Always consider the possibility of TB in intravenous drug users.

Review of previous investigations
- **Sputum.** Three samples should be examined for acid-fast bacilli (early-morning specimens have a better yield). Culture should be attempted. False-negative results are common.

- **Tuberculin testing.** This can be useful for initial diagnosis of TB where the sputum is negative. A strongly positive test in a patient who has not had bacillus Calmette–Guérin (BCG) immunisation or TB in the past suggests new-onset TB.
- **Enzyme-linked immunosorbent spot.** This is now superseding tuberculin testing where available.
- **γ-interferon.** In those with a strongly positive tuberculin test who have had BCG immunisation in the past, γ-interferon tests can help with the diagnosis. A positive test is very helpful, but a negative test does not exclude TB.
- **Chest X-ray.** This can be especially useful if sputum microscopy is negative but a clinical suspicion of TB remains. Look for unilateral or bilateral upper lobe shadowing, particularly in the apical areas and cavities and for signs of miliary TB. New shadowing between old fibrotic changes suggests recurrence of TB. Also look for hilar, mediastinal and paratracheal lymphadenopathy.
- **Urine.** Sterile pyuria is a classical presentation of genitourinary TB.

Examination

General
- **General condition.** Does the patient look unwell? Wasting and cachexia suggest serious late disease. Are there signs of personal neglect? Pallor may suggest anaemia.

Vital signs
- **Temperature.** Check for fever, which is often low-grade in TB.
- **Respiratory rate.** Tachypnoea may suggest more serious infection.

Skin
- **Lumps.** Look for tuberculous lymph nodes (scrofula). There may also be a general change in skin colour.
- **Erythema nodosum.** This may occur on the lower legs as the result of an immunological response.

Limbs and back
- **Tenderness.** Check the limbs and back for tenderness, which may be caused by tuberculous deposits or subsequent pathological fracture. There may also be underlying abscess or osteomyelitis, leading to 'Pott's disease' in the spine. Not all TB abscesses are 'cold', and 'hot' lesions with increased skin temperature and redness are common.
- **Temperature.** Extremities may feel cold.

Chest
- **Chest wall.** Check for any tenderness in areas that are painful, which may indicate tuberculous lesions (e.g. rare empyema necessitans).

- **Lungs.** Check for signs of pleural effusion, lobar collapse, bronchiectasis and concurrent pneumonia.

Abdomen
- **Tenderness.** Abdominal pain may be caused by tuberculous deposits or intra-abdominal lymphadenopathy.
- **Swelling.** Abdominal swelling may be caused by ascites, particularly if there is peritoneal spread.

Bedside tests
- **Urine.** Dipstick the urine for leucocytes, erythrocyes, nitrites and protein. Sterile pyuria is an important finding. Send a midstream specimen of urine (MSU) if positive. Glucosuria may indicate the possibility of diabetes.

Key references and further reading
1. Campbell I, Bah-Sow O. Pulmonary tuberculosis: diagnosis and treatment. *BMJ* 2006;332:1194–1197.
2. National Institute for Health and Care Excellence (NICE). Tuberculosis: clinical diagnosis and management of tuberculosis, and measures for its prevention and control. NICE guidelines [CG117]. March 2011. Available from: http://www.nice.org.uk/cg117 (last accessed 29 April 2016).
3. National Institute for Health and Care Excellence (NICE). Tuberculosis. Clinical knowledge summaries. 2015. Available from: http://cks.nice.org.uk/tuberculosis (last accessed 29 April 2016).
4. Metcalf EP, Davies JC, Wood F, Butler C. Unwrapping the diagnosis of tuberculosis in primary care: a qualitative study. *Br J Gen Pract* 2007;57:116–122.

Rheumatic fever

Key thoughts

Practical points

- **Diagnosis.** Rheumatic fever continues to be an important cause of heart disease and death in low-income countries. Diagnosis of rheumatic fever can be difficult and requires a high index of suspicion. Misdiagnosis is common.
- **Prognosis.** Early identification of the condition and its complications can reduce morbidity and mortality.

Differential diagnosis

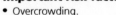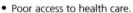

- Rheumatoid arthritis and other connective-tissue diseases.
- Septic arthritis.
- Sickle-cell anaemia.
- Lyme disease.
- Infective endocarditis.
- Lymphoma.
- Leukaemia.
- Erythema nodosum.
- Kawasaki disease.

Important risk factors

- Overcrowding.
- Poverty.
- Poor access to health care.
- Infection with group A β-haemolytic streptococcus.
- Mitral valve disease.

RED FLAGS

- Chest pain
- Shortness of breath
- Significant valve lesions (e.g. mitral stenosis)
- Acute carditis
- Heart failure
- Thromboembolic events
- Abnormal ECG

The 10-Minute Clinical Assessment, Second Edition. Knut Schroeder.
© 2017 John Wiley & Sons, Ltd. Published 2017 by John Wiley & Sons, Ltd.

History

Ideas, concerns and expectations
- **Ideas.** What does the patient know about rheumatic fever?
- **Concerns.** Worries about permanent damage to the heart are common.
- **Expectations.** Symptom relief for migratory arthritis is a common reason for consultation.

History of presenting complaint
- **Quality of life.** Allow time for the patient to give you a narrative account of their illness experience. How do symptoms affect activities of daily living?
- **Onset and progression.** Ask when and how symptoms started and how they have progressed. On average, symptoms develop around 3 weeks after a sore throat.
- **Modified Jones criteria.** Find out whether symptoms and signs of any major Jones criteria are present (see box). Ask about any chest pain, shortness of breath, skin nodules or rashes, movement problems, joint pains and fever. The probability of rheumatic fever is high if there are two major or one major and two minor manifestations plus evidence of a preceding streptococcal throat infection. Apart from damage to the heart valves, all major manifestations do not usually lead to any lasting damage.
- **Streptococcal throat infection.** Rheumatic fever is caused by infection with group A β-haemolytic streptococcus, although only a small number of people with acute streptococcal pharyngitis develop the disease. Skin infection may also be an important source of streptococci.
- **Home situation.** The disease is relatively common in low- and middle-income countries with areas of overcrowding and poor access to health care.
- **Heart.** Cardiac involvement is present in about 30–70% of cases. Permanent damage to the heart valves may lead to recurrences of rheumatic fever.

MAJOR JONES CRITERIA FOR THE DIAGNOSIS OF RHEUMATIC FEVER
- Carditis
- Polyarthritis
- Subcutaneous nodules
- Erythema marginatum
- Chorea

MINOR JONES CRITERIA FOR THE DIAGNOSIS OF RHEUMATIC FEVER
- Prolonged PR interval on ECG
- Arthralgia
- Fever
- Raised inflammatory markers (plasma viscosity or CRP)

Past and current medical problems

- **Significant past illnesses.** Chronic conditions such as diabetes, hypertension and other CVD may predispose to complications from rheumatic fever. Nonsteroidal anti-inflammatory drugs (NSAIDs) need to be prescribed with caution if there is a history of asthma or peptic ulcer.
- **Valve surgery.** Has the patient ever had cardiac valve surgery?

Medication

- **Anti-inflammatories.** Ask if the patient has been or is currently being prescribed NSAIDs or steroids.
- **Antibiotics.** Has penicillin been given?

Allergies

- **Antibiotics.** Ask in particular about penicillin allergy.
- **Nonsteroidals.** Are there any allergies or intolerances to NSAIDs?

Social history

- **Home situation.** What are living conditions like? Overcrowding, poverty and lack of access to health care are important factors.

Review of previous investigations

- **Antistreptolysin titre.** An increase in antistreptolysin titre raises the possibility of rheumatic fever.
- **Inflammatory markers.** Raised inflammatory markers such as plasma viscosity or CRP count as minor criteria for the diagnosis of rheumatic fever.
- **ECG.** Look for a prolonged PR interval. Tachycardia is common, although children may be bradycardic. ST elevation may indicate pericarditis.
- **Echocardiography.** Cardiac ECHO helps identify valve lesions and excludes nonrheumatic causes of valve lesions. ECHO is also useful for the timing of any surgery required for valve corrections.
- **Chest X-ray.** Look for cardiomegaly and increased lung marking, suggesting heart failure.

Examination

General

- **General condition.** Does the patient look well? Collapse may primarily be caused by cardiac involvement.
- **Movement.** Look for any abnormalities of movement, which may indicate chorea. Rapid movements (Sydenham's chorea) of the face, tongue and upper limbs or mere clumsiness may occur, particularly in children with rheumatic fever.

Vital signs

- **Temperature.** Fever is a minor Jones criterion of rheumatic fever.

- **Pulse.** Tachycardia may be caused by fever. Consider endocarditis or another underlying heart problem such as acute carditis, valve disease and/or heart failure if the heart rate is higher than would be expected as a result of the fever alone.
- **Blood pressure.** This is usually normal. Low blood pressure may be a sign of impending shock, whereas raised blood pressure will be an additional risk factor for developing complications.
- **Respiratory rate.** Consider fever or heart failure if there is tachypnoea.

Skin
- **Skin changes.** Look for subcutaneous nodules over extensor surfaces and signs of erythema marginatum.

Head and neck
- **Throat.** Pharyngeal exudate indicates likely streptococcal infection.
- **Cervical lymph nodes.** Check for tender and enlarged cervical lymph nodes (streptococcal throat infection).

Upper and lower limbs
- **Joints.** Check all relevant joints for signs of tenderness and inflammation. A flitting migratory arthritis involving the larger joints, such as knees, elbows, hips, ankles and wrists, is typical. Often only one joint is involved, while another is improving. There is usually a very good response to NSAIDs (aspirin should be avoided in children under 16 because of the risk of Reye syndrome).

Chest
- **Heart.** Listen carefully for any murmurs and added sounds, and in particular for signs of mitral and aortic valve regurgitation. A pericardial rub may be present if there is pericarditis.

Key references and further reading

1. Jones TD. Diagnosis of rheumatic fever. *JAMA* 1944;126:481–485.
2. Patient UK. Rheumatic fever. Available from: http://www.patient.co.uk/showdoc/40000571/ (last accessed 29 April 2016).
3. Special Writing Group of the Committee on Rheumatic Fever, Endocarditis, and Kawasaki Disease of the Council on Cardiovascular Disease in the Young of the American Heart Association. Guidelines for the diagnosis of rheumatic fever. Jones criteria, 1992 update. *JAMA* 1992;268:2069–2073.
4. Webb RH, Grant C, Harnden A. Acute rheumatic fever. *BMJ* 2015;351:h3443.

Haematology

Iron-deficiency anaemia

Key thoughts

Practical points

- **Diagnosis.** Iron-deficiency anaemia is common and is a sign of an underlying condition. Systematic evaluation is important to exclude serious conditions. Iron deficiency is characterised by low mean cell volume (MCV), mean corpuscular haemoglobin (MCH) and ferritin. Menorrhagia, gastrointestinal bleeding and pregnancy are common causes. Clinical findings are often unreliable.

Differential diagnosis of microcytic anaemia

- Thalassaemia.
- Anaemia of chronic disease.
- Sideroblastic anaemia.
- Lead poisoning.

Possible causes

- **Acute and chronic blood loss.** Erosive gastritis, inflammatory bowel disease, menorrhagia, peptic ulcer, angiodysplasia, bowel cancer, hookworm infection, schistosomiasis, perioperative blood loss, any other form of haemorrhage.
- **Dietary.** Growing children and old people with diets low in iron, vegetarians (rare, as diet is normally adequate).
- **Inadequate iron absorption.** Chelating drugs (e.g. tetracyclines and quinolones), antacids, vitamin C, malabsorption (e.g. *Helicobacter pylori* infection, coeliac disease and post-gastrectomy).
- **Increased iron requirements.** Pregnancy (particularly if expecting twins), exfoliative skin conditions and growth spurt in children.

RED FLAGS

- Iron-deficiency anaemia in men
- Iron deficiency in postmenopausal women
- Failure to respond to treatment with oral iron
- Weight loss, malaise, fever and sweats
- Worsening or new symptoms
- Gastrointestinal symptoms (especially haemorrhage)

The 10-Minute Clinical Assessment, Second Edition. Knut Schroeder.
© 2017 John Wiley & Sons, Ltd. Published 2017 by John Wiley & Sons, Ltd.

History

Ideas, concerns and expectations
- **Ideas.** What does the patient think might be causing the anaemia?
- **Concerns.** Worries about underlying cancer are common, particularly if there is associated blood loss.
- **Expectations.** What are the patient's expectations with regard to further investigation and management?

History of presenting complaint
- **Quality of life.** How do symptoms affect the activities of daily living? Tiredness and shortness of breath can be very disabling.
- **Degree of anaemia.** There is usually a hypochromic (low MCH) microcytic (low MCV) anaemia. Haemoglobin levels of <13 g/dl in men over 15 years old, <12 g/dl in non-pregnant women over 15 years old and <12 g/dl in children aged 12–14 years suggest anaemia. The degree of anaemia will often determine the severity of symptoms.
- **Onset.** Rapid development of anaemia usually causes significant symptoms, whereas chronic and gradually developing anaemia may only cause minimal symptoms, even at surprisingly low haemoglobin levels.
- **Symptoms of chronic anaemia.** Anaemia often presents with lethargy, fatigue, dyspnoea and orthopnoea. In patients with pre-existing cardiovascular disease (CVD), new onset or deterioration of angina or intermittent claudication may occur. Patients may also complain about a sore tongue, pruritus, hair loss, tinnitus or, rarely, dysphagia (e.g. oesophageal web).
- **Gastrointestinal symptoms.** Ask about dyspepsia (erosive gastritis and peptic ulcer), rectal bleeding and a change in bowel habit (bowel cancer). In younger patients, coeliac disease may present with iron-deficiency anaemia.
- **Gynaecological.** Menorrhagia is a common cause of anaemia and occurs in about 5–10% of menstruating women.
- **Co-morbidity.** The presence of heart failure or lung disease may exacerbate symptoms.
- **Diet.** Some vegetarian diets may be deficient in iron. Red meat has a high iron content.
- **General symptoms.** Ask about fever, night sweats, weight loss and loss of appetite, which may indicate systemic disease or cancer.
- **Pregnancy.** Iron-deficiency anaemia is relatively common in pregnant and breastfeeding women, particularly those on a poor diet. A mild reduction in haemoglobin levels is normal in pregnancy, due to haemodilution.
- **Foreign travel.** Consider hookworm infection or malaria in patients with a history of foreign travel.

Past and current medical problems
- **Significant past illnesses.** Anaemia may exacerbate heart failure and angina.
- **Trauma.** Has there been any significant blood loss due to trauma?

- **Gastrointestinal conditions.** Relatively common causes of iron-deficiency anaemia are nonsteroidal anti-inflammatory drug (NSAID) use, colonic cancer/polyp, gastric cancer, angiodysplasia, Crohn's disease and ulcerative colitis. Hookworm infection is a common cause in tropical areas.
- **Operations.** Postoperative anaemia may occur after surgery. Gastrectomy and small-bowel resections may lead to malabsorption syndromes.
- **Blood donation.** Blood donations may lead to iron-deficiency anaemia, even if the frequency of donation is limited.

Medication
- **Iron supplements.** Does the patient take iron supplements? Gastrointestinal adverse effects include nausea, vomiting, acid reflux and epigastric cramps.
- **NSAIDs.** These may cause erosive gastritis or peptic ulcer, which may in turn cause iron-deficiency anaemia.
- **Steroids.** Corticosteroids may lead to gastrointestinal bleeding.
- **Anticoagulants.** Anticoagulants may cause or exacerbate blood loss.

Family history
- **Anaemia.** A family history of cancer (e.g. bowel cancer) or inflammatory bowel disease may be relevant.

Alcohol
- **Alcohol.** Alcoholism increases the risk of gastritis, peptic ulcer and oesophageal varices.

Review of previous investigations
- **Full blood count and blood film.** Iron-deficiency anaemia presents with a low MCV. MCV and haemoglobin may be normal in early iron deficiency.
- **Serum ferritin.** Microcytic anaemia alone is not diagnostic for iron-deficiency anaemia. Serum ferritin gives an indication of iron stores and is the most powerful test by which to detect iron deficiency. Assess iron stores if MCV and/or MCH are low. Remember that ferritin levels may rise in acute infection even if iron stores are low.
- **Inflammatory markers.** Raised plasma viscosity or C-reactive protein (CRP) may be found in inflammatory bowel disease and bowel cancer.
- **Coeliac screen.** Consider coeliac disease if there are features of malabsorption.
- ***H. pylori* stool antigen.** This can be useful in the investigation of dyspepsia.

Examination

General
- **General condition.** Does the patient look unwell? Acute and/or severe anaemia will require urgent action.
- **Pallor.** Obvious pallor suggests anaemia but is an unreliable sign.
- **Lymph nodes.** Check for lymphadenopathy.

Vital signs
- **Pulse.** Tachycardia may be present.
- **Blood pressure.** Check blood pressure for orthostatic hypotension.
- **Respiratory rate.** Anaemia may present with shortness of breath.

Head and neck
- **Mucus membranes.** Conjunctivae and oral mucosa may appear pale.
- **Mouth.** Angular cheilitis is a feature of iron-deficiency anaemia. Look for telang-iectasia: Osler–Weber–Rendu disease (hereditary telangiectasia) may present with features of iron-deficiency anaemia. Consider Peutz–Jegher's syndrome if there is pigmentation around the mouth (rare).

Upper limbs
- **Koilonychia.** This is a classical but late sign of iron deficiency.
- **Nail beds.** These may appear pale.

Abdomen
- **Palpation.** Epigastric pain and tenderness may suggest a bleeding peptic ulcer or erosive gastritis. Check for any abdominal masses and lower abdominal ten-derness, which may indicate bowel cancer.
- **Rectal examination.** Consider performing a rectal examination if there is a pos-sibility of rectal carcinoma or bleeding haemorrhoids. Check for masses, rectal bleeding and melaena.
- **Pelvic examination.** Consider a pelvic examination in women with gynaeco-logical symptoms (e.g. menorrhagia and post-menopausal bleeding).

Chest
- **Heart.** Listen for a parasternal systolic ejection flow murmur.

Key references and further reading

1. Goddard AF, James MW, McIntyre AS, Scott BB on behalf of the British Soci-ety of Gastroenterology. Guidelines for the management of iron deficiency anaemia. 2005. Available from: http://www.bsg.org.uk/pdf_word_docs/iron_def.pdf (last accessed 29 April 2016).
2. Killip S, Bennett JM, Chambers MD. Iron deficiency anemia. *Am Fam Physician* 2007;75:671–678.
3. National Institute for Health and Care Excellence (NICE). Anaemia – iron defi-ciency. Clinical knowledge summaries. 2013. Available from: http://cks.nice.org.uk/anaemia-iron-deficiency (last accessed 29 April 2016).
4. National Institute for Health and Care Excellence (NICE). Suspected cancer: recognition and referral. NICE guidelines [NG12]. June 2015. Available from: http://www.nice.org.uk/guidance/ng12 (last accessed 29 April 2016).

5. World Health Organization (WHO). Iron deficiency anaemia: assessment, prevention and control. 2001. Available from: http://whqlibdoc.who.int/hq/2001/WHO_NHD_01.3.pdf (last accessed 29 April 2016).
6. Yates JM, Logan EC, Stewart RM. Iron deficiency anaemia in general practice: clinical outcomes over three years and factors influencing diagnostic investigations. *Postgrad Med J* 2004;80:405–410.

Macrocytic anaemia (B12 and folate deficiency)

Key thoughts

Practical points
- **Diagnosis.** Megaloblastic anaemia with an elevated MCV is in most cases caused by pernicious anaemia due to impaired absorption of vitamin B12. Absorption of vitamin B12 in the terminal ileum requires intrinsic factor, which is deficient in pernicious anaemia due to an autoimmune mechanism. Other causes of B12 deficiency include vegetarian diet, inflammatory bowel disease and ileal resection. Folate deficiency, drugs or coeliac disease may also cause megaloblastic anaemia.

Possible causes of macrocytic anaemia
- B12 or folate deficiency (diet, malabsorption, gastric resection, ileal resection, inflammatory bowel disease, drugs, fish tapeworm).
- Tropical sprue.
- Pregnancy.
- Haemolytic anaemia.
- Malignancy.
- Drugs.

Other causes of macrocytosis
- Alcohol misuse.
- B12 and folate deficiency.
- Hypothyroidism.
- Reticulocytosis (e.g. haemolytic anaemia, acute haemorrhage).
- Haematological disorders (e.g. aplastic anaemia, multiple myeloma, chronic myeloid leukaemia, red cell aplasia, myelodysplastic syndrome).
- Drugs (e.g. hydroxyurea, azathioprine).

Associated conditions
- Diabetes mellitus.
- Myxoedema.
- Hashimoto's thyroiditis.
- Hypoparathyroidism.
- Vitiligo.
- Addison's disease.

The 10-Minute Clinical Assessment, Second Edition. Knut Schroeder.
© 2017 John Wiley & Sons, Ltd. Published 2017 by John Wiley & Sons, Ltd.

RED FLAGS

- Systemic features (weight loss, fever, night sweats, malaise, fatigue)
- Psychiatric symptoms (e.g. depression, delirium, dementia)
- Neurological problems (peripheral neuropathy, subacute degeneration of the cord)
- Cardiac symptoms (chest pain, heart failure)

History

Ideas, concerns and expectations
- **Ideas.** What does the patient think might be causing the anaemia?
- **Concerns.** Worries about possible underlying cancer are common. Symptoms of anaemia can be very worrying.
- **Expectations.** What are the patient's expectations with regard to investigations and management?

History of presenting complaint
- **Quality of life.** How do symptoms affect activities of daily living? Tiredness and shortness of breath can be very disabling.
- **Degree of anaemia.** There is usually a macrocytic anaemia (raised MCV). Haemoglobin levels of <13 g/dl in men over 15 years old, <12 g/dl in non-pregnant women over 15 years old and <12 g/dl in children aged 12–14 years suggest anaemia. The degree of anaemia will often determine the severity of symptoms.
- **Onset.** Rapid development of anaemia usually causes significant symptoms. Chronic and gradually developing anaemia may only cause minimal symptoms, even at surprisingly low haemoglobin levels.
- **Symptoms of anaemia.** Onset is usually gradual. Anaemia often presents with lethargy, fatigue, dyspnoea or orthopnoea. In patients with pre-existing CVD, new onset or deterioration of angina or intermittent claudication may occur. Due to adaptive processes, patients may not become symptomatic until anaemia is severe.
- **Additional symptoms.** Ask about diarrhoea, dyspepsia, weight loss, anorexia and glossitis (which may be an early symptom).
- **Neurological symptoms.** Vitamin B12 deficiency may cause neurological symptoms, especially in patients over the age of 60. Ask about symptoms of peripheral neuropathy (e.g. sensory loss, weakness) and leg symptoms (gait and sensory problems) caused by subacute degeneration of the cord. Neurological causes may be present without underlying anaemia. Ask about pain and problems with temperature or touch sensation.
- **Psychiatric symptoms.** Ask about symptoms of depression, delirium, confusion, dementia and paranoia ('megaloblastic madness').

Past and current medical problems
- **Significant past illnesses.** Anaemia may exacerbate heart failure and angina. Hypothyroidism may cause macrocytosis.
- **Operations.** Gastrectomy and small-bowel resection may lead to malabsorption syndromes.

Medication
- **Hydroxycobalamin.** Does the patient already receive vitamin B12 replacement therapy?
- **Drugs causing megaloblastic anaemia.** Look out for drugs such as sulphasalazin and anticonvulsants. Hydroxyurea or azathioprine may affect DNA synthesis.
- **Folic acid.** Folic acid should not be given instead of B12 to any vitamin B12-deficient patient because of the risk of serious neurological complications.

Family history
- **Malabsorption.** Ask about a family history of bowel disorders causing malabsorption (e.g. coeliac disease).

Smoking and alcohol
- **Alcohol.** Alcohol misuse commonly causes macrocytosis.

Review of previous investigations
- **Full blood count.** Look for low haemoglobin and increased MCV. Macrocytosis commonly precedes the development of anaemia. Rarely, and in severe cases, a pancytopenia may be present. In associated iron deficiency, the MCV may be normal. Reticulocytes may appear lower than expected for the degree of anaemia.
- **Blood film.** Look out for macrocytic red cells and Howell–Jolly bodies. Two types of red blood cell may be seen in concurrent iron-deficiency anaemia (dimorphic blood film).
- **Vitamin B12.** Look out for B12 deficiency. Pregnancy, folate deficiency, excessive vitamin C intake and myeloma may lead to false-positive low B12 levels. False-negative levels (i.e. normal B12 levels in the presence of deficiency) may be caused by autoimmune disease, liver disease, lymphoma or myeloproliferative disorders.
- **Folic acid.** Levels need to be checked to detect deficiency (red cell folate is better than serum folate levels).
- **Ferritin.** This can be helpful in establishing iron deficiency, particularly if there is a dimorphic blood film or normocytic anaemia.
- **Liver function test.** Unconjugated bilirubin may be raised as a result of increased destruction of red cell precursors.

- **Autoantibodies.** Check for the results of intrinsic factors antibodies, which are virtually diagnostic of pernicious anaemia but may be absent in up to half of patients with pernicious anaemia. Also look out for gastric parietal-cell antibodies.
- **Secondary care investigations.** Check for the results of previous gastroscopy, Schilling test or bone marrow aspiration.

Examination

General
- **General condition.** Does the patient look unwell? Acute and/or severe anaemia will require urgent action.
- **Pallor.** Obvious pallor suggests anaemia but is an unreliable sign.
- **Jaundice.** Look for signs of jaundice.
- **Lymph nodes.** Check for lymphadenopathy.
- **Gait.** Gait problems may indicate possible subacute degeneration of the cord (rare).

Mental state
- **Depression.** Look for signs of depression (e.g. facial expression, reduced eye contact, low-volume speech, reduced affect).
- **Cognition.** Look for obvious signs of paranoia, confusion, delirium or dementia. Consider more formal assessment if there are any abnormalities.

Vital signs
- **Temperature.** Check for a fever. An acute infection may trigger heart failure in patients with anaemia.
- **Pulse.** Resting or orthostatic tachycardia may be present.
- **Blood pressure.** Check blood pressure for orthostatic hypotension.
- **Respiratory rate.** Anaemia may present with shortness of breath.

Head and neck
- **Mucus membranes.** Conjunctivae and oral mucosa may appear pale.
- **Fundoscopy.** Check for optic atrophy.

Abdomen
- **Organs.** Hepatomegaly and splenomegaly may be present. Check for epigastric masses (e.g. gastric cancer).

Chest
- **Heart.** Listen for a parasternal systolic ejection flow murmur.
- **Lungs.** Severe anaemia may present with heart failure (fine basal inspiratory crackles).

Limbs

* **Neurology.** Check tone, power, sensation, coordination and reflexes. Reduced vibration and position sense are early signs of central nervous system (CNS) involvement. Ataxia, Babinski response and spasticity are late signs. Legs and feet are more commonly affected than the upper limbs.

Key references and further reading

1. Andres E, Loukili NH, Noel E et al. Vitamin B12 (cobalamin) deficiency in elderly patients. *CMAJ* 2004;171:251–259.
2. Gulden KD. Pernicious anemia, vitiligo, and infertility. *J Am Board Fam Pract* 1990;3:217–220.
3. Hoffbrand V, Provan D. ABC of clinical haematology: macrocytic anaemias. *BMJ* 1997;314:430.
4. National Institute for Health and Care Excellence (NICE). Anaemia – B12 and folate deficiency. Clinical knowledge summaries. 2015. Available from: http://cks.nice.org.uk/anaemia-b12-and-folate-deficiency (last accessed 29 April 2016).
5. Oh R, Brown DL. Vitamin B12 deficiency. *Am Fam Physician* 2003;67:979–986.

Bleeding disorders

Key thoughts

Practical points
- **Diagnosis.** Both haematological and general conditions may cause bruising and bleeding. Coagulopathies, abnormal platelet function and abnormal blood vessel walls are important causes. Very low platelet counts carry a high risk of intracranial haemorrhage.
- **Prognosis.** Haematological malignancies and severe systemic disease may present with bleeding problems.

Haematological causes
- Inherited coagulation disorders (e.g. haemophilia A, Christmas disease, von Willebrand's disease).
- Idiopathic thrombocytopenic purpura (ITP).
- Leukaemia.
- Myelodysplasia.
- Myelofibrosis with splenomegaly.

General causes
- Alcohol.
- Vitamin K deficiency (e.g. dietary, malabsorption).
- Liver disease.
- Drugs (e.g. anticoagulants, antiplatelet therapy, steroids).
- Renal failure.
- Shock.
- Meningococcal septicaemia and other sepsis.
- Systemic lupus erythematosus (SLE).
- Antiphospholipid syndrome.
- Nutritional (e.g. vitamin C deficiency).

RED FLAGS
- Bruising over face, neck or trunk
- Petechiae and/or purpura on the extremities or trunk
- Bleeding from multiple sites
- Sepsis
- Fever
- Systemic symptoms (weight loss, malaise, fatigue, fever, sweats)

The 10-Minute Clinical Assessment, Second Edition. Knut Schroeder.
© 2017 John Wiley & Sons, Ltd. Published 2017 by John Wiley & Sons, Ltd.

History

Ideas, concerns and expectations
- **Ideas.** What does the patient believe is the cause of the bruising or bleeding?
- **Concerns.** Bruising and bleeding symptoms can be extremely frightening for patients, who may fear a life-threatening underlying condition. Bruises can make patients self-conscious, particularly when other people comment on them.
- **Expectations.** Identifying the underlying cause of the symptoms is usually the priority for patients.

History of presenting complaint
- **Quality of life.** How does bruising affect day-to-day life?
- **Onset.** A long history of easy bruising may be the result of an inherited coagulation defect or of conditions such as von Willebrand's disease. A rapid onset is more common in acquired conditions. Idiopathic thrombocytopenia usually develops gradually in adults but may present acutely in children.
- **Pattern.** Does bruising appear in unusual areas that are not normally knocked during day-to-day activities? Unexpectedly large bruises in response to trauma may raise suspicions of underlying disease.
- **Type.** Petechiae usually indicate an underlying clotting disorder. Petechiae on the legs suggest more serious underlying disease.
- **Bleeding.** Patients may mention prolonged bleeding after dental treatment or minor trauma. Ask about haematuria, rectal bleeding, epistaxis and menorrhagia. Coagulation disorders may lead to both bruising and bleeding. Significant platelet disorders may also present with bleeding. Bleeding from a number of sites suggests underlying coagulopathy.
- **Mental health.** Are there any mental health problems or relationship issues? Always consider the possibility of non-accidental injury or self-inflicted bruising if the history is inconsistent or the pattern of bruising is suspicious.
- **Systemic symptoms.** Ask about weight loss, loss of appetite, night sweats, fever and malaise, which may suggest underlying serious disease, such as a haematological malignancy or SLE. Viral infection may precede the development of ITP.

Past and current medical problems
- **Bleeding disorder.** Ask about a personal history of bleeding disorder.
- **Surgery.** Have transfusions been required for past operations?
- **Chronic disease.** Consider in particular any liver and renal problems.

Medication
- **Anticoagulants.** Anticoagulants (e.g. warfarin, heparin) may lead to easy bruising and bleeding.
- **NSAIDs.** These can affect platelet function.
- **Corticosteroids.** Long-term steroid therapy may lead to thinning of the skin and cause easy bruising and petechiae.

- **Drugs triggering ITP.** Consider drugs such as quinine and sulphonamides.
- **Drugs causing liver problems.** A number of drugs can affect liver function and may lead to coagulation problems.
- **Herbal medicines and supplements.** Some herbal medicines and dietary supplements may have anticoagulant effects or may be contaminated with steroids.

Family history
- **Coagulation disorders.** Check whether there is a family history of any bruising or bleeding disorders.

Alcohol, smoking and recreational drugs
- **Alcohol.** Chronic alcohol misuse can directly affect platelet function and may affect coagulation through effects on the liver.
- **Drug misuse.** High-risk behaviour may lead to human immunodeficiency virus (HIV) or hepatitis infection, which can result in ITP or liver damage.

Review of previous investigations
- **Full blood count.** Look for anaemia and thrombocytopenia. All blood cell lines may be reduced in aplastic anaemia. Also search for evidence of myelodysplasia or haematological malignancy. Macrocytosis may indicate alcohol misuse.
- **Clotting screen.** The prothrombin time may be increased in treatment with anticoagulants, liver failure or vitamin K deficiency. An isolated prolonged activated partial thromboplastin time occurs with coagulation factor VIII, IX or XI deficiencies, heparin treatment, von Willebrand's disease and lupus anticoagulant. Combined abnormalities may be present in liver failure or vitamin K deficiency.
- **Liver function tests.** Check for changes related to liver failure or alcohol.
- **Urea and electrolytes.** Look out for renal failure and uraemia.
- **HIV/hepatitis C.** These should be considered in at-risk patients.
- **Bone marrow.** Look out for any results of bone marrow examinations, if indicated.
- **Gene analysis.** Genetic tests may be useful for the investigation of congenital disorders.

Examination

General
- **General condition.** Does the patient look unwell or in shock?
- **Pallor.** This may indicate aplastic anaemia or haematological malignancy.
- **Injuries.** Look out for any injuries that might indicate non-accidental injury or self-harm.
- **Lymph nodes.** Generalised lymphadenopathy may suggest haematological or other malignancy.
- **CNS bleeding.** Consider this if there are any CNS or retinal signs.

Vital signs
- **Pulse.** Check for tachycardia if there is acute bleeding, which may suggest significant blood loss.
- **Blood pressure.** Check blood pressure as a baseline. Postural hypotension may indicate hypovolaemia due to blood loss.

Skin
- **Bruises.** Assess and record the site, size and distribution of any bruises.
- **Petechiae and purpura.** Search for any petechiae, purpura and ecchymoses.
- **Liver disease.** Look for signs of chronic liver disease (e.g. jaundice, spider naevi, scratch marks)

Head and neck
- **Mouth.** Look for evidence of mucosal bleeding.
- **Sclerae.** Look for jaundice.
- **Facial rash.** A 'butterfly rash' may suggest SLE.
- **Fundoscopy.** Look for retinal bleeding if there is a suggestion of CNS bleeding.

Upper limbs
- **Palmar erythema.** This may suggest underlying liver disease due to alcohol or hepatitis.

Abdomen
- **Liver.** Hepatomegaly or hepatic tenderness suggests liver disease.
- **Spleen.** Splenomegaly or splenic tenderness may point towards malignancy or myelofibrosis.
- **Rectal examination.** Consider a rectal examination to check for rectal bleeding and melaena.

Key references and further reading

1. Bolton-Maggs PH, Pasi KJ. Haemophilias A and B. *Lancet* 2003;361:1801–1809.
2. Hampton KK, Preston FE. ABC of clinical haematology. Bleeding disorders, thrombosis, and anticoagulation. *BMJ* 1997;314:1026–1029.
3. Mannucci PM, Duga S, Peyvandi F. Recessively inherited coagulation disorders. *Blood* 2004;104:1243–1252.
4. National Institute for Health and Care Excellence (NICE). Bruising. Clinical knowledge summaries. 2010. Available from: http://cks.nice.org.uk/bruising (last accessed 29 April 2016).

Myeloma

Key thoughts

Practical points
- **Diagnosis.** Myeloma is more common in patients over 70 years of age. Symptoms are often vague, and physical examination may be entirely normal. Back pain, pathological fractures, nerve root compression and fatigue are common presenting features. Secondary amyloidosis and renal impairment may occur.

Differential diagnosis
- Chronic lymphocytic leukaemia.
- Amyloid light-chain (AL) amyloidosis.
- B-cell non-Hodgkin's lymphoma.
- Waldenström macroglobulinaemia.
- Solitary plasmacytoma.
- Monoclonal gammopathy of undetermined significance.

Risk factors
- Older age (>70 years).
- Afro-Caribbean ethnicity.
- Radiation exposure.
- Male sex.

RED FLAGS

- Bone pain
- Recurrent bacterial infections
- Spinal cord compression
- Pathological fracture
- Acute renal failure
- Hypercalcaemia
- Generalised itching
- Weight loss, night sweats, fever, tiredness, malaise
- Breathlessness
- Alcohol-induced pain
- Lymphadenopathy
- Splenomegaly
- Lytic lesions on X-ray
- Anaemia
- Symptomatic hyperviscosity

The 10-Minute Clinical Assessment, Second Edition. Knut Schroeder.
© 2017 John Wiley & Sons, Ltd. Published 2017 by John Wiley & Sons, Ltd.

History

Ideas, concerns and expectations
- **Ideas.** What does the patient think is causing the symptoms?
- **Concerns.** Fears about underlying cancer are often predominant.
- **Expectations.** Relief of bone pain is a common reason for consultation. Does the patient have particular views about future care?

History of presenting complaint
- **Quality of life.** Allow the patient time to tell you about all their symptoms in their own words. How has their quality of life been affected? Tiredness and bone pain can be very distressing and disabling.
- **General symptoms.** Fatigue in myeloma may be caused by anaemia, renal failure or persistent infection. Ask about weight loss, night sweats, fever, generalised itching, recurrent infections and lymphadenopathy. Dizziness, anorexia and malaise are common. Dehydration may be caused by proximale tubule dysfunction resulting from light-chain precipitation.
- **Back pain.** Back pain is a common presenting feature of myeloma and affects either a single or multiple bones. Bone pain may be precipitated or exacerbated by alcohol. Consider spinal cord compression or sudden vertebral collapse (due to infiltration of the spinal vertebra and pathological fracture) if back pain is associated with neurological features. The spine, ribs, long bones and shoulder may be affected, but extremities are usually spared.
- **Bruising.** Ask about any bruising or bleeding (e.g. nose bleeds).
- **Features of hypercalcaemia.** Hypercalcaemia is present in 30–50% of patients. Ask about nausea, vomiting, thirst, constipation, polydipsia, polyuria and confusion.
- **Signs of hyperviscosity syndrome.** Hyperviscosity may lead to visual disturbances, dizziness, headaches, mental changes, mucosal bleeding and heart failure. Transient ischaemic attacks (TIAs) and strokes may occur.
- **Immunosuppression.** Consider all myeloma patients as being immunosuppressed and look out for symptoms and signs of bacterial infection (e.g. respiratory infection, urinary tract infection).
- **Mental health.** Depression and anxiety are common in patients with myeloma.
- **Mobility.** Is mobility affected? Is there a need for input from a physiotherapist?
- **Amyloidosis.** Ask about features of secondary amyloidosis, such as shortness of breath (heart failure) and oedema (nephrotic syndrome).

Past and current medical problems
- **Immunisation.** Patients with myeloma should have an annual influenza immunisation.

- **Haematology.** Is the patient already under the care of a haematologist? Look out for recent clinic letters.

Medication
- **Analgesia.** What has been tried to treat bone pain? Is analgesia adequate? Are there any adverse effects? NSAIDs should be avoided because they reduce renal blood flow and may lead to renal failure.
- **Bisphosphonates.** These may help to reduce pain and bone complications.

Social history
- **Home.** Who else is at home? Try to identify any unmet needs and obtain baseline information to help plan future care.
- **Other services.** In patients with established myeloma, are the local hospice and social services already involved? Is there involvement from the wider multidisciplinary team?

Review of previous investigations
- **Full blood count.** Normocytic normochromic anaemia may be caused by bone marrow infiltration, renal failure or infection due to bone marrow suppression. Neutrophils tend to be normal, but there may be neutropenia. There may be rouleaux formation due to paraproteins. Platelets are usually normal, but thrombocytopenia may occur.
- **Inflammatory markers.** Plasma viscosity and CRP tend to be persistently raised.
- **Calcium.** Acute hypercalcaemia is common and may lead to renal damage.
- **Renal function.** Look for acute renal failure or chronic renal impairment, which may be caused by light-chain nephropathy and hypercalcaemia. Some patients with myeloma will require dialysis.
- **Uric acid.** This is often raised and may lead to acute gout.
- **Liver function tests.** Alkaline phosphatase is usually normal in uncomplicated myeloma, but raised levels may occur with pathological fractures. The prognosis is usually poor if albumin is low.
- **Serum immunoglobulins and protein electrophoresis.** The neoplastic plasma cells produce monoclonal immunoglobulin. Look for raised or suppressed immunoglobulin A, M and G (IgA, IgM and IgG) levels. There will be an M (monoclonal) band on electrophoresis.
- **Urine.** Check for the presence of light chains/Bence–Jones protein.
- **Radiography.** Lytic lesions may be found on routine plain X-rays (e.g. 'punched-out lesions' or 'pepper pot skull'). Diffuse osteoporosis may be present. Look out for pathological fractures and vertebral collapse.
- **Second-line investigations.** Look for the results of any second-line investigations, such as bone-marrow biopsy, isotope bone scan, skeletal survey, computerised tomograhpy (CT) scans, tissue biopsies or magnetic resonance imaging (MRI) scans.

Examination

General
- **General condition.** Patients tend to be reasonably well unless they are hyper-calcaemic or suffer from infection. Physical examination is often normal.

Vital signs
- **Temperature.** Look for signs of infection if there is fever.

Head and neck
- **Lymphadenopathy.** Swollen lymph nodes may occur but are unusual.

Musculoskeletal
- **Bone tenderness.** Check for bone pain and tenderness, which may suggest infiltration or pathological fracture.

Chest
- **Lungs.** Check for signs of respiratory infection.

Abdomen
- **Masses.** Hepatomegaly, splenomegaly and lymphadenopathy may be caused by secondary amyloidosis but are relatively rare.

Bedside tests
- **Urine.** Dipstick urine is not a reliable test for Bence–Jones proteinuria.

Key references and further reading
1. Alastair Smith A, Wisloff F, Samson D on behalf of the UK Myeloma Forum, Nordic Myeloma Study Group and British Committee for Standards in Haematology. Guidelines on the diagnosis and management of multiple myeloma. *Br J Haematol* 2005;132:410–451.
2. National Comprehensive Cancer Network (NCCN). Multiple myeloma. Clinical practice guidelines in oncology. 2008. Available from: http://www.nccn.org/professionals/physician_gls/PDF/myeloma.pdf (last accessed 29 April 2016).
3. National Institute for Health and Care Excellence (NICE). Haematological malignancy – suspected. Clinical knowledge summaries. 2009. Available from: http://cks.nice.org.uk/haematological-malignancy-suspected (last accessed 29 April 2016).
4. Weber DM, Dimopoulos MA, Moulopoulos LA et al. Prognostic features of asymptomatic multiple myeloma. *Br J Haematol* 1997;97:810–814.

Musculoskeletal

Soft-tissue injury

Key thoughts

Practical points

- **Diagnosis.** Soft-tissue injuries are common. It is important to establish the extent of injuries to ligaments, muscles and tendons and to record all findings carefully, particularly if there is a potential risk of a future medicolegal dispute.

Differential diagnosis

- Sprain (torn or overstretched ligament).
- Strain (overstretched or partially torn muscle or tendon).
- Rupture (overstretched and torn muscle or tendon).
- Haematoma or deep bruising resulting from blood collection within a muscle.
- Damage to major organs.
- Fractures.

Important risk factors

- Age.
- Frequent falls.
- Underlying medical conditions.

RED FLAGS

- Neurological deficit
- Distal underperfusion
- Bone pain suggesting fracture
- Severe pain
- Immediate significant swelling or bruising
- Grating or cracking noises at the site of injury

History

Ideas, concerns and expectations

- **Ideas.** Patients may wrongly believe that an X-ray will always be necessary for most injuries.
- **Concerns.** Explore any concerns about future ability to work, performance of daily routines or taking part in recreational activities.
- **Expectations.** Ask about expectations in terms of recovery time and type of treatment.

The 10-Minute Clinical Assessment, Second Edition. Knut Schroeder.
© 2017 John Wiley & Sons, Ltd. Published 2017 by John Wiley & Sons, Ltd.

History of presenting complaint

- **Quality of life.** How has the quality of life been affected by the injury? Are there any limitations in performing day-to-day activities (e.g. home, work, leisure)?
- **Circumstances.** Obtain details about the circumstances of the injury. Were there any witnesses? What type of force was involved? Is there any risk of contamination of the wound? Injuries at sports, work or home are common and often follow specific mechanisms.
- **Timing.** Ask about the timing of the injury. This will help decide whether a wound is suitable for primary closure. If not, surgical toilet and waiting until the wound is clean might be more appropriate.
- **Nature.** Knife injuries, punctures, glass injuries and blunt trauma are common. Find out what exactly caused the injury and how it happened. This will help decide whether there is the potential for damage to underlying or adjacent structures, such as bones or nerves, or whether foreign bodies might be embedded in the wound.
- **Severity.** Some bruising and swelling, pain at the extreme ends of movement and a stable joint suggest mild injury only. Muscle spasm is absent and there is no loss of function. Bruising, swelling, more pronounced pain, some possible joint instability and reduced ability of muscles to contract suggest moderate injury. In severe injury, swelling is significant, with severe pain at rest and considerably reduced function. In severe ligamentous injuries, there is usually marked laxity of joints. Severe spasm and loss of function are common in muscular injuries.
- **Function.** Ask about reduced motor function and sensory loss. Has any loss of function resulted in significant impairment or disability?
- **Sounds.** A popping sound at the time of injury suggests ligamentous injury (e.g. knee or Achilles tendon).
- **Management of the injury.** What has been tried so far? Ask about protection, rest, ice, compression, elevation and any rehabilitation.

Past and current medical problems

- **Previous injuries.** Ask whether there have been any previous injuries close to the new injury which might have left symptoms or signs. This is important for possible medicolegal disputes resulting from the new injury and to put any damage caused by the new injury into context.
- **Immune status.** Check tetanus immunisation status in case immunisation or a booster is necessary.

Medication

- **Anticoagulants.** Patients taking warfarin or aspirin are at higher risk of bleeding and developing a haematoma.
- **Steroids.** High-dose steroid treatment can mask symptoms, particularly in abdominal trauma.
- **Anti-inflammatory drugs and other analgesics.** Ask what has been tried (including topical preparations). What has been effective? Have there been any adverse effects?

Allergies
- **Antibiotics.** Ask about allergies to antibiotics in case these are needed for treatment of infection.
- **Other drugs, latex and plaster.** Consider allergies to any other medication that may need to be used (e.g. anaesthetic agents), as well as allergies to latex or plaster.

Social history
- **Home and family.** Does the injury have implications for day-to-day life? Are there dependent children that need looking after?
- **Work.** Are there any problems with regard to work as a result of the injury? If the injury was work-related, ask for details about the types of activity undertaken as part of the job and whether there are health and safety aspects that may need to be addressed in the future.
- **Leisure and hobbies.** Ask about any potential effect of the injury on hobbies and exercise. Has a hobby caused the injury?

Alcohol and other drugs
- **Alcohol and drugs.** Ask for details about alcohol and drug consumption. Could the injury have been alcohol-related?

Review of previous investigations
- **Radiology.** Obtain and check any previous X-ray films or reports around the injured body part. These will be helpful for comparison in case new X-rays are needed. If new X-rays or ultrasound scans have been obtained since the injury, look in particular for opaque foreign bodies and bone damage.

Examination

General
- **General condition.** Does the patient look well? Pallor may suggest significant blood loss.
- **Walking.** Is the patient able to bear weight? Are balance and gait normal?
- **Pain.** Assess the amount of pain the patient is in. Consider giving analgesia prior to further assessment to make the patient more comfortable and to reduce muscle spasm as a reaction to the injury.
- **Biomechanics.** Look for obvious predisposing factors (e.g. pes planus may predispose to ankle or Achilles tendon injuries).

Vital signs
- **Temperature.** Raised temperature suggests infection.
- **Pulse.** Tachycardia may be caused by significant blood loss, pain or infection. In case of abdominal injury, intra-abdominal blood loss may not be obvious, and tachycardia may be the only abnormal sign.

- **Blood pressure.** Check for postural hypotension, especially if there is blood loss.

Inspection of the injury
- **General appearance.** Note the appearance of the wound and whether it is obviously or potentially contaminated. Is there any tissue distortion?
- **Wound description.** Note the exact location, size and side of the wound. Gauge its apparent depth and try to describe any damage to surrounding tissues. Check whether the wound edges come together easily.
- **Bleeding and swelling.** Record the amount of bleeding and whether there is any swelling. If there is substantial bleeding, swelling and bruising, it is more likely that a significant blood vessel has been damaged. If a proximal tourniquet is needed to stop any blood loss, the wound may not be suitable for repair in a primary care setting or a basic casualty department. Rapid development of a knee effusion suggests haemarthrosis.
- **Dislocation.** Check for dislocated joints.

Palpation
- **Bones.** Check for bony tenderness and other signs of fracture.

Neurological examination
- **Sensation.** Check sensation distal to the injury and compare this with the normal side. Ensure that you check sensation prior to administration of local anaesthetics. Use a cotton wool ball rather than a pin prick to assess sensation in a child, as this is much less likely to cause immediate withdrawal. Loss of sensation may be patchy if nerve damage has been incomplete. Take your time when testing sensation and record your findings carefully.
- **Motor function.** Check distal motor function and make comparisons with the normal side. Any loss in motor function might be caused by a damaged muscle, nerve, tendon or bone, or it might be due to pain only. Motor function and range of movement can be checked after local anaesthetic has been given, as the pain relief may make this easier and less unpleasant for the patient.

Circulation
- **Check distal pulses.** Always check distal circulation in limb injuries. Even if a palpable pulse is present distal to an injury, damage to the blood vessel cannot be excluded. A palpable pulse can only confirm that blood supply is likely to be adequate at the time of the examination. An absent pulse may suggest vascular damage or pre-existing peripheral vascular disease.
- **Capillary return.** Checking capillary return is a fairly crude measure of circulation, as it may still be present even in severe injuries. Also check whether pulp contour returns after putting pressure on tissue distal to an injury.

Abdomen
- **Palpation.** A tender abdomen with guarding suggests intra-abdominal injury.

Key references and further reading

1. Andreasen TJ, Green SD, Childers BJ. Massive infectious soft-tissue injury: diagnosis and management of necrotizing fasciitis and purpura fulminans. *Plast Reconstr Surg* 2001;107:1025–1034.

2. National Institute for Health and Care Excellence (NICE). Sprains and strains. Clinical knowledge summaries. 2015. Available from: http://cks.nice.org.uk/sprains-and-strains (last accessed 29 April 2016).

3. Ogilvie-Harris DJ, Gilbart M. Treatment modalities for soft tissue injuries of the ankle: a critical review. *Clin J Sport Med* 1995:175–186.

Acute hot and swollen joint

Key thoughts

Practical points

- **Diagnosis.** Gout is a common cause of the hot and swollen joint. It is important to exclude septic arthritis because of the risk of permanent joint damage and mortality. Consider age and sex when weighing up other possible diagnoses, such as reactive arthritis and gonococcal arthritis (young people), gout (middle-aged men) and pseudogout (women in later life).

Possible causes

- Gout.
- Pseudogout.
- Reactive arthritis.
- Gonococcal arthritis.
- Rheumatoid arthritis.
- Inflammatory exacerbation of osteoarthritis.
- Septic arthritis.

Risk factors

- Viral infection.
- Diabetes mellitus.
- Recent joint surgery.
- Hip or knee prosthesis.
- Human immunodeficiency virus (HIV) infection.
- Rheumatoid arthritis.
- Recent intra-articular steroid injection.
- Malignancy.
- Alcoholism.

RED FLAGS

- Single hot joint
- Reluctance to move the joint
- Inability to bear weight
- Constitutional features such as fever, weight loss and malaise

---

The 10-Minute Clinical Assessment, Second Edition. Knut Schroeder.
© 2017 John Wiley & Sons, Ltd. Published 2017 by John Wiley & Sons, Ltd.

History

Ideas, concerns and expectations
- **Ideas.** What does the patient believe is the underlying cause of the joint problem? If gout is suspected or has been confirmed in the past, explore the patient's knowledge and beliefs about the diagnosis.
- **Concerns.** Septic arthritis is rare and can be very frightening, due to the often severe pain and the inability to move the affected joint. Older people may be concerned about potential loss of independence or having to move into alternative accommodation.
- **Expectations.** What are the patient's expectations with regard to further investigation and management?

History of presenting complaint
- **Quality of life.** How has the quality of life been affected? Which day-to-day activities are limited?
- **Onset and progression.** Septic arthritis (rare) and crystal arthropathies (gout, pseudogout) develop over a short period of time, whereas symptoms in osteoarthritis and rheumatoid arthritis progress more gradually. Consider the possibility of septic arthritis if there is sudden onset of pain, swelling or loss of function in a single joint in a patient with underlying inflammatory arthritis.
- **Recent trauma.** Haemarthrosis develops fast after an injury and can lead to a hot swollen joint. Consider traumatic synovitis if there is a delayed response. Be aware that human or animal bites may puncture the skin over a joint and result in septic arthritis.
- **Number of affected joints.** Gout and septic arthritis usually affect single joints (rarely multiple joints). In rheumatoid and reactive arthritis, more than one joint is usually involved.
- **Site.** Gout affects the metatarsophalangeal joint of the big toe in most cases, but other joints in the ankle, foot, knee, elbow, wrist and hand may also be involved. In people over 60 years of age, gout may present with more unusual patterns of joint involvement. Septic arthritis usually presents in the knee in adults and the hip in children, but any other joints may also be affected.
- **History of joint swelling.** A past history of gout, pseudogout or rheumatoid arthritis may point towards an acute inflammatory exacerbation of a chronic condition. Consider septic arthritis if these patients develop constitutional symptoms.

Important symptom patterns
- **Septic arthritis.** Septic arthritis is uncommon but important not to miss. Typical presentation is as a single, hot and painful joint, which can present in a similar way to gout. There is loss of function and patients are reluctant to bear weight on the joint. Fever, rigors and malaise may or may not be present. Older and immunocompromised people may present with nonspecific ill health. Risk factors include diabetes mellitus, steroid use, recent joint surgery, steroid joint

injections, skin infection, HIV infection, intravenous drug use and immunosuppression.

- **Recent infection.** Reactive arthritis (Reiter's syndrome) may occur after gastrointestinal or urinary infections. Urethral discharge may indicate gonococcal arthritis. Consider Lyme arthritis if there is erythema migrans, headache, myalgia, fever, malaise and a history of tick exposure in an endemic area. Septic arthritis may rarely occur as a result of dental sepsis.
- **Psoriasis.** Acute psoriatic arthritis can affect single joints and may resemble septic arthritis. Psoriatic skin lesions will usually be obvious.

Medication
- **Analgesia.** What has been tried so far? Ask about both prescription and over-the-counter medication. What has worked? Are there any adverse effects?
- **Steroids.** Systemic steroid treatment increases the risk of septic arthritis and may mask symptoms.
- **Anticoagulants.** Consider haemarthrosis in patients on anticoagulants.

Allergies
- **Antibiotics.** Check that there is no allergy to antibiotics.

Review of previous investigations
- **Full blood count.** The white cell count is usually raised in septic arthritis.
- **Inflammatory markers.** Raised plasma viscosity or C-reactive protein (CRP) indicates infection or severe inflammation but cannot distinguish between the two. This is useful for monitoring treatment response.
- **Glucose.** Diabetes predisposes to infection.
- **Uric acid.** This suggests gout if raised, but it may be normal during an acute attack.
- **Renal and liver function.** Renal or liver impairment may influence the choice of antibiotics.
- **Joint aspiration.** The absence of pus does not necessarily exclude infection. Check culture results and whether aspirate was examined for crystals.
- **Blood cultures.** These are useful for investigation of suspected sepsis but are usually only performed in secondary care.

Examination

General
- **General condition.** Does the patient look unwell?
- **Skin.** Look for gout tophi and skin nodules.

Vital signs
- **Pulse.** Tachycardia may be caused by fever or pain.
- **Fever.** Absence of fever does not exclude infection.
- **Blood pressure.** Check for postural hypotension.

Joint examination

- **Inspection.** Swelling, erythema and deformity may occur in acute inflammatory arthritis, gout and septic arthritis.
- **Palpation.** The joint will be tender and warm to the touch in inflammatory arthritis, gout and septic arthritis. Check for an effusion.
- **Movement.** Check whether active and passive movements are painful. Check and record range of movement. Is there joint instability?
- **Function.** Is the patient able to walk? Are other functions, such as getting dressed, affected?
- **Blood glucose.** Check for hyperglycaemia, as underlying diabetes increases the risk of septic arthritis.

Key references and further reading

1. Coakley G, Mathews C, Field M et al. on behalf of the British Society for Rheumatology Standards, Guidelines and Audit Working Group. BSR & BHPR, BOA, RCGP and BSAC guidelines for management of the hot swollen joint in adults. *Rheumatology* 2006;45:1039–1041.
2. Guidelines and a proposed audit protocol for the initial management of an acute hot joint. Report of a Working Group of the British Society for Rheumatology and the Research Unit of the Royal College of Physicians. *J R Coll Physicians* 1992;26:83–85.
3. Margaretten ME, Kohlwes J, Moore D, Bent S. Does this adult have septic arthritis? *JAMA* 2007;297:1478–1488.
4. National Institute for Health and Care Excellence (NICE). Knee pain – assessment. Clinical knowledge summaries. 2011. Available from: http://cks.nice.org.uk/knee-pain-assessment (last accessed 29 April 2016).
5. National Institute for Health and Care Excellence (NICE). Gout. Clinical knowledge summaries. 2015. Available from: http://cks.nice.org.uk/gout (last accessed 29 April 2016).
6. National Institute for Health and Care Excellence (NICE). Sprains and strains. Clinical knowledge summaries. 2015. Available from: http://cks.nice.org.uk/sprains-and-strains (last accessed 29 April 2016).
7. Siva C, Velazquez C, Mody A, Brasington R. Diagnosing acute monoarthritis in adults: a practical approach for the family physician. *Am Fam Physician* 2003;68:83–90.

Chronic musculoskeletal pain

Key thoughts

Practical points

- **Diagnosis.** Fibromyalgia and chronic fatigue syndrome are common and often debilitating. Generalised muscle aches are a frequent side effect of statins. Also consider less common causes of muscular pain, such as polymyalgia rheumatica (PMR), polymyositis, paraneoplastic syndrome and myopathies.
- **Patient concerns.** Take patients' concerns seriously and perform a thorough assessment.

Possible causes

- Fibromyalgia.
- Drugs (e.g. statins).
- Alcohol misuse.
- PMR.
- Chronic fatigue syndrome.
- Paraneoplastic syndrome.
- Rarely, polymyositis, dermatomyositis or myopathy due to other causes (metabolic, inherited).

RED FLAGS

- Localising/focal neurological signs
- Signs of inflammatory arthritis or connective-tissue disease
- Signs of cardiorespiratory disease
- Unintentional weight loss
- Lymphadenopathy

History

Ideas, concerns and expectations

- **Ideas.** Older patients often see muscular symptoms as a part of normal ageing and may present late.
- **Concerns.** Chronic muscle pains can be extremely frustrating for both patients and health professionals involved in their management. Patients may worry about chronic disability and persistent effects on their quality of life.
- **Expectations.** Expectations for a quick recovery may be unrealistic.

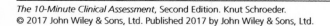

The 10-Minute Clinical Assessment, Second Edition. Knut Schroeder.
© 2017 John Wiley & Sons, Ltd. Published 2017 by John Wiley & Sons, Ltd.

History of presenting complaint

- **Quality of life.** How do muscular symptoms affect quality of life and daily activities (home, work, leisure)?
- **Onset and progression.** When did the pains start? Is the pain static or getting worse?
- **Exacerbating and relieving factors.** What makes the pain better or worse?
- **Site.** Consider using a pain drawing: an outline of the human body, both back and front, on which the patient marks the main areas of pain. In fibromyalgia, pain is often 'all over', with the lower back, neck and shoulders usually particularly affected.
- **Associated symptoms.** Ask about tiredness and stiffness. Has there been any weight loss? Is there muscle weakness? Ask about headaches, depression and problems with sleeping.
- **Trauma.** Is there a history of emotional or physical trauma? Repetitive overuse injury is common and can become chronic. Severe pain following trauma together with swelling may rarely suggest compartment syndrome due to haematoma, which needs urgent decompression to avoid irreversible muscle or nerve damage.
- **Infection.** Generalised muscular ache is common with viral infection but is usually self-limiting. Infectious mononucleosis (glandular fever) may cause muscle aches and tiredness, which can persist for weeks or months.
- **Constitutional symptoms.** Consider paraneoplastic syndrome if there is fever, weight loss, anorexia, sweats and malaise.
- **Response to treatment.** Proximal muscle pain with raised inflammatory markers that responds well to steroids is likely to be caused by PMR.

Common symptom patterns

- **Fibromyalgia.** Pain is usually widespread, with tender points in certain areas. There is an increased sensitivity to pain. Other symptoms are depression, fatigue, stiffness, feeling of swollen joints (without actual swelling), cognitive problems (word finding, memory), headache and sleep problems (which may exacerbate symptoms).
- **Chronic fatigue syndrome.** There is new onset of persistent or recurrent fatigue without obvious cause that severely affects activity levels and is worse after exercise (usually with a delay of 24 hours). Other problems include sleep problems, widespread muscle pains, headache, painful non-enlarged lymph nodes, cognitive problems (concentration, planning, word finding), malaise and palpitations.
- **PMR.** This is rare in people aged <50 years, and more commonly affects women than men. Symptoms include pain on active and passive movements of joints (mainly shoulders, hips and neck), tiredness, morning stiffness, weight loss, depression, joint effusions and mild fever. There is usually a dramatic response to systemic steroids.
- **Polymyositis.** Onset is slow over weeks and months, with steady progression. There is diffuse weakness in the proximal muscles, causing problems with

climbing steps, rising from a chair, combing hair and lifting objects; this may vary from week to week. Fine movement of the hands will not be affected. Muscle pain occurs only in a minority of patients. Polymyositis may be associated with malignancy (e.g. lung, breast, stomach, ovary).

- **Dermatomyositis.** In addition to proximal muscle weakness, there is arthralgia, fever, weight loss and malaise. Consider paraneoplastic syndrome (particularly in the elderly), as well as associated cardiac disease (e.g. arrhythmias), cardiomyopathy, gastrointestinal problems (ulcers and infections) and interstitial lung disease. Children may also be affected.
- **Temporal arteritis.** In older people, muscle aches in connection with headaches, intermittent or permanent visual loss or jaw claudication on chewing suggest temporal arteritis.
- **Hypothyroidism.** Chronic muscular pain is a feature of hypothyroidism. Ask about tiredness, cold intolerance, weight gain, constipation, depressive symptoms and menstrual disturbance.

Medication and other treatments
- **Recent medication usage.** Ask whether the muscle pains started after prescription of a new medication. Statins, particularly when taken with fibrates, commonly cause muscle pain and may in rare cases lead to rhabdomyolysis. Amiodarone and lithium can cause hypothyroidism, which in turn may lead to muscle aches. Steroids can cause myopathy.
- **Success of previous treatments.** Ask what has been tried and what has worked so far, including analgesics, antidepressants and steroids. Are any other health professionals involved? Ask about previous massage therapy, physiotherapy and transcutaneous electric nerve stimulation.

Social history
- **Travel.** Consider the possibility of a tropical disease such as malaria in any person who presents with muscle ache, general malaise and fever who has visited or lives in an endemic area.

Alcohol and drugs
- **Alcohol and drug use.** Alcohol and other recreational drugs can cause muscle weakness.

Review of previous investigations
- **Full blood count.** A normochromic anaemia is common in chronic diseases such as connective-tissue disorder. The white blood cell count and platelets may be elevated in rheumatoid disease. Leucopenia and thrombocytopenia occur in systemic lupus erythematosus (SLE).
- **Inflammatory markers.** Plasma viscosity and CRP are usually elevated in connective tissue diseases and vasculitis. They are often very high in temporal arteritis or PMR and can be useful in monitoring treatment.
- **Paul-Bunnell test/Monospot.** This may confirm infectious mononucleosis.
- **Renal function tests.** Check for renal involvement in rheumatic disease.

- **Liver function tests.** These may be abnormal in patients using statins.
- **Thyroid function tests.** A raised thyroid-stimulating hormone (TSH) indicates hypothyroidism.
- **Creatine kinase.** This is often raised in inflammatory myopathies, including polymyositis. It may also be raised in hypothyroidism.
- **Autoimmune profile, including rheumatoid arthritis latex.** This may be raised in rheumatoid arthritis and other connective-tissue disorders.
- **Urinalysis.** Proteinuria and/or haematuria occurs in renal disease, which may be caused by polyarteritis nodosa and SLE.
- **X-rays.** Recent or old X-ray reports may give clues about longstanding joint changes caused by rheumatoid arthritis.
- **Other tests.** Electromyography, muscle biopsy and imaging are second-line investigations, usually initiated by specialists

Examination

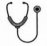

General
- **General condition.** Does the patient look unwell? Are there signs of serious underlying disease, such as cachexia or pallor?

Musculoskeletal
- **Walking.** Look for any obvious abnormality of posture or walking.
- **Pain.** Is there any obvious pain or stiffness when the patient moves or removes clothing?
- **Muscle wasting.** Look for any obvious muscle wasting, screening all the major muscle groups from head to toe.
- **Active movement.** Ask the patient to move all affected muscles actively, and look for pain, stiffness and range of movement.
- **Muscle palpation.** Check muscles for any warmth and tenderness. A nodular grainy feel may indicate polymyositis. Check trigger points for fibromyalgia.
- **Muscle strength.** Assess muscle strength in all relevant muscle groups and compare both sides. Pain and weakness may influence muscle strength. Check whether the weakness is in one limb, unilateral, proximal, distal or global. Proximal weakness is typical of polymyositis, whereas distal weakness is a feature of peripheral neuropathies.
- **Joint inflammation.** A symmetrical polyarthritis affecting the metacarpophalangeal (MCP) joints and wrists is often seen in rheumatoid disease.

Skin
- **Skin changes.** Look out for the blue/purple heliotrope rash of dermatomyositis (upper eye lids, face, upper trunk and knuckles, knees, shoulders, back and upper chest). Hypothyroid patients often have pale and dry skin.
- **Hands.** Check the nails for any nail-fold infarcts and erythema, which are signs of SLE and dermatomyositis. Fingers may be cold and discoloured in Raynaud's phenomenon, which occurs commonly in connective-tissue diseases.

Head and neck

- **Face.** SLE can cause a photosensitive erythematous rash that affects the cheeks and nose in a butterfly distribution. Periorbital oedema and thin eyebrows are common in hypothyroidism. The facial skin is often tight in systemic sclerosis (scleroderma), which is rare.
- **Eyes.** Red and painful eyes may result from iritis or episcleritis, as seen in connective-tissue disorders and Sjögren's disease.
- **Temporal arteries.** Tenderness and absent pulses in the temporal area suggest temporal arteritis.

Key references and further reading
1. Barraclough K, Liddell W, du Toit J et al. Polymyalgia rheumatica in primary care: a cohort study of the diagnostic criteria and outcome. *Fam Pract* 2008;25:328–333.
2. Bergman S. A general practice approach to management of chronic widespread musculoskeletal pain and fibromyalgia. Available from: https://www.arthritis researchuk.org/~/media/Files/Education/Hands-On/IP10-Jan-2003.ashx (last accessed 29 April 2016).
3. National Institute for Health and Care Excellence (NICE). Chronic fatigue syndrome/myalgic encephalomyelitis (or encephalopathy); diagnosis and management. NICE clinical guideline [CG53]. August 2007. Available from: http://www.nice.org.uk/guidance/cg53 (last accessed 29 April 2016).
4. National Institute for Health and Clinical Excellence (NICE). Polymyalgia rheumatica. Clinical knowledge summaries. 2013. Available from: http://cks.nice.org.uk/polymyalgia-rheumatica (last accessed 29 April 2016).
5. Saguil A. Evaluation of the patient with muscle weakness. *Am Fam Physician* 2005;71:1327–1336.
6. Smetana GW, Shmerling RH. Does this patient have temporal arteritis? *JAMA* 2002;287:92–101.

Polyarthralgia

Key thoughts

Practical points
- **Diagnosis.** Distinguish between inflammatory and mechanical joint problems. Common causes are osteoarthritis and rheumatoid arthritis.
- **Quality of life.** Assessment of the functional impact of joint pains and the quality of life is important for patient-centred care.

Possible causes
- Osteoarthritis.
- Rheumatoid arthritis.
- Reactive arthritis.
- Fibromyalgia.
- Ankylosing spondylitis.
- Bone tumours (rare).
- Vitamin D deficiency.

Risk factors
- Family history of arthritis.
- Manual occupations.
- Obesity.
- Previous joint trauma (accidents, sporting injuries).

RED FLAGS

- Hot and swollen joint with reluctance to move
- Pain at rest or at night
- Constitutional features, such as fever, weight loss and malaise
- Associated weakness

History

Ideas, concerns and expectations
- **Ideas.** Many people are unaware of the differences between osteoarthritis and rheumatoid arthritis. What does the patient know about arthritis?
- **Concerns.** People with joint symptoms may be worried about future disability or the prospect of joint replacement.
- **Expectations.** What is the desired level of functioning and pain relief?

The 10-Minute Clinical Assessment, Second Edition. Knut Schroeder.
© 2017 John Wiley & Sons, Ltd. Published 2017 by John Wiley & Sons, Ltd.

History of presenting complaint

- **Function and the quality of life.** How do the joint problems affect quality of life and mental well being? Go through a normal day and ask about activities such as getting up, washing, dressing, preparing food, working, looking after dependants and taking part in hobbies. How much is the patient bothered by any loss of function? Find out what level of function is desired (e.g. work, hobbies).

- **Pain.** Mechanical pain is worse with activity and on weight-bearing. Identify the site(s), character and radiation of pain and ask about aggravating and relieving factors. Remember that any joint pain may be referred pain from other joints (e.g. hip pain often radiates to the knee). Pain due to pressure on nerves may present with associated paraesthesia. Inflammatory pain often varies in intensity, tends to be worse in the mornings and improves with activity. In longstanding inflammatory joint conditions, there may also be mechanical pain due to joint damage. Structural bone pain (e.g. bony metastasis) may be constant and continue through the night.

- **Swelling.** Consider effusion or synovitis in inflammatory joint conditions and after trauma (traumatic effusion, haemarthrosis).

- **Stiffness.** Early-morning stiffness is the key symptom of inflammatory arthritis. Joint stiffness usually resolves within a few minutes in osteoarthritis but lasts for an hour or so in inflammatory arthritis. Locking or gelling suggests a mechanical problem. Constant stiffness may be caused by contracture or severe inflammation.

- **Pattern of joint involvement.** Symmetrical joint problems are more common in rheumatoid arthritis and PMR. Distal and proximal interphalangeal joints are involved in osteoarthritis. In inflammatory arthritis, the metacarpophalangeal and metatarsophalangeal joints are often affected. Arthritis in SLE tends to be asymmetrical. Monoarthritis indicates the possibility of septic arthritis, gout or rare bone tumours. Insidious onset of back pain without trauma may suggest an inflammatory cause, particularly in younger people and if associated with morning stiffness (consider ankylosing spondylitis).

- **Constitutional symptoms.** Ask about fever, fatigue, weight loss, night sweats and malaise, which may occur in inflammatory arthritis, septic arthritis or as part of a paraneoplastic syndrome.

- **Associated symptoms.** Joint pain can be linked to inflammatory bowel disease, such as Crohn's disease, ulcerative colitis or other acute bowel infections. Consider Reiter's syndrome if there is associated urethritis and conjunctivitis. Psoriatic arthritis may develop in patients suffering from psoriasis, and psoriatic lesions will usually be present.

Common symptom patterns

- **Osteoarthritis.** Osteoarthritis mainly affects the larger joints (hip, knee) and joints of the hand (carpometacarpal and distal interphalangeal). Heberden's nodes may have developed and patients may notice crepitus. Obesity and sedentary lifestyle are often associated. Ask about trauma and repetitive use of the joint in the past (occupational, sport).

- **Rheumatoid arthritis.** Features include symmetrical pain and swelling in at least three different joints for more than 6 weeks, early-morning stiffness and joint swelling in the hands (metacarpophalangeal joints, wrist or proximal interphalangeal joints).
- **Seronegative arthritis or connective tissue disease.** Ask about a history of psoriasis, urinary symptoms (Reiter's syndrome), bowel disorders (ulcerative colitis, Crohn's, bowel infections such as salmonella and shigella), streptococcal sore throat and anterior uveitis. There will usually be asymmetrical pain in a small number of large joints (also sacroiliitis). Photosensitive rashes, hair loss, Raynaud's, mouth ulcers and fatigue may also occur.

Medication
- **Analgesics and anti-inflammatory drugs.** What has been tried and has it been effective? Are there any adverse effects? Ask about adherence and taking patterns. Nonsteroidals are useful in patients without contraindications.
- **Steroids and disease-modifying antirheumatic drugs (DMARDs).** These are usually given under specialist supervision. Ask about adverse effects and other problems. Remember that steroids can mask other symptoms.
- **Drug monitoring.** If the patient is taking DMARDs, who monitors these in terms of regular blood tests and medication reviews? Have there been any recent problems with abnormal blood tests or adverse effects? Is the patient taking appropriate bone protection? Who is responsible for monitoring the need to step up or step down treatment?

Other treatments
- **Physiotherapy.** Upper and lower limb-strengthening exercises are part of first-line treatment. Have these been successfully tried?
- **Lifestyle interventions.** Weight loss can be useful for all forms of arthritis in overweight people. Has this been considered and tried?
- **Surgery.** Is there a history of joint surgery (e.g. functional corrections, joint replacement)?

Family history
- **Joint disease.** Ask about a family history of joint problems or autoimmune disorders.

Social history
- **Home.** How have the joint problems affected home life and work? Does the patient make use of mobility aids? Does the accommodation need modification (e.g. downstairs toilet)? What support network is available? How is the main carer coping, and what are *their* ideas, concerns and expectations?

Review of previous investigations
- **Specific rheumatological tests.** Remember that these can be falsely positive (e.g. in infection). Check whether tests for rheumatoid factor (rheumatoid

arthritis, only positive in one-third of patients, is a useful prognostic tool) or antinuclear antibodies (connective-tissue disease; have shown positive results in the past). Results are more meaningful if tests are performed in patients with a high pretest probability of rheumatological disease.

- **Unspecific inflammatory markers.** CRP or plasma viscosity will usually be raised in inflammatory conditions and can be helpful for monitoring the response to treatment.
- **Full blood count.** This may show anaemia of chronic disease in inflammatory arthritis. The full blood count needs to be monitored in patients on any medication that may cause haematological adverse effects (e.g. DMARDs).
- **Radiology.** X-rays are often unnecessary in inflammatory arthritis. There may be typical findings, such as joint space narrowing and osteophytes in osteoarthritis or erosions in rheumatoid arthritis. In non-inflammatory conditions such as osteoarthritis, imaging is usually not required to make a diagnosis but may be needed for preoperative assessment. A chest X-ray is useful as a baseline prior to starting methotrexate (risk of pulmonary fibrosis) and may show pleural effusion in severe rheumatoid arthritis.
- **Renal function.** Renal failure may be associated with inflammatory arthritis and can indicate drug adverse effects.
- **Liver function tests.** Many treatments prescribed for arthritis can cause liver abnormalities.
- **Urinalysis.** Proteinuria and/or haematuria suggests kidney involvement in rheumatological conditions.

Examination

General

- **General health.** Does the patient look unwell? Observe posture and gait. Is the patient in pain or breathless? Pallor may suggest anaemia of chronic disease. Are there signs of treatment complications (e.g. cushingoid features due to steroids)?

Vital signs

- **Temperature.** Fever may occur in inflammatory arthritis or sepsis.
- **Pulse.** There may be tachycardia due to pain or fever. Rheumatoid arthritis may occasionally cause conduction disturbances.
- **Blood pressure.** Blood pressure may be raised in renal involvement.
- **Respiratory rate.** Tachycardia may rarely be caused by lung conditions (e.g. fibrosis) associated with connective-tissue disease.

Joints

- **Site.** Check which joints are affected. Is distribution symmetrical or asymmetrical?
- **Inspection.** Look for abnormal curvature of the spine (indicating scoliosis or vertebral collapse). Check all relevant muscle groups for wasting and weakness. Nodules may be present on shins and elbows. Is there subluxation or deformity of joints (e.g. 'swan neck', 'boutonnière', 'ulnar deviation')? Look for nail-fold infarcts (vasculitis).

- **Palpation.** Check for synovial thickening (a soft and boggy feeling at the joint line) and effusion. Squeeze the metacarpophalangeal joints. Pain is common in rheumatoid arthritis. Is there evidence of Dupuytren's contracture (check for tendon thickening and painful contractures)?
- **Nonarticular pathology.** Differentiate between tenosynovitis and arthritis. Nonarticular pathology does not usually cause joint swelling, and any tenderness will be localised to tendon sheaths, bursae and other structures adjacent to the joint.
- **Range of movement.** Check the range of active and passive movements for all joints, including the neck and spine.
- **Function.** Assess function by asking the patient to perform some common tasks (combing hair, getting up from a chair, etc.). Test finer movements of the hands (e.g. writing, pincer grip, holding objects, undoing buttons, using a knife and fork).

Head and neck
- **Face.** Look for a butterfly rash, which may in rare cases suggest SLE. This usually spares the nasolabial folds, which distinguishes it from seborrhoeic dermatitis and rosacea.
- **Eyes.** Check for signs of anterior uveitis and episcleritis.
- **Lymph nodes.** Check for lymphadenopathy.

Chest
- **Lungs.** In rheumatoid arthritis, check for evidence of pleural effusion. Fine crackles may indicate pulmonary fibrosis due to methotrexate treatment.
- **Heart.** Pericarditis may occur in rheumatoid arthritis.

Abdomen
- **Splenomegaly.** This may occur in rheumatoid arthritis.

Legs
- **Neurology.** Check for signs of peripheral neuropathy in rheumatological disease.

Key references and further reading
1. American College of Rheumatology Ad Hoc Committee on Clinical Guidelines. Guidelines for the initial evaluation of the adult patient with acute musculoskeletal symptoms. *Arthritis Rheum* 1996;39:1–8.
2. Conaghan PG, Dickson J, Grant RL. Care and management of osteoarthritis in adults: summary of NICE guidance. *BMJ* 2008;336:502–503.
3. Doherty M, Dacre J, Dieppe P, Snaith M. The 'GALS' locomotor screen. *Ann Rheum Dis* 1992;51:1165–1169.
4. Luqmani R, Hennel S, Estrach C. British Society for Rheumatology and British Health Professionals in Rheumatology guidelines for the management of rheumatoid arthritis (the first two years). *Rheumatology* 2006;45:1167–1169.

5. National Institute for Health and Care Excellence (NICE). Rheumatoid arthritis in adults: management. NICE guidelines [CG79]. February 2009. Available from: http://www.nice.org.uk/guidance/cg79 (last accessed 29 April 2016).
6. National Institute for Health and Care Excellence (NICE). Rheumatoid arthritis. Clinical knowledge summaries. 2013. Available from: http://cks.nice.org.uk/rheumatoid-arthritis (last accessed 29 April 2016).
7. National Institute for Health and Care Excellence (NICE). Osteoarthritis: care and management. NICE guidelines [CG177]. February 2014. Available from: http://www.nice.org.uk/guidance/cg177 (last accessed 29 April 2016).
8. National Institute for Health and Clinical Excellence (NICE). Osteoarthritis. Clinical knowledge summaries. 2015. Available from: http://cks.nice.org.uk/osteoarthritis (last accessed 29 April 2016).

Neck pain

Key thoughts

Practical points

- **Diagnosis.** Neck pain is a frequent complaint in primary care. Muscular strain, chronic cervical disc degeneration and whiplash injury are common causes of chronic neck ache. In acute presentations, it is important to rule out serious complications such as cord compression, meningitis or subarachnoid haemorrhage.

Possible causes

- Muscular pain.
- Postural neck ache.
- Cervical spondylosis/osteoarthritis.
- Disc prolapse.
- Whiplash injury.
- Fibromyalgia.
- Rheumatoid arthritis.
- Malignancy (e.g. primary tumour, myeloma, metastases).
- Infection (e.g. tuberculosis (TB), osteomyelitis).
- Metabolic (e.g. severe osteoporosis with collapse, Paget's disease).
- Rarely, meningitis, malignancy, pathological fracture.

Risk factors

- Frequent falls.
- Postural hypotension.
- Certain sports (gymnastics, rugby).
- Road traffic accident.

> **RED FLAGS**
>
> - Systemic symptoms such as fever, night sweats or weight loss
> - History of inflammatory arthritis, cancer, infection, TB, HIV, immunosuppression, drug dependency
> - Very severe pain
> - History of high-speed injury
> - Onset age <30 years (congenital abnormalities of the spine)
> - Tenderness over a vertebral body
> - Night pain

The 10-Minute Clinical Assessment, Second Edition. Knut Schroeder.
© 2017 John Wiley & Sons, Ltd. Published 2017 by John Wiley & Sons, Ltd.

- Cervical lymphadenopathy
- Symptoms and signs of raised intracranial pressure
- Drop attacks
- History of neck surgery

History

Ideas, concerns and expectations

- **Ideas.** People often feel that whiplash injury may have damaged their cervical spine.
- **Concerns.** Chronic neck problems can be very worrying due to their effect on the quality of life and function.
- **Expectations.** Expectations about success of treatment for cervical spondylosis may be unrealistic.

History of presenting complaint

- **Quality of life.** Assess the effect of neck problems on the quality of life and day-to-day activities. Neck pain can be very disabling.
- **Onset.** Most patients with neck pain have chronic intermittent symptoms. In patients with cervical spondylosis or in young people, a sudden deterioration of symptoms and the development of neurological signs may suggest disc herniation.
- **Site.** Cervical spondylosis is common in the lower half of the neck, whereas rheumatoid arthritis tends to affect the upper part.
- **Severity.** Muscular pain and cervical spondylosis cause mild to moderate symptoms in most cases. Excruciating or worsening pain or intractable night pain suggest a more severe underlying cause – consider malignancy, infection or inflammation.
- **Injury.** A minor flexion injury or fall can cause acute cervical myelopathy in individuals over 60 years of age who have a narrow spinal canal. Neck pain is common after whiplash injury caused by a traffic accident. A turned head at the time of impact and high forces increase the risk of spinal damage.
- **Precipitating factors.** Poor posture, anxiety, depression and stress, as well as sporting and occupational activities, can all lead to neck pain. Neck pain is common in people who spend a lot of time in front of a computer.

Common symptom patterns

- **Cervical spondylosis.** Symptoms include neck pain which is worse on movement, retro-orbital or temporal pain (C1/C2), referred pain (suboccipital, between shoulders, upper limbs), cervical stiffness, balance problems and neurological symptoms (paraesthesia, weakness) in the upper limbs. Referred neck pain usually does not radiate below the elbow – if it does, it is likely to be nerve root pain or a peripheral nerve lesion. Impaired coordination of the hands, urinary symptoms, difficulties with tasks like buttoning clothes or gait disturbance suggests cervical myelopathy.

- **Whiplash injury.** A cervical spine X-ray is indicated after whiplash injury if there is inability to rotate the neck through 45° in both directions, if there are paraesthesiae and other neurological features and if the patient is not walking around.

Medication

- **Analgesia.** What has been tried, and what has been successful in relieving any symptoms? Ask in particular about commonly used analgesics and nonsteroidal anti-inflammatory drugs (NSAIDs), both prescribed and over-the-counter. Tricyclic antidepressants can be useful in chronic pain.

Review of previous investigations

- **Neck X-ray.** Most people with neck problems will not require imaging. Appearances consistent with cervical spondylosis do not always correlate with the clinical condition of the patient. In patients with rheumatoid arthritis, flexion and extension radiographs of the neck may reveal whether atlantoaxial subluxation is present.
- **Magnetic resonance imaging (MRI).** This will often be indicated if there are neurological abnormalities or other alarm features. MRI can be useful in distinguishing between intraspinal and extraspinal causes of neck pain. Intraspinal causes may include a prolapsed cervical disc, tumours, infection or syringomyelia and demyelinating disease. Extraspinal causes may include subarachnoid haemorrhage or carotid artery dissection.

Past and current medical problems

- **Osteoporosis.** A history of osteoporosis is a risk factor for vertebral collapse.
- **History of neck surgery.** Consider recurrence of underlying conditions and possible complications due to scarring.
- **Planned surgery.** In patients with cervical spine problems, intubation can be dangerous.

Social history

- **Home.** Ask about home circumstances and whether the neck problems affect family life or independence.
- **Work.** Are there any problems with work? Does work contribute to the neck problems?

Examination

General

- **General condition.** Is the patient well? Are there any obvious deformities? What is the posture like?
- **Gait.** Disturbed gait occurs with cervical myelopathy.

- **Hands.** Wasting of the hand muscles and clumsy hand movements suggest cervical myelopathy.

Inspection and palpation of the neck
- **Deformities.** Look for any obvious deformities.
- **Cervical spine.** Exquisite tenderness over a vertebral body may suggest a more serious underlying cause (e.g. tumour, fracture).
- **Cervical lymph nodes.** Swollen cervical lymph nodes suggest underlying infection or malignancy.

Neck movement
- **Lateral neck flexion.** This is one of the first movements lost in cervical spondylosis. In cervical radiculopathy, tilting the head to one side may relieve arm pain, which is usually worse than the neck pain.
- **Neck rotation and extension.** Both of these are limited in cervical spondylosis.
- **Neck flexion.** An electric shock-like pain down the arm on neck flexion suggests cervical myelopathy (Lhermitte's sign).
- **Adson manoeuvre.** Symptoms are reproduced by hyperextending the neck and turning the head towards the affected side in thoracic outlet syndrome.

Upper and lower limbs
- **Touch and pressure sensation.** Reduction in touch and pressure sensation suggests compression of the anterior spinothalamic tracts.
- **Pain and temperature sensation.** If pain and temperature sensation are reduced, consider lateral spinothalamic tract involvement.
- **Proprioception and vibration sense.** Check these in both hands and feet. They are reduced in compression of the posterior columns.
- **Coordination.** Clumsy hands can be seen with central cord injury. This may be due to chronic neck injury through repeated small insults.
- **Tone.** This is increased in upper motor neuron lesion.
- **Reflexes.** Reflexes are brisk below the level of stenosis. There may be clonus and the plantar response extensor.
- **Root level.** Try to determine the level of any lesion.
  - **C5 root.** Pain in shoulder and upper arm, deltoid weakness, diminished biceps reflex, sensory changes over deltoid.
  - **C6 root.** Pain in lateral arm and dorsal aspect of forearm, weakness in biceps, sensory changes in thumb and dorsal aspect of the hand, biceps or brachioradialis reflexes diminished or absent.
  - **C7 root.** Pain in forearm, middle and ring fingers, weakness of triceps and extensors of wrists and fingers, sensory deficit in index and middle finger, reduced triceps reflex.
  - **C8 root.** Pain in medial aspect of arm and forearm, weakness of intrinsic muscles of the hand, paraesthesia in ring and little fingers and along medial side of forearm, preserved arm reflexes.

Abdomen
- **Bladder.** Is there an enlarged bladder, suggesting bladder dysfunction?

Key references and further reading
1. Binder AI. Cervical spondylosis and neck pain. *BMJ* 2007;334:527–531.
2. Hoving JL, de Vet HC, Twisk JW et al. Prognostic factors for neck pain in general practice. *Pain* 2004;110:639–645.
3. National Institute for Health and Care Excellence (NICE). Neck pain – non-specific. Clinical knowledge summaries. 2015. Available from: http://cks.nice.org.uk/neck-pain-non-specific (last accessed 29 April 2016).
4. Stiell IG, Wells GA, Vandemheen KL et al. The Canadian C-spine rule for radiography in alert and stable trauma patients. *JAMA* 2001;286:1841–1848.
5. Vos C, Verhagen A, Passchier J, Koes B. Management of acute neck pain in general practice: a prospective study. *Br J Gen Pract* 2007;57:23–28.

Back pain

Key thoughts

Practical points
- **Diagnosis.** Back pain is the most common musculoskeletal reason for consultation in primary care. Mechanical back pain and sciatica due to disc prolapse are common. Occasionally, serious causes, such as bone metastases, myeloma, pancreatitis and aortic aneurysm, may present with back pain.
- **Prognosis.** Try to recognise and assess the level of disability and identify barriers to recovery.

Possible causes
- Mechanical back pain.
- Nerve root pain (sciatica).
- Rarely, cauda equina syndrome, metastasis (e.g. bone, breast, prostate), ankylosing spondylitis, abdominal aortic aneurysm, trauma (e.g. road traffic accident, riding injury), spondylolysis (young athletes, such as gymnasts and cricket players).

Risk factors
- Poor posture and working environment.
- Heavy lifting.
- History of cancer.
- Previous back problems.
- Immunosuppression.

RED FLAGS
- Saddle anaesthesia
- Perianal or perineal sensory loss
- Severe or progressive neurological deficit in the lower extremities
- Gait problems (e.g. foot drop)
- Loss of sexual function
- Bladder or bowel dysfunction
- Major motor weakness
- Sudden onset of severe central pain in the spine relieved by lying down
- Major trauma (e.g. road accident, fall from a height)
- Minor trauma in people with osteoporosis
- Age >50 years or <20 years

The 10-Minute Clinical Assessment, Second Edition. Knut Schroeder.
© 2017 John Wiley & Sons, Ltd. Published 2017 by John Wiley & Sons, Ltd.

- History of cancer
- Night-time pain disturbing sleep
- Constitutional symptoms, such as fever, night sweats and unexplained weight loss
- Immunosuppression
- Thoracic pain

History

Ideas, concerns and expectations

- **Ideas.** Ask what the patient believes to be the cause of the back pain. There are many myths about back pain, which will be worth exploring (see box).
- **Concerns.** Common concerns include serious underlying pathology, bone damage and disc prolapse. Also consider worries about disability, work and leisure activities.
- **Expectations.** What does the patient expect in terms of treatment (e.g. analgesia, a sick note, referral for physiotherapy, referral to a spinal specialist, or further investigation such as X-ray or MRI)? High expectations may lead to a negative attitude and reduced activity. Realistic expectations, use of self-help and increased patient knowledge about back pain are likely to improve outcome.

COMMON MYTHS ABOUT BACK PAIN

- Further testing is always necessary if there is no clear underlying diagnosis.
- An MRI scan or other diagnostic test is always needed.
- There is a standard cure for most causes of back or neck pain.
- Rest is the key to recovery from back pain.
- Exercise causes damage to the back.
- Long-term pain means that surgery will be needed.
- Work should be avoided if back pain is present.

Source: Department of Health. *The Musculoskeletal Services Framework.* Available from: http://webarchive.nationalarchives.gov.uk/20130107105354/ http://www.dh.gov.uk/prod_consum_dh/groups/dh_digitalassets/@dh/@en/do cuments/digitalasset/dh_4138412.pdf (last accessed 29 April 2016).

History of presenting complaint

- **Quality of life.** How does back pain affect the quality of life and day-to-day activities (home, work, leisure)?
- **Onset and progression.** Was onset acute or insidious? Acute back pain has a better prognosis than pain that has been present for over a year. Is the pain getting worse? What was the patient doing when the pain started? Ask about injury or trauma.

- **Site of pain.** Where exactly is the pain? Use of a body diagram may be helpful. Ill-defined unilateral or bilateral buttock pain suggests a disc lesion or sacroiliitis.
- **Severity.** Mechanical back pain is usually mild or moderately severe. Pain due to sciatica can be severe and disabling. Night pain disturbing sleep may suggest a serious underlying cause (e.g. cancer, infection).
- **Exacerbating factors.** Increased pain on bending forward suggests disc prolapse, degenerative problems or muscle pain. Pain on leaning back may indicate facet joint pain, spondylolysis or spondylolisthesis. The latter two conditions may be seen in people who play a lot of sports involving lower back extension and rotation (e.g. gymnastics, bowling, tennis, butterfly swimming). Pain on coughing or straining is often discogenic. Pain worse on exercise may be caused by spinal stenosis.
- **Radiation.** Radiation to one or both legs indicates nerve root pain. True sciatica radiates below the ankle.
- **Referred pain.** Ask about any gastrointestinal symptoms, such as dyspepsia (e.g. peptic ulcer, pancreatic disease) or genito-urinary symptoms (kidney pain).
- **Stiffness.** Stiffness is a main feature of ankylosing spondylitis. It is usually worse in the morning or after rest, lasts for at least 30 minutes and improves with activity.
- **Associated symptoms.** Ask about bladder or bowel problems, leg weakness and sensory disturbance (e.g. paraesthesia, saddle anaesthesia), which may, in rare cases, indicate cord compression. Check whether there is fever, weight loss and sweats, which suggests a more serious underlying cause (e.g. cancer, TB).
- **Trauma.** Consider traumatic damage to the spine if there is a history of a fall from a height or serious trauma, such as a car accident.
- **Lifestyle.** Obesity, sedentary lifestyle, heavy physical work, poor posture, prolonged standing in awkward positions and repetitive lifting or twisting can all contribute to the development and continuation of back pain. What has the patient done to relieve the pain to date?
- **Barriers to recovery.** Identify issues that predispose to chronic pain and disability (e.g. negative attitude to treatment, work-related issues such as compensation, mood disturbance).

Past and current medical problems
- **Back problems.** Ask about a history of back problems or back operations.
- **Cancer.** Consider the possibility of the back pain being caused by bone metastasis, particularly if there is underlying prostate, breast, thyroid, renal or uterine cancer.
- **Immunosuppression.** HIV infection and chemotherapy are risk factors for infection and cancer.
- **Infection.** Consider TB in at-risk groups.
- **Osteoporosis.** Severe osteoporosis may result in vertebral collapse.

Medication
- **Analgesia.** What medication has been tried and is currently being taken? What has been effective? Ask about over-the-counter medication. Have there been

any side effects? Are there any contraindications or cautions, such as asthma or peptic ulcer disease (NSAIDs)?
- **Steroids.** High-dose steroids can mask symptoms and may lead to osteoporosis.

Other treatments
- **Physical treatments.** Ask in particular about physiotherapy, osteopathy, chiropractic treatments and occupational therapists. Has a rheumatologist been consulted in the past? Has the patient contacted self-help organisations?

Allergies
- **Analgesics and anti-inflammatory drugs.** Ask about allergies to drugs commonly used for symptomatic treatment of back pain (e.g. NSAIDs).

Social history
- **Home.** How does the back pain affect home and family life? How are certain roles affected, such as being a parent or partner?
- **Work.** Ask about occupation and for details about routine work activities. Has the patient taken time off work? Does work contribute to back pain?
- **Social problems.** Chronic back pain may lead to depression and social withdrawal.

Review of previous investigations
- **Imaging.** Imaging is rarely required in the management of simple mechanical low back pain. Symptoms, pathology and radiological appearances correlate poorly, and imaging is only needed if a serious underlying cause is suspected. MRI can be useful in suspected nerve root compression or cancer.
- **Blood tests.** Blood tests are rarely required. Full blood count and inflammatory markers may be helpful if infection or inflammation is suspected. A myeloma screen may be helpful if symptoms are suggestive.

Examination

General
- **General physical condition.** Does the patient look unwell or in pain? Pallor, cachexia, jaundice or lymphadenopathy may suggest systemic disease.
- **Gait and mobility.** Observe the patient getting in and out of a chair and taking off/putting on clothes. Gait abnormalities suggest a potentially serious cause. Ask the patient to walk on heels and tiptoes, which is an easy way to check for weakness (especially foot drop).
- **Breasts.** Examine the breasts in women if pain might be caused by metastases from breast cancer.

Examination of the spine
- **Posture.** Assess posture and the level of shoulders and iliac crests. Look for any muscle wasting (nerve damage), structural abnormality (kyphosis, scoliosis, lordosis) or flexion deformity (vertebral collapse).

- **Tenderness.** Palpate the back for tenderness and muscle spasm. Focus on the paraspinal muscles, the spinal processes and the sacroiliac joints. The site of pain often corresponds with the site of the abnormality.
- **Cervical spine.** Check active and passive neck movements (flexion, extension, lateral flexion and rotation), assessing range of movement and pain. Repeat with gentle pressure on the skull.
- **Thoracic spine.** Check rotation and chest expansion (should be >5 cm).
- **Lumbar spine.** Check flexion, extension, lateral flexion and rotation. Pain on bending forward suggests disc prolapse (± neurological signs), annular tear or muscle strain. If leaning back causes pain, consider facet joint disorder, spondylolysis, spondylolisthesis or a sacroiliac disorder. Limitation of lower spine movements may rarely suggest ankylosing spondylitis.
- **Sacroiliac joints.** Palpate and press the joints. Flex one hip, while keeping the other extended.
- **Walking.** Claudicant pain eased by flexion raises the possibility of spinal stenosis.
- **Straight leg raising (SLR).** Poor SLR means poor prognosis and a probable disc lesion. Bending the knee during hip flexion should relieve the pain, and pressure in the popliteal region should worsen it (popliteal compression test). Placing the knee back in full extension during SLR and dorsiflexing the ankle can increase the pain in nerve root and sciatic nerve irritation (Lasègue's sign).

Lower limbs

- **Peripheral pulses.** Check circulation by palpating peripheral pulses.
- **Neurological assessment.** Check tone, sensation, power, coordination and reflexes, especially if indicated by the history. Significant weakness, particularly if unilateral, suggests nerve root involvement. If there is any abnormality, check for saddle numbness and loss of anal sphincter tone (cauda equine syndrome). Note the distribution of any paraesthesia or sensory loss. Check ankle and great toe dorsiflexion and knee and ankle reflexes (all can be affected in disc lesions). Progressive bilateral neurological signs and sphincter disturbance occur in central disc prolapse, cauda equina syndrome, cord compression and spinal vascular event.

Abdomen

- **Palpation.** Palpate the abdomen for tenderness (peptic ulcer) and masses (abdominal aortic aneurysm), if suggested by the history.
- **Rectal examination.** Consider rectal examination if the history suggests possible prostate cancer (back pain from metastasis).

Key references and further reading

1. Bratton R. Assessment and management of low back pain. *Am Fam Physician* 1999;60:2299–2306.
2. Department of Health. *The Musculoskeletal Services Framework.* Available from: http://webarchive.nationalarchives.gov.uk/20130107105354/http://

www.dh.gov.uk/prod_consum_dh/groups/dh_digitalassets/@dh/@en/docume
nts/digitalasset/dh_4138412.pdf (last accessed 29 April 2016).

3. Koes BW, van Tulder MW, Thomas S. Clinical review: diagnosis and treatment of low back pain. *BMJ* 2006;332:1430–1434.

4. National Institute for Health and Care Excellence (NICE). Back pain – low (without radiculopathy). Clinical knowledge summaries. 2015. Available from: http://cks.nice.org.uk/back-pain-low-without-radiculopathy (last accessed 29 April 2016).

5. National Institute for Health and Care Excellence (NICE). Sciatica (lumbar radiculopathy). Clinical knowledge summaries. 2015. Available from: http://cks.nice.org.uk/sciatica-lumbar-radiculopathy (last accessed 29 April 2016).

6. Speed C. ABC of rheumatology. Low back pain. *BMJ* 2004;328:1119–1121.

7. van Tulder M, Becker A, Bekkering T et al. on behalf of the COST B13 Working Group on Guidelines for the Management of Acute Low Back Pain in Primary Care. European guidelines for the management of acute non-specific low back pain in primary care. 2004. Available from: http://www.ncbi.nlm.nih.gov/pmc/articles/PMC3454540/pdf/586_2006_Article_1071.pdf (last accessed 29 April 2016).

Shoulder and arm problems

Key thoughts

Practical points
- **Diagnosis.** Shoulder pain is a common presentation in primary care. Pain often originates from the shoulder joint or adjacent structures, including ligaments, muscles and tendons. Also consider referred pain from the neck, heart or diaphragm.
- **Function.** Assess the effect of shoulder problems on the patient's life, including day-to-day activities at home, work and leisure.

Possible causes
- **Shoulder joint.** Arm overuse, rotator cuff disorders (impingement, tendinopathy, bursitis, tendonitis, tears), acromioclavicular joint problems, glenohumeral capsulitis ('frozen shoulder'), arthritis, traumatic dislocation.
- **Other.** Referred pain (neck, myocardial infarction (MI), gallbladder disease, subphrenic abscess), malignancy (apical lung cancer, metastases), PMR.

Risk factors
- Occupational (repetitive movements, vibration).
- Sports and exercise (throwing, swimming, rugby).
- Manual work.
- Trauma (e.g. dislocation).
- History of arthritis.

> **RED FLAGS**
>
> - Constitutional features, such as fever, weight loss, malaise
> - Significant trauma with risk of fracture or dislocation
> - Chest or abdominal pain (MI, abscess, gall bladder)
> - History of malignancy
> - Overlying skin erythema
> - Symptoms suggestive of PMR
> - Unexplained sensory or motor deficit
> - History of trauma or dislocation
> - Loss of shoulder contour and rotation (dislocation)
> - Acute severe pain with positive arm-drop test (rotator cuff tear)

The 10-Minute Clinical Assessment, Second Edition. Knut Schroeder.
© 2017 John Wiley & Sons, Ltd. Published 2017 by John Wiley & Sons, Ltd.

History

Ideas, concerns and expectations

- **Ideas.** Many people do not realise that shoulder or arm pain can have causes other than shoulder joint conditions. Find out what the patient believes to be the underlying problem.
- **Concerns.** Patients are often concerned about the pain, loss of function, home life and work.
- **Expectations.** Patients may have unrealistic expectations with regard to the speed of recovery.

History of presenting complaint

- **Quality of life.** Shoulder problems can severely limit daily routines and affect work and leisure activities. Sleep is commonly impaired. Ask about difficulties lifting or throwing (elevation), washing and wiping the bottom (internal rotation), putting on a coat and combing hair (external rotation). Explore whether there is depression or social withdrawal.
- **Onset.** Acute onset with a history of trauma suggests rotator cuff tear (which can be atraumatic in the elderly), fracture or dislocation. Gradual onset of true shoulder pain, building up to a maximum level over a short period of time, is consistent with frozen shoulder. The three phases of frozen shoulder are pain, stiffness and resolution.
- **Site of pain.** Deep joint pain and pain at the outer aspect of the upper arm associated with restriction of all movements is likely to be caused by adhesive capsulitis (frozen shoulder) or glenohumeral arthritis. Pain over the anterior upper biceps insertion is caused by anterior capsulitis. In frozen shoulder, there may be less severe pain at the end range of the movement. Rotator cuff pain is also felt in the upper aspect of the arm or deltoid region. Bilateral shoulder pain suggests an inflammatory cause, such as rheumatoid arthritis or PMR. Pain in the acromioclavicular joint suggests acromioclavicular joint disease. Is the dominant hand/arm affected?
- **Character.** A 'dead arm feeling' may occur with shoulder instability without dislocation. There is likely to be discomfort without obvious restriction of movement.
- **Radiation.** Ask for any symptoms in adjacent areas such as the axillae, upper limbs, neck and chest. In referred pain, shoulder movement is usually normal and does not change the character of the pain.
- **Night pain.** Is there difficulty sleeping on the affected side? Pain during the night may be caused by difficulty finding a comfortable sleeping position, but may also be caused by rotator cuff pain, nerve root pain or cancer.
- **Neurovascular compromise.** Is there poor circulation or numbness in the arm? Compression of the brachial plexus may result in thoracic outlet syndrome, which can cause numbness and pain in the hand, arm or shoulder. An underlying cervical rib, large muscles, poor posture or repetitive activities may be responsible. Ask about loss of muscle mass and sensory or motor symptoms.

- **Precipitating factors.** Is pain caused by a sports-related injury? Ask about any lifting of heavy loads, using the arms in awkward positions and prolonged elevation of the upper limbs, all of which can be associated with shoulder problems. Carrying a heavy rucksack for prolonged periods may cause painless trauma to the long thoracic nerve, which can lead to paralysis of the serratus anterior muscle, with subsequent winging of the scapula. Immobility is a risk factor for adhesive capsulitis (frozen shoulder) and may result from a stroke, cardiac disease, shoulder surgery or trauma.
- **Exacerbating and relieving factors.** Neck movement may reproduce pain originating from the cervical spine. Pain associated with overhead upper limb movements suggests rotator cuff tendinopathy.
- **Associated symptoms.** Cardiac pain can radiate to the shoulder. Ask about chest pain, shortness of breath and nausea. Proximal muscle pain and morning stiffness are features of PMR. Widespread joint pain may indicate inflammatory arthritis.
- **Previous shoulder injury.** Is there a history of injury, acute shoulder pain or shoulder instability? Check whether the shoulder joint has ever dislocated. Ask about past shoulder surgery.
- **Systemic symptoms.** Fever, night sweats, generalised joint pains, rashes and weight loss may all suggest a systemic underlying cause (cancer, inflammation, infection). Ask about a history of cancer. Have there been any unexplained deformities or masses? Ask about swollen lymph nodes. In smokers, consider apical lung cancer (Pancoast tumour) and metastases.
- **Dislocation.** This is usually caused by trauma, epileptic fit or electric shock. There tends to be severe acute and disabling pain, with significant weakness on elevation of the affected arm.

Past and current medical problems
- **Degenerative disorders.** Arthritis and cervical spondylosis can cause shoulder pain.
- **Diabetes.** Diabetes is associated with frozen shoulder.
- **Gallbladder disease.** Pain from the gall bladder or a subphrenic abscess may radiate to the shoulder.
- **Renal disease.** Renal disease can limit the range of drugs that can be used to treat shoulder problems.
- **Cancer.** A history of breast or lung cancer raises the possibility of a metastatic lesion. Mediastinal tumours may present with shoulder pain.

Medication
- **Pain relief.** Ask for details about past and current drug treatments. Has treatment been effective? Have there been adverse effects from any treatments? The severity of shoulder pain can be judged by the amount of analgesia required.

Other past treatments
- **Joint injections.** Have these been tried in the past, and were they successful?

- **Occupational therapy.** Occupational therapy may be useful in providing home aids, such as light weight irons, angled sponges for washing or special kitchen equipment.
- **Physiotherapy.** Has the patient had physiotherapy?

Social history
- **Home.** How is function affected, and which activities are limited?
- **Occupation and sporting activities.** Occupations such as plastering, hair dressing and construction work predispose to shoulder problems through heavy lifting and repetitive movements in awkward positions.
- **Work and hobbies.** Ask which specific activities are undertaken at work and as part of leisure activities (particularly sports). What have been the effects on these activities?

Alcohol and smoking
- **Smoking.** Consider the possibility of Pancoast tumour in current or previous smokers.
- **Alcohol.** Have there been any falls related to alcohol consumption that might have contributed to the shoulder problems?

Review of previous investigations
- **Blood tests.** These are rarely needed. A raised plasma viscosity may indicate PMR.
- **Ultrasound or MRI.** These are usually only necessary if there are 'red flag' symptoms or signs, or if there are other specific indications. Synovitis and structural shoulder problems may be detected by ultrasound or MRI.
- **X-ray.** Plain shoulder X-rays may show abnormalities of the glenohumeral or acromioclavicular joints. Chest X-ray may detect an apical lung carcinoma in referred shoulder pain, if suggested by the history.

Examination

General
- **General condition.** Does the patient look in pain? Look for posture and difficulties in taking off or putting on clothes.
- **Neck, axilla and chest wall.** Inspect for any obvious abnormality.
- **Lymph nodes.** Examine the axillae and neck for lymph nodes.

Cervical spine
- **Inspection.** Look for any obvious deformity.
- **Palpation.** Check for any vertebral or muscular tenderness.
- **Movement.** Limited range of movement of the cervical spine may indicate spinal problems.

Shoulder

- **Inspection.** Inspect the shoulder from all angles and look for posture, muscle wasting, scars, swelling, deformity, redness and symmetry. In shoulder dislocation, the arm will be held in a fixed position.
- **Palpation.** Palpate muscles, bony landmarks and joints for swelling, tenderness and crepitus. A tender acromioclavicular joint may suggest injury in younger people or osteoarthritis in older people. Crepitus on joint movement suggests pericapsulitis (frozen shoulder).
- **Global restriction of movement.** Pain arising from the shoulder joint can usually be reproduced by shoulder movements. This is common with frozen shoulder.
- **Abduction and elevation.** Restricted abduction due to pain is commonly caused by impingement or supraspinatus tendinitis. Poor active abduction with a preserved passive range of movement may occur with a large rotator cuff tear. Check from behind the patient for a painful arc between 70 and 120° during active abduction, which would suggest impingement. In case of a significant rotator cuff tear, the patient will be unable to support the weight of the affected arm if abducted to 90°. Pain on raising the arm from 90° (horizontal) to 180° (vertical) suggests osteoarthritis of the acromioclavicular joint.
- **External rotation.** External rotation may be reduced in frozen shoulder or infraspinatus tendonitis. Limited passive external rotation may suggest a glenohumeral problem, including osteoarthritis or locked posterior dislocation. In severe glenohumeral shoulder problems, there is global pain and restriction of all active and passive movements. If full external rotation is possible, frozen shoulder is unlikely.
- **Internal rotation.** Restriction of internal rotation is common with subscapularis tendinitis.
- **Flexion and extension.** Ask the patient to raise their arms to the front and behind them in order to assess flexion and extension.
- **Flexion and supination of the forearm.** Pain on resisted flexion or supination of the forearm is common with bicipital tendinitis and produces pain at the tip of the shoulder.
- **Power.** Weakness, rather than pain, is the main feature in neurological disorders.
- **Function.** This includes getting the hands comfortably behind the lower back and behind the head, which is important for washing and grooming.

Chest
- **Lungs.** Listen for chest signs if Pancoast tumour is a possibility.

Abdomen

- **Upper abdomen.** Palpate the upper abdomen if subdiaphragmatic pathology may be causing shoulder-tip pain.

Bedside tests
- **Urine glucose.** Check this to screen for diabetes (frozen shoulder).

Key references and further reading
1. Dias R, Cutts S, Massoud S. Frozen shoulder. *BMJ* 2005;331:1453–1456.
2. Luime J, Verhagen A, Miedema H et al. Does this patient have an instability of the shoulder or a labrum lesion? *JAMA* 2004;292:1989–1999.
3. Mitchell C, Adebajo A, Hay E, Carr A. Shoulder pain: diagnosis and management in primary care. *BMJ* 2005;331:1124–1128.
4. National Institute for Health and Care Excellence (NICE). Shoulder pain. Clinical knowledge summaries. 2015. Available from: http://cks.nice.org.uk/shoulder-pain (last accessed 29 April 2016).
5. Woodward TW, Best TM. The painful shoulder: part I. Clinical evaluation. *Am Fam Physician* 2000;61:3079–3088.
6. Woodward TW, Best TM. The painful shoulder: part II. Acute and chronic disorders. *Am Fam Physician* 2000;61:3291–3300.

Elbow problems

Key thoughts

Practical points
- **Diagnosis.** Lateral and medial epicondylitis are common and are mostly caused by overuse injury. Pain may also be referred from the neck or shoulder.
- **Function.** Elbow problems can be very disabling. Assess the impact of the problem on the patient's life.

Possible causes
- Overuse trauma, such as lateral epicondylitis (tennis elbow) or medial epicondylitis (golfer's elbow) – most commonly caused by do-it-yourself (DIY) projects.
- Referred pain from the neck or the shoulder.
- Olecranon bursitis.
- Dislocation of the radial head.
- Rarely, rheumatoid arthritis, gout, cubital tunnel syndrome, fracture of the elbow, septic arthritis.

> **RED FLAGS**
>
> - Injury to the median nerve
> - Malunion of fractures
> - Ulnar palsy
> - Chronic lateral or medial epicondylitis
> - Uncontrollable pain
> - Hot and swollen joint, suggesting sepsis
> - Constitutional features, such as fever, weight loss, malaise, night sweats
> - Significant trauma with risk of fracture or dislocation

History

Ideas, concerns and expectations
- **Ideas.** Patients may already have an idea of what is causing the elbow problems.
- **Concerns.** Patients will often worry about being able to carry on with work or continue with hobbies (e.g. sports, music).
- **Expectations.** What level of functioning is needed to continue with usual activities?

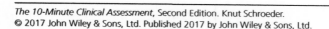

The 10-Minute Clinical Assessment, Second Edition. Knut Schroeder.
© 2017 John Wiley & Sons, Ltd. Published 2017 by John Wiley & Sons, Ltd.

History of presenting complaint
- **Quality of life.** How does the elbow problem affect the quality of life? Which activities are mainly affected?
- **Onset.** For how long have symptoms been present? Trauma and overuse injuries are usually of acute onset.
- **Character.** Diffuse pain is common in extensor tendinopathy or joint problems. Lateral and medial epicondylitis tend to be more localised. Aching pain is often caused by overuse injury, whereas a burning or tingling pain suggests nerve involvement.
- **Precipitating factors.** Ask about any recent changes in training or the use of the arms at work. Has any new equipment been used at work, at home (e.g. DIY projects) or when exercising? Has there been any recent trauma?
- **Exacerbating factors.** Elbow pain can range from minimal discomfort to excruciating pain. Ask what makes the pain worse (e.g. minor activities like lifting up a glass or repeated activities like hard manual work or playing tennis).
- **Neck and shoulder pain.** Consider referred pain if there are neck or shoulder problems, particularly if pain is persistent or related to posture.
- **Stiffness.** Is stiffness preventing movements like putting the hand to the mouth, combing the hair or washing?
- **Swelling.** Swelling occurs with bursitis, joint injury or trauma.

Past and current medical problems
- **Locomotor.** Ask about prior elbow dislocation or fracture and previous overuse injuries. Is there a history of cervical spondylosis?

Family history
- **Arthritis.** Ask about a family history of arthritis.

Medication
- **Analgesic and anti-inflammatory medication.** Check what drugs have been prescribed to date and whether they have been effective. Have there been any adverse effects (e.g. dyspepsia from NSAIDs or constipation from drugs containing codeine)?
- **Over-the-counter medication.** Paracetamol and NSAIDs (including topical preparations) are often bought over the counter, without prescription.

Allergies
- **Drugs.** Ask about any allergies to drugs used to treat locomotor problems.

Social history
- **Home.** How is the patient coping at home? Is any support needed with personal care, shopping, cooking or cleaning? Are any mobility or other aids required?

- **Occupation.** Ask for details about what activities are being performed at work and whether these might be implicated or affected. Repetitive occupations, such as bricklaying and carpentry, predispose to elbow problems.
- **Sports.** Ask in particular about racket sports, such as tennis, badminton and squash.

Examination

Inspection
- **Carrying angle.** Look from the front for the carrying angle and from the side for flexion deformity. Cubitus valgus and hypermobility may cause elbow pain and are common after non-union of a fractured lateral condyle.
- **Skin.** Look for scars, muscle wasting, psoriatic plaques, rashes, rheumatoid nodules and any swellings. A soft swelling at the posterior aspect of the elbow suggests olecranon bursitis.

Palpation
- **Pain.** Ask about any pain before starting to palpate the elbow.
- **Skin temperature.** Raised skin temperature may suggest infection or acute inflammation.
- **Elbow.** Palpate the elbow flexed at 90° with your thumb to feel for the head of the radius and the joint line. Feel for any swelling (suggesting joint effusion or bursitis) and fullness between the olecranon and the lateral epicondyle, which occurs in synovitis. Cubital tunnel syndrome is caused by pressure on the ulnar nerve as it traverses the elbow due to prolonged flexion in athletes and wheelchair users and during sleep. This is commonly associated with paraesthesia of the ring and little fingers. The soft tissues around the elbow are often affected by gout.
- **Epicondyles.** Check for lateral (tennis elbow) and medial (golfer's elbow) epicondylitis and look for evidence of bursitis.

Movement
- **Flexion and extension.** Assess the range of movement in the elbow joint, comparing both sides. Assess both active and passive movements and look for any reduction in flexion or extension. Passive limitation of extension suggests muscular flexion contracture or mechanical blockade. Pain on forced extension suggests olecranon impingement.
- **Pronation and supination.** Check both actively and passively and feel for any crepitus suggesting arthritis or fracture.

Function
- **Important elbow movements.** Check whether the patient is able to reach the mouth with the hand on the affected side – this is one of the most important movements. Also assess whether the hands can be moved behind the head.

Key references and further reading

1. National Institute for Health and Clinical Excellence (NICE). Olecranon bursitis. Clinical knowledge summaries. 2015. Available from: http://cks.nice.org.uk/olecranon-bursitis (last accessed 29 April 2016).
2. National Institute for Health and Care Excellence (NICE). Tennis elbow. Clinical knowledge summaries. 2015. Available from: http://cks.nice.org.uk/tennis-elbow (last accessed 29 April 2016).
3. Salzman KL, Lillegard WA, Butcher JD. Upper extremity bursitis. *Am Fam Physician* 1997;56:1797–1806, 1811–1812.
4. Sheps DM, Hildebrand KA, Boorman RS. Simple dislocations of the elbow: evaluation and treatment. *Hand Clin* 2004;20:389–404.
5. Smidt N, van der Windt DA. Tennis elbow in primary care. *BMJ* 2006;333:927–928.

Hand problems

Key thoughts

Practical points
- **Diagnosis.** Overuse injuries are common. Consider osteoarthritis and rheumatoid arthritis if there is joint pain and swelling. It is important not to miss scaphoid fracture if there is a history of injury.
- **Impact.** Hand problems can severely impact on daily activities and reduce the quality of life.

Important hand and wrist problems
- Tenosynovitis.
- Carpal tunnel syndrome.
- Osteoarthritis.
- Rheumatoid arthritis.
- Dupuytren's contracture.
- Avulsion fractures.
- Tendonitis.
- Mallet finger.
- Raynaud's phenomenon.
- Repetitive strain injury.
- Trigger finger.

RED FLAGS

- Severe loss of function
- Severe pain
- Systemic symptoms
- Tender scaphoid
- Joint destruction
- Hot and swollen joint, suggesting sepsis
- Constitutional features, such as fever, weight loss and malaise
- Significant trauma with risk of fracture or dislocation
- Numbness and paraesthesiae

History

Ideas, concerns and expectations
- **Ideas.** Patients will often have a good idea as to what might be causing the problem.

The 10-Minute Clinical Assessment, Second Edition. Knut Schroeder.
© 2017 John Wiley & Sons, Ltd. Published 2017 by John Wiley & Sons, Ltd.

- **Concerns.** People presenting with arthritis or trauma are often worried about future ability to carry out simple tasks with their hands. Fear of malignancy or embarrassment when shaking hands is common in people presenting with Dupuytren's contracture.
- **Expectations.** What level of function is needed with daily activities and hobbies?

History of presenting complaint in case of injury

- **Impact on daily activities.** How far do hand or wrist problems affect daily activities? Ask about daily living, work and leisure activities. Has the patient had to take time off work?
- **Symptoms.** What is the main problem? Pain is often caused by trauma, overuse or chronic musculoskeletal conditions.
- **Onset and progression.** For how long have problems been present? Is pain progressive?
- **Finger locking.** This is usually caused by trigger finger. Patients often describe a clicking sensation on straightening a finger, or locking of the finger during flexion in more severe cases.

Injuries

- **Nature of the injury.** Ask for details about how the injury happened and what types of force were involved. Pain in the presence of swelling and functional impairment makes underlying bone or joint damage likely.
- **Metacarpal bones.** The neck of the metacarpal can fracture as a result of a direct punch, usually leading to volar displacement of the head. Injury often involves the fifth metacarpal but can occur in any finger.
- **Proximal phalanges.** Direct blows to the finger can lead to spiral or transverse fracture, which is often more obvious when the fingers are flexed.
- **Middle phalanges.** Volar plate avulsion is a common injury and usually results from a hyperextension injury. It may be associated with a dislocation of the proximal phalangeal joint.
- **Distal phalanges.** Crush injuries are common. Mallet fingers are caused by a direct blow to the extended digit, with damage to the extensor tendon at its insertion to the base of the distal phalanx, leading to flexion deformity.
- **Thumb.** Bennet's fracture and dislocation is an oblique fracture of the base of the first metacarpal with dorsal dislocation or subluxation of the first metacarpal. An abduction injury to the thumb can lead to 'gamekeeper's' or 'skier's' thumb due to outward distraction of the thumb and an avulsion of the attachment of the ulnar collateral ligament, sometimes associated with a bony avulsion fracture.

Common symptom patterns

- **De Quervain's tendonitis.** Pain on moving the thumb and tenderness over first extensor compartments is suggestive of De Quervain's tendonitis. This occurs most commonly in women between the ages of 30 and 60 years and is not usually caused by injury or work.

- **Carpal tunnel syndrome.** Tingling in the tips of the thumb, index finger, middle finger and radial half of the ring finger, as well as the radial side of the palm and back of the hand, suggests carpal tunnel syndrome. This may be more severe at night, and patients often complain of clumsiness as they may have difficulties feeling objects they are trying to manipulate. There may, in addition, be pain and paraesthesia in the forearm, elbow and shoulder. In severe cases, there will be a reduced grip. Pain is often worse at night and may be relieved by shaking of the hand. Certain hand positions and activities may also exacerbate symptoms. Consider peripheral neuropathy, cervical spondylosis and thoracic inlet tumours in the differential diagnosis.
- **Osteoarthritis.** Features include a reduced range of movement, pain on joint movement, swelling and crepitus. Systemic features, such as fever and rash, are absent.
- **Rheumatoid arthritis.** The proximal interphalangeal and MCP joints and the wrists are commonly involved.
- **Dupuytren's contracture.** Features are painless lumps in the palm together with problems straightening the fingers. Ask about a positive family history. Risk factors include diabetes mellitus, smoking, excessive alcohol intake, insulin-dependent diabetes and the use of vibrating machinery.

Past and current medical problems
- **Chronic conditions.** Diabetes mellitus, rheumatoid arthritis, thyroid disease and pregnancy are all associated with carpal tunnel syndrome. Diabetes and rheumatoid arthritis also predispose to trigger finger.

Medication
- **Analgesia.** What has been tried and what has been effective in relieving any pain? Have there been any side effects?

Allergies
- **Drugs.** Are there any allergies to analgesic medication?

Social history
- **Home.** How far are home life and leisure activities affected?
- **Work.** Are the hand or wrist problems work-related? Do they affect work?

Examination

Inspection
- **Position and deformities.** Inspect the hand and wrist with palms up and down. Look for any obvious deformity, soft-tissue or joint swelling, muscle wasting and scars. Are any changes symmetrical or asymmetrical? The nail plane may be slanted in hand injuries, leading to malrotation of one or more fingers. Check whether the finger bends in a straight line on flexion or whether there is evidence of malrotation.
- **Nails.** Look for pitting or loose nails, which occur in psoriasis (psoriatic arthropathy). Is there evidence of nail-fold vasculitis?

- **Skin.** Inspect the skin for any thinning (may indicate long-term steroid use) or bruises. A rash may give diagnostic clues (e.g. in dermatomyositis).
- **Injury.** There may be a laceration or partial (abrasion) or complete loss of skin. Skin flaps are more likely to survive the wider their base is. Narrow flaps, or those with a distal base, are more likely to become necrotic.
- **Muscles.** Look for evidence of muscle wasting. In severe carpal tunnel syndrome, the first and second lumbricals, opponens pollicis, abductor pollicis brevis and flexor pollicis brevis are usually affected.
- **Lumps.** Ganglia can often be found around the dorsal or volar side of the wrist and only rarely cause pain. Giant-cell tumours of the tendon sheath occur most often on the flexor tendons adjacent to the distal interphalangeal joints. Heberden's nodes are hard or bony swellings that can develop in the distal interphalangeal joints and are associated with osteoarthritis.
- **Joints.** There may be bony swelling and deformity due to osteophytes at the distal interphalangeal joints (Heberden's nodes) or proximal interphalangeal joints (Bouchard's nodes) in osteoarthritis. Look for deformities resulting from rheumatoid arthritis, such as ulnar deviation, swan neck and boutonniere (fingers), Z-deformity (thumb) and 'piano key' deformity of the wrist. Check for muscle wasting and tendon rupture.

Palpation

- **Pulses.** Check radial pulses in both the wrists.
- **Muscle bulk.** Is there any wasting of the thenar and hypothenar muscle eminences (carpal tunnel syndrome)?
- **Skin and soft tissues.** Palpate both wrists bimanually and check both forearms for any rheumatoid nodules or psoriatic plaques on the extensor surfaces.
- **Joints.** Squeeze the MCP joints gently for any tenderness, which may suggest rheumatoid arthritis. If there is pain, assess each joint in turn for swelling and temperature.
- **Bones.** Check for bone tenderness, crepitus and deformity, all of which make bone injury more likely.
- **Scaphoid.** Check for tenderness in the 'anatomical snuffbox' if scaphoid fracture is a possibility. Pushing the thumb, index finger and middle finger towards the wrist may also cause pain in the scaphoid area, making fracture more likely.
- **First extensor compartment.** Tenderness over the first extensor compartment suggests De Quervain's tendinitis, particularly if associated with swelling.
- **Palmar fascia.** Feel for thickening of the palmar skin and painless lumps in the palmar fascia (Dupuytren's contracture).
- **Tinel's sign.** This is a sign of a compressed nerve in carpal tunnel syndrome. Percuss the median nerve over the wrist; this leads to paraesthesia in the fingertips in carpal tunnel syndrome.

Movement

- **Fingers.** Ask the patient to straighten the fingers fully. Any problems may indicate extensor tendon rupture (e.g. mallet finger), Dupuytren's contracture, joint disease or neurological damage. Assess flexion by asking the patient to tuck the fingers into the palm. Also check flexion in individual fingers, with all other fingers held straight. Any difficulties may indicate tendon or small joint problems. Impaired flexion of the proximal interphalangeal joint suggests damage to the flexor digitorum superficialis. Reduced flexion of the distal interphalangeal joint when the proximal joint is held fully straight occurs with damage to the flexor digitorum profundus. Stenosing tenosynovitis causes trigger finger, in which the fingers or the thumb stay in a bent position and straighten with a 'snap'. If severe, the finger may become locked in the bent position.

- **Wrist.** Assess wrist flexion and extension both actively and passively.
- **Power.** Assess the power of the median and ulnar nerves by abduction of the thumb and by asking the patient to spread the fingers apart.
- **Upper limb and neck.** Check for range of movement and tenderness in the upper limbs and the neck to help rule out referred pain.
- **Phalen's test.** Check for carpal tunnel syndrome by flexing the wrist for 1 minute, which results in paraesthesia.
- **Finkelstein's test.** Ask the patient to stretch the tendons of the first extensor compartment by firmly gripping the thumb in the palm. This causes pain in De Quervain's tendinitis.

Function

- **Power grip.** Assess power grip by asking the patient to grip two of your fingers.
- **Pincer grip.** Ask the patient to pinch your finger or to pick an object such as a coin from your palm in order to assess pincer grip, which is very important for many day-to-day activities.

Neurology

- **Sensation.** Is sensation normal and equal on both sides? Consider neurological involvement if it is abnormal. Touch the thumb and index finger web space lightly to assess radial nerve sensation. If a digital nerve is injured, this usually leads to sensory loss in the affected half of the finger pulp, and sweating will be absent. If a more proximal nerve is affected, this will lead to both motor and sensory dysfunction.

Key references and further reading

1. Arthritis Research UK. *Clinical Assessment of the Musculoskeletal System: A Guide for Medical Students and Healthcare Professionals.* 2011. Available from: https://www.arthritisresearchuk.org/~/media/Files/Education/Student%20Handbook%2011-2.ashx (last accessed 29 April 2016).
2. Burke FD, Ellis J, McKenna H, Bradley MJ. Primary care management of carpal tunnel syndrome. *Postgrad Med J* 2003;79:43–47.
3. Conaghan PG, Dickson J, Grant RL. Care and management of osteoarthritis in adults: summary of NICE guidance. *BMJ* 2008;336:502–503.
4. Hunter DJ, Felson DT. *Osteoarthritis. BMJ* 2006;332:639–642.
5. National Institute for Health and Care Excellence (NICE). Osteoarthritis. Clinical knowledge summaries. 2015. Available from: http://cks.nice.org.uk/osteoarthritis (last accessed 29 April 2016).

Hip pain

Key thoughts

Practical points
- **Diagnosis.** Osteoarthritis of the hip is common. Also consider spinal problems and hip fracture. Hip replacement is frequently performed.
- **Effect on life.** Pain and disability are often the principal clinical problems. Concern about the diagnosis is common.

Possible causes
- Osteoarthritis.
- Soft-tissue inflammation around the hip joint (e.g. trochanteric bursitis).
- Spinal problems.
- Hip fracture.
- Other forms of arthritis, such as rheumatoid arthritis, ankylosing spondylitis and psoriatic arthritis.
- Paget's disease.
- Avascular necrosis.
- Malignancy.
- Infection.

> **RED FLAGS**
>
> - Inability to bear weight
> - Trauma
> - Younger and older age groups
> - Progressive reduction in joint movement
> - History of cancer
> - Systemic symptoms, such as fever, malaise, weight loss
> - Uncontrollable pain
> - Hot and swollen joint, suggesting sepsis
> - Significant trauma with risk of fracture or dislocation
> - Progressive disability and dependency

History

Ideas, concerns and expectations
- **Ideas.** What is the patient's attitude to the hip problem and its potential cause? There are many myths around hip pain, which will often be worth exploring.

The 10-Minute Clinical Assessment, Second Edition. Knut Schroeder.
© 2017 John Wiley & Sons, Ltd. Published 2017 by John Wiley & Sons, Ltd.

Common misconceptions are that nothing can be done about hip pain, that exercise should be avoided and that surgery will always be successful.

- **Concerns.** Are there any fears about the prognosis and its implications for the patient's life? Concerns about ongoing pain and disability are common.
- **Expectations.** Explore expectations about investigations and future management.

Clinical features

- **Quality of life.** How does the hip pain affect the quality of life? Ask about problems with day-to-day activities, from getting up in the morning to personal care, household activities, work and leisure. How far can the patient walk if pushed, and what is the maximum comfortable walking distance? Formal standardised assessment tools are available for the assessment of joint pain, but these are often too time-consuming for routine clinical practice.
- **Site.** Hip pain is usually located in the groin or anterior/lateral thigh. It is easy to miss hip pain that is referred to the knee. Pain around the side or the back of the hip is unlikely to originate in the joint space. Buttock pain may result from hip pathology but more commonly originates from the lumbar spine.
- **Soft-tissue inflammation around the hip joint.** Consider trochanteric bursitis if there is pain over the trochanter rather than in the groin. The condition is usually self-limiting but may require anti-inflammatories or steroid injection in protracted or severe cases.
- **Radiation.** Hip pain can radiate to the groin, buttock or thigh, but not usually below the knee.
- **Referred pain.** Pain that originates from the lumbar spine is commonly misdiagnosed as hip pain. Pain from the third and fourth lumbar segments and involving the femoral nerve often radiates to the groin and the anterior aspect of the thigh.
- **Exacerbating factors.** Ask about activity-related pain and night pain, which are both common in osteoarthritis. If pain is constant and not related to position, consider serious underlying causes, such as fracture or cancer. Ask about early-morning pain and stiffness, which are features of rheumatoid arthritis. Inactivity stiffness is more common in osteoarthritis. Rarely, a snapped iliopsoas tendon may cause a painful 'clunk' in the groin when the hip moves from extension to flexion. A torn acetabular labrum leads to pain in the groin on rotatory movements of the hip, which may feel unstable or give way.
- **Associated symptoms.** Limp is common with hip disorders. Crepitus and 'bony swelling' are associated with osteoarthritis.
- **Range of movement.** The range of movement is often reduced in arthritis.
- **Injury.** Ask about any falls and injuries to the hip, which raise the possibility of fracture. Stress fractures may occur in athletes. Pain due to injury is usually worse on movement and relieved by rest. Fractures are more common in elderly women, and there is usually an inability to bear weight.
- **Treatment aids.** Is the patient aware of the potential advantages of losing weight, appropriate footwear, shock-absorbing insoles and regular exercise, particularly if there is underlying osteoarthritis?

- **Mental health.** Ask about symptoms of depression and anxiety, which are common in people with arthritis. Fears about disability and reduced mobility can affect mood and motivation, and the ability to cope with day-to-day life.
- **Infection.** Fever and systemic symptoms are usually (but not always) present if there is underlying infection (rare). Always consider the possibility of infection in immunocompromised patients (e.g. HIV, oral steroids, chemotherapy).

Past and current medical problems
- **Osteoarthritis.** Is there a history of arthritis?
- **Cancer.** Consider the possibility of bony metastasis if there is a history of cancer (e.g. breast, prostate).
- **Obesity.** Weight change can significantly improve symptoms of osteoarthritis.

Medication
- **Analgesics and anti-inflammatories.** What drugs have been used for symptom relief? Ask about prescribed oral drugs, topical preparations and over-the-counter medication. Have they been effective? Are there any adverse effects?

Other treatments
- **Past treatments.** Ask about local steroid injections, weight reduction, modification of mechanical factors, exercise, physiotherapy, arthroscopy, joint washout and debridement, joint replacement and osteotomy.
- **Use of aids.** Are appliances such as sticks or walking frames being used? Are they used safely and correctly? Is a bath stool available?

Involvement of other health professionals
- **Specialist input.** Has there been any contact with musculoskeletal specialists in the past? Are follow-up arrangements in place?
- **Physiotherapy.** Has physiotherapy been tried, and if so, was it successful?

Investigation findings
- **X-rays.** These are not usually necessary for diagnosis of osteoarthritis but will be helpful in preoperative assessment and for investigation of possible hip fracture. Loss of interbone distance, subchondral sclerosis and cysts and marginal osteophytes suggest osteoarthritis. Many people have radiological changes without symptoms.
- **Blood tests.** Rheumatoid-factor titres or raised inflammatory markers such as plasma viscosity or CRP are often normal in osteoarthritis but may be raised in rheumatoid arthritis.

Social history
- **Home.** Ask whether symptoms affect daily activities, such as getting in and out of bed or into a bath, getting dressed, putting on shoes and foot care.
- **Independence.** Is the patient able to live independently? If not, are suitable care arrangements in place? Ask about any help at home, such as meals on wheels, home help and occupational therapy.

Examination

General
- **General condition.** Does the patient look unwell or in pain? Would they be fit for surgery?

Vital signs
- **Temperature.** If suggested by the history, increased temperature may point to infection or severe inflammation.
- **Pulse.** Heart rate is increased in fever and severe pain. Arrhythmias may predispose to falls and subsequent hip fractures.
- **Blood pressure.** Postural hypotension may lead to falls. Uncontrolled blood pressure may require treatment prior to hip operations.

Inspection
- **Gait.** A limp may suggest osteoarthritis, hip fracture or avascular necrosis. Inability to bear weight may indicate hip fracture or septic arthritis, although an undisplaced fracture may not necessarily stop the patient from walking.
- **Muscles.** Look for wasting of the gluteal muscle from behind with the patient standing. Are there any scars overlying the hip, indicating previous hip surgery?
- **Skin.** Psoriatic skin lesions suggest the possibility of psoriatic arthritis, which commonly affects the hip.
- **Trendelenburg test.** Ask the patient to stand on each leg alone. If the pelvis remains level or rises, the test is negative. The test is abnormal if the pelvis dips on the contralateral side, which suggests damage to the superior gluteal nerve, with resulting paralysis of the gluteus medius and minimus muscles.
- **Walking.** A waddling gait indicates muscle weakness, whereas a limp is often caused by pain or severe hip disease.
- **Leg length.** If the leg appears shortened, measure and record the distance from the anterior superior iliac crest to the medial malleolus of the ankle on the same side. Consider a fractured neck of femur in an externally rotated and shortened leg.
- **Deformity.** With the patient lying flat on the back, look for any obvious flexion deformity of the hip.

Hip joint assessment
- **Swelling.** Bony and soft-tissue articular swelling suggest osteoarthritis.
- **Numbness.** Check for numbness over the lateral aspect of the thigh, which may indicate meralgia paraesthetica due to entrapment of the femoral nerve.
- **Greater trochanter.** Palpate over the greater trochanter. If tender, consider trochanteric bursitis or hip fracture.
- **Pain on movement.** Pain and joint tenderness may suggest inflammatory arthritis. Pain in the groin on rotatory movements of the hip may indicate a torn acetabular labrum.

- **Flexion and extension.** A painful 'clunk' when moving the hip (with the knee fixed at 90°) from extension to flexion may suggest a snapped iliopsoas tendon. Painful passive hip flexion may indicate inflammation of the psoas muscle. Consider psoas abscess if there is pain and spasm of the psoas muscle with consequent flexion of the hip (rare).
- **Rotation.** Pain and restriction on internal rotation suggest osteoarthritis (test with the hip flexed at 90°). If full internal rotation is possible, significant osteoarthritis is unlikely. Pain on rotatory movements of the hip may also occur with a torn acetabular labrum.
- **Thomas's test.** Perform Thomas's test to check for a fixed flexion deformity of the hip. To ensure that the normal lumbar lordosis is removed, keep one hand under the patient's back. Then fully flex one hip and observe the opposite leg. Fixed flexion deformity of the hip is likely if the opposite leg lifts off the couch.

Lower spine
- **Inspection.** Look for any obvious spinal abnormalities (e.g. scoliosis).
- **Palpation.** Palpate the lower back. Tenderness over the lower spine may indicate a spinal cause for the pain.
- **Specific tests.** Check the straight-leg raise and the femoral stretch test to diagnose any problems with the sciatic or femoral nerve.

Key references and further reading
1. Conaghan PG, Dickson J, Grant RL. Care and management of osteoarthritis in adults: summary of NICE guidance. *BMJ* 2008;336:502–503.
2. Department of Health. *The Musculoskeletal Services Framework.* Available from: http://webarchive.nationalarchives.gov.uk/20130107105354/http://www w.dh.gov.uk/prod_consum_dh/groups/dh_digitalassets/@dh/@en/documents/ digitalasset/dh_4138412.pdf (last accessed 29 April 2016).
3. Hamer A. Pain in the hip and knee. ABC of rheumatology. *BMJ* 2004;328: 1067–1069.
4. Lohmander LS, Roos EM. Clinical update: treating osteoarthritis. *Lancet* 2007;370:2082–2084.
5. National Institute for Health and Care Excellence (NICE). Osteoarthritis: care and management. NICE guidelines [CG177]. February 2014. Available from: http://www.nice.org.uk/guidance/cg177 (last accessed 29 April 2016).
6. National Institute for Health and Care Excellence (NICE). Osteoarthritis. Clinical knowledge summaries. 2015. Available from: http://cks.nice.org.uk/ osteoarthritis (last accessed 29 April 2016).

Groin problems

Key thoughts

Practical points
- **Diagnosis.** Groin pain may arise from any of the underlying structures, including the inguinal region, bone, genitalia and abdomen. Inguinal hernia is common. Osteoarthritis of the hip often presents with groin pain.

Possible causes
- Groin/adductor strain (e.g. Gilmore's groin).
- Lower abdominal muscle strain.
- Osteoarthritis of the hip.
- Inguinal hernia.
- Orchitis or other testicular problems.
- Abscess or sebaceous cyst.
- Palpable lymph nodes.
- Metastatic cancer.
- Saphena varix.
- Rarely, psoas abscess, abdominal aortic aneurysm or lymphoma.

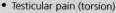
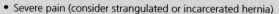

RED FLAGS

- Severe pain (consider strangulated or incarcerated hernia)
- Testicular pain (torsion)
- Past history of cancer
- Systemic features (fever, weight loss, malaise, fatigue and sweats)

History

Ideas, concerns and expectations
- **Ideas.** What does the patient think is causing the problem?
- **Concerns.** Patients with osteoarthritis are often concerned about the effect on their quality of life and the possible need for hip replacement.
- **Expectations.** What are the patient's expectations with regard to further investigation or management?

History of presenting complaint
- **Quality of life.** How do the groin problems affect the quality of life? Which day-to-day activities are mainly affected?

The 10-Minute Clinical Assessment, Second Edition. Knut Schroeder.
© 2017 John Wiley & Sons, Ltd. Published 2017 by John Wiley & Sons, Ltd.

- **Onset.** When and how did the pain start? Relatively acute onset of discomfort together with swelling suggests inguinal hernia. Acute onset of groin pain in boys or young men suggests possible testicular torsion. Osteoarthritis causes chronic and slowly progressive pain.
- **Progression.** Is the pain getting better or worse, or staying the same? Pain in osteoarthritis may vary from day to day and from week to week but tends to worsen over months and years. Inguinal hernia often presents with a dragging pain that gets worse as the day progresses. Chronic progressive pain that is not related to exercise raises suspicion of bone metastases or osteomyelitis, particularly if associated with systemic symptoms.
- **Pattern of pain.** Intermittent pain may be caused by a labral tear or osteoarthritis of the hip, which is commonly felt as groin or knee pain.
- **Injury.** Is there a history of injury or a fall? If so, consider hip fracture or slipped femoral epiphysis.
- **Associated symptoms.** If there is additional back pain, the groin pain could be the result of an L1–2 or L5–S1 nerve root lesion. If there is an infection in the leg on the affected side, it might be caused by tender lymphadenopathy. Has there been any blood in the urine, suggesting renal colic?
- **Systemic symptoms.** Consider the possibility of cancer or systemic illness if there is fever, night sweats, weight loss or general malaise.
- **Sports and exercise.** Are symptoms exercise-related? Ask about the type of exercise, recent injuries and the amount of training each week. Groin strain is common in kicking sports, such as football and rugby. Traumatic osteitis pubis syndrome, adductor longus strain, rectus abdominis strain and hernias are relatively common. In high-impact sports, consider stress fracture.
- **Sexually-transmitted infections (STIs).** Lymphadenopathy in the groin may be caused by an STI, such as gonorrhoea or syphilis. If suspected, ask about any unprotected sex with new or existing partners in the past 6 months and whether there have been any genital ulcers. Ask about vaginal or urethral discharge.
- **Intestinal obstruction.** Consider intestinal obstruction if there is abdominal pain, vomiting, absolute constipation and abdominal distension (e.g. incarcerated hernia).

Past and current medical problems
- **Cardiovascular disease (CVD).** Consider the possibility of referred pain from an abdominal aortic aneurysm if there is an increased risk of CVD (e.g. smoking, diabetes, raised cholesterol, family history, high blood pressure) or if the patient is known to have an aneurysm (uncommon, but important not to miss). Ask about any cardiovascular problems when you are considering the patient's fitness for an operation.
- **Lung disease.** Chronic lung conditions, such as chronic obstructive pulmonary disease (COPD) or asthma, may increase anaesthetic risks if an operation is needed.
- **Arthritis.** Arthritis of the hip is common. Ask about a history of osteoarthritis or rheumatoid arthritis and establish which other joints have been affected.

- **Renal colic.** Renal colic is often recurrent.
- **Hernia.** Has there been a previous hernia repair?

Medication
- **Analgesia.** What has been tried so far and what has been effective? Ask about prescribed and over-the-counter medications.

Allergies
- **Analgesia.** Ask about allergies to analgesics and anti-inflammatory medication.

Social history
- **Home.** Are there any problems with day-to-day life at home? If there is disabling pain, is additional support needed with shopping, cooking or childcare?
- **Work.** Is work affected? Has the problem been made worse by any work activities, such as heavy lifting (e.g. hernia)?

Examination

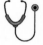

General
- **General condition.** Does the patient look unwell (e.g. systemic illness or strangulated hernia)?
- **Posture.** Consider psoas abscess (rare) if the patient is holding the hip in flexion.

Groin
- **Inspection.** Look for lumps in the groin and elsewhere.
- **Groin palpation.** Locate the position of any lump and assess the temperature, shape, size, tension and composition to determine whether the likely content of the swelling is solid, fluid or gaseous. A localised reducible swelling that is worse on coughing or straining with or without tenderness is likely to be caused by a femoral or inguinal hernia or a saphena varix. Try to distinguish between a femoral (below and lateral to pubic tubercle) and inguinal (above and medial to pubic tubercle) hernia, as the former has a higher risk of strangulation. Hernia is unlikely if it is possible to 'get above' the swelling and feel the upper border. There is no need to differentiate between direct and indirect inguinal hernias during initial assessment. Check for groin tenderness (e.g. ischaemia, infection, lymphadenopathy, strangulated hernia, testicular torsion, epididymo-orchitis, psoas abscess).
- **Squeeze test.** Ask the patient to bend the knees, put your fist between the knees and then ask the patient to squeeze the knees together. If this reproduces groin pain, then adductor pathology is likely.
- **Resisted sit-up.** Lower abdominal pathology or Gilmore's groin (soft-tissue injury in kicking sports) often prevents the patient from doing a sit-up from the supine position.

Abdominal examination
- **Palpation.** Palpate the abdomen for any masses that might directly or indirectly lead to raised intra-abdominal pressure, such as an enlarged bladder, chronic intestinal obstruction, pregnancy or an enlarged prostate. Tenderness in the right iliac fossa may suggest appendicitis. Check for evidence of an abdominal aortic aneurysm. Palpate the kidneys for size and tenderness. A renal stone may present with colicky groin pain.
- **Rectal examination.** Prostatitis can cause groin pain and may be revealed by a tender and enlarged prostate gland on rectal examination.
- **Bimanual vaginal examination.** In women, consider searching for an ovarian swelling (ovarian carcinoma).
- **Scrotum and testes.** Carefully palpate the testes and epididymes in male patients, as testicular torsion, testicular cancer, epididymitis and varicocele can all cause groin pain. Is the lump separate from the testis? Cystic swellings (e.g. due to hydrocele) may transilluminate, whereas solid tumours and most hernias will not. Varicoceles often feel like a 'bag of worms' and are more common on the left side. Consider testicular cancer in any testicular lump. In children and adolescents, always consider the possibility of testicular torsion.

Locomotor
- **Spine.** Assess the lower spine if referred pain is a possibility.
- **Hips.** Assess movement in the hips. Painful internal rotation suggests osteoarthritis.

Key references and further reading
1. Dawson C, Whitfield H. ABC of urology. Urological malignancy – III: renal and testicular carcinoma. *BMJ* 1996;312:1146–1148.
2. Jenkins J, O'Dwyer P. Inguinal hernias. *BMJ* 2008;336:269–272.
3. McIntosh A, Hutchinson A, Roberts A, Withers H. Evidence-based management of groin hernia in primary care – a systematic review. *Fam Pract* 2000;17:442–447.
4. Sepulveda L, Gorgala T, Lage J et al. Undescended testis presenting as incarcerated inguinal hernia in adults: a rare case and literature review. *Curr Urol* 2014;7:214–216.

Leg pain and/or swelling

Key thoughts

Practical points
- **Diagnosis.** Deep venous thrombosis and cellulitis are relatively common and should be considered in every patient with leg pain. Arterial disease is likely if cardiovascular risk factors and intermittent claudication are present.

Possible causes of leg pain and swelling
- Cellulitis.
- Deep venous thrombosis.
- Baker's cyst.
- Varicose veins.

Possible causes of leg swelling only
- Dependent oedema (heart failure, liver failure, nephrotic syndrome).
- Medication (e.g. calcium channel blockers).
- Hypothyroidism.
- Pelvic mass.
- Lymphoedema.

Possible causes of leg pain only
- Sciatica and other radicular pain.
- Varicose veins.
- Muscular strain or injury.
- Arterial disease.
- Spinal claudication.

Risk factors for deep venous thrombosis

- Major surgery within 4 weeks.
- Long-distance travel.
- Obesity.
- Pregnancy.
- Previous deep venous thrombosis.
- Combined oral contraceptive pill.
- Hormone replacement therapy.
- Immobilisation of lower extremities due to plaster or paresis.
- Confinement to bed for more than 3 days.
- Active cancer.

The 10-Minute Clinical Assessment, Second Edition. Knut Schroeder.
© 2017 John Wiley & Sons, Ltd. Published 2017 by John Wiley & Sons, Ltd.

Risk factors for arterial disease

- Smoking.
- Hypertension.
- Diabetes mellitus.
- Obesity.
- Hyperlipidaemia.
- Physical inactivity.
- Family history of CVD.

RED FLAGS

- Unilateral pain and calf tenderness
- Risk factors for deep venous thrombosis
- Swelling of the entire leg
- Collateral superficial veins

History

Ideas, concerns and expectations

- **Ideas.** Patients are often unaware of the potentially life-threatening complications of undiagnosed and untreated deep venous thrombosis.
- **Concerns.** Patients are often concerned about the long-term effects on quality of life. They may worry about having to take anticoagulants ('rat poison'). Another common – and usually unjustified – fear is that the leg may need to be amputated.
- **Expectations.** Why has the patient come to see you? Common reasons for consultation are symptom relief and finding an underlying cause. Patients and carers may become very worried about leg oedema and often expect a course of diuretics for treatment, which for dependent oedema is often not appropriate or required.

History of presenting complaint

- **Quality of life.** How do the leg problems affect the quality of life? Which day-to-day activities have been affected? Ask for details about the maximum distance the patient can walk (on a level surface and uphill).
- **Site.** Consider deep venous thrombosis if there is calf pain. Trochanteric pain is commonly caused by trochanteric bursitis or fibromyalgia. In posterior thigh and buttock pain, consider sciatica and, rarely, spondylolisthesis, facet joint arthropathy, sacroiliitis and piriformis syndrome. Alternating buttock pain and waking with back pain during the second half of the night may rarely be symptoms of ankylosing spondylitis. Pain in the lateral upper thigh may be caused by meralgia paraesthetica and often presents together with a tingling or burning sensation in people who are obese or diabetic.

- **Leg swelling.** Pain combined with leg swelling points towards infective or vascular pathology. In any unilateral swelling, consider deep venous thrombosis, cellulitis, bursitis around the knee and, less commonly, venous or lymphatic obstruction due to malignancy. In older people, some mild postural and intermittent ankle oedema at the end of the day or in hot weather can be regarded as normal. Generalised or more severe oedema suggests a systemic cause, such as heart failure, hypoalbuminaemia (e.g. liver cirrhosis) or nephrotic syndrome. The early stages of lymphatic obstruction usually cause a painless swelling of insidious onset. Consider a ruptured Baker's cysts after an injury.
- **Infection.** Are there symptoms of infection? Cellulitis can cause a painful hot leg with or without swelling. There may or may not be a fever. A mild fever may occur in deep venous thrombosis.
- **Exacerbating and relieving factors.** Pain on standing which is relieved by lying down is a feature of varicose veins. There may be associated itching, together with varicose eczema and venous ulcers. Severe referred leg pain or shooting pains dependant on position suggest a disc lesion (sciatica). Predictable pain on exercise that is relieved by rest and that worsens while going uphill suggests intermittent claudication due to arterial disease. Patients with arterial disease often sleep with their leg hanging out of the bed. Pain associated with weakness that worsens going downhill may be caused by spinal claudication.
- **Injury.** Sporting activities predispose to muscle and tendon injuries and to bursitis, which may present as calf swelling. Bleeding into the calf muscle due to injury can cause unilateral leg swelling, and there is usually an obvious temporal association. Trauma to the gluteal region can cause piriformis syndrome. Pain and swelling that increase together point towards infective or vascular pathology.
- **Associated symptoms.** Shortness of breath (especially when exertional or on lying down) and fatigue suggest heart failure. Always consider the possibility of pulmonary embolism if shortness of breath is associated with unilateral leg swelling.
- **Physical measures.** Ask whether leg elevation has been tried to reduce leg swelling. Compression stockings can be effective in relieving mild ankle oedema, but they have to be the right size.

Past and current medical problems

- **Deep venous thrombosis.** Ask specifically about a past history of thrombosis or pulmonary embolus. Is the patient taking warfarin?
- **CVD.** Intermittent claudication is more likely if there is a history of CVD. Ask about risk factors such as diabetes, smoking and hypercholesterinaemia. Heart failure can be subtle in the elderly but usually causes a certain degree of shortness of breath on exertion, as well as tiredness.
- **Arthritis.** Consider ruptured Baker's cyst.
- **Hypothyroidism.** Hypothyroidism may cause myxoedema.
- **Renal disease.** Nephrotic syndrome with renal failure is an important but rare cause of leg oedema due to proteinuria.

- **Lymphoedema.** This is usually chronic, and there will be a long history.
- **Malabsorption.** Inflammatory bowel disease may cause oedema due to hypoalbuminaemia.
- **Liver failure.** Failed protein synthesis in liver failure can lead to hypoalbuminaemia.
- **Cancer.** Leg swelling may result from obstruction of lymphatic and venous drainage in lymphoma, prostate or other disseminated cancer. Cancer increases the risk of deep venous thrombosis.

Medication
- **Aspirin.** Is the patient already taking aspirin for peripheral vascular disease?
- **Beta blockers.** Beta adrenoceptor blockers can cause intermittent claudication in patients with underlying arterial disease.
- **Analgesia.** What has been tried? What has been effective? Have there been any adverse effects?
- **Steroids.** Oral steroids may lead to oedema.
- **Calcium channel blockers.** These can cause ankle swelling not responsive to diuretics.
- **Diuretics.** If the patient is taking diuretics, ask about frequency of urine and any resulting inconvenience. Check whether there has been dizziness or falls (postural hypotension).

Social history
- **Home, work and social life.** What are the effects of leg problems on roles at home and at work?

Review of previous investigations
- **D-dimer.** Near-patient tests are available. A negative test is helpful in excluding deep venous thrombosis.
- **Full blood count.** Look for any evidence of anaemia (e.g. possible malignancy). The white cell count may be raised in infection.
- **Plasma viscosity.** Raised inflammatory markers may suggest infection or, rarely, malignancy.
- **Creatinine and electrolytes.** Assess renal function.
- **Liver function tests.** Check for signs of liver disease and hypoalbuminaemia.
- **Thyroid function tests.** Hypothyroidism is associated with leg swelling and heart failure.
- **Fasting glucose and lipids.** Consider these in view of possible peripheral vascular disease, cardiac failure, hypertension or obesity. Hyperlipidaemia is a feature of nephrotic syndrome.
- **Arteriogram or venogram.** These can be useful in an investigation of vascular causes.

Examination

General
- **General condition.** Does the patient look unwell?
- **Generalised oedema.** This may rarely indicate a systemic cause. Fingers and face may be puffy in nephrotic syndrome.

Vital signs
- **Temperature.** Fever may indicate cellulitis or systemic illness. A low-grade fever may also occur in deep venous thrombosis.
- **Pulse.** There may be tachycardia in extensive deep venous thrombosis (particularly when associated with a pulmonary embolus) and in heart failure. Bradycardia occurs in hypothyroidism.
- **Blood pressure.** Raised blood pressure is a risk factor for peripheral vascular disease. Severe hypertension may precipitate heart failure. Check for postural hypotension, particularly if the patient is taking diuretics.
- **Respiratory rate.** Tachypnoea may suggest pulmonary embolus (due to deep venous thrombosis) or heart failure.

Legs
- **Skin changes.** Check for erythema and raised skin temperature (cellulitis). Look for changes of chronic venous disease (e.g. varicose eczema and venous ulcers) and evidence of trauma. In contrast to venous ulcers, arterial ulcers are painful.
- **Leg circumference.** Measure thigh and calf circumferences (10 cm below the tibial tuberosity) in both legs to compare sides and as a baseline.
- **Knees.** Is there evidence of bursitis or effusion?
- **Ankles.** Check for pitting ankle oedema (firm pressure for 5–10 seconds may be required to detect mild ankle oedema). Non-pitting oedema occurs in lymphoedema and myxoedema.
- **Veins.** Venous dilation may occur in deep venous thrombosis. Look for swollen and locally tender veins, which may indicate superficial thrombophlebitis.
- **Pulses.** Check pulses in both legs to assess arterial circulation, which may be compromised as a result of arterial emboli, peripheral vascular disease or compartment syndrome.
- **Neurology.** Check tone, power, sensation, coordination and reflexes in both legs if you suspect neuropathic pain, which can occur together with calf pain in systemic illness.

Chest
- **Auscultation.** Basal crackles and added sounds may be heard in congestive cardiac failure. Also check for pleural effusion.

Abdomen
- **Palpate the liver.** Tender or non-tender hepatomegaly is a sign of heart failure.

- **Masses.** Palpate the abdomen for any masses that might cause leg oedema via venous obstruction. Ascites can be found in nephrotic syndrome and liver disease, both of which can lead to hypoalbuminaemia.
- **Rectal and pelvic examination.** Consider a rectal examination to palpate the prostate and check for masses if there is a possibility of bowel or, in men, prostatic carcinoma. In women, consider a pelvic examination to check for gynaecological cancers.

Bedside tests
- **D-dimer.** A negative result effectively rules out deep venous thrombosis in patients with low or moderate clinical probability.
- **Urinalysis.** Glycosuria may suggest diabetes with renal complications. Look for proteinuria, which may rarely suggest renal disease.
- **Wells score.** Score one point for each of the following: active cancer, paralysis/paresis/recent plaster immobilisation, recent confinement to bed for 3 days or more, localised tenderness along the deep venous system, swelling of the entire leg, calf swelling >3 cm more than in the nonsymptomatic leg, pitting oedema greater than on the asymptomatic leg, collateral superficial veins and previously documented deep venous thrombosis. Subtract two points if an alternative cause is more likely. The risk of deep venous thrombosis is *likely* if the score is two points or more and *unlikely* if the score is one point or less.

Key references and further reading

1. Fancher TL, White RH, Kravitz RL. Combined use of rapid d-dimer testing and estimation of clinical probability in the diagnosis of deep vein thrombosis: systematic review. *BMJ* 2004;329:821–824.
2. Goodacre S, Sutton AJ, Sampson FC. Meta-analysis: the value of clinical assessment in the diagnosis of deep venous thrombosis. *Ann Intern Med* 2005;143:129–139.
3. National Institute for Health and Care Excellence (NICE). Deep venous thrombosis. Clinical knowledge summaries. 2013. Available from: http://cks.nice.org.uk/deep-vein-thrombosis (last accessed 29 April 2016).
4. Oudega R, Moons KGM, Hoes AW. Limited value of patient history and physical examination in diagnosing deep vein thrombosis in primary care. *Fam Pract* 2005;22:86–91.
5. Oudega R, Hoes AW, Moons KGM. The Wells rule does not adequately rule out deep venous thrombosis in primary care patients. *Ann Intern Med* 2005;143:100–107.
6. Scottish Intercollegiate Guidelines Network (SIGN). Diagnosis and management of peripheral arterial disease. October 2006. Available from: http://www.sign.ac.uk/pdf/sign89.pdf (last accessed 29 April 2016).
7. Wells PS, Anderson DR, Bormanis J et al. Value of assessment of pre-test probability of deep-vein thrombosis in clinical management. *Lancet* 1997; 350:1795–1798.

Knee pain

Key thoughts

Practical points

- **Diagnosis.** Knee pain is common, particularly in connection with twisting sport injuries (especially meniscal tears) and osteoarthritis (in people over 50 years of age). Accurate diagnosis can be difficult, and the combination of findings from the history and from different tests on examination is more useful than individual findings alone.
- **Quality of life.** Establish the effect of knee pain on home life, work and leisure activities.

Possible causes

- Osteoarthritis in the knee.
- Referred pain from the hip.
- Patellofemoral tracking problems.
- Knee injury (e.g. meniscal tear, anterior cruciate ligament (ACL) rupture).
- Patellar tendinitis.
- Iliotibial band syndrome.
- Gout.
- Reiter's syndrome.
- Rheumatoid arthritis.
- Pseudogout.
- Septic arthritis.

Risk factors

- History of arthritis.
- Exercise.
- Injury.
- Gout.

RED FLAGS

- Acute locking
- Severe swelling
- Giving way
- Pain at night
- Inability to bear weight
- Uncontrollable pain

The 10-Minute Clinical Assessment, Second Edition. Knut Schroeder.
© 2017 John Wiley & Sons, Ltd. Published 2017 by John Wiley & Sons, Ltd.

- Hot and swollen joint, suggesting sepsis
- Mass or swelling
- Constitutional features, such as fever, weight loss, malaise
- Significant trauma with risk of fracture or dislocation

History

Ideas, concerns and expectations
- **Ideas.** Many myths surround arthritis, such as:
  - Nothing can be done about it.
  - You mustn't exercise if you have it.
  - Only elderly people get it.
  - Surgery always makes you better.
  - The only options are paracetamol and surgery.
  - You can't work if you have it.

  Source: Department of Health. *The Musculoskeletal Services Framework.* Available from: http://webarchive.nationalarchives.gov.uk/20130107105354/http://www.dh.gov.uk/prod_consum_dh/groups/dh_digitalassets/@dh/@en/documents/digitalasset/dh_4138412.pdf (last accessed 29 April 2016).
- **Concerns.** Anxieties about work and exercise are common. Older people may be concerned about the potential loss of independence.
- **Expectations.** Are there any expectations with regard to investigations and treatment? Are there any expectations with regard to staying off or returning to work?

History of presenting complaint
- **Quality of life.** How does the knee pain affect quality of life? What daily activities are mainly affected? Ask about home, work and leisure.
- **Onset.** Osteoarthritis causes chronic pain, usually in the medial compartment of the knee, and may lead to the development of a varus abnormality. Acute injury-related knee pain is usually immediate. Dull and nonspecific pain in the anterior knee that gradually gets worse may be caused by patellofemoral syndrome (chondromalacia patellae). This is often felt either medially, laterally or superiorly to the patella or in the retropatellar region. It is often made worse by climbing up or down stairs, and pain may continue at night. Spontaneous onset of severe pain in the absence of trauma suggests infection, pathological fracture or osteonecrosis.
- **Site.** Patellofemoral pain is the most common cause of anterior knee pain. Pain at the level of the knee joint points towards femorotibial or meniscal pathology. Pain just above or below the medial joint line is often caused by a medial collateral ligament injury. Pain over the patella suggests patellofemoral disease. Hip and spinal problems commonly present with referred pain to the knee. A rheumatological cause is more likely if other joints are also affected. Consider more serious trauma or another underlying cause if there is night pain.

- **Injury.** Knee injuries due to sport are common. Is there a history of previous knee injury? Ask in detail about the direction of any forces. Twisting injuries often cause meniscal injuries, particularly if associated with swelling. A 'pop' or 'snap' at the time of injury suggests ligament or meniscal rupture. Consider intra-articular fractures if there has been a fall from a height or any serious trauma. Red-flag symptoms after knee injury include difficulty in bearing weight, severe swelling and locking. Meniscal tears may occur without a clear history of trauma.

- **Swelling.** Any swelling that develops within 2 hours of an injury has a relatively high chance of being the result of an anterior cruciate ligament tear or patellar dislocation with resulting haemarthrosis. Other common causes of haemarthrosis are meniscal tear and intra-articular fracture. With a capsular tear, an effusion may disperse into the surrounding tissues. Delayed swelling (within 6–24 hours) is more likely to be due to effusion (e.g. caused by a meniscal tear).

- **Locking and giving way.** Knee instability may be caused by muscle weakness, a medial meniscal tear or loose bodies (e.g. osteoarthritis, osteochondritis dissecans). There may be a feeling of catching, giving way or locking, which is often associated with pain and swelling. Chronic instability may be caused by an old rupture of the anterior cruciate ligament.

- **Kneeling.** Chronic kneeling (e.g. in carpet layers) can cause swelling and inflammation of the bursae around the knee. The infrapatellar (kneeling on haunches – 'clergyman's knee') and prepatellar (kneeling on all fours on a hard surface – 'housemaid's knee') bursae are most commonly affected.

- **Running.** Running-related anterior shin pain is common, and is often caused by medial tibial stress syndrome (MTSS) or exercise-induced compartment syndrome, which may overlap. Lateral knee pain due to iliotibial band syndrome is commonly caused by overuse or by increasing running mileage too quickly.

- **Associated symptoms.** Acute arthritis in an inflamed knee joint should particularly be suspected if there is no history of injury. Urinary symptoms and conjunctivitis suggest Reiter's syndrome. A history of STI may indicate gonococcal arthritis.

- **Septic arthritis.** Consider septic arthritis if there is severe nontraumatic knee pain in association with a hot and swollen joint. There is usually a lack of ability to bend the knee and to bear weight. Systemic symptoms, including fever and malaise, are common. There may be an obvious source of infection, such as endocarditis or an infected injection site. Septic arthritis may develop on the basis of existing arthritis.

INDICATIONS FOR KNEE X-RAYS (OTTAWA KNEE RULE) IN ACUTE INJURY

- Injury due to trauma
- Age >55 years
- Tenderness at the head of the fibula or the patella
- Inability to bear weight for four steps
- Inability to flex the knee to 90°

Review of previous investigations

- **Full blood count and inflammatory markers.** These are rarely indicated. A raised white cell count and inflammatory markers such as plasma viscosity suggest infection or acute inflammation.
- **Rheumatoid factor.** This may be positive in rheumatoid arthritis.
- **X-rays.** Past X-rays may show evidence of arthritis. Look out for chondrocalcinosis, suggesting pseudogout. If the patient has already been seen in an emergency department after injury, X-rays may already have been taken to exclude fracture.

Past and current medical problems

- **Arthritis.** Osteoarthritis and rheumatoid arthritis are common causes of knee pain. Check which other joints are affected.
- **Past injuries.** Past knee injuries or operations can accelerate the development of arthritis.
- **Gout.** A history of gout suggests a possible gout attack (medication and alcohol are common precipitating factors).

Medication

- **Analgesia and anti-inflammatory medication.** What has been tried, and has it worked? Ask about NSAIDs, non-opioid analgesics, compound analgesics, local injections, osteoporosis treatment and antidepressants. Also consider over-the-counter medications.
- **Steroids.** Is the patient on steroid treatment? Steroids may mask symptoms, particularly in septic arthritis.

Allergies

- **Analgesics and antibiotics.** Ask about allergies to any medication that might need to be used to treat knee pain and possible infection.

Social history

- **Home.** How has home life been affected? Particularly in the elderly, consider any problems that threaten independence.
- **Work.** How far have the knee problems affected work? Are work activities responsible for any of the knee symptoms?

Examination

General inspection

- **General condition.** If the patient looks unwell, consider septic arthritis (rare). Is there an obvious limp or muscle wasting?

Vital signs

- **Temperature.** This may be raised in septic arthritis but is usually normal in other forms of arthritis.

Inspection
- **Deformities.** Varus deformity is common in osteoarthritis, whereas rheumatoid arthritis usually leads to valgus deformity.
- **Dimples around the patella.** Disappearance of the dimples around the patella suggests an effusion.
- **Bony prominences.** Osteophytic changes occur in osteoarthritis.

Palpation
- **Swelling.** Feel for a swelling behind the knee. This may indicate a popliteal cyst (Baker's cyst).
- **Tenderness.** If the knee is tender then it is probably the source of the knee pain, but if examination is normal, consider a cause elsewhere. Check the joint line, patellofemoral joint, collateral ligaments and popliteal fossa.
- **Temperature.** Differences in temperature between the knees suggest inflammation or infection.
- **Patella.** Relatively sudden onset of pain and tenderness at the inferior patellar pole suggests patellar tendinopathy, which is commonly caused by sports involving jumping. A mild effusion around the patella together with medial or lateral patellar tenderness of gradual onset is indicative of patellofemoral syndrome.
- **Joint line.** Joint-line tenderness with the knee flexed at 90° may suggest meniscal injury or osteoarthritis.
- **Suprapatellar pouch.** Occasionally, loose bodies (e.g. in osteoarthritis) may be palpable.
- **Lateral knee.** Discomfort over the lateral femoral epicondyle may be caused by iliotibial band syndrome resulting from overuse (e.g. running or rowing).
- **Tibia.** Medial periosteal pain and tenderness are common at the junction between the middle and the lower third of the tibia in running-related injuries. If unilateral, consider stress reaction or fracture of the tibia due to injury. This frequently goes undiagnosed, as X-rays may be negative for up to 6 weeks. If there is a transient reproducible tender swelling on exercise, consider a (rare) muscle hernia (e.g. tibialis anterior).
- **Effusion.** There is no need to do any tests if there is obvious swelling. Otherwise, check for patellar tap and perform the massage test.

Movement
- **Range of movement.** Check active and passive flexion and extension, comparing both sides.
- **Passive knee flexion.** Pain around the joint line on full passive knee flexion may suggest menisceal injury. Clicking and crepitus may occur in cartilage damage resulting from osteoarthritis or patellofemoral syndrome.

Posterior cruciate ligament
- **Posterior sag and drawer test.** Looking from the side, check for a posterior sag or step-back of the tibia and perform the posterior drawer test, which, if positive, suggests posterior cruciate ligament damage.

Anterior cruciate ligament

- **Anterior draw test.** With the knee flexed at 90°, perform the anterior draw test to check for anterior cruciate ligament laxity.
- **Lachman's test.** Flex the knee to 20–30° with the patient supine and pull the top of the tibia to detect injuries of the anterior cruciate ligament. This test is more sensitive and specific than the anterior draw test. Support the knee, as otherwise the quadriceps will inhibit movement.

Collateral ligaments

- **Collateral ligaments.** Flex the knee to 15–30° and alternately stress the joint lines on the two sides by applying force to the lower tibia.

Menisci

- **McMurray's test.** Perform internal and external rotation with the knee flexed at different angles. Pain with or without a palpable clunk suggests a possible meniscal lesion. This test can be difficult to perform – as an alternative, ask the patient to squat down: this is difficult and painful in the presence of a meniscal tear. A negative clinical examination in a patient who is symptomatic does not necessarily exclude menisceal pathology, and MRI scanning may be required.

Patella

- **Clarke's test.** Compress the patella into the femoral groove and ask the patient to extend the knee against resistance. Pain suggests patellofemoral syndrome, which is the commonest cause of anterior knee pain in athletes.
- **Patellar apprehension test.** Flex the extended knee to 30° while applying pressure to the medial side of the patella. Check for patellar movement and reluctance from the patient to follow the movement.

Function

- **Gait and getting up from a chair.** Observe the patient getting up from the sitting position and walking around the room.
- **Functional tests.** Other functional tests include duck-walking, squatting, jumping on one leg and running on the spot.

Examination of other structures

- **Hip.** As a minimum, check hip flexion and internal rotation, as knee pain can be caused by pain referred from the hip (commonly, osteoarthritis).
- **Spine.** The back is another possible source of knee pain. Test the range of movement in the lower spine and perform a straight-leg raise and femoral stretch test, if indicated.

Key references and further reading

1. Calmbach WL, Hutchens M. Evaluation of patients presenting with knee pain: part II. Differential diagnosis. *Am Fam Physician* 2003;68:917–922.

2. Department of Health. *The Musculoskeletal Services Framework.* Available from: http://webarchive.nationalarchives.gov.uk/20130107105354/http://www.dh.gov.uk/prod_consum_dh/groups/dh_digitalassets/@dh/@en/documents/digitalasset/dh_4138412.pdf (last accessed 29 April 2016).

3. Hamer A. Pain in the hip and knee. ABC of rheumatology. *BMJ* 2004; 328:1067–1069.

4. Jackson JL, O'Malley PG, Kroenke K. Evaluation of knee pain in primary care. *Ann Int Med* 2003;139:575–588.

5. National Institute for Health and Care Excellence (NICE). Knee pain – assessment. Clinical knowledge summaries. 2011. Available from: http://cks.nice.org.uk/knee-pain-assessment (last accessed 29 April 2016).

6. Scholten RJ, Deville WL, Opstelten W et al. The accuracy of physical diagnostic tests for assessing meniscal lesions of the knee: a meta-analysis. *J Fam Pract* 2001;50:938–944.

7. Solomon DH, Simel DL, Bates DW et al. Does this patient have a torn meniscus or ligament of the knee? Value of the physical examination. *JAMA* 2001;286:1610–1620.

8. Stiell IG, Greenberg GH, Wells GA et al. Derivation of a decision rule for the use of radiography in acute knee injuries. *Ann Emerg Med* 1995;26:405–413.

9. Stiell IG, Wells GA, McDowell I et al. Use of radiography in acute knee injuries: need for clinical decision rules. *Acad Emerg Med* 1995;2:966–973.

Foot and ankle problems

Key thoughts

Practical points
- **Diagnosis.** Pain arising from skin, muscles, tendons and joints of the feet is common, particularly in obese people and sportspeople. Consider underlying conditions such as diabetes, CVD, gout and arthritis.
- **Prognosis.** Foot problems can impact severely on the patient's life and are an important risk factor for falls in the elderly.

Possible causes
- **Skin lesions.** Corns, calluses, ulcers, blisters, fungal or bacterial infections.
- **Ligaments and tendons.** Achilles tendinitis, plantar fasciitis, ankle sprain.
- **Joints.** Hallux valgus, gout, rheumatoid arthritis.
- **Ischaemia.** Peripheral vascular disease, embolism.
- **Polyneuropathy.** Diabetes, rarely vasculitis.

Risk factors
- Inadequate footwear.
- Obesity.
- Exercise.
- Advancing age.
- Diabetes.
- Poor foot care.

RED FLAGS

- Inability to walk and bear weight
- Bruising
- Trauma with risk of fracture
- Hot and swollen joint, suggesting sepsis
- Constitutional features, such as fever, weight loss, malaise
- Severe pain (particularly bone pain)
- Significant trauma with risk of fracture or dislocation
- Numbness and paresthaesiae

The 10-Minute Clinical Assessment, Second Edition. Knut Schroeder.
© 2017 John Wiley & Sons, Ltd. Published 2017 by John Wiley & Sons, Ltd.

History

Ideas, concerns and expectations

- **Ideas.** Does the patient have any thoughts as to what might be causing the foot problem?
- **Concerns.** Patients often worry about future quality of life if there is a risk that foot problems will become chronic. People with diabetes may fear that they will need amputation at some stage in the future.
- **Expectations.** What are the expectations in terms of investigation, treatment and prognosis?

History of presenting complaint

- **Quality of life.** How does the foot problem affect quality of life? Even relatively minor foot problems can be disabling, particularly for active sportspeople or the elderly. Ask about problems with activities such as walking and running.
- **Onset.** Acute onset is often a result of injury or overuse, whereas problems caused by plantar fasciitis or arthritis are usually chronic.
- **Site.** The site of the pain will in many cases give the diagnosis away. Check whether pain is diffuse or localised. Problems above the foot (e.g. knee, hip, spine) may result in foot pain due to postural adjustments. Similarly, poor foot posture or foot pain can lead to pain in the ankles, knees, hips and back.
- **Severity.** How severe is the pain? Is it getting worse? The inability to bear weight is suggestive of serious injury or fracture.
- **Ankle injury.** The most common injury to the ankle is an inversion sprain with the foot in plantar flexion, damaging the lateral ligament complex. There may be associated bony injury.
- **Serious causes.** Continuous pain day and night associated with systemic symptoms suggests possible osteomyelitis or a tumour (rare).
- **Skin.** Ulcers may be caused by diabetic neuropathy, peripheral vascular disease or poor venous return. Tinea is common and can be very troublesome.
- **Occupation and sports.** Ask for details about work activities and exercise regimens. Has there been a recent sporting injury? Is footwear adequate (e.g. running shoes)?
- **Self-management.** Have stretching or strengthening exercises been tried? Has an adequate period of rest been achieved? Does the patient wear any insoles or soft soles that might help improve symptoms? When were running shoes last changed?

Common symptom patterns

- **Plantar fasciitis.** A stabbing pain in the base of the heel (not the sides) when it first hits the floor in the morning that eases after walking suggests plantar fasciitis. This is often precipitated by a change in footwear, increased walking or a change in posture and is relieved by rest.

- **Heel pad pain.** Heel-pad pain is usually of more rapid onset. Pain is dull and bruise-like and is felt over the heel fat pad, and it does not alter with stretching of the fascia. This is usually caused by injury, such as a fall or other mild trauma to the heel.
- **Calcaneal stress fracture.** Consider calcaneal stress fracture if there is gradual onset of crescendo pain over the calcaneus, which commonly occurs in road runners who increase their workload by more than 10% each week or who use inadequate footwear.
- **Achilles tendinitis or rupture.** Insidious onset of pain and swelling over the achilles tendon suggests achilles tendinopathy. A sharp snap in the tendon on exertion or during a sudden unexpected movement suggests partial or complete Achilles tendon rupture.
- **First metatarsophalangeal (MTP) joint.** Gout often manifests itself via pain and tenderness of the first MTP joint. During an acute attack, this can become so sensitive that patients may not be able to tolerate a blanket over this joint during the night.
- **Forefoot pain.** Consider problems due to hallux valgus or rigidus, metatarsal stress fractures, rheumatoid arthritis or L5/S1 nerve root lesions. Morton's neuroma is commonly overlooked and usually presents with burning or shooting pain in the second or third interdigital space.
- **Neurological symptoms.** Nerve entrapment may cause a burning and, particularly, nocturnal pain associated with sensory disturbance and decreased sensation distally.

Past and current medical problems
- **Diabetes.** Foot problems are common in diabetes and may be caused by micro- or macrovascular damage, as well as by diabetic neuropathy. Ask about thirst, polyuria and tiredness if diabetes has not been diagnosed but is a possibility.

Medication
- **Analgesics and anti-inflammatory drugs.** Ask whether any medication has been tried and whether it has been effective. Have there been any adverse effects? Also consider any over-the-counter medications and topical preparations.

Other treatments
- **Physiotherapy.** Physiotherapy can be effective for many foot conditions.
- **Surgery.** Ask about any previous operations on the affected foot.

Social history
- **Home.** Have the foot problems affected home life in any way?
- **Work.** Is work affected, or has work caused the problem?
- **Leisure and sports.** Which activities have been affected? What is the desired level of function?

Review of previous investigations
- **Inflammatory markers.** Raised inflammatory markers, such as plasma viscosity, suggest infection or inflammation.
- **Uric acid.** Uric acid may be normal during an acute attack of gout, and people with high uric acid may be asymptomatic.
- **X-rays.** Look out for old or recent X-rays that might help with establishing the underlying diagnosis.

Examination

General
- **Pain.** Is the pain localised or diffuse, covering a wide area?
- **Weight bearing.** Consider fracture, infection or other serious conditions if the patient is not weight-bearing.
- **Obesity.** Obesity is a major risk factor for foot problems.

Vital signs
- **Fever.** Any fever may suggest cellulitis, osteomyelitis (rare) or septic arthritis (rare).

Gait
- **Gait cycle.** Look for the normal gait cycle of heel strike, stance and toe off.

Foot inspection
- **Footwear.** Examine the patient's footwear for any asymmetrical or abnormal wear and tear of the sole, for presence of special insoles and for evidence of poor fit.
- **Achilles tendon.** From behind, look for any swelling or thickening of the Achilles tendon.
- **Alignment of the hindfoot.** Abnormalities of the ankle or subtalar joint may lead to a varus or valgus deformity.
- **Midfoot.** Observe the arch position of the midfoot when standing. A dropped arch in a normal person should disappear when standing on tiptoes. There may be excessive pronation of the ankle and a flat arch of the foot in plantar fasciitis. A high arched foot (pes cavus) may rarely suggest a neurological cause, such as muscular dystrophy or peripheral nerve lesions. Central causes include Friedreich's ataxia and cerebral palsy. Check the base of the spine for a hairy patch, which may suggest spina bifida occulta.
- **Plantar surface.** Look at the underside of the foot for callus formation. Erythema is not usually present in plantar fasciitis and may suggest infection, fracture or inflammatory conditions. Take particular care in diabetic patients and check for diabetic neuropathy and ulcers.
- **Toes.** Check alignment of the toes and look for any joint swelling, clawing or callus formation, which may suggest subluxation (partial dislocation) of the MTP

joints. Bunions, calluses, corns and hammer toes are often affected by poorly fitting shoes.

- **Nails.** Look for ingrowing toenails and any nail changes that might indicate psoriasis.

Palpation

- **Skin temperature.** Raised skin temperature over the forefoot or ankle may suggest gout, inflammation or infection (rare).
- **Pulses.** Check dorsalis pedis and tibialis posterior pulses to assess circulation.
- **Achilles tendon.** The Achilles tendon often becomes tight in plantar fasciitis, leading to reduced dorsiflexion of the ankle and big toe compared with the other side. Check for tenderness and swelling, which may indicate partial or complete rupture.
- **Heel.** Tenderness along any part of the plantar fascia is suggestive of plantar fasciitis, especially if located medially to the calcaneal insertion. Tenderness is best located when the fascia is put under tension by dorsiflexing the big toe. Squeezing of the sides of the heel should be free of pain in plantar fasciitis. Granulomata may be palpable along the medial edge of the fascia. A tender heel in all aspects together with erythema suggests calcaneal stress fracture.
- **Ankle.** After an ankle injury, check for bone tenderness over the navicular bone, the base of the fifth metatarsal at the insertion point of the peroneus brevis and the tip or posterior edge of the lower 6 cm of either the medial or the lateral malleolus. Tenderness over any of these spots may indicate a fracture or serious ligament damage, which could require an X-ray (Ottawa ankle rules).
- **Fifth metatarsal base.** Injury to the fifth metatarsal base may mimic ankle sprain.
- **Midfoot.** Tenderness and pain in the midfoot can be caused by gout or pseudogout, or by L5 nerve root lesions. Gout does not always present as joint inflammation in this area and may be misdiagnosed as cellulitis.
- **MTP joints.** Gently squeeze across the MTP joints. Any tenderness may suggest inflammatory arthritis.
- **First MTP joint.** Check for redness and inflammation, which may indicate acute gout.

Movement

- **Subtalar joint.** Check inversion and eversion at the subtalar joint, both actively and passively, as well as with and without plantar flexion.
- **Ankle and big toe.** Assess dorsi and plantar flexion for both joints. Passive dorsiflexion of the toes causes pain in plantar fasciitis, as this stretches the fascia.
- **Achilles tendon.** Squeeze the calf with the patient lying face down and with feet over the end of the couch. Plantar flexion of the foot occurs if the tendon is intact. In case of rupture, there may only be a small flicker of the foot (Thompson's test).

Knees, hips and spine

- **Inspection.** Briefly inspect joints above the foot for any abnormalities. Has the foot problem caused a change in posture?
- **Palpation.** Check for any tenderness in the knee, hip or spine.
- **Movement.** Check range of movement in the knees, hips and spine, particularly if the foot pain might be referred pain from these structures, or in case the foot pain has caused compensatory changes in any of the higher joints.

Key references and further reading

1. Bachmann LM, Kolb E, Koller MT et al. Accuracy of Ottawa ankle rules to exclude fractures of the ankle and mid-foot: systematic review. *BMJ* 2003; 326:417.
2. Cole C, Seto C, Gazewood J. Plantar fasciitis: evidence-based review of diagnosis and therapy. *Am Fam Physician* 2005;72:2237–2242.
3. Irving DB, Cook JL, Young MA, Menz HB. Obesity and pronated foot type may increase the risk of chronic plantar heel pain: a matched case-control study. *BMC Musculoskelet Disord* 2007;8:41.
4. Menz HB, Morris ME. Footwear characteristics and foot problems in older people. *Gerontology* 2005;51:346–351.
5. National Institute for Health and Care Excellence (NICE). Plantar fasciitis. Clinical knowledge summaries. 2015. Available from: http://cks.nice.org.uk/plantar-fasciitis (last accessed 29 April 2016).
6. National Institute for Health and Care Excellence (NICE). Sprains and strains. Clinical knowledge summaries. 2015. Available from: http://cks.nice.org.uk/sprains-and-strains (last accessed 29 April 2016).

Gout

Key thoughts

Practical points

- **Diagnosis.** Gout may present as asymptomatic hyperuricaemia, acute gout, intercritical gout or chronic tophaceous gout. The first metatarsophalangeal joint is the most commonly affected, but gout may also involve other joints, such as the midtarsal joints, ankle, knee, small hand joints, wrists and elbows. Onset is usually acute, with a peak at 24 hours.

Differential diagnosis

- Calcium pyrophosphate deposition disease (pseudogout).
- Osteoarthritis.
- Inflammatory arthritis.
- Septic arthritis (rare).

Important risk factors

- Male sex.
- Past history of gout.
- High alcohol intake.
- Drugs (e.g. thiazide diuretics).
- Obesity.
- Hypertension.
- Coronary heart disease (CHD).
- Diabetes mellitus.
- Diet high in meat or seafood.
- Chronic renal disease.
- Raised triglycerides.
- Myeloproliferative disorders.

RED FLAGS

- Uncontrollable pain
- Joint destruction
- Constitutional features, such as fever, weight loss or malaise
- Renal failure

The 10-Minute Clinical Assessment, Second Edition. Knut Schroeder.
© 2017 John Wiley & Sons, Ltd. Published 2017 by John Wiley & Sons, Ltd.

History

Ideas, concerns and expectations
- **Ideas.** What does the patient know about gout and its possible precipitating factors? How does the patient feel about taking medication for treatment or prophylaxis of an acute gout attack?
- **Concerns.** Worries about joint damage and future disability are common.
- **Expectations.** What are the expectations with regard to symptom control and future management?

History of presenting complaint
- **Quality of life.** Gout can be extremely disabling. Frequent and severe attacks can significantly impair the quality of life.
- **Onset and duration.** Pain tends to develop rapidly over 24 hours, usually starting during the night. Occasionally, there are preceding twinges in the affected joint. Attacks tend to last for 7–10 days.
- **Severity.** The pain of acute gout is severe. Patients may be unable to tolerate a blanket over the affected joint during the night.
- **Site.** The classical clinical presentation is podagra, with acute inflammation of the first MTP joint, particularly if this is the first attack. Other commonly affected joints include the knee, ankle, elbow, wrist and fingers.
- **Precipitating factors.** Ask particularly about alcohol excess, trauma, exercise or starvation prior to the attack. Consider any of the other possible risk factors.
- **Associated symptoms.** Fever and malaise are common, and it may be difficult to distinguish between gout and septic arthritis.
- **Frequency.** Has the patient suffered from similar attacks in the past? Two or more attacks of gout in the past year may be an indication for lifelong prophylactic therapy.
- **Tophi.** In chronic gout, ask about any swellings over the Achilles tendon and around the elbow and finger joints (tophi).

Past and current medical problems
- **Gout.** There is frequently a history of previous gout attacks.
- **Chronic renal disease.** Ask about a history of kidney problems, particularly if associated with renal failure or renal transplant.
- **Renal stones.** Uric acid calculi may lead to renal colic.
- **Hypertension.** Raised blood pressure increases the risk of gout when it affects renal function.
- **Complications of hyperuricaemia.** High serum urate is a risk factor for acute coronary syndrome and can occur in diabetes mellitus, stroke, pre-eclampsia, lipid abnormalities, secondary amyloid and HIV infection.
- **Heart failure.** Colchicine (used for treatment of acute gout) has vasoconstrictor effects, and its use and the use of steroids may be limited if there is a history of heart failure.

- **Myeloproliferative/lymphoproliferative disorders.** These predispose to gout attacks, due to high cell turnover.

Family history
- **Family history of gout.** A positive family history may indicate a genetic predisposition to gout (disorders of purine metabolism).

Medication and other treatments
- **Drugs.** Diuretics (especially thiazides), low-dose aspirin, ethambutol and cytotoxics can all increase serum urate and provoke acute attacks of gout.
- **Gout treatments.** Ask in particular about whether colchicine, NSAIDs and steroids have been effective in the past for the treatment of acute attacks. Is allopurinol being taken for prevention?
- **Other treatments.** Have simple analgesia and ice packs been tried? In obese people, has weight loss been recommended and attempted?
- **Adverse effects and intolerance.** Ask about previous adverse reactions to drugs used for the management of gout. Common adverse effects of allopurinol include nausea, alopecia and abnormal liver function tests. Colchicine may cause diarrhoea, nausea and vomiting.
- **Other medication.** Allopurinol may interact with oral anticoagulants, theophylline and azathioprine.

Alcohol
- **Alcohol consumption.** Excessive alcohol intake increases the risk of gout.

Review of previous investigations
- **Serum urate.** The higher the serum urate, the higher the risk of an acute gout attack. Urate levels often fall during an acute attack, and a normal urate does not exclude the diagnosis of gout. Many people remain asymptomatic even if uric acid is raised.
- **Full blood count.** The white cell count may be moderately raised during an acute attack. If the white cell count is markedly raised, consider septic arthritis (rare). The blood count is also likely to be abnormal in myeloproliferative disorder.
- **Inflammatory markers.** The plasma viscosity may rise during an acute attack.
- **Liver function tests.** Abnormal liver function tests may be caused by alcohol misuse or might be a side effect of allopurinol.
- **Renal function.** Drug doses may need altering if renal function is poor. All patients with a diagnosis of gout should also have lifelong monitoring of renal function.
- **Blood pressure, fasting glucose and lipid profile.** These will give an indication of cardiovascular risk.
- **Joint aspiration.** Detecting urate crystals in a joint aspirate confirms the diagnosis of gout, but this is not commonly performed in practice.

Examination

General inspection
- **General condition.** Does the patient look unwell?

Vital signs
- **Temperature.** This may be raised in gout attacks, usually when larger joints are involved. Consider the possibility of septic arthritis (rare).
- **Blood pressure.** Hyperuricaemia is associated with raised blood pressure. Rarely, postural hypotension may be present in sepsis.

Joint examination
- **Inspection.** During a gout attack, the affected joint tends to be red, hot and swollen, and the presentation may resemble that of septic arthritis. The overlying skin may peel once the inflammation subsides. Gout may be polyarticular.
- **Palpation.** There is usually severe tenderness even to light touch.

Skin
- **Tophi.** Look for gout tophi if there is a history of persistent hyperuricaemia and recurrent attacks of gout. The most common sites for tophi are the pinna, Achilles tendon, olecranon bursa and small joints of the hands and feet.
- **Alcohol.** Look out for alcohol-related changes, such as jaundice, spider naevi and palmar erythema, as alcohol is a risk factor for gout.

Bedside test
- **Protein.** Proteinuria may indicate renal problems caused by chronic gout.

Key references and further reading

1. Jordan KM, Cameron JS, Snaith M et al. on behalf of the British Society for Rheumatology and British Health Professionals in Rheumatology Standards, Guidelines and Audit Working Group (SGAWG). British Society for Rheumatology and British Health Professionals in Rheumatology guideline for the management of gout. *Rheumatology* 2007;46(8):1372–1374.
2. National Institute for Health and Care Excellence (NICE). Gout. Clinical knowledge summaries. 2015. Available from: http://cks.nice.org.uk/gout (last accessed 29 April 2016).
3. Underwood M. Clinical review: diagnosis and management of gout. *BMJ* 2006;332:1315–1319.
4. Zhang W, Doherty M, Pascual E et al.; EULAR Standing Committee for International Clinical Studies Including Therapeutics. EULAR evidence based recommendations for gout. Part I: diagnosis. Report of a task force of the Standing Committee for International Clinical Studies Including Therapeutics (ESCISIT). *Ann Rheum Dis* 2006;65:1301–1311.

Osteoporosis

Key thoughts

Practical points

- **Diagnosis.** Osteoporosis is characterised by decreased bone density. It is often underdiagnosed, particularly in elderly post-menopausal women. Most patients are asymptomatic, but the condition may present with bone fractures that occur after only minimal trauma.
- **Risk factors.** It is important to identify modifiable risk factors, in order to establish fracture risk and to guide management.

Important risk factors

- Immobility.
- History of previous fracture.
- Drug therapy (e.g. steroids, depot progestogens).
- Malabsorption (e.g. coeliac disease).
- Bone-marrow disorders.
- Renal disease.
- Low body mass index (BMI) (<18.5 kg/m²).
- Family history of osteoporosis and hip fracture.
- Smoking.
- Hyperthyroidism.
- Oestrogen deficiency.
- Low calcium intake.
- Alcohol intake of more than 14 units per week for women and more than 21 units per week for men.
- Rheumatoid arthritis.
- Lack of weight-bearing physical activity.
- Bone tumour.

Risk assessment tools, such as FRAX or Qfracture, are available to assess osteoporotic fracture risk more formally. For details, see NICE and NOGG guidelines referenced at the end of this chapter.

> **RED FLAGS**
>
> - Premature menopause
> - Osteoporosis in a man
> - Pain suggesting fracture
> - Recurrent fractures

The 10-Minute Clinical Assessment, Second Edition. Knut Schroeder.
© 2017 John Wiley & Sons, Ltd. Published 2017 by John Wiley & Sons, Ltd.

- Risk of falling or a history of falls
- Back pain
- Neurological symptoms

History

Ideas, concerns and expectations
- **Ideas.** What is the patient's understanding of osteoporosis and its causes?
- **Concerns.** Explore any concerns about the diagnosis and management of osteoporosis. Fears about future fractures, disability and side effects from treatment are common.
- **Expectations.** Ask about expectations and attitudes with regard to treatment and fracture risk.

History of presenting complaint
- **Quality of life.** Most patients with osteoporosis are asymptomatic, but fractures are an important complication that can severely reduce the quality of life in terms of pain and reduced function. Explore the impact of any fractures on daily activities.
- **Pain.** Ask about any pain in the wrists, hips and spine, which may suggest fracture. Pain is usually constant and made worse by putting stress on a particular bone. Have there been any previous fractures?
- **External factors.** Ask about periods of immobility, low levels of physical activity and low calcium intake. Low body weight is also associated with osteoporosis.
- **Internal factors.** Kidney problems, as well as gastrointestinal and bone marrow disorders, may lead to osteoporosis.
- **Alcohol and smoking.** Cigarette smoking and alcohol misuse are associated with osteoporosis. Stopping smoking can reduce the fracture rate in post-menopausal women.
- **Drugs causing osteoporosis.** Consider steroids, anticonvulsants, long-term heparin therapy and depot progesterone injections for contraception. Ask about anabolic steroid misuse in athletes and body builders.

Common presenting patterns
- **Vertebral fracture.** Fracture may occur spontaneously or after minimal trauma, such as coughing, sneezing or lifting. Pain due to vertebral fractures may range from very mild or even asymptomatic to very severe and is often made worse by movement.
- **Hip fracture.** This often results from moderate trauma, such as a fall. Pain can be mild but is often severe. Hip fracture carries a high risk of complications, such as reduced mobility, disability, move into care and death.
- **Wrist fracture.** Ask about pain in the wrists, which can occur after trying to break a fall. Long-term morbidity due to wrist fractures is rare.

- **Back pain.** Chronic back pain may be caused by osteoporotic vertebral collapse. Other causes of pathological vertebral fracture include hyperparathyroidism, osteomalacia and malignancy.
- **Falls.** Ask about any falls, which are a major risk factor for the development of fractures in osteoporosis. Have any measures been put into place to prevent falls, such as removal of environmental hazards?

Past and current medical problems
- **Endocrine.** Consider oestrogen deficiency in menopausal women, women with amenorrhoea and women with premature menopause. Hypogonadism and hyperthyroidism may also cause osteoporosis.
- **Malabsorption.** Gastrointestinal conditions, such as coeliac disease, primary biliary cirrhosis and small-bowel resection, may cause osteoporosis due to malabsorption.

Family history
- **Osteoporosis.** Establish whether there is a history of osteoporosis or fractures (osteoporosis may not have been diagnosed) in first-degree relatives.

Medication
- **Prophylaxis and treatment of osteoporosis.** Ask about calcium, vitamin D supplements and hormone replacement therapy, which are commonly used for prophylaxis but are insufficient for the treatment of osteoporosis. Are bisphosphonates, selective oestrogen receptor modulators or more specialist drugs such as calcitonin being used for the treatment of osteoporosis?
- **Adverse effects and adherence.** Check whether there are any adverse effects and whether medication is being taken as prescribed. Bisphosphonates can lead to potentially severe oesophageal irritation (particularly if not taken correctly) and other adverse effects.

Social history
- **Home.** If there is pain due to fracture, ask whether any activities at home are being affected.
- **Diet in childhood.** Poor diet in childhood and adolescence and anorexia nervosa predispose to the development of osteoporosis.
- **Nutrition.** Ask for details about dietary habits. Adequate nutrition is important in the prevention of osteoporosis. Is the diet low in calcium?
- **Exercise.** Regular weight-bearing exercise of more than 30 minutes a day helps reduce the risk of osteoporosis.

Review of previous investigations
- **Bone mineral density.** Check for any reports from dual-energy X-ray absorptiometry (DEXA), quantitative CT scan or peripheral ultrasound. DEXA scan of the hips and spine is precise, useful for diagnosis and can help in monitoring the

efficacy of drugs. Peripheral measurements can help identify osteoporosis but are less sensitive.

- **Blood tests.** Review any results of full blood count, plasma viscosity, TSH, urea and electrolytes, bone and liver function tests, which are usually normal in osteoporosis. Look for results of oestrogen/follicle-stimulating hormone (FSH)/luteinising hormone (LH)/testosterone if the hormone status is unclear.
- **Myeloma.** If myeloma is a possibility, have tests for serum paraproteins/urine Bence–Jones protein and/or a bone scan been performed?

Examination

General
- **General condition.** Try and gauge general fitness and alertness. Is there evidence of malnutrition, weight loss or poor dentition? Are there any cushingoid features?
- **BMI.** Measure weight and height to calculate BMI.
- **Risk of falling.** Are there any features that increase the risk of falls, such as parkinsonism, poor eye sight, inadequate footwear or a need for mobility aids?

Head and neck
- **Ears.** In the elderly, check ears for wax and briefly assess hearing. Loss of hearing increases the risk of falling.
- **Eyes.** Are there any visual problems that might increase the risk of falling?

Locomotor
- **Gait.** Look for any obvious problems with walking, sitting down and getting up from a chair, which may suggest hip fracture. Are there any obvious balance problems that increase the risk of falling?
- **Posture.** Stooped posture and increased kyphosis suggest osteoporotic changes in the spine. Are there any deformities? Is there any obvious loss of height (e.g. suggested by poorly fitting clothes)?
- **Hips.** Examine the hips if there have been any previous fractures or a recent fall.
- **Wrists.** Examine the wrists for swelling and function.
- **Spine.** Any pain in the spine is usually the result of vertebral collapse. Check for point tenderness and deformity.

Key references and further reading

1. Kanis JA. Diagnosis of osteoporosis and assessment of fracture risk. *Lancet* 2002;359:1929–1936.
2. National Institute for Health and Care Excellence (NICE). Osteoporosis: assessing the risk of fragility fracture. NICE guidelines [CG146]. August 2012. Available from: http://www.nice.org.uk/guidance/cg146 (last accessed 29 April 2016).

3. National Institute for Health and Care Excellence (NICE). Osteoporosis – prevention of fragility fractures. Clinical knowledge summaries. 2015. Available from: http://cks.nice.org.uk/osteoporosis-prevention-of-fragility-fractures (last accessed 29 April 2016).

4. National Osteoporosis Guideline Group (NOGG). Osteoporosis: clinical guideline for prevention and treatment. Executive summary, updated January 2016. Available from: http://www.shef.ac.uk/NOGG/NOGG_Executive_Summary.pdf (last accessed 29 April 2016).

5. National Osteoporosis Society. www.nos.org.uk.

6. Poole KES, Compston JE. Clinical review: osteoporosis and its management. *BMJ* 2006;333:1251–1256.

Neurology

Headache

Key thoughts

Practical points

- **Diagnosis.** Headache can have many causes, and a diagnosis can often be made based on the history alone. Tension headaches and migraines are common. A small proportion of patients may have headaches with a sinister underlying cause (e.g. subarachnoid haemorrhage (SAH), temporal arteritis, meningitis or brain tumour).

Possible causes

- Tension headache.
- Migraine.
- Chronic daily headache.
- Analgesic rebound headache.
- Cervical spondylosis.
- Trigeminal neuralgia.
- Cluster headache.
- Rarely, brain tumour, intracranial bleed or stroke (including cerebral venous thrombosis), meningitis or encephalitis, temporal arteritis, neuralgia and other causes of facial pain, primary acute angle-closure glaucoma, idiopathic intracranial hypertension.

> **RED FLAGS**
>
> - Severe persistent headache of acute onset
> - Sudden change in previously stable headache
> - Early-morning headache (although also common with migraine)
> - 'Thunderclap' headache – rapid time to peak headache intensity
> - Nausea and vomiting (although common in migraine)
> - Fever
> - Night-time awakening
> - Non-blanching rash (meningitis)
> - Recent head trauma (within past three months)
> - Retro-orbital pain
> - Neck stiffness
> - Jaw claudication (temporal arteritis)
> - Neurological findings, such as hemiparesis, cranial nerve abnormalities or hemianaesthesia, drowsiness
> - Cough headache or headache when bending over, laughing or straining

The 10-Minute Clinical Assessment, Second Edition. Knut Schroeder.
© 2017 John Wiley & Sons, Ltd. Published 2017 by John Wiley & Sons, Ltd.

- Postural headache that is worse when lying down
- Headache triggered by exercise
- Human immunodeficiency virus (HIV) infection
- History of cancer

History

Ideas, concerns and expectations
- **Ideas.** What does the patient think the underlying problem is? What does the headache 'mean' for the patient? There is a common belief that high blood pressure causes headache.
- **Concerns.** Fears about the possibility of brain tumour or meningitis are common.
- **Expectations.** Common reasons for headache consultations are symptom control, the need for reassurance, further investigation and referral. Patients often expect to have their blood pressure checked.

History of presenting complaint
- **Quality of life.** Allow the patient time to explain their symptoms in their own words. How does the headache affect activities of daily living? Migraine can be very disabling, whereas tension headache usually allows most activities to be carried out as normal.
- **Character and spread.** What does the patient mean by 'headache'? Headache may be related to conditions affecting underlying structures, such as teeth or ears. Tension headache is usually unilateral but can be frontal, temporal or occipital. Vascular headache is usually unilateral. Trigeminal neuralgia involves only the skin division of the trigeminal nerve. In cluster headache, there is excruciating piercing pain in and around the eye and on other parts of the face, lasting anything from 45 minutes to 3 hours.
- **Nature and quality.** Headache tends to be band-like in tension headache and throbbing in migraine. Piercing pain is a feature of cluster headaches.
- **Onset.** Headache starting in childhood is often vascular in origin. Tension headache develops over hours to days and then stays constant. Migraine usually develops over several hours and is chronic intermittent. Pain in cluster headache reaches full force rapidly within a few minutes. New onset of severe headache in normally asymptomatic adults should raise suspicion of meningitis or intracranial bleed.
- **Severity.** Estimate severity on a scale of 0–10, with 0 being no pain and 10 the worst pain ever. In migraine, people often lie still in a darkened room, whereas an individual with cluster headache will be unable to remain still and will pace around during an attack. Headache worsening over time suggests organic disease. Consider SAH or cluster headache if there is sudden onset of severe pain.

- **Frequency and temporal pattern.** In chronic daily headache, there may be more than 15 episodes each month, whereas migraines tend to occur less often. Patterns may help with the diagnosis, so consider asking the patient to complete a headache diary. Longstanding intermittent headaches are usually not serious, but consider abscess or tumour if progressive. Vascular headaches and trigeminal neuralgia tend to be episodic, lasting from minutes (cluster headache, trigeminal neuralgia) to hours (migraine). Cluster headaches are episodic. Consider organic origin, such as sinus disease or tumour, if pain is constant. Patients are usually completely well in between episodes in migraine, whereas residual headaches are common with tension headache.
- **Sleep.** Headache affecting sleep raises suspicions of an intracranial lesion or cluster headache.
- **Associated symptoms.** Aura and transient focal neurological symptoms occur in migraine. Consider an intracranial lesion if there are persistent neurological features, such as photophobia, seizures, syncope or visual symptoms. Fever may be a sign of meningitis, particularly if associated with a rash. An intracranial tumour may lead to weight loss. Consider temporal arteritis if there is acute visual loss. Cranial autonomic symptoms, such as a red eye, drooping of the eyelid, runny nose or facial sweating, suggest cluster headache.
- **Precipitating factors.** Exercise and other trigger factors may bring on migraines. Headache worse on bending forward or when coughing may suggest an intracranial lesion. Jaw claudication and pain on brushing hair occur in temporal arteritis. Ask about any recent head trauma, which can lead to SAH, particularly in the elderly.
- **Relieving factors.** Lying down in a darkened room often helps in migraine. Do simple analgesics help? Exercise sometimes relieves tension headache.
- **Mental health.** Headaches are common in depression and may in themselves cause low mood and anxiety.

Common symptom patterns

- **Chronic tension-type headache.** There are usually 15 or more days with headache in a month for at least 6 months, which are bilateral, pressing or tightening in quality and of mild or moderate intensity. The headache does not prohibit activities and is not aggravated by routine physical activity. No more than one additional clinical feature (nausea, photophobia or phonophobia) should be present (there should be no vomiting).
- **Chronic daily headache.** This takes several years to develop from the original pattern of episodic headache. Headache may be migraine-like and patients tend to be severely affected by chronic pain, with reduced quality of life.
- **Migraine.** There is moderate to severe, throbbing and mostly unilateral headache, which is exacerbated by physical activity. Nausea, vomiting, photophobia and phonophobia are common. Attacks occur once to four times per month and last for 4–72 hours, separated by pain-free intervals. The typical attack has different phases: prodrome, aura, headache resolution and recovery. The key feature is the impact on daily activities. Quality of life is often severely

reduced, and there may be difficulties with employment, household jobs and leisure activities.

- **Cluster headache.** Patients are often male, aged >30 years with a positive alcohol history. There is no aura, and pain is severe and of sudden onset. The headache peaks within 10–15 minutes, is unilateral around the eyes, boring and stabbing in nature (as if 'the eye is pushed out'). Patients commonly complain about watery eyes, runny nose, facial sweating, restlessness and agitation. There is usually scalp and facial tenderness, and the patient may contemplate suicide. Periodicity is the most important feature, and there are typically one or two cluster periods per year, lasting 2–3 months each. Remission may last for around 2 years. During clusters, headaches are frequent (one to eight per day) and last 15–180 minutes.
- **Temporal arteritis.** This usually affects patients over 50 years of age. Headache is variable and persistent. Symptoms are often worse at night and accompanied by scalp and muscle tenderness, jaw claudication and malaise. Headache can be very severe and may be associated with weight loss, visual disturbance, proximal myalgia and visual-field defects.
- **Meningitis.** Headache is usually progressive over hours and associated with fever, nausea $\pm$ vomiting and possibly reduced consciousness. Patients are usually unwell and may present with photophobia and a rash.
- **Intracranial lesion.** A history of malignancy suggests possible brain metastases. Personality changes occur with frontal lobe tumours. Other features include a change in behaviour, reduced alertness, fits, focal neurological signs, signs of systemic disease (abscess) and papilloedema.
- **SAH.** There is usually (but not always) sudden onset of severe headache, occasionally (in 30–50% of aneurysmal SAHs) preceded by prodromal (warning) headaches over a few hours to a few months. Other features are seizures, nausea/vomiting, meningeal irritation (neck stiffness, low back pain, bilateral leg pain), photophobia and visual changes. There may also be lost or reduced consciousness, global neurological abnormalities, cranial nerve compression (oculomotor, abducens, monocular vision loss) or motor deficits.

Medication
- **Analgesics.** Analgesia abuse can cause headaches. Good response to triptans is diagnostic of migraine.
- **Oral contraceptive.** The combined oral contraceptive can exacerbate migraine.
- **Other drugs.** Many drugs can cause headaches (e.g. antihypertensives, antidepressants).

Family history
- **Migraine.** Migraine often runs in families.

Social history
- **Home.** What activities of daily living have become difficult or impossible? What has been the effect on other family members?

- **Work.** Have any days at work been lost due to headaches? Does work cause headaches?

Alcohol, smoking and recreational drugs
- **Alcohol.** Alcohol consumption may lead to headaches the following day.

Review of previous investigations
- **Inflammatory markers.** A raised plasma viscosity can be found in temporal arteritis, malignancy and infection.
- **Imaging.** Has the patient undergone brain imaging before (e.g. magnetic resonance imaging (MRI), computerised tomography (CT))?

Examination

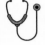

General
- **General appearance.** Does the patient look unwell?
- **Level of consciousness.** Most people will be well apart from the headache. A reduced level of consciousness may rarely be found if there is a serious underlying cause, such as meningitis, intracranial bleed or tumour. Check for any evidence of disorientation, dysphasia, dysarthria or confusion.
- **Gait and balance.** Any abnormalities will usually be obvious and may suggest intracranial pathology.

Vital signs
- **Temperature.** Fever suggests a nonspecific viral illness or, rarely, meningitis.
- **Pulse.** Tachycardia may occur with fever and severe pain. A slow heart rate can be a sign of an intracranial space-occupying lesion.
- **Blood pressure.** Raised blood pressure is a rare cause of headache (usually only if very high), but patients will usually expect measurement of blood pressure. Raised blood pressure may make other causes of headache, such as migraines, more difficult to treat. Some drugs for headache can affect blood pressure, and some antihypertensives can cause headaches.
- **Respiratory rate.** Tachypnoea may indicate pain or infection, whereas respiratory depression can be a sign of intracranial tumour.

Skin
- **Petechiae.** Screen for petechiae and purpuric rash as signs of meningitis (rare).

Head and neck
- **Neck movements.** Consider cervical spondylosis or meningitis if there is pain on neck movement or obvious neck stiffness.
- **Temporal arteries.** If indicated, palpate the temporal arteries for tenderness and swelling. Scalp tenderness may result from temporal arteritis.

- **Photophobia.** Photophobia (test with a pen-torch) is common in migraine but may also suggest meningitis or SAH.
- **Pupils.** Check pupillary reactions and eye movements, which may be abnormal if there is underlying organic disease. Consider acute glaucoma in the elderly if there is a fixed wide pupil with reduced visual acuity and associated nausea and abdominal pain (rare).
- **Fundi.** Ophthalmoscopy is mandatory. Check for papilloedema as a sign of raised intracranial pressure in SAH, brain tumour or idiopathic intracranial hypertension in young obese women (may be the only abnormal sign). Briefly check the retina for haemorrhages (e.g. SAH).
- **Visual fields.** These may be impaired in temporal arteritis or stroke.
- **Visual acuity.** Check briefly with newsprint or, more formally, with a Snellen's chart.
- **Cranial nerves.** Check the cranial nerves, particularly if any abnormalities are suggested by the history. Look in particular for evidence of ptosis, ophthalmoplegia, nystagmus or Horner's.
- **Carotid arteries.** Listen for bruits if a stroke is suspected.

Limbs
- **Neurology.** Consider testing tone, power, sensation, coordination and reflexes, especially if suggested by the history.
- **Kernig's sign.** Extend the flexed knee with the hip in flexion and the patient lying supine if you suspect meningitis. Pain suggests a positive test (indicating meningeal irritation).

Key references and further reading
1. Al-Shahi R, White PM, Davenport RJ, Lindsay KW. Subarachnoid haemorrhage. *BMJ* 2006;333:235–240.
2. British Association for the Study of Headache (BASH). Guidelines for all healthcare professionals in the diagnosis and management of migraine, tension-type headache, cluster headache, medication-overuse headache. Third edition. 2010. Available from: http://www.bash.org.uk/wp-content/uploads/2012/07/10102-BASH-Guidelines-update-2_v5-1-indd.pdf (last accessed 29 April 2016).
3. Fuller G, Kaye C. *Headaches. BMJ* 2007;334:254–256.
4. Headache Classification Sub-Committee of the International Headache Society. The international classification of headache disorders. *Cephalgia* 2004; 24(Suppl. 1):1–160.
5. Kavanagh S. Diagnosing acute headache. In: *MPS UK Casebook 3.* The Medical Protection Society, London; 2003.
6. Loder E, Rizzoli P. Tension type headache. *BMJ* 2008;336:88–92.
7. National Institute for Health and Care Excellence (NICE). Headaches in over 12s: diagnosis and treatment. NICE guidelines [CG150]. September 2012. Available from: http://www.nice.org.uk/guidance/cg150 (last accessed 29 April 2016).

8. National Institute for Health and Care Excellence (NICE). Headache. Clinical knowledge summaries. 2013. Available from: http://cks.nice.org.uk/headache-assessment (last accessed 29 April 2016).
9. Scottish Intercollegiate Guidelines Network (SIGN). Diagnosis and management of headaches in adults. SIGN guideline 107. November 2008. Available from: http://www.sign.ac.uk/pdf/qrg107.pdf (last accessed 29 April 2016).

Transient ischaemic attack and stroke

Key thoughts

Practical points
- **Diagnosis.** Transient ischaemic attacks (TIAs) and strokes are common and frequently occur as a result of a thromboembolic event. Haemorrhagic stroke is less common. Consider other causes in more unusual cases (e.g. space-occupying lesion, hypoglycaemia).
- **Prognosis.** Particularly in settings where TIA clinics and stroke units are available, early diagnosis and management save lives and prevent disability.

Differential diagnosis

- Ischaemic or haemorrhagic stroke.
- Migraine.
- Hypoglycaemia.
- Intracranial space-occupying lesion.
- Subdural haemorrhage.
- Partial seizures (simple or complex).
- Lower motor neurone lesions (e.g. Bell's palsy).
- Temporal arteritis and other forms of vasculitis.
- Cerebral hypoperfusion.
- Transient global amnesia.

Important risk factors for ischaemic stroke

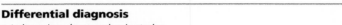

- Atrial fibrillation.
- Hypertension.
- Family history of stroke.
- Smoking.
- Diabetes.
- Hyperlipidaemia.
- Obesity.
- Oral contraceptive pill in women at risk.
- Lack of exercise.

> **RED FLAGS**
>
>
> - Severe headache
> - Neck stiffness

The 10-Minute Clinical Assessment, Second Edition. Knut Schroeder.
© 2017 John Wiley & Sons, Ltd. Published 2017 by John Wiley & Sons, Ltd.

- Visual loss
- Malignant hypertension
- Reduced consciousness
- Neurological deficit
- Swallowing problems

History

Ideas, concerns and expectations
- **Ideas.** What does the patient think is wrong? What does the patient know about stroke and TIA?
- **Concerns.** Many people with stroke or TIA are very worried about the diagnosis, and fears about future disability and death are common.
- **Expectations.** Patients and relatives may have unrealistic expectations about the speed and extent of recovery.

History of presenting complaint
- **Communication problems.** Find out whether there are any communication problems (e.g. dysphasia) and, if appropriate, try to obtain additional information from a person close to the patient.
- **Onset.** Acute stroke usually presents with sudden onset of focal neurological symptoms, such as hemiparesis, with or without evidence of cortical deficits, dysphasia or visual field loss.
- **Risk factors.** Important risk factors include previous stroke or TIA, diabetes, hypertension and atrial fibrillation. Consider using the ABCD (age, blood pressure, clinical features and duration of symptoms) scoring system in the assessment of acute TIA (see box). A score of 5 or 6 in people with TIA indicates a high risk of stroke.
- **Weakness.** Ask about the extent of any weakness. Motor weakness is usually one-sided, although the face, arms and legs may be affected with different degrees of severity.
- **Vision.** Visual-field defects are common and may cause significant distress and disability, particularly if vision in the other eye is already poor. Diplopia may occur due to the involvement of ocular muscles.
- **Speech.** Ask about any speech problems. These can be very distressing and can severely affect the quality of life.
- **Swallowing.** It is important to check for swallowing problems, because of the risk of aspiration. Ask about dribbling and difficulties with throat clearance.
- **Dizziness.** This is a common symptom in posterior circulation events and may lead to fears of falling and fears over leaving the house.
- **Gait problems.** Gait problems may result from hemiparesis or ataxia (involvement of the cerebellum).
- **Associated symptoms.** Ask about any chest pain or shortness of breath. Myocardial infarction may have caused stroke through an intramural thrombus

that has produced an embolus. Depression is common and symptoms of depression may not be mentioned unless asked for. Urinary incontinence is common, and is often secondary to brain damage and poor mobility.

- **Quality of life.** Allow patients and carers time to explain their symptoms and problems in their own words. How has the quality of life been affected? How do symptoms affect the activities of daily living? Ask in particular about problems with mobility and personal care.

ABCD SCORING SYSTEM

- **Age.** <60 years = 0, ≥60 years = 1
- **Blood pressure.** Systolic blood pressure >140 mmHg or diastolic blood pressure ≥90 mmHg = 1
- **Clinical features.** Unilateral weakness = 2, speech disturbance without weakness = 1, other = 0
- **Duration of symptoms.** >60 minutes = 2, 10–59 minutes = 1, <10 minutes = 0

Past and current medical problems

- **Significant past illnesses.** Ask about atrial fibrillation, diabetes, hypertension and any form of cardiovascular disease (CVD). Does the patient have any other known conditions that might cause stroke, such as cerebral aneurysm, clotting disorder, vasculitis or metastasis from malignancy? Is there a history of migraine?
- **Trauma.** Ask about recent head injury, particularly in the elderly.

Medication

- **Aspirin.** Does the patient already take aspirin?
- **Anticoagulants.** Warfarin is likely to be prescribed if there is atrial fibrillation. Consider acute haemorrhagic stroke if there is over-anticoagulation.
- **Oral contraceptive and hormone replacement therapy.** In older women, and particularly those who smoke and have other risk factors, oestrogens may contribute to the development of stroke.
- **Psychotropic medication.** Antidepressants and other psychoactive substances may affect the mental state examination and may cause postural hypotension, which can lead to transient neurological symptoms.

Allergies

- **Drugs.** Ask about allergies or intolerances to any drugs that might need to be prescribed for acute treatment and future prevention of stroke (e.g. aspirin, anti-hypertensives, lipid-lowering medication).

Family history

- **Stroke.** Ask about a family history of stroke, CVD, migraine and other relevant conditions.

Social history
- **Home.** Stroke can be very disabling. Find out which activities of daily living have been affected. Ask in particular about all areas of personal care, mobility and essential tasks of day-to-day life. What is the home environment like? Are there any carers, and what is their health? Depression in carers is often underdiagnosed.
- **Domestic and marital relationships.** Stroke can have a significant negative impact on relationships. Ask about any relationship and family problems and how they affect the patient's life. Are there any dependants about whom the patient is concerned?
- **Driving.** Driving usually needs to be discontinued for at least 4 weeks if there are multiple TIAs or if there is visual-field loss. Check current regulations with the relevant driving authorities and advise the patient accordingly. Regulations for heavy goods vehicle drivers may be stricter.

Alcohol, smoking and recreational drugs
- **Alcohol.** Ask about past and present alcohol intake, as excess alcohol may contribute to the development of stroke.
- **Smoking.** Record past and current smoking status and calculate the number of pack years (= (number of cigarettes smoked per day × number of years smoked)/20).
- **Recreational drugs.** Ask about the use of cocaine and ecstasy, both of which can increase the risk of stroke.

Review of previous investigations
- **Full blood count.** This may show significant anaemia or polycythaemia, both risk factors for stroke.
- **Inflammatory markers.** Raised plasma viscosity is not uncommon and may indicate infection or inflammation.
- **Urea and electrolytes and liver function tests.** Check these before starting any medication that might affect renal and liver function (e.g. angeotensin-converting enzyme (ACE) inhibitors and statins). Clotting may be reduced in chronic liver disease.
- **Glucose.** Is the patient diabetic? Diabetes is an important risk factor for cerebrovascular disease. Hypoglycaemia may directly cause stroke-like symptoms.
- **Cholesterol.** Raised cholesterol is an important risk factor for stroke.
- **Clotting studies.** If the patient has atrial fibrillation, is there evidence of over-anticoagulation?
- **Syphilis.** Rarely, neurosyphilis may present with stroke-like features.
- **Electrocardiogram (ECG).** Look for evidence of atrial fibrillation, which is an important risk factor for thromboembolic stroke.
- **Chest X-ray.** There may be cardiomegaly due to hypertension. Also look for evidence of a large atrium, which may increase the risk of embolic stroke.
- **CT or MRI.** Is there evidence of large artery infarcts, small-vessel disease or haemorrhage?
- **Carotid and vertebral artery duplex.** Look for significant stenosis.

Examination

General
- **General condition.** Does the patient look unwell?
- **Consciousness.** Is the patient alert and orientated? If not, do a more formal mental state examination.
- **Speech.** Is there evidence of dysphasia or dysarthria?
- **Gait.** If the legs are affected, people with stroke may present with the typical gait. Is there evidence of ataxia?

Vital signs
- **Pulse.** Check rate and rhythm. An irregularly irregular pulse suggests atrial fibrillation.
- **Blood pressure.** Stroke is more common in hypertension. Stroke in itself can also lead to an acute rise in blood pressure, which is often left untreated initially as it tends to drop during the recovery phase.
- **Respiratory rate.** Abnormal breathing patterns may occur in stroke.

Skin
- **Injuries.** Look for any injuries that might have occurred due to a fall.
- **Pressure ulcers.** In people with established strokes, pressure ulcers may develop as a result of hemiparesis or hemiplegia and subsequent mobility problems.

Head and neck
- **Facial weakness.** Look for dropping of the angle of the mouth and facial nerve weakness. Frowning is usually preserved in stroke but not in peripheral facial nerve palsy.
- **Eyes.** Check vision and ocular movements. Check the fundi for papilloedema or retinal haemorrhages (raised intracranial pressure or haemorrhage).
- **Cranial nerves.** Check the cranial nerves for any other abnormalities.
- **Carotid bruit.** The presence of carotid bruit supports the diagnosis of ischaemic stroke.
- **Swallowing.** Are there obvious signs of poor swallowing (e.g. dribbling)? Look for dense facial weakness. There may be a 'wet' voice. Test swallowing with teaspoons full of water (but not if you are admitting to hospital in acute TIA or stroke). Does this provoke coughing? Are there difficulties with throat clearance?

Upper and lower limbs
- **Neurology.** Start by looking for a pronator drift. Check tone, power, sensation, coordination and reflexes for signs of hemiparesis and other abnormalities. If it is safe to do so, watch the patient walk. Weakness is initially flaccid before it becomes spastic. Contralateral sensory loss is also common. Lacunar infarcts may cause pure or mixed motor and sensory signs, as well as ataxia, impaired cognition and reduced consciousness.

- **Peripheral vascular disease.** Check pulses in all limbs, particularly the legs. Are there any signs of peripheral vascular disease?

Chest
- **Heart.** Check for an irregularly irregular heart beat as a sign of atrial fibrillation. Check for murmurs or added sounds that might suggest structural valvular heart disease.

Abdomen
- **Palpation.** Check for any organomegaly and masses. A pulsating upper or central abdominal mass may in rare cases suggest abdominal aortic aneurysm (more common in patients with CVD).

Bedside tests
- **Stick test for glucose.** Raised blood glucose suggests diabetes. Check for hypoglycaemia.

Key references and further reading

1. Giles MF, Rothwell PM. Risk prediction after TIA: the ABCD system and other methods. *Geriatrics* 2008;63:10–13.
2. Goldstein LB, Simel DL. Is this patient having a stroke? *JAMA* 2005;293:2391–2402.
3. National Institute for Health and Care Excellence (NICE). Stroke and transient ischaemic attack in over 16s: diagnosis and initial management. NICE guidelines [CG68]. July 2008. Available from: http://www.nice.org.uk/guidance/cg68 (last accessed 29 April 2016).
4. National Institute for Health and Care Excellence (NICE). Stroke and TIA. Clinical knowledge summaries. 2013. Available from: http://cks.nice.org.uk/stroke-and-tia (last accessed 29 April 2016).
5. Royal College of Physicians (RCP). National clinical guidelines for stroke. September 2012. Available from: https://www.rcplondon.ac.uk/file/1299/download?token=mcyQFjEq (last accessed 29 April 2016).

Head injury in adults

Key thoughts

Practical points
- **Diagnosis.** Look out for features indicating skull fracture or intracranial bleed. Always consider the possibility of non-accidental injury.
- **Prognosis.** Features such as an open head wound and dangerous mechanism of injury suggest serious head injury.
- **Management.** Evaluate whether the patient can safely be managed at home or whether close observation in hospital or even referral to a neurosurgical unit is needed. Decide whether immediate CT of the brain and the cervical spine is required. If there is evidence of cervical spine injury, it is important to fully immobilise the cervical spine prior to further assessment.

Complications
- Open head wound.
- Intracranial bleed.
- Shock.
- Multitrauma.

RED FLAGS

- Reduced Glasgow Coma Scale (GCS) score <13
- GCS score <15, 2 hours after initial assessment
- Open or depressed skull fracture
- Sign of basal skull fracture
- Seizures
- Focal neurological deficit
- Persistent vomiting
- Retrograde amnesia for more than 30 minutes prior to the impact
- Dangerous mechanism of injury
- Alcohol or drug intake
- Signs of physical trauma to the head and neck

History

Ideas, concerns and expectations
- **Ideas.** What does the patient think has led to the head injury?
- **Concerns.** Fears about brain damage are common.

The 10-Minute Clinical Assessment, Second Edition. Knut Schroeder.
© 2017 John Wiley & Sons, Ltd. Published 2017 by John Wiley & Sons, Ltd.

- **Expectations.** People with minor head injury often expect admission to hospital or brain scanning, which may not be indicated.

History of presenting complaint
- **Quality of life.** How have symptoms affected any activities so far?
- **Mechanism of injury.** Find out exactly what happened and at what times. Establish whether there has been a dangerous mechanism of injury (e.g. pedestrians or cyclists struck by a motor vehicle, occupants ejected from a motor vehicle, a fall from a height of over 1 m or down five or more stairs). Axial loads to the head (e.g. diving injuries, high-speed motor vehicle collisions, rollover motor accidents, bicycle collisions or accidents involving motorised recreational vehicles) may result in serious injury to the head and spine.
- **Safety of cervical spine assessment.** Check whether it will be safe to examine the cervical spine, which will be the case if the individual was involved in a simple rear-end motor vehicle collision but is sitting comfortably, has been walking around since the injury and has no midline tenderness of the spine and if there is delayed onset of neck pain. A definitive diagnosis of cervical spine injury is needed prior to any surgery.
- **Neck pain.** Any neck pain suggests possible injury to the cervical spine.
- **Focal neurological symptoms.** Ask about any focal neurological symptoms, such as problems with vision, hearing, swallowing, movements, muscle strengths, sensation or coordination.
- **Features of serious head injury.** Suspect serious head injury if there has been more than one episode of vomiting, persistent severe headache, drowsiness or post-traumatic seizure.
- **Skull fracture.** Is there an obvious open wound on the skull? Is there evidence of a depressed skull fracture?
- **Amnesia.** Find out how much the patient can remember about the events preceding the head injury. Amnesia of events more than 30 minutes prior to impact suggests serious head injury.
- **Non-accidental injury.** Consider the possibility that a head injury might have been caused by non-accidental injury (e.g. domestic violence, violent crime).
- **Additional unexplored issues.** Ask the patient if there are any other problems or issues that you have not covered but which might be important.
- **Head injury advice.** Check whether any head injury advice has already been given, particularly if you plan to discharge the patient home. An example is available in NICE guideline 65.

Past and current medical problems
- **Clotting disorders.** A patient with a history of bleeding or clotting disorders or who is currently taking anticoagulants is at higher risk of intracranial haemorrhage.
- **Chronic diseases.** Ask about any chronic diseases that might affect management (including surgery), such as asthma, diabetes, epilepsy and heart disease.

Medication
- **Analgesics.** Have any analgesics been taken?
- **Chronic diseases.** Ask about regular medication and check for drugs that might affect symptoms or management, such as beta blockers, diabetic drugs, anticonvulsants, psychotropic drugs and diuretics.

Allergies
- **Drugs.** Ask in particular about allergies to any drugs that might be needed for the management of head injury (e.g. analgesics, antibiotics, drugs used in anaesthesia), in case surgery is required.

Social history
- **Home.** People with head injury should usually only be discharged home if there is someone suitable to supervise them and monitor the clinical condition.

Alcohol, smoking and recreational drugs
- **Alcohol.** Was alcohol involved in the injury? There is a higher risk of complications if the patient is intoxicated.
- **Drugs.** Is there a history of drug misuse?

Examination

General
- **Level of consciousness.** Describe the three components of the GCS (eye opening, verbal response and motor response) at every assessment, as well as in all communications and in every note, in addition to giving the total score. If the GCS is <8, then this is an indication to involve an anaesthesist or critical care physician early. Any deteriorating conscious level during or after the initial assessment suggests serious head injury. Any patient who is being assessed for discharge home needs to have a GCS of 15.
- **Screen for trauma.** Look for any evidence of other trauma, as suggested by the history. Copious bleeding into the mouth may require intubation.
- **Airways, breathing and circulation (ABC).** Ensure that ABC is adequate prior to further assessment.

Vital signs
- **Temperature.** Any fever may suggest wound infection.
- **Pulse.** Tachycardia may be caused by pain or intravascular fluid depletion. Raised intracranial pressure may lead to bradycardia.
- **Blood pressure.** Raised intracranial pressure can lead to raised or low blood pressure. Postural hypotension indicates fluid depletion (also consider the possibility of additional intra-abdominal injury).
- **Respiratory rate.** Reduced respiratory rates or abnormal breathing patterns (e.g. Cheyne–Stokes breathing) may occur in raised intracranial pressure.

Head and neck

- **Skull fracture.** Inspect the head for any signs of open or depressed skull fracture.
- **Ears.** Haematotympanum or leakage of cerebrospinal fluid (CSF) suggests fracture of the base of the skull. Also look for evidence of bruising over the mastoids (Battle's sign).
- **Nose.** Consider fracture of the base of the skull if there is leakage of CSF.
- **Eyes.** Look for periorbital ecchymosis (panda eyes), which may occur in fracture of the base of the skull. Check pupil size and reactivity, which may be abnormal in raised intracranial pressure.
- **Cranial nerves.** Check for any evidence of a focal neurological deficit.
- **Cervical spine.** If it is safe to do so (see earlier), check for midline tenderness, which suggests possible cervical spine injury.
- **Neck rotation.** Unless there is the possibility of serious spinal injury, check whether the patient is able to actively rotate the neck by 45° to both sides.

Skin

- **Signs of injury.** Look for any signs of injury or clues suggesting non-accidental injury.

Upper and lower limbs

- **Movements.** Check for spontaneous limb movements. Is there any obvious asymmetry?

Chest

- **Inspection.** Look for chest injury. Are breathing pattern and depth of inspiration normal?
- **Lungs.** Check air entry to exclude pneumothorax. Percuss and listen to the lungs for evidence of haemothorax.

Abdomen

- **Inspection.** Look for any obvious injuries.
- **Palpation.** Feel for any masses and tenderness that might suggest intra-abdominal injury.

Bedside tests

- **Blood oxygen saturation.** Check for evidence of hypoxia.

Key references and further reading

1. National Institute for Health and Care Excellence (NICE). Head injury: triage, assessment, investigation and early management of head injury in infants, children and adults. NICE guidelines [CG65]. September 2007. Available from: http://www.nice.org.uk/guidance/cg56 (last accessed 29 April 2016).

2. National Institute for Health and Care Excellence (NICE). Head injury. Clinical knowledge summary. 2009. Available from: http://cks.nice.org.uk/head-injury (last accessed 29 April 2016).
3. National Institute for Health and Care Excellence (NICE). Head injury: assessment and early management. NICE guidelines [CG176]. January 2014. Available from: http://www.nice.org.uk/guidance/cg176 (last accessed 29 April 2016).
4. Smits M, Dippel D, de Haan G et al. External validation of the Canadian CT head rule and the New Orleans Criteria for CT scanning in patients with minor head injury. *JAMA* 2005;294;1519–1525.

Suspected or confirmed brain tumour

Key thoughts

Practical points
- **Diagnosis.** Early diagnosis may allow a cure or the planning of adequate palliative care. Brain tumour may be primary or metastatic. Early features can be very subtle.
- **Prognosis.** Prognosis depends on the type of tumour and the timing of the diagnosis.
- **Disability.** Brain tumours can lead to significant disability. Assessment of current problems and care needs is important in improving the quality of life.

Differential diagnosis
- Primary malignant brain tumour, including gliomas (particularly astrocytoma) and meningiomas.
- Lymphoma (common in HIV infection).
- Acoustic neuroma.
- Benign tumours.
- Metastasis.
- Sarcoidosis.
- Tuberculosis.
- Cerebral abscess.
- Cerebral aneurysm.
- Stroke.
- Vasculitis.
- Encephalitis.
- Multiple sclerosis.

RED FLAGS

- Progressive focal and nonfocal neurological deficit
- New-onset seizures in adults
- Nerve palsies
- Exposure to ionising radiation
- Unilateral sensorineural deafness
- Progressive headache, particularly if posture-related
- Features suggestive of raised intracranial pressure, such as vomiting and drowsiness

The 10-Minute Clinical Assessment, Second Edition. Knut Schroeder.
© 2017 John Wiley & Sons, Ltd. Published 2017 by John Wiley & Sons, Ltd.

- Pulse-synchronous tinnitus
- Blackouts
- Unexplained cognitive impairment, behavioural disturbances or mental slowness
- Systemic features (e.g. weight loss, fever, night sweats, malaise, fatigue)

History

Ideas, concerns and expectations

- **Ideas.** People with 'benign' brain tumours may wrongly believe that their prognosis must be good.
- **Concerns.** Fears about future disability and death are common. Functional impairment resulting from a brain tumour can cause a lot of distress and anxiety. People with brain tumour may also be fearful of having to receive help from support services and are often worried about finance issues.
- **Expectations.** Symptom relief, explanation of symptoms, diagnosis, investigation and specialist referral are common reasons for consultation.

History of presenting complaint

- **Quality of life.** Allow the patient time to explain their symptoms in their own words. How do symptoms affect activities of daily living and the quality of life in general?
- **Headache.** Many people who have a brain tumour present with headache. This is often of gradual onset and gets progressively worse. It may be worse in the morning and on coughing.
- **Symptoms of raised intracranial pressure.** Ask about headaches, nausea, vomiting, irritability, drowsiness, seizures and fatigue.
- **Focal neurological symptoms.** Ask about weakness and other focal sensory or motor signs. Is there blurred vision or a visual-field defect? Check for new-onset tinnitus and unilateral sensorineural hearing loss (acoustic neuroma).
- **Fits.** Any-new onset partial or generalised seizure in patients over 18 without preceding head injury may be caused by a brain tumour.
- **False localising signs.** New-onset double vision (third nerve palsy) or double vision on lateral gaze (sixth nerve palsy) may be caused by raised intracranial pressure leading to descent of the brain and traction on these structures at the base of the brain. A stroke-like presentation may be caused by acute bleeding into a tumour.
- **Nonfocal neurological symptoms.** Ask about memory problems, confusion, change in personality and problems with walking.
- **General symptoms.** Weight loss, lack of energy, night sweats and low-grade fever are suggestive of malignancy.
- **Symptoms of underlying primary cancers.** Ask about cough and smoking history (lung cancer). Have there been any breast lumps (breast cancer)? Are

there any dark moles anywhere on the body that have changed in size or colour, or that itch or bleed (melanoma)? Has there been a change in bowel habit or rectal bleeding (colorectal cancer)? Are there any new-onset urinary symptoms, such as frequency or haematuria, which might suggest a urological cancer?

- **Foreign travel.** Ask about recent foreign travel. Consider schistosomiasis and malaria, as these may cause headaches with central nervous system (CNS) symptoms. Cysticercosis may be caused by contaminated water or by ingestion of uncooked meat. Has there been exposure to tuberculosis (tuberculous meningitis)?
- **Additional unexplored issues.** Ask the patient if there are any other problems or issues that you have not covered but which might be important.

Past and current medical problems
- **Significant past illnesses.** List any significant medical problems that might be relevant to management (e.g. perioperative risk), such as hypertension, diabetes, asthma and CVD.
- **Surgery.** Has there been any past operation for brain tumour or another form of cancer?

Medication
- **Analgesics.** Codeine is commonly used for the treatment of headaches. Ask if there have been any adverse effects.
- **Dexamethasone.** This is commonly used to reduce the oedema surrounding brain tumours.
- **Anticonvulsants.** These may be used to prevent fevers if the tumour involves the hippocampus or cerebral cortex.

Other treatments
- **Treatment for brain tumour.** Has the patient had any treatment in the form of surgery, chemotherapy or radiation?

Allergies
- **Analgesics and antibiotics.** Ask about any allergies to drugs, particularly those that might need to be used in the management of symptoms caused by brain tumour.

Family history
- **Cancer.** Ask in particular about a family history of cancer.

Social history
- **Home.** Ask about any impairment affecting activities of daily living, including washing, dressing, shopping, general mobility and leisure. Is there a current or future need for home care, nursing home placement, hospice referral, district nurse input or involvement of social services?

- **Domestic and marital relationships.** How have the symptoms or the diagnosis affected relationships with close people? People with brain tumours may experience sexual problems and may welcome exploration and discussion of these.
- **Carers.** Are there any carers? If so, are they in need of further support? Are their needs being assessed and addressed? Do they suffer from carer strain?
- **Work.** Has work been affected? Is the patient aware of any benefits that they might be able to claim?

Alcohol, smoking and recreational drugs

- **Alcohol.** High alcohol consumption in the past is a risk factor for liver problems and some cancers.
- **Smoking.** Consider the possibility of lung cancer in a patient with a strong smoking history.

Review of previous investigations

- **Neuroimaging.** Look out for results of any recent brain scans, such as CT or MRI.
- **Histology.** Has a tissue diagnosis already been made?

Examination

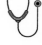

General

- **General condition.** Cachexia and pallor suggest malignancy.
- **Gait.** Look for evidence of unsteadiness and assess general mobility.
- **Consciousness.** Check the level of alertness. Coma may occur in the later stages of raised intracranial pressure.
- **Mental state.** Are there signs of depression or dementia?

Vital signs

- **Temperature.** Fever suggests infection or inflammation.
- **Pulse.** Bradycardia may be a sign of raised intracranial pressure. Tachycardia is caused by fever or severe pain.
- **Blood pressure.** Brain tumours can lead to both arterial hypertension and reduced blood pressure.
- **Respiratory rate.** Breathing patterns may be affected by raised intracranial pressure.

Head and neck

- **Pupils.** Look for ipsilateral or unequal dilatation of the pupils (sign of raised intracranial pressure).
- **Visual fields.** Check visual fields to confrontation.
- **Fundi.** Check the fundi for evidence of papilloedema, but remember that the absence of papilloedema does not exclude the possibility of a brain tumour.

- **Hearing.** Any new-onset unilateral sensorineural deafness may be caused by a brain tumour or acoustic neuroma.

Chest

- **Heart and lungs.** Check heart and lungs for any obvious problems to assess perioperative risk. Consider primary lung cancer if there are any suspicious signs.

Abdomen

- **Liver.** Check for hepatomegaly, although metastases are usually difficult to detect clinically.

Upper and lower limbs

- **Neurology.** Test tone, power, sensation, coordination and reflexes. Focal abnormalities may give clues about the location of a tumour.

Key references and further reading

1. Buckner JC, Brown PD, O'Neill BP et al. Central nervous system tumors. *Mayo Clin Proc* 2007;82:1271–1286.
2. National Institute for Health and Care Excellence (NICE). Brain tumour – suspected. Clinical knowledge summaries. 2012. Available from: http://cks.nice.org.uk/brain-tumour-suspected (last accessed 29 April 2016).
3. National Institute for Health and Care Excellence (NICE). Suspected cancer: diagnosis and referral. NICE guidelines [NG12]. June 2015. Available from: http://www.nice.org.uk/guidance/ng12 (last accessed 29 April 2016).
4. Soffietti R, Cornu P, Delattre JY et al. EFNS Guidelines on diagnosis and treatment of brain metastases: report of an EFNS Task Force. *Eur J Neurol* 2006;13(7):674–681.

Tremor

Key thoughts

Practical points
- **Diagnosis.** Benign essential tremor is common. Try to establish the underlying cause (e.g. Parkinson's, hyperthyroidism), which is likely to have distinguishing features.
- **Impact.** Tremor can be very distressing and may severely impair the quality of life.

Differential diagnosis
- Benign essential tremor.
- Intention tremor.
- Postural tremor.
- Alcoholism.
- Hyperthyroidism.
- Parkinson's disease.
- Drug-induced tremor.
- Drug withdrawal (e.g. sedatives, antidepressants, recreational drugs).
- Rarely, cerebellar tremor, multiple sclerosis, metabolic encephalopathy, poisoning.

> **RED FLAGS**
>
> - Disabling effect on daily life
> - Suspected Parkinson's disease
> - Alcohol or drug misuse
> - Systemic features (weight loss, malaise, fever, night sweats, anorexia)
> - Signs of raised intracranial pressure
> - Additional neurological features

History

Ideas, concerns and expectations
- **Ideas.** Identify thoughts about possible underlying diagnoses. How does the patient feel about the tremor?
- **Concerns.** Patients are often worried about the possibility of Parkinson's disease and any social stigma that may be attached to it.

The 10-Minute Clinical Assessment, Second Edition. Knut Schroeder.
© 2017 John Wiley & Sons, Ltd. Published 2017 by John Wiley & Sons, Ltd.

- **Expectations.** What are the expectations about prognosis and success of management in both patient and carers?

History of presenting complaint
- **Quality of life.** How does the tremor affect the quality of life? Which day-to-day activities have become more difficult or impossible to carry out?
- **Description and location of tremor.** Find out what is meant by 'tremor' and which body parts are affected. Tremor is often most noticeable in the hands, but it may also affect other body parts, such as the head, face, vocal cords, legs and trunk. Unilateral tremor is common in Parkinson's disease, whereas essential tremor is usually bilateral.
- **Characteristics.** A fine regular tremor confined to the outstretched hands and fingers suggests metabolic disease, such as hyperthyroidism. A coarse generalised tremor that occurs at rest or with movement can be seen in sudden alcohol withdrawal. The diagnosis is confirmed if ingestion of alcohol reduces the tremor.
- **Other symptoms.** Are there symptoms of hyperthyroidism, such as feeling hot and sweaty, weight loss or palpitations? Ask about symptoms of anxiety (e.g. palpitations, social phobia) in an otherwise well patient. Are there features of Parkinson's disease, such as frequent falls, bradykinesia or rigidity? If the patient is well, with no other symptoms, and the tremor is made worse by stress, benign essential tremor is likely.
- **Multifactorial cause.** There may be more than one cause for tremor, particularly in older patients.

Common presenting patterns
- **Postural tremor.** If the tremor occurs only when the limb is moved against gravity, consider essential tremor, physiologic tremor, metabolic causes, alcohol or drug withdrawal, psychogenic causes or drug-induced tremor.
- **Resting tremor.** This may suggest Parkinson's disease, multiple-systems atrophy, drug-induced tremor or progressive supranuclear palsy. Resting tremor alleviated by movement suggests Parkinson's disease.
- **Kinetic tremor.** Tremor during any kind of movement suggests a cerebellar lesion.
- **Intention tremor.** Benign essential tremor is often familial and affects hands and voice while sparing the lower limbs. Intention tremor is common; it is absent when the limb is at rest. Stress and excitement can make intention tremor worse.

Medication
- **Prescribed drugs.** Lithium, beta agonists and withdrawal of prescribed opiates or sedatives can cause tremor. Other drugs that may induce tremor include fluoxetine, caffeine, metoclopramide, theophylline and sodium valproate.
- **Drug treatment for tremor.** Have any drugs been tried in the past to treat the tremor? Ask in particular about prescriptions for beta adrenoceptor blockers, sedatives and drugs used for the treatment of Parkinson's disease.

Family history

- **Essential tremor.** A positive family history is common in essential tremor.

Alcohol and drugs

- **Alcohol.** Benign essential tremor often improves with small doses of alcohol. Tremors caused by drug withdrawal or anxiety can also be improved by alcohol, but higher amounts are usually needed.
- **Drugs.** Opiate withdrawal may cause tremor.

Social history

- **Home.** How does the tremor affect home life? Many people feel embarrassed about the tremor and may have become anxious about taking part in social activities.
- **Work.** Ask if the patient is currently working. How far is the work affected by the tremor? Has the patient been exposed to toxins, such as heavy metals or methyl bromide?

Review of previous investigations

- **Full blood count.** Check for signs of anaemia and infection.
- **Thyroid function tests.** Look for evidence of hyperthyroidism.
- **Liver function tests.** Are there signs of liver disease?
- **Glucose.** Is the patient diabetic? Tremor may occur during hypoglycaemic episodes.

Examination

General

- **General appearance.** Does the patient look unwell? If well, suspect benign essential tremor or anxiety. If there is obvious mask-like facies, rigidity, shuffling gait, postural instability or bradykinesia, consider Parkinson's. If the patient sweats and looks uncomfortable, consider hyperthyroidism or anxiety.
- **Breath.** Is there a smell of alcohol? Suspect this particularly in middle-aged and elderly men who live alone and have developed a postural tremor.
- **Signs of alcohol misuse.** Look for jaundice, palmar erythema, scratch marks and spider naevi.

Vital signs

- **Pulse.** Irregularly irregular pulse suggests atrial fibrillation, which is a cardiovascular complication of hyperthyroidism. Anxiety and drug withdrawal may cause tachycardia.
- **Blood pressure.** Raised blood pressure may suggest essential hypertension or anxiety.

Head and neck

- **Sclera.** Inspect the sclerae for signs of jaundice (alcoholic liver disease).
- **Nystagmus.** Check the eyes for nystagmus, which may indicate cerebellar disease.

Upper and lower limbs

- **Hand tremor.** Can you see the tremor? Look for 'pill-rolling' tremor of Parkinson's. Tremor in hyperthyroidism may only be seen with a sheet of paper put on the outstretched hands. Test for intention tremor by asking the patient to hold a glass of water – often, both hands will be used to avoid spilling.
- **Signs of Parkinson's disease.** Check for bradykinesia and cogwheel rigidity.

Check for cerebellar dysfunction

- **Gait.** Is there any evidence of an abnormal 'cerebellar' gait? Look out for the 'shuffling' gait of Parkinson's and difficulties with initiation of movement.
- **Coordination.** Check finger–nose, dysdiadochokinesis and heel–shin test (cerebellar disease).
- **Speech.** Dysarthria may occur as a result of alcohol ingestion and cerebellar disease.

Key references and further reading
1. Bhidayasiri R. Differential diagnosis of common tremor syndromes. *Postgrad Med J* 2005;81:756–762.
2. National Institute for Health and Care Excellence (NICE). Parkinson's disease in over 20s: diagnosis and management. NICE guidelines [CG35]. June 2006. Available from: http://www.nice.org.uk/guidance/cg35 (last accessed 29 April 2016).
3. National Institute for Health and Care Excellence (NICE). Parkinson's disease. Clinical knowledge summaries. 2014. Available from: http://cks.nice.org.uk/parkinsons-disease (last accessed 29 April 2016).
4. Pahwa R, Lyons KE. Essential tremor: differential diagnosis and current therapy. *Am J Med* 2003;115:134–142.
5. Smaga S. Tremor. *Am Fam Physician* 2003;68:1545–1553.

Motor neurone disease

Key thoughts

Practical points
- **Diagnosis.** Symptoms and signs in early motor neurone disease (MND) may be subtle but usually progress steadily. Key findings include the combination of lower and upper motor neuron dysfunction with weak, atrophic and fasciculating muscles plus increased tone and hyperreflexia.
- **Prognosis.** MND carries a poor prognosis and there is no cure. It is important to exclude other treatable causes of muscular weakness that may present in a similar way.
- **Symptom control.** Good symptom control is essential to help improve the quality of life in people with MND.

Differential diagnosis

- Amyotrophic lateral sclerosis (ALS).
- Progressive muscular atrophy.
- Progressive bulbar palsy.
- Primary lateral sclerosis.
- ALS plus syndromes with additional extrapyramidal signs, dementia or cerebellar features.
- Benign cramp-fasciculation syndrome.
- Degenerative spinal disease.
- Motor neuropathies.
- Myasthenia gravis.
- Polymyositis.
- Lead poisoning.
- Hyperparathyroidism.

Risk factors

- Increasing age.
- Family history of ALS.
- Male gender.

RED FLAGS

- Speech problems
- Pneumonia due to aspiration
- Immobility and disability
- Involvement of respiratory muscles

The 10-Minute Clinical Assessment, Second Edition. Knut Schroeder.
© 2017 John Wiley & Sons, Ltd. Published 2017 by John Wiley & Sons, Ltd.

- Depression
- Complications of immobility (e.g. skin infections, ulcers, bed sores)

History

Ideas, concerns and expectations
- **Ideas.** What does the patient know about MND? Explore ideas about the condition and its management. Do they have any preferences with regard to end-of-life care?
- **Concerns.** The diagnosis can be completely overwhelming, and people may suddenly feel alone. Fears about increasing disability, loss of independence and dying are common. Affected individuals often worry about the effect their illness will have on their and their family's quality of life.
- **Expectations.** People with MND may be desperate to achieve a cure. Common reasons for consultation are help with symptom relief and maintenance of independence, as well as support in obtaining help from other agencies.

History of presenting complaint
- **Quality of life.** Allow the patient time to explain their symptoms in their own words. How are quality of life and daily activities being affected?
- **Weakness.** Patients may present because of difficulties with day-to-day tasks like unscrewing bottle tops, holding plates or turning keys. Involvement of the proximal muscles often shows itself through increasing difficulties with activities like writing or combing hair. People with lower limb symptoms may describe dragging of one leg or problems with tripping.
- **Limb symptoms.** In ALS, initial symptoms usually include muscle wasting, weakness and fasciculation, as well as stiffness. Symptoms start in the limbs in most cases, and less commonly in the bulbar muscles. Distribution of weakness is often asymmetrical at the beginning and may only affect one limb to start with.
- **Bulbar symptoms.** Ask about changes in speech, which may become more difficult to understand or slurred, particularly when the patient is tired. People close to the patient may notice the development of nasal speech, which can result from involvement of the soft palate. Bulbar muscles may become spastic, which will give the speech a tighter quality. Hoarseness will be present if the vocal cords are affected. Problems with swallowing usually develop after the development of dysarthria, and it may take much longer for patients to finish a meal. Chewed food may start to leak from the mouth and liquid may be regurgitated. Patients often begin to lose weight once problems with food intake develop. Communication may become difficult.
- **Physical disabilities.** Getting up from a chair or climbing stairs will often be difficult. Patients may become unable to walk, talk or eat. If the upper limbs are involved, patients will become unable to look after themselves (e.g. washing, toileting, feeding). If the axial muscles are affected, head drop and a stooped

position may be prominent, and turning in bed may become difficult or impossible. Getting to the toilet in time may be tricky, leading to incontinence, which may not be mentioned by the patient unless they are asked about it directly.

- **Accompanying symptoms.** Tiredness and lethargy are common and may become disabling. Emotional lability is common, causing affected people to cry or laugh inappropriately. Intellect is not usually affected, although dementia may develop in a small number of sufferers.
- **Anxiety and depression.** Check for symptoms of depression. Such problems are common and may severely reduce the quality of life. Is the patient already taking antidepressants? Ask about sleep disturbances and pain, which may affect mood considerably. Is there a treatable underlying reason for any pain?
- **Breathing problems.** Involvement of the respiratory muscles is usually a late feature but may occur early in the disease. Ask about shortness of breath on exertion or at rest. Has the patient started to use more pillows at night, to maintain a more upright position? Ask about unrefreshing sleep, morning headaches and increased day-time sleepiness. Cough may also be present.
- **Additional unexplored issues.** Ask if there are any other problems or issues that you have not covered but which are important to the patient.

Past and current medical problems

- **Significant past illnesses.** Are there any other current medical problems that need attention?
- **Other professionals.** Find out whether any other health professionals or agencies are involved in the patient's care. A neurologist should normally be involved from the outset. Physiotherapists and speech therapists may help to increase the patient's quality of life.

Medication

- **Riluzole.** This antiglutaminergic drug may prolong survival. Ask about common adverse effects, such as tiredness, nausea and diarrhoea.
- **Analgesics.** Check about current use of analgesics and level of pain control. Are there any adverse effects?
- **Herbal and over-the-counter drugs.** Ask whether any medication is being purchased over the counter, without prescription.

Family history

- **MND.** Is there a family history of MND?

Social history

- **Home.** Ask for details about the home situation. Who else lives with the patient? Are there any dependants? Ask the patient to list any problems with day-to-day life. Are any outside carers involved? Has the home already been assessed by other agencies, such as social services or an occupational therapist? Are there any financial problems?

- **Work.** Has work been affected? Is a sick note needed?
- **Driving.** Driving may not be affected in the early stages, but the appropriate driving licensing authorities should be informed at diagnosis.

Review of previous investigations
- **Electromyography.** Evidence of muscle denervation and reinnervation may be suggestive of ALS and may involve regions of the spinal cord which are not yet affected clinically.
- **MRI or CT.** Head scans may help exclude any structural intracranial lesions.
- **Muscle biopsy.** This is sometimes used to exclude inflammatory myopathy.
- **Creatine kinase.** This may be elevated to 2 or 3 times the normal level in about 50% of people with ALS.
- **Serum electrophoresis.** A small number of individuals with ALS show a serum paraprotein band.
- **Liver function tests.** These need to be monitored monthly for the first 3 months and quarterly after starting riluzole therapy.

Examination

General
- **General condition.** General debility and cachexia may indicate problems with adequate fluid and food intake.
- **Communication.** Severe communication problems will usually be obvious.

Skin
- **Pressure ulcers.** If the patient's mobility is reduced, ask about and look for any evidence of pressure ulcers in relevant areas (e.g. hips, sacrum, ankles, elbows).

Head and neck
- **Cranial nerves.** Look in particular for any bulbar symptoms, such as speech and swallowing problems.
- **Head drop.** This may be caused by weakness of the neck extensor muscle and is relatively common.
- **Mouth.** Look for tongue wasting, weakness and fasciculation (indicating lower motor neurone involvement). Tongue movement may be slow, due to spasticity.
- **Jaw jerk.** A brisk jaw jerk suggests upper motor neurone bulbar involvement.
- **Frontal release signs.** Grasp reflex and palmomental reflex may be present.

Limbs
- **Muscles.** Check for lower motor neurone features, such as muscle wasting, weakness, fasciculation, stiffness and brisk reflexes (indicating upper motor neurone involvement). Fasciculation alone is uncommon and may be entirely benign in the absence of muscle weakness.

- **Sensation.** There is no sensory loss.
- **Plantar response.** These may be upgoing if there is upper motor neurone involvement.

Chest
- **Respiratory muscles.** These are often affected in the later stages, causing death through respiratory failure about 3–5 years after onset.

Abdomen
- **Abdominal wall.** Look for any paradoxical movement of the abdominal wall during breathing, which may indicate diaphragmatic weakness.

Key references and further reading

1. Department of Health. End of life care strategy: promoting high quality care for adults at the end of their life. July 2008. Available from: https://www.gov. uk/government/publications/end-of-life-care-strategy-promoting-high-quality-care-for-adults-at-the-end-of-their-life (last accessed 29 April 2016).
2. Motor Neurone Disease Association. www.mndassociation.org.
3. Nageshwaran S, Davies LM, Rafi I, Radunovic A. Motor neurone disease. *BMJ* 2014;349:g4052.
4. Royal College of Physicians (RCP). Long-term neurological conditions: management at the interface between neurology, rehabilitation and palliative care. National guidelines number 10. March 2008. Available from: https://www. rcplondon.ac.uk/file/1611/download?token=4aB87zLp (last accessed 29 April 2016).
5. The Scottish Motor Neuron Disease Research Group. The Scottish Motor Neuron Disease Register: a prospective study of adult onset motor neuron disease in Scotland. *Methodology, demography and clinical features of incident cases in 1989. J Neurol Neurosurg Psychiatr* 1992;55:536–541.

Peripheral neuropathy

Key thoughts

Practical points
- **Diagnosis.** Peripheral neuropathy is relatively common and can severely impair the quality of life. In most cases, symptoms develop slowly over several months. There are many potential underlying causes, and diagnosis can be challenging. Diabetic and nutritional neuropathies (including alcohol) are common.

Possible causes
- Diabetes mellitus.
- Alcohol misuse (with or without vitamin B1 deficiency).
- Vitamin B12 deficiency.
- Drugs (e.g. phenytoin, nitrofurantoin, vincristin, isoniazid, gold and excess amounts of vitamin B6/pyridoxine).
- Trauma.
- Cervical spondylosis.
- Malignancy.
- Metabolic causes (e.g. hypothyroidism, liver failure, renal failure).
- HIV infection.
- Heavy metal poisoning (e.g. lead, mercury).
- Guillain–Barré syndrome/acute inflammatory demyelinating polyneuropathy (AIDP).
- Hereditary causes (e.g. Charcot–Marie–Tooth disease).
- Other (e.g. leprosy, syphilis, lymphoma, amyloidosis, sarcoidosis, paraneoplastic, haematological malignancy).

RED FLAGS
- Features suggesting cancer
- Signs of cord compression
- Abnormal perineal sensation
- Urinary or bowel symptoms

History

Ideas, concerns and expectations
- **Ideas.** What does the patient think may be causing the peripheral neuropathy?

The 10-Minute Clinical Assessment, Second Edition. Knut Schroeder.
© 2017 John Wiley & Sons, Ltd. Published 2017 by John Wiley & Sons, Ltd.

- **Concerns.** People who develop paraesthesiae are often worried about multiple sclerosis (MS) and future disability.
- **Expectations.** Common reasons for consultation include reassurance, exclusion of MS, further investigation and referral to a specialist.

History of presenting complaint

- **Quality of life.** How have symptoms affected the quality of life and the activities of daily living? Neuropathies can be very distressing and disabling.
- **Description of symptoms.** Find out whether the main problem is disturbed sensation (suggesting sensory loss) or a feeling of weakness (implying a motor lesion). People with sensory loss usually describe a perception of 'numbness' or complete loss of feeling, whereas positive symptoms may include itching, prickling, buzzing and burning sensations. Tingling and buzzing paraesthesia may be caused by dorsal column lesions. Spinothalamic problems may lead to pain, which can show different qualities.
- **Onset and progression.** Relapsing/remitting symptoms point towards MS, whereas gradual deterioration can be found in mononeuropathies. Peripheral neuropathy tends to start distally and then moves proximally with time. Carpal tunnel syndrome tends to be worse at night and may disturb sleep; it improves with hand-shaking, and symptoms tend to be less severe during the day. Focal migraines, epilepsy and TIAs often present with symptoms of sudden onset and quick resolution. Prolonged paraesthesiae suggest stroke or a space-occupying lesion.
- **Site and extent.** Does the area of paraesthesia follow a particular nerve distribution? Has there been any recent injury to this nerve that could explain the symptoms? Spinal problems usually cause patterns that are less well localised. In cord compression, symptoms are present below the level of the lesion. In disc prolapse, symptoms tend to be confined to a nerve root (dermatome). Glove and stocking distribution can be found in polyneuropathy. A symmetrical peripheral neuropathy caused by Guillain–Barré syndrome is rare but important (potentially life-threatening, due to the respiratory muscles being affected).
- **Exacerbating and relieving factors.** Changes in posture and neck movement may exacerbate symptoms caused by pressure on nerve roots due to cervical spondylosis, injury or spinal tumour. Wrist flexion and extension tend to exacerbate symptoms in carpal tunnel syndrome.
- **Trigger factors.** Ask about any preceding trauma (e.g. neck or spinal injury). Repetitive activity and peripheral nerve compression may precipitate symptoms.
- **Other neurological symptoms.** Symptoms such as bowel and bladder problems, muscle weakness, pain and loss of balance or coordination may indicate a CNS lesion. Consider cauda equina syndrome if there is leg pain, unsteadiness, urinary urgency and frequency, bowel dysfunction or loss of perineal sensation. Accompanying visual symptoms may suggest optic neuritis due to MS. Vertigo, nausea, diplopia and ataxia may occur with brain stem syndrome.
- **Systemic illness.** Check for features of systemic illness (e.g. metabolic, vasculitic or connective-tissue conditions). Ask about weight change, musculoskeletal

symptoms, tiredness, fever and rashes. Polydipsia and polyuria together with tiredness may occasionally suggest new-onset diabetes mellitus as the cause of the neuropathy.

Past and current medical problems
- **Significant past illnesses.** Ask about a history of systemic disease (e.g. diabetes, stroke, inflammatory conditions or MS).
- **Trauma.** Old fractures may lead to hyperostosis or reactive neuroma, which can cause symptoms after some delay.
- **Operations.** Nerves may get damaged during surgery.
- **Anxiety.** Anxiety and panic attacks may lead to hyperventilation, which is a common cause of paraesthesiae.

Family history
- **Hereditary disease.** Problems that have been present since childhood may represent a hereditary neuropathy.

Medication
- **Drug history.** A variety of drugs may cause peripheral neuropathy, including metronidazole, phenytoin, isoniazid and nitrofurantoin, as well as drugs used for cancer treatment.
- **Treatment.** Have any treatments (e.g. antidepressants) been tried to help with symptomatic relief (e.g. paraesthesiae)?

Social history
- **Home.** Are activities of daily living affected in any way?
- **Work.** Ask about any problems at work.

Alcohol, smoking and recreational drugs
- **Alcohol.** Alcohol misuse can lead to neurotoxicity.
- **Smoking.** Smoking is a risk factor for lung cancer, which can lead to isolated neuritis or secondary neuropathy (paraneoplastic syndrome).
- **Drugs.** Drug misuse can cause neuropathic pain and sensory disturbances.

Review of previous investigations
- **Full blood count.** Macrocytosis may point towards alcohol misuse, hypothyroidism or vitamin B12/folate deficiency. Normochromic normocytic anaemia may suggest chronic disease.
- **Inflammatory markers.** Plasma viscosity or C-reactive protein (CRP) is raised in connective-tissue disease, infection and paraproteinaemia.
- **Urea and electrolytes.** Is there evidence of renal failure?
- **Blood glucose.** Check for evidence of diabetes.
- **Liver function tests and gamma-glutamyl transpeptidase (GGT).** If these are raised, it may indicate alcoholic liver disease and alcoholic neuropathy.

- **Calcium.** Both hypo- and hypercalcaemia may cause paraesthesiae (consider hyperparathyroidism, myeloma and sarcoidosis).
- **Thyroid tests.** Hypothyroidism may lead to myxoedema, which can present with neuropathy or carpal tunnel syndrome.
- **Vitamin B12 and folate.** Check for deficiencies.
- **Protein electrophoresis.** Abnormalities may suggest paraproteinaemia, myeloma or amyloidosis.
- **Nerve conduction studies.** These may be helpful in identifying peripheral nerve lesions.
- **Imaging.** Have any X-rays or other imaging studies been carried out? A normal chest X-ray will help exclude sarcoidosis or significant lung tumour. MRI scans of the brain can be helpful in ruling out a CNS lesion.

Examination

General
- **General condition.** Cachexia and poor general health may result from underlying cancer, renal failure, infection, diabetes or a connective-tissue disease.
- **Anxiety.** Sweaty palms, fidgeting and poor eye contact may suggest anxiety with hyperventilation during panic attacks.
- **Gait.** Check balance. A foot-drop gait or the inability to stand on heels or tip-toes suggests distal weakness. Balance problems on eye closure (Romberg's test) point towards vibration and proprioceptive sensory problems in the spinal cord or peripheral nerves.

Limbs
- **Neurology.** Check tone, power, sensation, coordination and reflexes of all limbs if you suspect a systemic neurological cause. Test for saddle anaesthesia, if indicated.
- **Main area of paraesthesia.** Carefully outline the area(s) involved by testing pin-prick and light-touch sensation. Check whether there is a difference between light-touch/pain sensation and position/vibration sense (dissociated sensory loss). Dissociated sensory loss occurs in spinal cord or occasionally in mid-brain lesions.
- **Other paraesthetic areas.** Test other areas for any sensory changes. Mononeuritis multiplex may suggest diabetes mellitus, malignancy or amyloidosis.
- **Wasting.** Inspect relevant muscles for evidence of wasting, particularly around the area of paraesthesia. Is there any fasciculation?
- **Power.** Test individual muscle groups for signs of weakness.
- **Reflexes.** Reflexes will be reduced or absent in lower motor neurone lesions.
- **Joints.** Joint swelling and deformity suggest rheumatoid disease or systemic lupus erythematosus (SLE).

Bedside tests

- **Glucose.** Check glucose levels for evidence of diabetes.
- **Urinalysis.** This may show renal involvement in diabetes, paraproteinaemia, vasculitis and connective-tissue disease.

Key references and further reading

1. Aring A, Jones D, Falko J. Evaluation and prevention of diabetic neuropathy. *Am Fam Physician* 2005;71:2123–2128.
2. Dyck PD, Dyck JB, Grant IA, Fealey RD. Ten steps in characterizing and diagnosing patients with peripheral neuropathy. *Neurology* 1996;47:10–17.
3. Hughes R. Peripheral neuropathy. *BMJ* 2002;32:166–169.
4. Leger JM, Behin A. Multifocal motor neuropathy. *Curr Opin Neurol* 2005; 18:567–573.
5. National Institute for Health and Care Excellence (NICE). Diabetic foot problems: prevention and management. NICE guidelines [NG19]. August 2015. Available from: http://www.nice.org.uk/guidance/ng19 (last accessed 29 April 2016).
6. Stojkovic T. Peripheral neuropathies: the rational diagnostic process. *Rev Med Intern* 2006;27:302–312.

Multiple sclerosis

Key thoughts

Practical points
- **Diagnosis.** MS can present in many different ways. An individual suspected of having MS should be referred to a specialist neurology service. Clinically isolated syndromes include, for example, optic neuritis, transverse myelitis and brain stem syndrome.
- **Pattern of MS.** Differentiate between relapsing/remitting MS, secondary progressive MS and primary progressive MS.

Differential diagnosis
- Diabetic neuropathy.
- Malignancy.
- HIV.
- Tuberculosis.
- Rarely, SLE, sarcoidosis, syphilis.

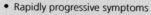

> **RED FLAGS**
>
> - Rapidly progressive symptoms
> - Severe disability
> - Mental health problems

History

Ideas, concerns and expectations
- **Ideas.** The patient may have already developed various ideas as to what might be wrong. This can help with the diagnosis, but may also point towards any myths about MS and other conditions that they hold, which may be worth exploring.
- **Concerns.** Concerns about the possibility of cancer, losing a job or impending disability are common.
- **Expectations.** People with symptoms of MS will usually expect an explanation as to what is wrong, referral to a specialist and some indication as to how problems may be managed in the future.

History of presenting complaint
- **Onset and progression.** When did the symptoms start, and how have they progressed since? In relapsing/remitting MS, symptoms will be intermittent, with

The 10-Minute Clinical Assessment, Second Edition. Knut Schroeder.
© 2017 John Wiley & Sons, Ltd. Published 2017 by John Wiley & Sons, Ltd.

phases of good health or remission followed by sudden onset of new symptoms. In about half of those with relapsing/remitting MS, secondary progressive MS develops within the first year of the illness, with gradually worsening symptoms and less frequent remissions. Primary progressive MS affects 10–15% of people with MS.

- **Past symptoms.** Presentation of MS may be unusual and may go almost unnoticed by the patient. Ask specifically about any previous symptoms that might be related.
- **Visual symptoms.** Consider optic neuritis if there is unilateral pain on eye movements followed by loss of vision or visual blurring, which may result in optic atrophy. Double vision is common.
- **Sensory symptoms.** Explore whether there have been any sustained episodes of numbness or paraesthesiae anywhere on the body. Patients commonly describe unpleasant sensations of tingling, twisting, tearing, pulling, burning or tightness. Pain and thermal perception may also be involved. Ask about loss of sensation in the legs and changes in taste or smell.
- **Motor symptoms.** Facial weakness may be caused by Bell's palsy. Ask about any other weaknesses or motor symptoms.
- **Cognitive impairment.** Visual and auditory attention may be reduced. Some people with MS may not be able to follow every detail during the assessment, even if there is no obvious disability. Try to be straightforward, check that the patient has understood, back up what you say or ask with written material and reinforce any messages, if necessary.
- **Associated symptoms.** Ask about tiredness, symptoms of depression, cognitive impairment, sexual problems and problems with bladder control. Swallowing problems suggest bulbar involvement.

Impact on the quality of life

- **Quality of life.** MS can affect numerous body systems. Many people with MS live an almost trouble-free life, but some may suffer significant disabilities, affecting all aspects of their lives, as well as those of their families.
- **Activity.** Ask in more detail about which activities are affected by any symptoms. Consider work, family roles, leisure, shopping, community activities, washing and dressing, getting about and control of the environment (e.g. opening windows, switching appliances on and off, using the phone). Can the patient walk unaided for 100 m or more?
- **Impairments.** Ask about problems with tiredness, speech and communication, food and fluid intake, bladder and bowel control, control over movement, vision and eye problems, sexual function, partnership relations and 'getting on' in social situations. If there is sexual dysfunction, consider contributing factors, such as depression, anxiety, adverse medication effects and muscle spasms.
- **Emotional state.** Try to assess the patient's need for emotional support. How are relationships with people close to them? Depending on the type of support required, you may be able to meet this need directly or you might have to refer to a suitable resource.

- **Autonomy.** People with MS should play an active part in making decisions in all aspects of their health care. Find out what, if any, information has been given about their condition and whether they feel they have a choice in making decisions. Do they know how and where to obtain further help?
- **Carers.** Try to find out about the physical and emotional health and well being of family members and carers. What information have they received? Are they in need of further help? Are they willing and able to support the patient in personal activities of daily living, such as dressing and toileting? Is the patient happy to accept such help?
- **Services involved.** Find out details about any services that may have already been involved, such as specialist neurological rehabilitation teams, occupational therapists, physiotherapists and social services or home care.

Common symptom patterns
- **Brain stem syndrome.** Consider this if there are neurological symptoms, including nausea, vertigo, unsteady gait, cranial nerve palsies, cerebellar signs and internuclear ophthalmoplegia (consisting of slow or incomplete adduction of one eye, with nystagmus in the other).
- **Transverse myelitis.** Ask about any numbness or weakness in the arms, legs or trunk associated with urinary or bowel problems (this is a neurological emergency).

Past and current medical problems
- **Significant past illnesses.** Ask about any other relevant medical problems that need monitoring or that might affect MS.
- **Immunisation.** People with MS should be offered immunisation against influenza. There is no evidence to suggest that vaccinations increase the risk of relapse.

Medication
- **Analgesics.** Is pain relief needed? If the patient already takes analgesic medication, is this effective? Are there any adverse drug effects?
- **Interferon beta or glatiramer acetate.** Have either of these been used for the treatment of MS? If so, what has been the response? Have there been any adverse effects?
- **Any other treatment for MS.** Have any other drugs or treatments been used for the management of MS? Ask about over-the-counter medication and complementary medicine.

Allergies
- **Drugs.** Ask about allergies to any drugs that might be used in the management of MS or related conditions.

Social history
- **Home.** Ask about the home situation, including housing, access to the home, driving, current level of independence and finances.

- **Work.** Is the patient currently in employment? Has work been affected in any way?

Review of previous investigations

- **Evoked potentials.** The visual evoked potential is most commonly used to aid diagnosis.
- **MRI.** Periventricular lesions and discrete white-matter abnormalities are common. The size and number of lesions does not necessarily correlate with disease activity and progression.
- **Cerebrospinal fluid.** Total protein and immunoglobulins may be raised (oligoclonal bands).

Examination

General

- **General condition.** Does the patient look tired or depressed? Is there evidence of malnutrition? Is the patient in pain?
- **Mobility.** Is there obvious spasticity? Look out for gait and balance abnormalities. Is there tremor or ataxia?
- **Speech.** Check for dysarthria or other speech problems that might be helped by referral to a speech therapist.
- **Equipment.** If there are mobility problems, are mobility aids and other equipment available, appropriate and in good working order?

Skin

- **Pressure sores.** Check relevant areas for any pressure sores, especially if the patient uses a wheelchair or has significantly reduced mobility.

Head and neck

- **Lhermitte's phenomenon.** An electrical sensation on neck flexion suggests cervical cord inflammation.
- **Eyes.** Look for optic neuritis or atrophy and check eye movements.
- **Cranial nerves.** Check the cranial nerves for any abnormalities and focus on any problem areas.

Limbs

- **Neurology.** Check tone, power, sensation, coordination and reflexes, focusing on areas suggested by the history.

Chest

- **Lungs.** Check for signs of chest infection.

Abdomen

- **Bladder.** Check for a palpable bladder, which may suggest urinary retention.

Bedside tests
• **Urine dipstick.** Look for any evidence of urinary tract infection.

Key references and further reading

1. Murray TJ. Diagnosis and treatment of multiple sclerosis. *BMJ* 2006;332:525–527.
2. National Institute for Health and Care Excellence (NICE). Multiple sclerosis: management of multiple sclerosis in primary and secondary care. NICE guidelines [CG8]. November 2003 Available from: http://www.nice.org.uk/guidance/cg8 (last accessed 29 April 2016).
3. National Institute for Health and Care Excellence (NICE). Multiple sclerosis in adults: management. Nice guidelines [CG186]. October 2014. Available from: http://www.nice.org.uk/guidance/cg186 (last accessed 29 April 2016).
4. National Institute for Health and Care Excellence (NICE). Multiple sclerosis. Clinical knowledge summaries. 2015. Available from: http://cks.nice.org.uk/multiple-sclerosis (last accessed 29 April 2016).
5. Polman CH, Reingold SC, Edan G et al. Diagnostic criteria for multiple sclerosis: 2005 revisions to the 'McDonald Criteria'. *Ann Neurol* 2005;58:840–846.

Gynaecology

Combined oral contraception

Key thoughts

Practical points
- **Special groups.** Be aware of issues around prescribing in women who fall into special groups because of age or comorbidities.
- **Examination.** There is usually no need for breast or vaginal examination, unless prompted by the history.
- **Information.** Any information given during the consultation should be backed by providing an appropriate patient information leaflet. Tailor advice and information to the women's knowledge and preferences.

Cautions
- Age <16.
- Age >35.
- Breastfeeding.
- Inflammatory bowel disease.
- Drugs interacting with the combined oral contraception.
- Hypertension.
- Migraine without focal aura or controlled with 5-HT$_1$ agonist.
- Smoking.
- Family history of venous thromboembolism or arterial disease.
- Diabetes.
- Obesity.
- Long-term immobilisation.

> **CONTRAINDICATIONS**
>
> - Pregnancy (perform pregnancy test if cycles are not regular)
> - Pre-existing cardiovascular disease (CVD)
> - Age over 50 years
> - Migraine with preceding focal aura, or severe migraine lasting over 72 hours despite treatment, or migraines treated with ergot derivatives
> - Severe or multiple risk factors for arterial disease or venous thromboembolism
> - Heart disease associated with pulmonary hypertension or embolus
> - Transient ischaemic attacks (TIAs)
> - Liver disease
> - Undiagnosed vaginal bleeding
> - Breast or genital tract carcinoma

The 10-Minute Clinical Assessment, Second Edition. Knut Schroeder.
© 2017 John Wiley & Sons, Ltd. Published 2017 by John Wiley & Sons, Ltd.

History

Ideas, concerns and expectations

- **Ideas.** Women may not appreciate that additional protection against sexually transmitted infections (STIs) may be required. Is the patient aware of how combined oral contraception works and the risks and benefits of taking it? Does she have any preferences with regard to contraception? Are there any issues around coercion or exploitation?
- **Concerns.** Worries about thromboembolic disease or cancer due to the pill are common. Has the patient used the pill in the past?
- **Expectations.** Why has the patient come to see you now?

History of presenting complaint

- **Need for contraception.** Try to explore gently why contraception is needed now, and whether there are any particular issues that might affect prescribing.
- **Age <16 years.** Try to persuade the patient to inform her parents. Assess competence by satisfying yourself that she will understand your advice. In particular, consider prescribing only if she is likely to begin or continue to have sexual intercourse with or without contraceptive treatment or if her health is likely to suffer.
- **Alternative contraception.** Is the patient aware of alternatives to combined oral contraception? Consider discussing long-acting progestogen contraceptives (LARCs) and non-oral hormonal methods, such as the patch. Non-oral progetogen-only methods include injectable preparations, implants and intrauterine devices. Non-hormonal non-oral methods include intrauterine devices containing copper and barrier methods.
- **Cautions and contraindications.** The health risks attributable to the pill in otherwise healthy women are small. Make sure you cover the previously mentioned main cautions and contraindications when discussing the pill.
- **Starting regimens.** Check guidance such as the British National Formulary (www.bnf.org) when starting regimens and when changing to the combined oral contraceptive pill from another form of contraception or after childbirth, abortion or miscarriage. Combined oral contraception should normally be started on the first day of the period, but can be started on up to day 5 of the cycle (check the manufacturer's instructions for individual preparations).
- **Risks.** Is the patient aware of risks such as venous thromboembolism, breast cancer and cervical cancer? The pill should be discontinued 6 weeks prior to major elective surgery, any surgery to the legs and surgery which involved prolonged immobilisation.
- **Benefits.** Does the patient appreciate the protective effects of the combined pill on ovarian and endometrial cancer? Other desired beneficial effects include lighter and less painful periods. Combined oral contraception can improve acne.
- **Adverse effects.** Mention important adverse effects, such as nausea, vomiting, headache, changes in body weight, fluid retention, changes in libido and

depression. Spotting or unscheduled bleeding may occur, particularly in early cycles.

- **Reduced effectiveness.** Make sure the patient knows what to do when she misses a pill. Make her aware that vomiting and diarrhoea can affect absorption.
- **Sexual and menstrual history.** Ask about the date of the last menstrual period, the current risk of pregnancy and any new partner(s) in the past 6 months. Is there a history of abnormal smears?
- **STI.** Is the patient aware of the risk of STIs and the need to use condoms for protection? Does she have symptoms of STI, such as vaginal discharge, intermenstrual bleeding or dyspareunia?

Past and current medical problems

- **Significant past or ongoing illnesses.** Consider in particular a history of CVD, venous thromboembolism, thrombophilia, liver disease, migraine or hyperlipidaemia.

Medication

- **Antibiotics.** Broad-spectrum antibiotics lead to reduced absorption of the combined oral contraceptive pill. Women prescribed a short course (<3 weeks) of a non-liver enzyme-inducing antibiotic should be advised to use additional contraception while taking the antibiotic and for 7 days after the antibiotic is stopped. If this takes them to their 'pill-free week', they should not take their usual 7-day break, but should start a new pill packet the day after finishing the old one.
- **Drug interactions.** Ask about any prescription drugs and check their potential for interaction (www.bnf.org). The effectiveness of both combined and progestogen-only pills can be considerably reduced by drugs that induce hepatic enzymes, such as carbamazepine, griseofulvin, phenytoin, St John's Wort, topiramate and rifampicin.

Family history

- **First-degree relatives.** Ask in particular about family history in a first-degree relative of early venous or arterial disease, liver conditions or breast cancer.

Alcohol, smoking and recreational drugs

- **Smoking.** Use of combined oral contraception by women <35 years who smoke is not recommended. Heavy smoking (over 20 cigarettes per day) in a woman of any age is a significant caution.

Review of previous investigations

- **Liver function tests.** Are there any abnormalities that suggest underlying liver disease?
- **Cervical smear.** Has the patient had regular smears in the past? Were any of them abnormal?

Examination

General
- **Weight and height.** Measure weight and height to calculate body mass index (BMI).

Vital signs
- **Blood pressure.** Check for hypertension and monitor any changes. The combined oral contraceptive is not usually recommended if blood pressure is consistently >140 mmHg systolic and/or 90 mmHg diastolic.

Key references and further reading
1. Beral V, Hermon C, Kay C et al. Mortality associated with oral contraceptive use: 25 year follow up of cohort of 46 000 women from Royal College of General Practitioners' oral contraception study. *BMJ* 1999;318:96–100.
2. British National Formulary. www.bnf.org.
3. Faculty of Family Planning and Reproductive Health Care Clinical Effectiveness Unit. First prescription of combined oral contraception. October 2003. Available from: http://jfprhc.bmj.com/content/29/4/209.full.pdf (last accessed 29 April 2016).
4. Guillebaud J. *Contraception Today* (5th edition). Martin Dunitz, London, New York; 2004.
5. National Institute for Health and Care Excellence (NICE). Contraception – assessment. Clinical knowledge summaries. 2012. Available from: http://cks.nice.org.uk/contraception-assessment (last accessed 29 April 2016).
6. National Institute for Health and Care Excellence (NICE). Contraception – combined hormonal methods. Clinical knowledge summaries. 2014. Available from: http://cks.nice.org.uk/contraception-combined-hormonal-methods (last accessed 29 April 2016).

Menorrhagia

Key thoughts

Practical points
- **Epidemiology.** Menorrhagia is a common presentation in both primary and secondary care.
- **Diagnosis.** No obvious cause is found in about half of cases.
- **Prognosis.** If there is no intermenstrual or postcoital bleeding, the risk of a sinister cause is relatively small.

Possible causes
- Idiopathic.
- Fibroids.
- Endometriosis.
- Adenomyosis.
- Endometrial polyps.
- Hypothyroidism.
- Copper intrauterine contraceptive devices (IUCDs).
- Anticoagulants.
- Coagulation disorders.
- Endometrial cancer.

Risk factors for endometrial cancer
- Tamoxifen.
- Unopposed oestrogen therapy.
- Polycystic ovary syndrome (PCOS).
- Obesity.

> **RED FLAGS**
>
> - Age >40
> - Anaemia
> - Failed medical treatment
> - Persistent intermenstrual bleeding
> - Abnormal smear
> - Severe dysmenorrhoea
> - Pressure symptoms
> - Abdominal pain between periods

The 10-Minute Clinical Assessment, Second Edition. Knut Schroeder.
© 2017 John Wiley & Sons, Ltd. Published 2017 by John Wiley & Sons, Ltd.

History

Ideas, concerns and expectations
- **Ideas.** What does the patient believe is the cause of the heavy menstrual bleeding? Does she have any preferences with regard to treatment?
- **Concerns.** The patient may be worried about underlying endometrial cancer or that she will need a hysterectomy.
- **Expectations.** The patient may in the first instance want symptomatic relief – heavy periods can severely affect the quality of life, particularly if they are also painful.

History of presenting complaint
- **Quality of life.** How far does heavy menstrual bleeding affect the quality of life and daily routines?
- **Onset and progression.** For how long have the patient's periods been heavy? Are the problems getting worse?
- **Severity.** How heavy is the bleeding? Does the patient pass clots? Is there flooding? Ask about the number of pads or tampons used per day. Does she have to get up at night to change? Menorrhagia is defined as losing more than 80 ml of blood per cycle, but this is difficult to quantify in routine practice.
- **Duration and frequency of periods.** How long do periods usually last? How frequently do they occur (first day of cycle to first day of the next)? Excessive blood loss in regular cycles is the most common presentation. Regular cycles suggest that ovulation takes place. Dysfunctional uterine bleeding may occur in ovulatory as well as anovulatory cycles. Anovulatory cycles are more common just after the menarche and in the perimenopause.
- **Other bleeding.** Is there any postcoital or intermenstrual bleeding?
- **Dysmenorrhoea.** Are periods painful? If they are, then nonsteroidal anti-inflammatory drugs (NSAIDs), such as mefenamic acid or ibuprofen, may help. In non-painful menorrhagia, tranexamic acid may be taken during the period for a maximum of 4 days.
- **Pain.** Is there any pelvic pain or dyspareunia between periods? Are there any pressure symptoms?
- **Contraception.** Is there a need for contraception at the moment? What, if any, methods are currently being used? Periods may appear heavier after stopping the combined pill. Is the patient using the IUCD?

Past and current medical problems
- **Chronic conditions.** NSAIDs should be used with caution in women suffering from asthma or dyspepsia.
- **Gynaecological problems.** Is there a history of fibroids?
- **Contraindications for the oral contraceptive pill.** Check for contraindications for the combined pill, including liver disease, history of deep venous thrombosis, thrombophilia, focal migraines, raised blood pressure and smoking in women over 35 years of age.

- **Anaemia.** Is there a history of iron-deficiency anaemia or platelet disorders?

Medication
- **Oral contraceptive pill.** The combined oral contraceptive pill may be effective in reducing menstrual blood loss.
- **Past treatments.** Has the patient ever had treatment for menorrhagia in the past? Ask about non-hormonal treatment, such as NSAIDs and antifibrinolytics. Tranexamic acid is an effective first-line treatment. Hormonal treatments include progestogens (both oral and intrauterine), combined oestrogen/progestogens, danazol, gestrinone and gonadotropin-releasing hormone (GnRH) analogues.

Social history
- **Social factors.** Stress or a new sexual relationship may make a woman more conscious of her periods.

Review of previous investigations
- **Smear.** Look up past cervical smear results. Is the patient up to date with her cervical smears?
- **Full blood count.** This should always be carried out. Is there evidence of anaemia?
- **Thyroid function, female hormones and coagulation screen.** These tests are not routinely indicated in the assessment of menorrhagia, unless suggested by the presence of other symptoms.
- **Transvaginal ultrasound.** Look out for any structural abnormalities.
- **Hysteroscopy and endometrial biopsy.** These suggest that the patient has already been assessed in secondary care. Were there any abnormalities?

Examination

General
- **General condition.** Does the patient look pale or unwell (anaemia)?

Vital signs
- **Pulse.** Tachycardia may be caused by anaemia.
- **Blood pressure.** Check for postural hypotension.

Abdomen
- **Masses.** Palpate the abdomen for any obvious masses.
- **Bimanual examination.** If appropriate, assess the size and consistency of the uterus and adnexae. An enlarged uterus suggests fibroids. Are extrauterine fibroids palpable? Check for other pelvic masses and tenderness.
- **Speculum examination.** Check the cervix for any abnormalities and perform a smear test if it is due.

Key references and further reading

1. National Institute for Health and Care Excellence (NICE). Heavy menstrual bleeding: assessment and management. NICE guidelines [CG44]. January 2007. Available from: http://www.nice.org.uk/guidance/cg177 (last accessed 29 April 2016).

2. National Institute for Health and Care Excellence (NICE). Menorrhagia. Clinical knowledge summaries. 2015. Available from: http://cks.nice.org.uk/menorrhagia (last accessed 29 April 2016).

3. Protheroe J. Modern management of menorrhagia. *J Fam Plann Reprod Health Care* 2004;30:118–122.

Amenorrhoea

Key thoughts

Practical points
- **Diagnosis.** Differentiate between primary and secondary amenorrhoea. Always search for an underlying cause. The endometrium requires four withdrawal bleeds annually or continuous progestogen protection to remain healthy. Always consider the possibility of pregnancy.

Possible causes
- Physiological (e.g. pregnancy, lactation, menopause).
- PCOS.
- Excessive weight loss.
- Medication.
- Chronic illness.
- Excessive exercise.
- Hypothyroidism.
- Premature ovarian failure.
- Uterine cervical stenosis.
- Intrauterine adhesions.
- Androgen-secreting tumour.
- Hypopituitarism or hyperprolactinaemia.
- Chromosomal causes, such as in Turner's syndrome (primary amenorrhoea).

> ### RED FLAGS
> - Virilisation
> - Delayed puberty
> - Adolescent over 16 years of age (primary amenorrhoea)
> - No obvious underlying cause
> - Hyperprolactinaemia
> - Suspected premature ovarian failure with confirmatory raised follicle-stimulating hormone (FSH)
> - Weight loss, malaise, fever or anorexia

History

Ideas, concerns and expectations
- **Ideas.** What does the patient think is causing her periods to be absent?

The 10-Minute Clinical Assessment, Second Edition. Knut Schroeder.
© 2017 John Wiley & Sons, Ltd. Published 2017 by John Wiley & Sons, Ltd.

- **Concerns.** The patient may be concerned about the possibility of pregnancy or about not being 'normal'.
- **Expectations.** Diagnosis of the underlying cause and advice about fertility are common reasons for consultation.

History of presenting complaint
- **Quality of life.** Allow the patient time to tell you about her lack of periods in her own words. How is her life affected? How much does amenorrhoea bother her?
- **Menstrual history.** Has the patient ever had a period? When was the last period? Ask about onset of menarche and frequency and duration of previous periods.
- **Obstetric history.** Has the patient ever been pregnant?
- **Contraception and pregnancy.** What contraception has the patient used lately? Could she be pregnant? Pregnancy is the most common cause of secondary amenorrhoea. A delayed return of periods is common after stopping the combined oral contraceptive pill ('post-pill amenorrhoea').
- **Weight change.** Has there been any change in the patient's weight lately? If her BMI is <20, then regular periods are unlikely. Amenorrhoea may also occur if more than 15% of body weight is lost over a relatively short period of time. Weight loss may be caused by anorexia nervosa, acute illness or excessive exercise. Endocrine disorders may cause excessive weight gain.
- **Exercise.** Excessive or high-intensity exercise (e.g. professional sportswomen) can cause amenorrhoea.
- **Premature ovarian failure.** Ask about vaginal dryness and hot flushes.
- **PCOS.** Hirsutism and acne may suggest PCOS.
- **Galactorrhoea.** Milk secretion from the breasts may occur due to hyperprolactinaemia.
- **Thyroid disease.** Ask about any weight changes, heat or cold intolerance, tremor or development of coarser features.
- **Mental health.** Severe emotional problems due to stress, divorce or bereavement may lead to menstrual changes and amenorrhoea. Check for symptoms of depression or anxiety.
- **Additional unexplored issues.** Ask the patient if there are any other problems or issues that you have not covered which might be important.

Past and ongoing medical problems
- **Chronic illness.** Ask about a history of heart disease, renal conditions or diabetes, all of which can cause amenorrhoea.
- **Gynaecological.** Ask in particular about any gynaecological operations. Has the patient ever received radiotherapy to the abdomen, pelvis or head?

Medication
- **Contraception.** Oral progestogens, as well as depot preparations and the levonorgestrel-releasing intrauterine device, can lead to amenorrhoea.

- **Chemotherapy.** Has the patient ever received chemotherapy?
- **Dopaminergic drugs.** Does the patient take any dopaminergic drugs which might lead to hyperprolactinaemia (e.g. haloperidol, phenothiazines, metoclopramide, domperidone, clozapine or cimetidine)?

Family history
- **Premature menopause.** Ask about a family history of premature ovarian failure.

Social history
- **Home.** Are there any problems at home that might be connected to or affected by the amenorrhoea? Primary amenorrhoea is more common where a woman's sisters also have late-onset menstruation.

Alcohol, smoking and recreational drugs
- **Alcohol.** Excessive alcohol consumption may lead to amenorrhoea.
- **Smoking.** Smoking may contribute to amenorrhoea.

Review of previous investigations
- **Pregnancy test.** Has the patient done a pregnancy test lately? A pregnancy test is essential in the assessment of amenorrhoea.
- **Reproductive hormones.** Raised FSH and luteinising hormone (LH) suggest onset of the menopause (if of appropriate age), premature ovarian failure (in younger women) or resistant ovary syndrome. Testosterone may be raised in PCOS. Consider pituitary adenoma if there is hyperprolactinaemia.
- **Thyroid function.** Is there any evidence of thyroid disease?
- **Pelvic ultrasound scan.** Look for evidence of any masses or polycystic ovaries.
- **Karyotyping.** In primary amenorrhoea, karyotyping may reveal chromosomal abnormalities such as Turner's syndrome (45,X) or XXX syndrome (rare).

Examination

General
- **Height and weight.** Calculate BMI. Is there evidence of anorexia nervosa?
- **Turner's syndrome.** Look for features of Turner's syndrome, such as webbed neck and short stature.

Skin
- **Signs of androgen excess.** Look for acne, hirsutism and acanthosis, which all indicate androgen excess, possibly due to PCOS.
- **Signs of thyroid disease.** Hyperthyroidism can cause amenorrhoea. There may be fine tremor and tachycardia.

Head and neck
- **Visual fields.** Check visual fields if you suspect a pituitary tumour.

Chest
- **Breasts.** Consider breast examination if there is a history of galactorrhoea. Be aware that breast examination may falsely raise levels of prolactin.
- **Heart.** Check the pulse rate and rhythm. Atrial fibrillation may suggest hyperthyroidism. Bradycardia can occur in anorexia nervosa.

Abdomen
- **Palpation.** Check for any obvious abdominal tumours.
- **Genitals.** Look for any abnormalities. Is there clitoromegaly?
- **Pelvic examination.** Check for any adnexal and other pelvic masses. Pelvic examination is not appropriate in young girls who are not sexually active.

Bedside tests
- **Pregnancy test.** Always consider the possibility of pregnancy before carrying out any other investigations.

Key references and further reading

1. Hamilton-Fairley D, Taylor A. Anovulation. *BMJ* 2003;327:546–549.
2. Master-Hunter T, Heiman DL. Amenorrhoea: evaluation and treatment. *Am Fam Physician* 2006;73:1374–1387.
3. National Institute for Health and Care Excellence (NICE). Amenorrhoea. Clinical knowledge summaries. 2014. Available from: http://cks.nice.org.uk/amenorrhoea (last accessed 29 April 2016).

Breast lumps

Key thoughts

Practical points
- **Epidemiology.** The majority of breast lumps seen in primary care are of benign nature. In pre-menopausal women, most lumps will have resolved a week after the next period. Around 1% of breast cancers occur in men.
- **Prognosis.** Early diagnosis and referral of suspected cases of breast cancer are important in reducing morbidity and mortality.

Possible causes
- Fibroadenoma.
- Cyst.
- Carcinoma.
- Abscess.
- Lipoma.

RED FLAGS

- History of previous breast cancer
- New discrete breast lump that persists after the next period (age ≥30 years) or that presents after the menopause
- Skin nodule
- Ulceration
- Skin distortion
- Recent nipple retraction or distortion (<3 months)
- Nipple eczema
- Asymmetrical nodularity persisting at review after menstruation
- Persistently refilling or recurrent cyst
- Persistent pain in post-menopausal women
- Severe mastalgia
- Strong family history of breast cancer
- Abscess
- Nipple discharge in post-menopausal women, particularly if bloodstained or troublesome and associated with a lump
- Enlarged axillary lymph nodes

The 10-Minute Clinical Assessment, Second Edition. Knut Schroeder.
© 2017 John Wiley & Sons, Ltd. Published 2017 by John Wiley & Sons, Ltd.

History

Ideas, concerns and expectations
- **Ideas.** What does the patient think is causing the lump? Does she have any particular views about future investigation and treatment (this will usually be more important for follow-up consultations)?
- **Concerns.** Worries about breast cancer are extremely common.
- **Expectations.** Why has the patient come to see you? Reassurance and diagnosis are common reasons for consultation.

History of presenting complaint
- **Quality of life.** Allow the patient time to tell you how her symptoms fit into the context of her life.
- **Breast lump.** Any discrete lump, particularly in women over 30 years of age, may indicate breast cancer. Discrete lumps in women under 30 are less likely to be malignant.
- **Duration and progression.** When did the patient first notice the lump, and how has it developed over time?
- **Site.** Which breast is affected? Most breast cancers occur in the upper outer quadrant.
- **Relationship to menstrual cycle.** Are any changes of symptoms related to the menstrual cycle (suggesting hormonal involvement)?
- **Nipple discharge.** Nipple discharge may occur for a variety of reasons, including intraductal papilloma, duct ectasia, infection, pregnancy, menopause and hyperprolactinaemia (e.g. hypothyroidism, pituitary adenoma), and can also be physiological. Nipple discharge in women aged <50 with bilateral discharge sufficient to stain clothes or discharge that is bloodstained needs to be taken seriously. In women over 50, any nipple discharge should raise suspicions. Consider the possibility of pituitary adenoma if there is headache or visual-field defect.
- **Skin.** Are there any overlying skin changes?
- **Pain.** Breast pain is common and is often benign. Ask about severity and whether pain has responded to wearing a well-supported bra or use of medication.
- **Shape.** Has the breast changed size or shape recently? Is there new asymmetry?

Past and current medical problems
- **Menstrual history.** Ask about age at menarche, regularity and age at menopause, if relevant.
- **Children.** Ask for details about number of children, age at the birth of the first child and if any or all of the children were breastfed.
- **Past breast problems.** Is there a history of breast problems or breast cancer?
- **Operations.** Has there been any surgery to the breast, ovaries or uterus?
- **Other significant conditions.** Ask about any other disease that might be relevant for future management, such as diabetes and heart disease.

Medication
- Hormone replacement therapy and the combined pill. These are weak risk factors for breast cancer.

Family history
- **Gynaecological cancer.** Ask about a family history of breast or ovarian cancer.

Alcohol, smoking and recreational drugs
- **Smoking.** Smoking increases the risk of breast cancer.

Review of previous investigations
- **Breast imaging.** Check for reports of previous imaging, including ultrasound and mammogram.
- **Prolactin.** Prolactin levels can be useful in the initial workup for women with galactorrhoea.
- **Thyroid function.** Hypothyroidism may be caused by pituitary adenoma.
- **Skull X-ray or computerised tomography (CT) of the head.** These may have been undertaken as part of an assessment for possible pituitary adenoma.

Examination

General
- **General condition.** Does the patient look unwell? Cachexia, pallor and jaundice suggest malignancy. Ideally, examine the patient with a chaperone present or offer another opportunity for review if one is not available.

Vital signs
- **Temperature.** Check for fever if there is a suggestion of underlying breast tissue infection.

Breasts
- **Shape and skin changes.** Look for asymmetry, deformity or skin change. Is there any puckering of the skin or dimpling when the arms are elevated? Are there any ulcers or patches of eczema? Is there nipple distortion?
- **Lumps.** Examine all quadrants of the breast, particularly the central aspect. Determine whether a lump is discrete or part of an area of nodularity. Describe size, margins and consistency, and whether it is fixed to the skin or to underlying tissues. Tender and symmetrically lumpy breasts usually have benign causes. Is the lump tender?
- **Nipple discharge.** Look out for any nipple discharge, noting the colour and whether it comes from a single or multiple ducts. Is it spontaneous or does it occur after expression from a single or multiple ducts? Is there an underlying lump?

Axillae
• **Palpation.** Check both axillae for lymphadenopathy.

Bedside tests
• **Discharge.** Check any nipple discharge for haemoglobin using a dipstick.
• **Pregnancy test.** Consider performing a pregnancy test if pregnancy is a possibility.

Key references and further reading

1. Barton MB, Harris R, Fletcher SW. The rational clinical examination. Does this patient have breast cancer? The screening clinical breast examination: should it be done? How? *JAMA* 1999;282:1270–1280.
2. National. Institute for Health and Care Excellence (NICE). Breast cancer – suspected. Clinical knowledge summaries. 2009. Available from: http://cks.nice.org.uk/breast-cancer-suspected (last accessed 29 April 2016).
3. National Institute for Health and Care Excellence (NICE). Early and locally advanced breast cancer: diagnosis and treatment. NICE guidelines [CG80]. February 2009. Available from: http://www.nice.org.uk/guidance/cg80 (last accessed 29 April 2016).
4. National Institute for Health and Care Excellence (NICE). Familial breast cancer: classification, care and managing breast cancer and related risks in people with a family history of breast cancer. NICE guidelines [CG164]. June 2013. Available from: https://www.nice.org.uk/guidance/cg164 (last accessed 29 April 2016).
5. National Institute for Health and Care Excellence (NICE). Suspected cancer: recognition and referral. NICE guidelines [NG12]. June 2015. Available from: http://www.nice.org.uk/guidance/ng12 (last accessed 29 April 2016).
6. Scottish Intercollegiate Guidelines Network (SIGN). Treatment of primary breast cancer. Guideline 134. September 2013. Available from: http://www.sign.ac.uk/pdf/SIGN134.pdf (last accessed 29 April 2016).
7. Twoon M, Ng NYB, Thomoson SE. 10-minute consultation: breast lumps. *BMJ* 2014;349:g5275.

Loss of libido

Key thoughts

Practical points
- **Diagnosis.** Loss of libido is common. It can be difficult to pick up the signals that women give out if they or their partners are concerned about their loss of desire.
- **Your attitude.** Many health professionals find it difficult to talk about sexual matters, which may hinder an effective clinical assessment.

Possible causes
- Domestic problems.
- Relationship issues.
- Postpartum loss of desire.
- Medical problems.
- Dyspareunia.
- Mental health problems (e.g. anxiety, depression).

> **RED FLAGS**
>
> - Relationship problems
> - Depression (including postnatal depression)
> - Weight loss, malaise, fever, anorexia, lymphadenopathy
> - Possibility of undiagnosed physical illness
> - Domestic violence

History

Ideas, concerns and expectations
- **Ideas.** What does the patient believe is the reason for her having lost interest in sex? Many women and their partners feel that 'there must be a physical cause' or that 'lack of hormones' may be to blame.
- **Concerns.** The patient may worry about the future of her relationship.
- **Expectations.** The patient may just want an opportunity to talk about her loss of libido. Is she or her partner expecting a 'quick fix', like some form of 'script'?

History of presenting complaint
- **Quality of life.** Many women find it difficult to bring up loss of libido in the consultation and may start by talking about an unrelated minor issue. They may

The 10-Minute Clinical Assessment, Second Edition. Knut Schroeder.
© 2017 John Wiley & Sons, Ltd. Published 2017 by John Wiley & Sons, Ltd.

feel ashamed, embarrassed or frightened that they will be misjudged. Have a high index of suspicion if patients say they have 'difficulties' in their relationship or are 'too tired'. Find out about the story behind their lack of interest. They may present in other ways, such as being unable to tolerate various forms of contraception. They may also complain of vaginal, pelvic or abdominal pain.

- **Feelings.** How do the patient and her partner feel about the lack of libido? Resentment, frustration, anger and unhappiness are common feelings and may affect the relationship and wider family.
- **Onset.** Has lack of libido always been a problem? If of acute onset, have there been any traumatic events? Consider bereavement or the possibility of sexual assault.
- **Home situation.** The couple may live in accommodation that is not conductive to sexual activity. The bedroom may not be soundproof, which can cause stress if teenagers or parents share a house. Smaller children may wander into the bedroom at night, which can make it difficult for women to relax and enjoy sex.
- **Relationship problems.** These commonly cause a reduction in libido, and indeed the patient may be pushed by her partner to seek advice. Try to see her by herself, and ask about how she is getting on with her partner. Is her partner loving and understanding? Does she find her partner attractive? Have the couple discussed the problem? Have there been arguments about it? Is the couple heading for break-up?
- **Beliefs.** Certain beliefs can affect sexual desire. Some women feel that it is 'unnatural' to have sex once they have children. Others may think that sex is 'dirty'.
- **Menstrual history.** Menorrhagia may lead to anaemia, which in turn can cause exhaustion, with a reduced sex drive. Heavy periods can also be very disruptive in themselves. Menopausal symptoms, such as hot flushes, tiredness, vaginal dryness and night sweats, may affect a woman's libido.
- **Sexual activity and sexuality.** If appropriate, you may want to ask for details about the patient's sex life. There may be a lot of focus on the act itself, without attention being paid to creating the right environment. Her partner may have erectile problems, which can make her feel that he is no longer physically attracted to her. Does she feel her partner might be having an affair? She may be unsure about her own sexuality. Does she avoid any sexual activities?
- **Mental health.** Depression and anxiety are common and often lead to reduced sex drive. Is the patient happy with her appearance? Does she feel disfigured by any form of surgery or injury, or due to childbirth? The way she feels and thinks may be affected by early life experiences (e.g. bullying, violence, abusive parents).
- **Pain.** Ask whether sex hurts. Vaginismus can cause discomfort, as can any other cause of dyspareunia, such as ovarian cysts, pelvic inflammatory disease, endometriosis and vaginal infections. Is there any generalised pain, for example due to arthritis?

- **Postcoital bleeding.** Postcoital bleeding suggests STI or more serious pathology.
- **Past management.** Have the couple sought help before? Have they ever seen a psychosexual counsellor?
- **Additional unexplored issues.** Ask the patient whether there are any other problems or issues that you have not covered which might be important.

Past and ongoing medical problems
- **Surgery.** Has the patient had any pelvic or other surgery that mgiht affect her libido?
- **Medical problems.** Are there any chronic conditions, such as hypothyroidism or diabetes?
- **Obstetric problems.** Have there been any physical or emotional problems resulting from childbirth?

Medication
- **Psychoactive medication.** Hypnotics, sedatives and antidepressants can significantly affect sex drive.
- **Antihypertensives.** Antihypertensive medication may lead to reduced libido in both men and women.
- **Oral contraception.** Hormonal treatments for contraception can influence sexual desire.

Social history
- **Home and work.** Is the patient overworked or stressed?
- **Exercise.** Regular exercise may help with relaxation and energy levels.

Alcohol, smoking and recreational drugs
- **Alcohol.** Moderate alcohol use may stimulate sex drive, whereas alcohol misuse may lead to reduced libido.
- **Drugs.** Is there a history of drug misuse?

Review of previous investigations
- **Full blood count.** This may be indicated if there is the possibility of anaemia, perhaps due to menorrhagia.
- **Thyroid function.** This is usually only helpful if other features of thyroid disease are present.
- **Vaginal swabs.** Check for evidence of STI.

Examination

General
- **General condition.** Look for signs of depression, poor general health, thyroid disease and anaemia.

Abdomen

- **Palpation.** Palpate the abdomen for tenderness and masses.
- **Vaginal examination.** Consider a vaginal examination only if you feel it is appropriate and prompted by the history. In most cases, it can safely be deferred, particularly if it would be unduly embarrassing or distressing for the patient. Vulval eczema or candidiasis will usually be easy to treat.

Key references and further reading

1. Arunakumari PS, Walker S. 10-minute clinical consultation: reduced sexual desire in women. *BMJ* 2009;339:b2371.
2. National Institute for Health and Care Excellence (NICE). Menopause. Clinical knowledge summaries. 2015. Available from: http://cks.nice.org.uk/menopause (last accessed 29 April 2016).
3. Segraves RT. Management of hypoactive sexual desire disorder. *Adv Psychosom Med* 2008;29:23–32.
4. Segraves R, Woodard T. Female hypoactive sexual desire disorder: history and current status. *J Sex Med* 2006;3:408–418.
5. Wylie K, Daines B, Jannini EA et al. Loss of sexual desire in the postmenopausal woman. *J Sex Med* 2007;4:395–405.

Polycystic ovary syndrome

Key thoughts

Practical points

- **Epidemiology.** PCOS is one of the most common endocrine disorders affecting women during their reproductive years. About 20% of women have polycystic ovaries, and half of these experience some symptoms of PCOS.
- **Diagnosis.** The main symptoms are irregular or absent periods (oligomenorrhoea), excessive weight gain and hyperandrogenism. No single feature is diagnostic on its own.

Diagnostic features

- **Menstruation.** Irregular and usually prolonged menstrual cycles.
- **LH and FSH.** LH > FSH (FSH is usually normal, and LH is usually at least twice the level of FSH).
- **Total testosterone.** Usually raised.
- **Sex hormone-binding globulin (SHBG).** Reduced in slim women.
- **Serum prolactin.** Raised in 15% of women with PCOS.
- **Ferritin.** Low in a high proportion of women.
- **Family history.** Late-onset diabetes and premature balding in male relatives.

Differential diagnosis

- Androgen-producing tumours.
- Thyroid disorders.
- Cushing's syndrome.
- Acromegaly.

> **RED FLAGS**
>
> - Rapidly progressing hirsutism
> - Virilisation
> - Suspected Cushing's syndrome
> - Serum testosterone raised >4.5 nmol/l
> - Severe acne
> - Weight loss, fever, anorexia, malaise

The 10-Minute Clinical Assessment, Second Edition. Knut Schroeder.
© 2017 John Wiley & Sons, Ltd. Published 2017 by John Wiley & Sons, Ltd.

History

Ideas, concerns and expectations
- **Ideas.** What does the patient believe is causing her symptoms?
- **Concerns.** Infertility and change in facial appearance due to hair growth are common causes of concern.
- **Expectations.** A common reason for consultation is assessment for infertility. What does the patient expect in terms of further investigation and/or referral?

History of presenting complaint
- **Quality of life.** How far is quality of life affected by the symptoms? Infertility, menstruation problems and hirsutism can all be very distressing.
- **Menstrual cycle.** Irregular and prolonged cycles are commonly caused by failure of ovulation, which makes it difficult for the patient to conceive. Problems often start at menarche but may also develop after pregnancy or on stopping the pill.
- **Obesity.** Obesity is common in women with PCOS (around 50%). There is an association between PCOS and diabetes in later life, particularly in women who are obese (BMI >30 kg/m²).
- **Ethnicity.** PCOS is more common in certain ethnic groups, such as women from Asian communities.
- **Skin.** Hirsutism and acne are common in PCOS.
- **Miscarriage.** Patients with PCOS have an increased risk of miscarriage in the first trimester, particularly if there is a raised basal LH level. Obese women who enter pregnancy with a raised BMI are at higher risk of developing gestational diabetes requiring insulin.
- **Amenorrhoea.** Women with amenorrhoea should have a withdrawal bleed at least every 3 months because of the effects of unopposed oestrogens on the endometrium. This may be achieved with progesterone given for 1 week every 3 months.
- **Previous and current management.** What treatments have been tried? The oral contraceptive pill depresses ovarian testosterone production. Cyproterone acetate is particularly effective in managing hyperandrogenic signs, such as acne and hirsutism. Has the patient ever taken metformin to reduce insulin levels (this has the secondary effect of reducing the level of testosterone)? Diet and exercise are important additional management options.
- **Fertility.** Monthly ovulation can be helped by clomifene citrate (an antioestrogen).
- **Contraindications for the oral contraceptive pill.** Check for contraindications for the combined pill, including liver disease, severe obesity, history of deep venous thrombosis, thrombophilia, focal migraines, raised blood pressure and smoking in women over 35 years of age.

Past and current medical problems
- **Liver and renal disease.** Metformin should be avoided in women with pre-existing liver or renal disease.

- **Metabolic syndrome.** The metabolic syndrome is present in 25–50% of women with PCOS.

Medication
- **Metformin.** Metformin is effective in reducing testosterone levels and regulating menstrual cycles, particularly in obese women. Adverse effects, such as taste disturbance and gastrointestinal problems, are common. Indications to stop metformin temporarily are the need for a general anaesthetic, likelihood of drinking more than 8 units of alcohol during a 24-hour period and pregnancy.
- **Iron supplements.** Iron deficiency is common and should be corrected, particularly if pregnancy is planned.

Family history
- **Diabetes.** Ask about a family history of late-onset diabetes and PCOS. Is there a history of premature balding in male relatives? Also ask about a history of premature coronary artery disease or hypertension.

Social history
- **Relationship.** Relationship difficulties may arise from fertility problems.

Review of previous investigations
- **Reproductive hormones.** Blood levels of total testosterone, LH and insulin are usually raised. Also check results of FSH. Oestradiol E_2 and prolactin are usually normal but may be modestly elevated. SHBG is often reduced, particularly in slim women. Almost half of all women with PCOS do not show any hormone abnormality. If the patient menstruates, blood should be taken between days 2 and 5 of the cycle. There may be no hormone abnormality in about a third of women. The diagnosis may be masked in women taking the combined oral contraceptive pill, who usually have suppressed gonadotropin and testosterone levels.
- **Full blood count.** This may show anaemia due to iron deficiency.
- **Ferritin.** Low ferritin may be caused by raised levels of insulin-like growth factors (IGFs) in response to hyperinsulinaemia, which inhibit the production of transferrin and lead to reduced iron absorption.
- **Renal and liver function.** Check liver and renal function before starting metformin.
- **Lipid profile.** There is an increased risk of hyperlipidaemia, particularly in obese women.
- **Ovarian ultrasound.** The appearance of the ovaries on transvaginal ultrasound is the least reliable and reproducible diagnostic assessment for PCOS. Polycystic ovaries show up as enlarged ovaries with more than 10 cysts of 2–8 mm diameter around a thicker outer ovarian stroma, but this may be found in 15–20% of normal women, particularly in their later reproductive years.

Examination

General
- **General condition.** Does the patient look unwell or depressed?
- **Virilisation.** Deep voice, increased muscularity and clitoromegaly are not features of PCOS. If these are seen, a possible underlying virilising tumour needs to be considered.
- **Weight and height.** Look for truncal obesity and calculate the BMI. Beware that some women with PCOS have normal BMI, are not hirsute and do not have acne.

Vital signs
- **Blood pressure.** There is an increased risk of hypertension.

Skin
- **Hirsutism.** There will often be changes in the scalp hairline towards a more male pattern distribution, with a 'peak' on the frontal scalp hairline and development of lanugo-type hair on either side of the midline. Increased hair growth may also be visible around the sideburns, the upper lip, underneath the point of the jaw, on the midline of the lower abdomen and on the back of the neck.
- **Skin.** Look for acne and postpubertal acne. Acanthosis nigricans may be present in about 1 in 10 women with PCOS, particularly in skin folds at the back of the neck.

Abdomen
- **Palpation.** Check for any obvious masses or tenderness.
- **Pelvic examination.** Check for any pelvic masses and assess the cervix via speculum examination.

Bedside tests
- **Glucose.** Screen for hyperglycaemia.

Key references and further reading
1. Azziz R, Woods KS, Reyna R et al. The prevalence and features of the polycystic ovary syndrome in an unselected population. *J Clin Endocrinol Metab* 2004;89:2745–2749.
2. Balen AH, Rutherford AJ. Managing anovulatory infertility and polycystic ovary syndrome. *BMJ* 2007;335:663.
3. Broekmans FJ, Fauser BC. Diagnostic criteria for polycystic ovarian syndrome. *Endocrine* 2006;30(1):3–11.
4. Curran DR, Moore C, Huber T. Clinical inquiries. What is the best approach to the evaluation of hirsutism? *J Fam Pract* 2005;54:465–467.

5. National Institute for Health and Care Excellence (NICE). Polycystic ovary syndrome. Clinical knowledge summaries. 2013. Available from: http://cks.nice.org.uk/polycystic-ovary-syndrome (last accessed 29 April 2016).
6. The Rotterdam ESHRE/ASRM-Sponsored PCOS consensus workshop group. Revised 2003 consensus on diagnostic criteria and long-term health risks related to polycystic ovary syndrome (PCOS). *Hum Reprod* 2004;19:41–47.

Suspected ovarian cancer

Key thoughts

Practical points
- **Diagnosis.** Symptoms of ovarian cancer are often vague, and a high index of suspicion is needed for early diagnosis.
- **Prognosis.** Ovarian cancer is the leading cause of death from gynaecological malignancy in women.

Differential diagnosis
- Fibroids.
- Pyometrium.
- Benign ovarian cysts.
- Endometrial cancer.
- Large cervical cancer.
- Primary peritoneal cancer.
- Fallopian tube cancer.

RED FLAGS

- Progressive abdominal pain and swelling
- Feeling of being full and bloated
- Change in bowel or bladder function
- Irregular vaginal bleeding
- Family history of ovarian cancer
- Systemic features (weight loss, malaise, fatigue, sweats, anorexia)
- Indigestion and nausea
- Late menopause
- Unexplained back or abdominal pain
- Nulliparity
- Ascited and/or pelvic mass

History

Ideas, concerns and expectations
- **Ideas.** What does the patient believe is the cause of her symptoms?
- **Concerns.** Worries about cancer are common. They are often prompted by reading articles about ovarian cancer in magazines and newspapers or by the diagnosis of cancer in a relative or friend.

The 10-Minute Clinical Assessment, Second Edition. Knut Schroeder.
© 2017 John Wiley & Sons, Ltd. Published 2017 by John Wiley & Sons, Ltd.

- **Expectations.** Why is the patient presenting now? Reasons for consultation include referral, further investigation and simple reassurance.

History of presenting complaint
- **Quality of life.** Invite the patient to tell you about her symptoms in her own words. How do they affect day-to-day life?
- **Pain.** Abdominal pain may occur with ovarian cancer but is usually a late feature. Even large ovarian tumours may stay painless for a long time. Pain is often of gradual onset and progressive.
- **Abdominal swelling.** Consider the possibility of ovarian cancer in any women presenting with progressive abdominal swelling or bloating. Swelling may be caused by the tumour itself or by ascites.
- **Systemic symptoms.** Ask about weight loss, fatigue, sweats, fevers and loss of appetite.
- **Change in bowel habit.** An ovarian mass may cause bowel symptoms.
- **Urinary symptoms.** These may be caused by pressure from the tumour on adjacent structures or local metastasis. Urinary frequency is a common symptom.
- **Back pain.** New-onset and unexplained back pain may be caused by direct pressure from the tumour or metastasis.
- **Dyspareunia.** Ask about any pelvic pain during sex.
- **Post-menopausal bleeding.** What is the patient's menopausal status? Bleeding after the menopause is caused by vaginal, cervical, endometrial or ovarian cancer in about 10% of cases.
- **Nausea and vomiting.** This may be caused by spread of intra-abdominal tumour affecting the upper abdomen and omentum.

Past and current medical problems
- **Significant past illnesses.** Ask about any heart, lung or neck problems in case laparoscopy or laparotomy is indicated.
- **Operations.** Has the patient had any operations in the past (consider adhesions)?

Medication
- **Analgesics.** What pain relief has been tried? What has been effective? Have there been any adverse effects?
- **Hormone replacement therapy.** This slightly increases the risk of ovarian cancer.
- **Combined oral contraceptive pill.** This reduces the risk of ovarian cancer.

Family history
- **Cancer.** Ask about a family history of ovarian or breast cancer.

Social history
- **Domestic and marital relationships.** Abdominal tumours may cause dyspareunia, which can adversely affect sexual relationships.

- **Work.** Have symptoms affected the patient's ability to work? Is a sick note needed?

Review of previous investigations
- **Full blood count and plasma viscosity.** Check for anaemia and raised inflammatory markers.
- **Imaging.** Abdominal ± transvaginal ultrasound scanning is a first-line investigation for suspected ovarian cancer and is likely to detect cysts or an ovarian mass. A recent negative scan makes ovarian cancer less likely, but an initial ultrasound may be normal in the early stages of cancer. Ovarian cysts in pre-menopausal women are usually ovulatory. Also look out for any results of recent CT or MRI scans.
- **Cancer antigen (Ca)125.** This can be a marker of epithelial endometrial cancer but is neither a sensitive nor a specific test. It is not routinely performed as a screening test for ovarian cancer. Ca124 is often normal in the early stages of cancer and may be raised in conditions other than cancer (e.g. endometriosis, pelvic inflammatory disease, renal conditions, liver disease and heart problems).

Examination

General
- **General condition.** Is the patient unwell or cachectic?

Vital signs
- **Blood pressure.** Check for hypertension, in case an operation is needed.

Head and neck
- **Lymph nodes.** Check for any cervical or supraclavicular lymph nodes.

Chest
- **Chest auscultation.** Check heart and lungs for any obvious abnormalities, to exclude any operative risks.

Abdomen
- **Palpation.** Feel the abdomen for any palpable mass and tenderness, particularly in the lower abdomen.
- **Pelvic examination.** Perform a bimanual pelvic examination and examine the cervix. Pelvic masses can be difficult to feel, particularly if they are small, and a normal examination does not rule out cancer.
- **Rectal examination.** Rectal examination may be helpful in further assessment of an ovarian mass detected by bimanual pelvic examination.

Key references and further reading

1. Evans J, Ziebland S, McPherson A. Minimizing delays in ovarian cancer diagnosis: an expansion of Andersen's model of 'total patient delay'. *Fam Pract* 2007;24:48–55.
2. Friedman GD, Skilling JS, Udaltsova NV, Smith LH. Early symptoms of ovarian cancer: a case-control study without recall bias. *Fam Pract* 2005;22:548–553.
3. Goff BA, Mandel LS, Melancon CH, Muntz HG. Frequency of symptoms of ovarian cancer in women presenting to primary care clinics. *JAMA* 2004;291:2705–2712.
4. Hamilton W, Menon U. Ovarian cancer. *BMJ* 2009;339:b4650.
5. National Institute for Health and Care Excellence (NICE). Ovarian cancer: recognition and initial management. NICE guidelines [CG122]. April 2011. Available from: http://www.nice.org.uk/guidance/cg122 (last accessed 29 April 2016).
6. National Institute for Health and Care Excellence (NICE). Ovarian cancer. Clinical knowledge summaries. 2013. Available from: http://cks.nice.org.uk/ovarian-cancer (last accessed 29 April 2016).
7. Scottish Intercollegiate Guidelines Network (SIGN). Management of epithelial ovarian cancer. Guideline 135. November 2013. Available from: http://www.sign.ac.uk/pdf/sign135.pdf (last accessed 29 April 2016).

Obstetrics

Routine antenatal care

Key thoughts

Practical points
- **Diagnosis.** Look out for any clinical and/or social factors that might affect the health of mother and/or baby.
- **Information.** Give relevant information, with an opportunity to discuss issues and ask questions.

Important risk factors from past pregnancies
- **Antenatal.** Recurrent miscarriage, rhesus isoimmunisation or other significant blood group antibodies, uterine surgery, grand multiparity.
- **Perinatal.** Pre-term birth, severe pre-eclampsia, HELLP (haemolysis, elevated liver enzymes and low platelets) syndrome or eclampsia, antenatal or postpartum haemorrhage, stillbirth or neonatal death, small-for-gestational-age infant (below 5th centile), large-for-gestational-age infant (above 95th centile), baby weighing below 2.5 kg or above 4.5 kg, congenital abnormality (structural or chromosomal).
- **Post-natal.** Puerperal psychosis.

RED FLAGS

- Symptoms of pre-eclampsia (headache, vision problems, new epigastric pain, vomiting, breathlessness, sudden oedema)
- Obesity or underweight
- Women aged 40 years and older
- Vulnerable women, such as teenagers
- Lack of social support
- Chronic disease (e.g. severe asthma, cardiovascular disease (CVD) (including hypertension), renal problems, endocrine disorders, diabetes requiring insulin, haematological disorders, autoimmune disorders, epilepsy)
- Psychiatric disorders
- Malignant disease
- Drug misuse
- Human immunodeficiency virus (HIV) or hepatitis B infection

The 10-Minute Clinical Assessment, Second Edition. Knut Schroeder.
© 2017 John Wiley & Sons, Ltd. Published 2017 by John Wiley & Sons, Ltd.

History

Ideas, concerns and expectations
- **Ideas.** Seek the views, beliefs and values of the woman, her partner and her family in relation to her care and that of her baby at all times. Make sure she understands any information you provide.
- **Concerns.** Provide an opportunity to discuss any concerns or ask questions. Pregnancy is a major life event, and the woman may be worried about impending motherhood.
- **Expectations.** Make sure that any information and care given is culturally appropriate and addresses the woman's needs.

Suggested issues to cover at the booking visit
- **Quality of life.** Allow the woman time to tell you how the pregnancy fits into the context of her life. Is this a 'planned' pregnancy? Have there been difficulties conceiving?
- **Symptoms of pregnancy.** Does the woman suffer from pregnancy symptoms (e.g. extreme tiredness, nausea or hyperemesis gravidarum) which need addressing or treating? Headaches are common, often caused by caffeine withdrawal. Always consider the possibility of ectopic pregnancy if there is abdominal pain ± vaginal bleeding.
- **Information about care.** Offer the woman information based on the current available evidence. Support her in making informed decisions about her and the baby's care. Include information about where she will be seen and who will be involved in her care.
- **Information about lifestyle.** If this is her first contact with a health care professional, give the woman specific information on:
  - **Folic acid supplements.** These should be given until 14 weeks of gestation.
  - **Food hygiene.** Include information on how to reduce the risk of a food-acquired infection (unpasteurised milk, certain soft-mould cheeses, raw eggs and poultry, pâté, uncooked meals and meat, raw shellfish), vitamin A toxicity (liver and liver products) and methylmercury ingestion (shark, swordfish, marlin).
  - **Lifestyle.** Provide information on smoking cessation, recreational drug use and alcohol consumption.
  - **Antenatal screening.** Include guidance on the risks, benefits and limitations of screening tests.
- **Vitamin D deficiency.** Is the woman aware of the importance to her own and her baby's health of maintaining adequate vitamin D stores during pregnancy and whilst breastfeeding? Women are particularly at risk if they:
  - are of South Asian, African, Caribbean or Middle Eastern family origin;
  - have limited exposure to sunlight;
  - eat a diet particularly low in vitamin D;
  - have a pre-pregnancy body mass index (BMI) above 30 kg/m^2.

- **Screening for haematological conditions.** Is there a history of haematological disorders? Offer all women screening for sickle-cell diseases and thalassaemias as early as possible in pregnancy (ideally by 10 weeks).
- **Screening for foetal abnormalities.** Does the woman have any views on screening for foetal abnormalities? If available, offer the 'combined test' (nuchal translucency, beta-human chorionic gonadotrophin, pregnancy-associated plasma protein A) to screen for Down's syndrome at between 11 weeks 0 days and 13 weeks 6 days. Offer the most clinically and cost-effective serum screening test (triple or quadruple test) for women who book later in pregnancy, at between 15 and 20 weeks.
- **Screening for gestational diabetes.** Screen for gestational diabetes, particularly if risk factors are present. Offer testing for gestational diabetes if BMI is above 30 kg/m^2, if the woman had a previous macrosomic baby weighing 4.5 kg or above, if she has a personal or family history of gestational diabetes or if she has a family origin with a high prevalence of diabetes (South Asian, black Caribbean, Middle Eastern).
- **Antenatal information.** Has the woman received any information about her antenatal care so far? Make sure you cover:
  - where she will be seen and by whom;
  - the likely number, timing and content of antenatal appointments;
  - the availability of participant-led antenatal classes and breastfeeding workshops;
  - her right to accept or decline a test.
- **Mental health.** Depression during pregnancy is common. Ask about the woman's mood and whether there are any particular stressors. Always be aware of the possibility of domestic abuse or inability to cope with the additional stress of pregnancy.
- **Genital mutilation.** Identify women who have undergone genital mutilation (continues to be performed in some cultural settings).
- **Additional unexplored issues.** Always ask the woman if there are any other problems or issues that you have not covered but which might be important.

16-week appointment

- **Screening results.** Review and record the results of any screening tests that were offered at the booking visit.
- **Pre-eclampsia.** Warn the woman about symptoms of pre-eclampsia and advise her to seek immediate medical advice if should she develop any (including after delivery of the baby):
  - severe headaches (increasing frequency, unrelieved by regular analgesics);
  - vision problems (blurred vision, flashing lights, double vision, floating spots);
  - persistent new epigastric pain or pain in the right upper quadrant;
  - vomiting;
  - breathlessness;
  - sudden swelling of the face, hands or feet.

- **Influenza vaccination.** Offer influenza vaccination if the woman has not already been vaccinated in the current flu season.
- **Scan.** If the woman wishes to have a foetal anomaly scan at 18–20 weeks, discuss this with her and give her specific information about the scan.

Medication

- **Prescribed medication.** Ask about any prescribed medication and assess the benefits versus the risks of treatment (see www.bnf.org for information on safe prescribing in pregnancy). If the decision is to continue treatment, make sure the smallest effective dosage is used.
- **Herbal and over-the-counter drugs.** Does the woman use any medication bought over-the-counter, without prescription?

Social history

- **Home.** What is the woman's home situation? Does she have a supportive partner? Does she have any children? What ages are they? How will the new baby fit into the current family setup?
- **Work.** What type of work does the woman have? Does day-to-day work involve heavy lifting?

Alcohol, smoking and recreational drugs

- **Alcohol.** Alcohol misuse may result in maternal ill-health and may harm the foetus, particularly if the woman drinks heavily or binge-drinks.
- **Smoking.** Smoking is dangerous for both mother and foetus, with an increased risk of miscarriage, placental abruption and pre-term delivery. Offer smoking-cessation advice to all smokers.
- **Recreational drugs.** If the woman is a drug user, consider other health risks to her and her baby, including HIV and hepatitis B infection and sexually transmitted infections (STIs), as well as social and financial problems.

Review of previous investigations

- **Rubella.** Is the woman's rubella status known?
- **Blood group and rhesus D status.** The woman may need anti-D prophylaxis in the future if she is rhesus-negative and develops vaginal bleeding, depending on gestational age.
- **Full blood count.** This is important as a baseline, as anaemia may develop during pregnancy as a result of iron deficiency.
- **Blood glucose and HbA1c.** Diabetic control needs to be monitored in all diabetic women.
- **Haemoglobinopathies and red cell alloantibodies**. These often form part of the routine antenatal screening programme.
- **Hepatitis B, HIV and syphilis.** These tests should be offered to all pregnant women.

- **Chlamydia.** Inform women younger than 25 years about the high prevalence of chlamydia infection in their age group and give details of the local National Chlamydia Screening Programme, if appropriate.
- **Down's syndrome.** Screening for Down's syndrome should be discussed and offered.
- **Ultrasound.** Ultrasound scanning is useful for gestational age assessment and to detect structural abnormalities.

Examination

General
- **Height and weight.** Measure height and weight and calculate BMI.

Vital signs
- **Blood pressure.** Record booking blood pressure as a baseline. A raised baseline blood pressure may put the woman at higher risk of pre-eclampsia.

Abdominal examination
- **Palpation.** Check fundal height, although this is only a crude measure for foetal size. Is there any tenderness?
- **Foetal heart sound.** Listen for foetal heart sounds using a Pinard stethoscope, unless a handheld ultrasound (Doppler) machine is available. In early pregnancy, foetal heart rate (FHR) is typically in the 160s. Near term, FHR ranges from 110 to 160.
- **Symphysis–fundal height:** At 25 weeks, measure and plot symphysis–fundal height to identify small- or large-for-gestational-age infants.

Bedside tests
- **Urine dipstick.** Test urine for proteinuria, glucose, leucocytes and nitrites and offer screening for asymptomatic bacteriuria at every visit.

Key references and further reading
1. National Institute for Health and Care Excellence (NICE). Antenatal care for uncomplicated pregnancies. NICE guidelines [CG 62]. March 2008. Available from: http://www.nice.org.uk/guidance/cg62 (last accessed 29 April 2016).
2. National Institute for Health and Care Excellence (NICE). Hypertension in pregnancy: diagnosis and management. NICE guidelines [CG107]. August 2010. Available from: http://www.nice.org.uk/guidance/cg107 (last accessed 29 April 2016).
3. National Institute for Health and Care Excellence (NICE). Antenatal care – uncomplicated pregnancy. Clinical knowledge summaries. 2011. Available from: http://cks.nice.org.uk/antenatal-care-uncomplicated-pregnancy (last accessed 29 April 2016).
4. O'Keane V, Marsh. MS. Depression during pregnancy. *BMJ* 2007;334:1003–1005.

Bleeding in early pregnancy

Key thoughts

Practical points
- **Diagnosis.** Bleeding in early pregnancy is common (about 25% of pregnancies) and can happen for various reasons.
- **Prognosis.** Assume that any woman of childbearing age who presents with abdominal pain and vaginal bleeding may have an ectopic pregnancy until proven otherwise.

Possible causes
- Physiological – no cause found.
- Miscarriage or threatened miscarriage.
- Ectopic pregnancy.
- Trophoblastic disease.
- Conditions of the cervix, including polyp, friable cervix and cervical cancer.
- Subchorionic haemorrhage.

Risk factors for miscarriage
- Age >30 years (increased risk if age >35 years).
- Multiple pregnancies.
- Alcohol abuse.
- Illicit drug use.
- Smoking.
- Uncontrolled diabetes.
- Uterine surgery or abnormalities, such as incompetent cervix.
- Connective-tissue disorders, including systemic lupus erythematosus (SLE) and antiphospholipid antibodies.

> **RED FLAGS**
>
> - Abdominal or pelvic pain, particularly if severe and lateral to the midline
> - Vaginal bleeding, with or without clots
> - Dizziness, fainting or syncope
> - Shoulder-tip pain
> - Passage of tissue
> - Rectal pressure or pain on defecation
> - Postural hypotension

The 10-Minute Clinical Assessment, Second Edition. Knut Schroeder.
© 2017 John Wiley & Sons, Ltd. Published 2017 by John Wiley & Sons, Ltd.

History

Ideas, concerns and expectations
- **Ideas.** What does the patient think is causing the bleeding?
- **Concerns.** The woman is likely to be worried about possible miscarriage.
- **Expectations.** The woman may expect referral for further assessment and investigation.

History of presenting complaint
- **Quality of life.** Allow the woman time to tell you in her own words about the bleeding. Bleeding in pregnancy is often benign but can be very distressing.
- **Last menstrual period.** Check and record the date of the last menstrual period to help estimate the gestational age. Was the last period normal?
- **Pregnancy test.** When did the woman have a positive pregnancy test?
- **Pain.** Is there associated pain? In early pregnancy, up to about 14 weeks, consider the possibility of ectopic pregnancy, particularly if the pain preceded the bleeding. How severe is the pain? Colicky or constant pain in early pregnancy points towards possible ectopic pregnancy, particularly if it is lateral to the midline.
- **Nature of the bleed.** What is the colour and consistency of the loss? It can be difficult to distinguish blood clots from products of conception. Has the bleeding stopped or is it ongoing?
- **Severity.** How heavy is the bleeding? Is it spotting, like a period or heavier than a period? Blood loss due to ectopic pregnancy is usually lighter than that from miscarriage and may be very dark ('prune juice').
- **Previous bleeding.** Does the woman have a history of miscarriage?
- **Emotional state.** How does the woman feel emotionally? Does she need further support?

Past and ongoing medical problems
- **Significant past illnesses.** Does the woman suffer from any chronic illness that might be relevant, in case she needs an operation?

Medication
- **Regular drugs.** Does the woman take any regular drugs that it is important to know about, in case she requires surgery?

Social history
- **Home situation.** Does the woman have a supportive partner or other relatives?

Review of previous investigations
- **Ultrasound.** Has the woman had any ultrasound scans in this pregnancy to check the viability of the foetus?
- **Blood group and rhesus status.** Are these known? In rhesus-negative women, anti-D immunoglobulin may need to be given.

Examination

General
- **General condition.** Does the woman look unwell or pale?

Vital signs
- **Temperature.** Consider septic abortion if there is fever, particularly if associated with malodorous vaginal discharge.
- **Pulse.** A heart rate >100 beats per minute suggest impending shock or severe anxiety.
- **Blood pressure.** Blood pressure will usually be maintained unless blood loss is significant.

Abdomen
- **Palpation.** Check for guarding, tenderness and signs of peritonism. Unilateral lower abdominal tenderness suggests possible ectopic pregnancy in women <14 weeks pregnant.
- **Bimanual vaginal examination.** This is not usually necessary or useful at the first assessment if the woman is going to be referred to an early pregnancy assessment unit. Be aware that pelvic examination can cause rupture of an ectopic pregnancy or massive haemorrhage in underlying placenta praevia. If you decide to examine, check whether the uterus is of appropriate size for dates. The cervical os in a multiparous woman should only admit the tip of a finger. There may be cervical excitation in ectopic pregnancy.
- **Speculum.** Check whether the os is open. Are any products of conception visible? Is the bleeding coming from the uterus or the cervix itself?

Bedside tests
- **Pregnancy test.** Perform a pregnancy test in every woman of childbearing age who presents with abdominal pain and vaginal bleeding.

Key references and further reading
1. Murray H, Baakdah H, Bardell T, Tulandi T. Diagnosis and treatment of ectopic pregnancy. *CMAJ* 2005;173:905–912.
2. National Institute for Health and Care Excellence (NICE). Ectopic pregnancy and miscarriage: diagnosis and clinical management. NICE guidelines [CG154]. December 2012. Available from: https://www.nice.org.uk/guidance/cg154 (last accessed 29 April 2016).
3. National Institute for Health and Care Excellence (NICE). Ectopic pregnancy. Clinical knowledge summaries. 2013. Available from: http://cks.nice.org.uk/ectopic-pregnancy (last accessed 29 April 2016).
4. National Institute for Health and Care Excellence (NICE). Miscarriage. Clinical knowledge summaries. 2013. Available from: http://cks.nice.org.uk/miscarriage (last accessed 29 April 2016).

5. Royal College of Obstetricians and Gynaecologists (RCOG). Placenta praevia, placenta praevia accrete and vasa praevia: diagnosis and management. Green-top guideline no. 27. January 2011. Available from: https://www.rcog.org.uk/globalassets/documents/guidelines/gtg_27.pdf (last accessed 29 April 2016).

Abdominal pain in pregnancy

Key thoughts

Practical points
- **Diagnosis.** Try to establish whether abdominal pain is pregnancy-related or has other causes. Different conditions predominate in different trimesters. Always consider ectopic pregnancy in early pregnancy, particularly if risk factors are present. Think of pre-term labour in the later stages.
- **Prognosis.** Abdominal pain in pregnancy should be considered serious until proven otherwise. Signs of maternal shock or reduced foetal heart rate should prompt transfer to hospital.

Possible causes
- Urinary tract infection.
- Constipation.
- Braxton Hicks contractions.
- Round ligament pain.
- Threatened or actual miscarriage.
- Ectopic pregnancy.
- Pre-term labour.
- Acute abdomen due to either appendicitis, hernia, gastric ulcer, inflammatory bowel disease or other causes.
- Pre-eclampsia.
- Placental abruption.
- Uterine rupture.
- Red degeneration of a fibroid.
- Ovarian cyst.

Risk factors for ectopic pregnancy
- Previous ectopic pregnancy.
- History of infertility.
- Previous fallopian tube surgery.
- Endometriosis.
- Salpingitis.
- Pelvic inflammatory disease due to chlamydia infection.
- Increasing maternal age.
- Smoking.
- Progesterone intrauterine contraceptive device.

The 10-Minute Clinical Assessment, Second Edition. Knut Schroeder.
© 2017 John Wiley & Sons, Ltd. Published 2017 by John Wiley & Sons, Ltd.

RED FLAGS

- Associated vaginal bleeding
- Absent foetal activity
- Systemic illness
- Tachycardia
- Peritonism
- Features of pre-eclampsia

History

Ideas, concerns and expectations
- **Ideas.** Does she have any thoughts as to what might be causing the pain?
- **Concerns.** The woman's prime concern is often that she will lose the pregnancy. Problems during previous pregnancy may cause considerable worries about recurrence. She may worry and feel guilty that her own behaviour and lifestyle may have affected the pregnancy.
- **Expectations.** She will usually want reassurance, as well as swift further investigation and treatment, if appropriate.

History of presenting complaint
- **Quality of life.** Allow her time to explain in her own words how she experiences the pain and what it means to her. How has the pain affected her day-to-day life?
- **Last menstrual period.** Check and record the date of her last menstrual period, in order to calculate the gestation. Was the last period normal?
- **Pregnancy test.** When did she have a positive pregnancy test?
- **History of the current pregnancy.** Are there any unexplored issues with regard to this pregnancy? Multiple pregnancy increases the risk of pre-term labour.
- **Trauma.** Both minor and major abdominal trauma may lead to placental abruption.
- **Vaginal bleeding.** If present, what is the colour and consistency of her blood loss? It can be difficult to distinguish blood clots from products of conception. Has the bleeding stopped or is it ongoing?
- **Vaginal discharge.** Consider pre-term labour if there is vaginal discharge or a bloodstained 'show' together with uterine contractions. In addition, there may be a sudden watery discharge, suggesting premature rupture of membranes.
- **Urinary symptoms.** Due to urinary stasis and vesicoureteric reflux, urinary tract infection is common in pregnancy, and typical symptoms such as frequency of urine or dysuria may be absent. Consider pyelonephritis if there is loin pain in association with fever, nausea, vomiting and malaise.
- **Bowel symptoms.** Constipation is a common problem in pregnancy and may present with lower back pain. Haemorrhoids may cause rectal bleeding.

- **Foetal movements.** Take any reduction in foetal movements seriously.
- **Emotional state.** How does the woman feel emotionally? Does she need further support?

Common symptom presentations

- **Round ligament pain.** Mild intermittent chronic pain in the groin or around the symphysis pubis is commonly round ligament pain and is harmless.
- **Ectopic pregnancy.** Severe colicky or constant pain in early pregnancy points towards ectopic pregnancy, particularly if it is lateral to the midline and associated with vaginal bleeding.
- **Braxton Hicks contractions.** In later pregnancy, from 24 weeks onwards, mild niggling pains indicate Braxton Hicks contractions.
- **Pre-term labour.** Pre-term labour may be the cause of pain if uterine contractions are regular with increasing pressure in the lower back or perineum.
- **Urinary tract infection.** Consider urinary tract infection if there is groin or suprapubic pain, which may radiate into the loin, particularly when associated with urinary symptoms and malaise.
- **Placental abruption.** Constant and severe pain together with a rigid uterus and vaginal bleeding suggests placental abruption.
- **Appendicitis.** Acute appendicitis is the most common nonobstetric cause of pain in pregnancy. Pain may be felt above the right iliac fossa due to the uterus displacing the appendix upwards towards the right upper quadrant.
- **Pre-eclampsia.** Consider pre-eclampsia if there is epigastric pain in association with headaches, oedema, visual disturbance, raised blood pressure and proteinuria.

Past and ongoing medical problems

- **Obstetric and gynaecological problems.** One or more previous caesarean sections increase the risk of uterine rupture, which in some cases may occur before the onset of labour. Uterine fibroids may twist (torsion) or degenerate, leading to abdominal pain.
- **STI.** Chlamydia infection may cause pelvic inflammatory disease.
- **Abdominal surgery.** Appendicitis and cholecystitis can be ruled out if the woman has had appendicectomy or cholecystectomy. Any abdominal surgery may lead to adhesions.
- **Ovarian cyst.** Does the woman have a known ovarian cyst?

Medication

- **Regular drugs.** Does the woman take any regular drugs that it is important to know about, in case she requires surgery?

Social history

- **Home situation.** Does she have a supportive partner or other relatives?

Smoking

- **Smoking history.** Smoking increases her risk of pre-term labour.

Review of previous investigations

- **Ultrasound.** Has she had any ultrasound scans in this pregnancy to check the viability of the foetus? Has the foetus grown normally?
- **Blood group and rhesus status.** In rhesus-negative women, anti-D immunoglobulin may need to be given if there is bleeding.

Examination

General

- **General condition.** Does she look unwell or pale? Is she in severe pain? Consider abdominal cramps if she is rolling around in pain. Peritonism causes patients to lie very still with their knees bent.
- **Oedema.** Consider pre-eclampsia if there is leg or generalised oedema.

Vital signs

- **Temperature.** Consider urinary tract infection or pyelonephritis if there is a fever.
- **Pulse.** A heart rate >100 beats per minute suggest impending shock or severe anxiety. Shock that is out of proportion to vaginal bleeding indicates placental abruption.
- **Blood pressure.** Check for postural hypotension. Blood pressure will usually be maintained unless there is significant blood loss. Consider pre-eclampsia if blood pressure is raised.

Abdomen

- **Palpation.** Check for guarding, tenderness and signs of peritonism. Unilateral lower abdominal tenderness suggests ectopic pregnancy in women <14 weeks pregnant. Are there any masses? Consider appendicitis if there is tenderness over McBurney's point. Check fundal height, lie, presentation and foetal heart rate. A rigid tender uterus suggests placental abruption or uterine rupture.
- **Foetal heart rate.** Check foetal heart sounds using a Pinard stethoscope or, preferably, a handheld ultrasound (Doppler), if available.
- **Bimanual vaginal examination.** This is not usually necessary at the first assessment if the woman is going to be referred to an early pregnancy assessment unit. Be aware that pelvic examination can cause rupture of an ectopic pregnancy or massive haemorrhage in underlying placenta praevia. If you examine, check whether the uterus is of appropriate size for dates. The cervical os in a multiparous woman should only admit the tip of a finger. There may be cervical excitation in ectopic pregnancy. Also, vaginal examination should not be performed in primary care if there is suspected premature rupture of membranes.
- **Speculum.** Check whether the cervical os is open. Are any products of conception visible? Is any bleeding coming from the uterus or the cervix itself?

Limbs

- **Reflexes.** Reflexes may be brisk in pre-eclampsia.

Bedside tests
- **Pregnancy test.** Perform a pregnancy test in every woman of childbearing age who presents with abdominal pain and vaginal bleeding.
- **Urine dipstick.** Consider pre-eclampsia if there is proteinuria. Check for nitrites, leucocytes, blood and protein (urinary tract infection).

Key references and further reading

1. Albert H, Godskesen M, Westergard J. Prognosis in four syndromes of pregnancy-related pelvic pain. *Acta Obstet Gynecol Scand* 2001;80:505–510.
2. Gray J, Wardrope J, Fothergill DJ. Abdominal pain, abdominal pain in women, complications of pregnancy and labour. *Emerg Med J* 2004;21:606–613.
3. Mol BW, Hajenius PJ, Engelsbel S et al. Should patients who are suspected of having an ectopic pregnancy undergo physical examination? *Fertil Steril* 1999;71:155–157.
4. National Institute for Health and Care Excellence (NICE). Ectopic pregnancy. Clinical knowledge summaries. 2013. Available from: http://cks.nice.org.uk/ectopic-pregnancy (last accessed 29 April 2016).
5. National Institute for Health and Care Excellence (NICE). Miscarriage. Clinical knowledge summaries. 2013. Available from: http://cks.nice.org.uk/miscarriage (last accessed 29 April 2016).

Pre-eclampsia

Key thoughts

Practical points

- **Epidemiology.** Pre-eclampsia is the most common medical complication of pregnancy.
- **Diagnosis.** Early identification of key risk factors is important in preventing eclampsia, which may develop in about 1% of women with pre-eclampsia and is life-threatening.
- **Prognosis.** Severe pre-eclampsia can cause serious complications and even death in both the mother and the baby. The risk is greatly reduced if pre-eclampsia is diagnosed and treated early. The only 'cure' is delivery of the baby.

Risk factors and indications for specialist referral

- Primigravida.
- 10 years or more since the birth of the last baby.
- Previous pre-eclampsia.
- Age under 20 or over 35 years.
- Multiple pregnancy with twins or triplets.
- Obesity.
- Family history of pre-eclampsia.
- Hypertension prior to pregnancy.
- Diabetes.
- SLE.
- Chronic kidney disease.

RED FLAGS

- Severe headaches
- Blurred vision and other visual problems
- New epigastric or right upper quadrant pain
- Vomiting
- Breathlessness
- Sudden swelling of face, hands or feet
- Vaginal bleeding
- New hypertension
- New proteinuria
- Malaise
- Reduced foetal movements
- Foetus small for gestational age

The 10-Minute Clinical Assessment, Second Edition. Knut Schroeder.
© 2017 John Wiley & Sons, Ltd. Published 2017 by John Wiley & Sons, Ltd.

History

Ideas, concerns and expectations
- **Ideas.** What does the woman know about the symptoms and signs of pre-eclampsia? Does she understand the implications of delayed detection and treatment?
- **Concerns.** Is she worried about the outcome of the pregnancy for any particular reason?
- **Expectations.** Why has she come to see you?

History of presenting complaint
- **Quality of life.** Allow her time to explain her symptoms in her own words. How far has day-to-day life been affected?
- **Onset.** Pre-eclampsia develops after 20 weeks of pregnancy.
- **Blood pressure and proteinuria.** Check whether blood pressure and urine have been monitored and whether there have been abnormal readings in the past. Knowing her booking blood pressure is important, as a substantial rise from a low pressure may be significant, even if the absolute level would not raise concerns.
- **Symptoms of pre-eclampsia.** Pre-eclampsia may be entirely asymptomatic. Ask about headaches (increasing frequency and unrelieved by regular analgesics), blurred vision and other visual problems, such as flashing lights, double vision and floating spots. Is there persistent new epigastric pain or pain in the right upper quadrant? Has she vomited? Is she breathless? Malaise is common. Ask about leg swelling, which also occurs in normal pregnancies but usually worsens in pre-eclampsia. Also ask about any swelling of the face or hands.
- **HELLP syndrome.** HELLP stands for 'haemolysis, elevated liver enzymes and low platelets'. Is this suggested by any of the woman's recent blood tests?
- **Specialist input.** Has she already been referred to and seen a specialist for further assessment and management? Relevant letters and reports in the case notes may provide useful information.
- **Foetal health.** Does she feel foetal movements? Is the infant small for gestational age? Pre-eclampsia poses an increased risk of stillbirth.
- **Bleeding.** Severe placental haemorrhage is an important complication.

Past and ongoing medical problems
- **Chronic conditions.** Women with pre-existing hypertension, kidney disease, diabetes or antiphospholipid antibodies should normally be referred for further specialist assessment and shared care.

Medication
- **Antihypertensives.** Does she take any blood pressure-lowering medication?
- **Aspirin and calcium.** These may help prevent pre-eclampsia in some women.

Review of previous investigations
- **Full blood count.** Look out for low platelets (HELLP).
- **Liver function tests.** Raised live function tests suggest liver involvement (HELLP).
- **Renal function.** Look out for any deterioration in renal function and raised creatinine.

Examination

General
- **General condition.** Does she look unwell? Is there any clinical evidence that she may have had a stroke? Is she vomiting? Does she look puffy?

Vital signs
- **Blood pressure.** Normal blood pressure is below 140/90 mmHg. Higher readings (particularly if >160/100 mmHg) or a substantial rise in blood pressure from a booking pressure +90 mmHg will require urgent action. Most women with high blood pressure in pregnancy do not have pre-eclampsia but are at risk.

Head and neck
- **Eyes.** Check for papilloedema.

Chest
- **Lungs.** Check for signs of pulmonary oedema.

Abdomen
- **Epigastrium.** Check for epigastric tenderness.
- **Bleeding.** Is there evidence of vaginal blood loss?
- **Foetal heart.** Check foetal heart rate, either with a Pinard stethoscope or, preferably, with a handheld ultrasound (Doppler).
- **Uterus.** Is there uterine tenderness or evidence of contractions?

Upper and lower limbs
- **Oedema.** Check for peripheral oedema in the hands or feet.
- **Reflexes.** Look out for hyperreflexia with brisk tendon reflexes.

Bedside tests
- **Urine dipstick.** Check for proteinuria $\geq$ '+' (300 mg/l) on dipstick testing.

Key references and further reading
1. Duckitt K, Harrington D. Risk factors for pre-eclampsia at antenatal booking: a systematic review of controlled studies. *BMJ* 2005;330:565–567.
2. Lelia D, Meher S, Abalos E. Management of pre-eclampsia. *BMJ* 2006;332: 463–468.

3. Milne F, Redman C, Walker J et al. The preeclampsia community guideline (PRE-COG): how to screen for and detect onset of pre-eclampsia in the community. *BMJ* 2005;330:576–580.

4. National Institute for Health and Care Excellence (NICE). Antenatal care: uncomplicated pregnancy. Clinical knowledge summaries. 2011. Available from: http://cks.nice.org.uk/antenatal-care-uncomplicated-pregnancy (last accessed 29 April 2016).

Urology and renal medicine

Suspected urinary tract infection in women

Key thoughts

Practical points
- **Quality of life.** Urinary symptoms can be very bothersome and can severely affect quality of life.
- **Diagnosis.** Important causes are urinary tract infection, other bladder conditions and sexually transmitted infections (STIs).
- **Prognosis.** Most urinary tract infections are uncomplicated, but in severe or prolonged symptoms it is important to identify serious underlying causes (e.g. cancer, pyelonephritis).

Differential diagnosis
- Urinary tract infection.
- STI.
- Renal stone disease.
- Cancer.
- Pregnancy.
- Menopausal vaginal atrophy.

Important risk factors
- Sexual intercourse ('honeymoon cystitis').
- Structural urological disease.
- Wiping the bottom from back to front.

> ### RED FLAGS
>
> - Possibility of pregnancy
> - Recurrent or persistent symptoms
> - Haematuria
> - Systemic symptoms

History

Ideas, concerns and expectations
- **Ideas.** What does she believe to be the underlying cause?
- **Concerns.** Worries about cancer or STI are common.

The 10-Minute Clinical Assessment, Second Edition. Knut Schroeder.
© 2017 John Wiley & Sons, Ltd. Published 2017 by John Wiley & Sons, Ltd.

- **Expectations.** Many women will mainly come for symptom relief but may also expect further investigation.

History of presenting complaint
- **Quality of life.** What has been the effect of symptoms on her quality of life and day-to-day activities?
- **Frequency.** Most people urinate on average around six times a day.
- **Dysuria and urgency.** Lower urinary tract symptoms such as dysuria and urgency are common in cystitis and urethritis.
- **Strangury.** Ask about painful and slow urination, which is caused by muscular spasms of the bladder or urethra.
- **Haematuria.** Haematuria is common in urinary tract infection and usually settles with antibiotic therapy. Haematuria may also occur with renal stones, bladder cancer and schistosomiasis and will often require further investigation for confirmation of the diagnosis.
- **Pain.** Suprapubic pain is common in cystitis. Also ask about lower abdominal and loin pain, which can have bladder as well as renal causes.
- **Offensive urine.** Urine often has an offensive smell in urinary tract infection.
- **Systemic symptoms.** Fever, vomiting, rigors in association with loin pain, haematuria and general malaise may indicate pyelonephritis, particularly if these symptoms develop quickly.
- **Pregnancy.** Ascending infection is more common in pregnancy. Pregnancy limits the choice of antibiotics.
- **Travel.** Consider the possibility of schistosomiasis if the patient has been swimming in freshwater lakes where schistosomiasis is endemic.
- **Vaginal discharge.** Consider STI or vaginitis with *Trichomonas* or *Candida albicans* if there is vaginal discharge or a history of unprotected sexual intercourse with an infected partner. Has there been a recent change of partner? Ask about any vulval inflammation.

Past and current medical problems
- **Urinary tract infections.** Consider the possibility of bladder stones, hydronephrosis, atonic bladder or cancer if there are recurrent urinary tract infections.
- **Diabetes.** Recurrent urinary tract infections are more common in people with diabetes.
- **Interstitial cystitis.** This may be present if there is urinary urgency, frequency or pain for at least 6 months without the diagnosis of an underlying cause.
- **Surgery.** Ask about any past surgery (e.g. laparotomy, pelvic floor repair).

Medication
- **Antibiotics.** Have any antibiotics been taken recently for urinary tract infection or other infections? If so, have they been effective? Prematurely stopped courses of antibiotics may have led to resistance of organisms.

- **Oral contraceptive.** If the patient takes the combined oral contraceptive pill, make her aware that this may become less effective if she decides to take antibiotics and that she will need to take extra precautions (7-day rule).
- **Other treatments.** Ask about fluid intake, analgesics and use of alkaline salts (potassium citrate, bicarbonate of soda).

Allergies
- **Antibiotics.** Ask about allergies to antibiotics that are commonly used for the treatment of urinary tract infections, such as trimethoprim and nitrofurantoin.

Family history
- **Bladder cancer.** Is there a family history of bladder cancer?

Social history
- **Occupation.** Is the patient exposed to any occupational toxins that are risk factors for bladder cancer (e.g. some dyes)?

Alcohol and smoking
- **Smoking.** There is an increased risk of bladder cancer in people who smoke.

Review of previous investigations
- **Urine microscopy and culture.** Check for urinary tract infections and sensitivities. Urinary tract infection (especially when low-grade) may be present in the presence of normal urine microscopy. If the history is suggestive of infection, treatment may be worthwhile even if a midstream urine microscopy and culture are negative.
- **STIs.** Check whether the patient has been screened for STIs, particularly if symptoms are recurrent or unusual.
- **Blood tests.** A raised white cell count and inflammatory markers may show signs of infection. Abnormal urea and electrolytes may indicate underlying renal disease or electrolyte abnormality. Raised blood glucose will indicate diabetes. Blood tests are not usually needed in uncomplicated urinary tract infection but can be helpful if symptoms are persistent or serious.

Examination

General
- **General condition.** Suspect pyelonephritis if she is generally unwell.

Vital signs
- **Temperature.** Fever suggests infection, which may be high and persistent in pyelonephritis.

Abdomen
- **Tenderness.** Palpate the abdomen for any suprapubic tenderness. Loin tenderness may suggest pyelonephritis.
- **Masses.** Check for any renal masses that might indicate tumour.

Bedside tests
- **Urine dipstick.** The presence of leucocytes, nitrite and red blood cells suggests urinary tract infection. The validity of dipstick testing is still debated, as a negative dipstick cannot reliably rule out an infection when the pre-test likelihood is high.
- **Pregnancy test.** Always perform a pregnancy test if there is a possibility that she might be pregnant. Early pregnancy commonly presents with features suggestive of urinary tract infection.
- **Blood glucose.** Test the blood or urine for glucose in recurrent urinary tract infections.

Key references and further reading

1. Bent S, Nallamothu BK, Simel DL et al. The rational clinical examination: does this woman have an acute uncomplicated urinary tract infection? *JAMA* 2002;287:2701–2710.
2. Car J. Urinary tract infection in women: diagnosis and management in primary care. *BMJ* 2006;332:94–97.
3. Fahey T, Webb E, Montgomery AA, Heyderman RS. Clinical management of urinary tract infection in women: a prospective cohort study. *Fam Pract* 2003;20:1–6.
4. Hanno PM. The diagnosis of interstitial cystitis revisited: lessons learned from the National Institutes of Health interstitial cystitis database study. *J Urol* 1999;161:553–557.
5. Little P, Turner S, Rumsby K et al. Developing clinical rules to predict urinary tract infection in primary care settings: sensitivity and specificity of near patient tests (dipsticks) and clinical scores. *Br J Gen Pract* 2006;56:606–612.
6. National Institute for Health and Care Excellence (NICE). Urinary tract infection (lower) – woman. Clinical knowledge summaries. 2015. Available from: http://cks.nice.org.uk/urinary-tract-infection-lower-women (last accessed 29 April 2016).

Lower urinary tract symptoms in men

Key thoughts

Practical points
- **Quality of life.** Urinary symptoms can be very bothersome and may severely affect quality of life.
- **Diagnosis.** Benign prostatic hyperplasia is common but can be impossible to distinguish from prostatic cancer on clinical grounds alone. Both may coexist, but benign prostatic hyperplasia does not predispose to cancer.

Possible causes
- Drugs (e.g. diuretics).
- Cystitis.
- Urethritis.
- Nocturnal polyuria.
- Benign prostatic hyperplasia.
- Diabetes mellitus.
- Sexually transmitted disease (urethritis and prostatitis).
- Urethral stricture.
- Renal stone disease.
- Prostate cancer.
- Bladder, rectal and renal cancer.

Important risk factors
- Family history of prostate cancer at a young age.
- Age.

> **RED FLAGS SUGGESTING POSSIBLE CANCER**
>
> - Persistent microscopic or macroscopic haematuria
> - Pelvic pain
> - Systemic symptoms, including fever, weight loss and night sweats
> - Bone pain
> - Severe symptoms affecting the quality of life
> - Incontinence
> - Unexplained erectile dysfunction or bone or back pain
> - Persistent dysuria with negative cultures
> - Persistent sterile pyuria or recurrent urinary infections
> - Abnormal rectal examination
> - Raised prostate-specific antigen (PSA)

The 10-Minute Clinical Assessment, Second Edition. Knut Schroeder.
© 2017 John Wiley & Sons, Ltd. Published 2017 by John Wiley & Sons, Ltd.

History

Ideas, concerns and expectations
- **Ideas.** What does the patient think is causing the urinary symptoms?
- **Concerns.** The principal worry in men with lower urinary tract symptoms is prostate cancer. Lower urinary tract symptoms are often under-reported, and it is worth asking about these opportunistically.
- **Expectations.** Why has he come to see you? Common reasons for consultation are exclusion of prostate cancer and treatment of symptoms.

History of presenting complaint
- **Quality of life.** In what way is quality of life affected, and what are the most bothersome symptoms?
- **Onset.** Acute onset of symptoms is common in infection, whereas chronic symptoms point towards benign prostatic hyperplasia or cancer, particularly if symptoms are progressing.
- **Voiding symptoms.** Symptoms such as hesitancy, poor or intermittent flow and straining indicate outflow obstruction.
- **Storage and post-micturition symptoms.** Ask about incontinence, urgency, frequency, nocturia, intermittency, terminal dribbling and a feeling of incomplete emptying. Consider calculating the International Prostate Symptom Score (IPSS; see http://patient.info/doctor/international-prostate-symptom-score-i-pss). Frequency and nocturia are common in diabetes. Incontinence and chronic retention may occur in neurological disease.
- **Nocturnal polyuria.** How often does the patient have to get up at night to urinate? Nocturia may be the only presenting feature in early congestive heart failure. Ask about fluid intake (type of fluid and timing) and consider diabetes, adverse drug effects, heart failure and neurological disease.
- **Urine volume.** Ask about times and volumes of bladder emptying. A flow-volume chart drawn up over a few days may provide useful information about the pattern and severity of urinary problems. A standard kitchen jug specially bought for the purpose can be useful in recording urine volumes. If more than one-third of urine is passed at night, this may suggest nocturnal polyuria rather than bladder outflow obstruction.
- **Haematuria.** Haematuria may suggest renal stone disease, haemorrhagic cystitis or urological cancer.
- **Pain.** Is there any pelvic, perineal or lower back pain, which may occur in metastatic prostate cancer? Ask about any bone pain anywhere in the body.
- **Sexual function.** Explore any problems with sexual function, such as erectile dysfunction, loss of libido or premature/delayed ejaculation. Is there any pain on ejaculation or haematospermia?
- **Self-management.** Has fluid restriction and a reduction in caffeine-containing drinks been tried or considered?
- **Associated features.** Systemic symptoms, such as weight loss, fever and night sweats, may indicate cancer.

Past and current medical problems
- **Urological disease.** Ask about any previous urological problems. Renal stones commonly recur.
- **Systemic disease.** Chronic conditions, such as diabetes, multiple sclerosis and heart failure, may cause urological symptoms.

Medication
- **Diuretics.** Diuretics commonly cause frequency of urine and nocturia.
- **Warfarin or aspirin.** These drugs by themselves do not cause haematuria, but they may contribute to early presentation of urological cancers.
- **Antimuscarinic drugs.** Drugs such as amitriptyline may cause lower urinary tract symptoms.
- **Alpha 1 blockers and 5-α-reductase inhibitors.** Have these been used in the past or is the patient taking these at the moment? Ask about how effective the treatment is and whether there have been any adverse effects.

Other treatments
- **Urological treatments.** Ask about any previous urological operations or interventions.

Allergies
- **Antibiotics.** Ask about any allergies to antibiotics that might need to be used for the treatment of infection.

Family history
- **Urological disease.** Ask about a family history of urological or renal disease.

Social history
- **Nature of past and present occupations.** Occupational exposure to toxins may contribute to the development of bladder cancer (e.g. industrial dyes).
- **Domestic and marital relationships.** Are there any relationship problems resulting from the nocturia or erectile dysfunction?

Alcohol, smoking and recreational drugs
- **Smoking.** Smoking is a risk factor for bladder cancer.

Review of previous investigations
- **Blood.** Check for results from a full blood count (infection, cancer) and renal function. Check for previous hyperglycaemia (diabetes).
- **Imaging.** Are results available from previous ultrasound, computerised tomography (CT) or intravenous urogram imaging?

- **PSA.** A PSA that is raised for the patient's age or is rising may indicate prostate cancer. Other reasons for an elevated PSA include infection (prostatitis can elevate PSA for 4 weeks following treatment), ejaculation, digital rectal examination and vigorous exercise within the preceding 2 days.
- **Urine culture and microscopy.** Persistent dysuria with negative cultures may occur in bladder cancer or tuberculosis.

Examination

General
- **General condition.** General malaise may suggest infection. Consider malignancy if the patient looks cachectic.

Abdomen
- **Genitals.** Check for a tight phimosis or meatal stenosis.
- **Palpation.** Check for any loin or abdominal masses that might have a urological origin. A palpable bladder suggests urinary retention.
- **Rectal examination.** A nodular, enlarged or firm prostate may indicate prostatic hypertrophy or cancer. Be aware that digital rectal examination lacks sensitivity and specificity and may be entirely normal even if prostate cancer is present.

Lower back
- **Spine.** Examine the spine for range of movement and tenderness if there is a history of back pain. Always consider the possibility of cord compression or metastasis from prostate cancer if symptoms are severe or persistent.

Bedside tests
- **Urinalysis.** Check urine for blood, glucose, protein, leucocytes and nitrites.

Key references and further reading
1. Bosch JL, Hop WC, Kirkels WJ, Schroder FH. The International Prostate Symptom Score in a community-based sample of men between 55 and 74 years of age: prevalence and correlation of symptoms with age, prostate volume, flow rate and residual urine volume. *Br J Urol* 1995;75:622–630.
2. Hamilton W, Sharp D. Symptomatic diagnosis of prostate cancer in primary care: a structured review. *Br J Gen Pract* 2004;617–621.
3. Hamilton W, Sharp D, Peters TJ, Round AP. Clinical features of prostate cancer before diagnosis: a population-based case control study. *Br J Gen Pract* 2006;56:756–762.
4. National Institute for Health and Care Excellence (NICE). Urinary tract infection (lower) – men. Clinical knowledge summaries. 2014. Available from: http://cks.nice.org.uk/urinary-tract-infection-lower-men (last accessed 29 April 2016).

5. National Institute for Health and Care Excellence (NICE). Suspected cancer: recognition and referral. NICE guidelines [NG12]. June 2015. Available from: http://www.nice.org.uk/guidance/ng12 (last accessed 29 April 2016).
6. Wilt TJ, Thompson IM. Clinical review: clinically localised prostate cancer. *BMJ* 2006;333:1102–1106.

Urinary incontinence

Key thoughts

Practical points
- **Diagnosis.** Try and identify the underlying cause and assess bladder function.
- **Prognosis.** Differentiate between benign and serious underlying conditions.
- **Quality of life.** Urinary incontinence can be very distressing and may severely affect the quality of life. Explore the effect of symptoms on the patient's daily routines.

Differential diagnosis
- Urge incontinence.
- Overflow incontinence.
- Stress incontinence.

Important risk factors
- In women, vaginal delivery with damage to the pelvic floor.
- Underlying renal disease.
- Urinary tract infection.
- Neurological disease.
- Older age.
- Cognitive impairment.
- Enlarged prostate in men and pelvic tumours in women.

RED FLAGS
- Microscopic haematuria, if aged >50 years
- Recurrent or persistent urinary tract infection associated with haematuria, if aged >40 years
- Severely impaired quality of life
- Progressive symptoms
- Haematuria
- History of cancer
- Raised PSA in men
- Persistent bladder or urethral pain
- Faecal incontinence
- Suspected neurological disease
- Previous pelvic cancer surgery
- Previous continence surgery
- Previous pelvic radiation therapy

The 10-Minute Clinical Assessment, Second Edition. Knut Schroeder.
© 2017 John Wiley & Sons, Ltd. Published 2017 by John Wiley & Sons, Ltd.

- Urogenital fistulae
- Suspected malignant mass

History

Ideas, concerns and expectations
- **Ideas.** What does the patient think is causing incontinence?
- **Concerns.** Many patients find it difficult to mention incontinence unless the problem is severe.
- **Expectations.** Why has the patient come to see you? Help with improving symptoms and specialist referral are common reasons for consultation.

History of presenting complaint
- **Quality of life.** Incontinence can be extremely distressing and may severely impact on home life, work and social interaction.
- **Onset and duration.** When did the problems start and how quickly did they develop? Are urinary symptoms getting worse?
- **Incontinence.** How much urine is lost involuntarily? What are the circumstances in which incontinence occurs? Does the patient have to use pads or other continence aids? How many do they get through in 24 hours?
- **Urinary symptoms.** Find out which urinary symptoms are most bothersome. Ask about frequency of micturition during the day and at night and how often the patient is incontinent. Is there any warning? Is there any pain or discomfort on passing urine? Has the patient noticed any blood in the urine?
- **Fluid intake.** What types and quantities of fluid are being consumed, and at what times? Alcohol- and caffeine-containing drinks can cause urgency and problems with incontinence.
- **Bowels.** Constipation and, in particular, faecal impaction can lead to urinary incontinence.
- **Mobility.** Problems with mobility (e.g. due to arthritis) can make it difficult for people to get to the toilet in time.
- **Obstetric history (in females).** How many vaginal deliveries has the patient had? Were there any obstetric problems at the time (e.g. instrumental delivery)?
- **Use of continence aids.** Disposable pads and washable pants are often used initially. Find out what products the patient has tried. Pocket-size urinals that fold away into a hard plastic case are available. Penile sheaths can be useful unless the penis is very small or the patient suffers from confusion. Intermittent self-catheterisation may be helpful if bladder emptying is incomplete. Indwelling urethral catheters may also be used, but they carry an increased risk of infection.

Common symptom patterns
- **Stress incontinence.** Is there involuntary leakage of urine on effort or exertion or on sneezing or coughing? Prostatectomy is a common reason for stress

incontinence in men. Consider a structural abnormality if there is evidence of urine infection, such as a vaginal or rectal prolapse, urethral stricture, stone disease or a bladder diverticulum. Check for evidence of an enlarged prostate and bladder or prostate cancer in men.

- **Urge incontinence.** Ask about storage symptoms, such as urgency, frequency, urge incontinence and nocturia. Overactive bladder presents with a triad of frequency, urgency and nocturia. It occurs in men in the absence of obstruction and is often mistaken as being caused by prostate enlargement. Detrusor instability may also be secondary to obstruction and can cause urge incontinence. Are there voiding symptoms, such as hesitancy, poor stream or terminal dribble? Problems may result from an enlarged prostate or a neurological cause, such as stroke, diabetic neuropathy, Parkinson's, Alzheimer's or spinal cord disease.
- **Overflow incontinence.** Nocturnal incontinence together with a tense bladder may suggest high-pressure chronic retention due to obstructive uropathy. In low-pressure chronic retention, there tends to be much less bladder discomfort. Neurological conditions, such as multiple sclerosis and spinal disease, may cause a hypotonic bladder.

Past and current medical problems

- **Urogenital problems.** Ask about any personal history of urogenital problems, particularly any structural abnormalities.
- **Diabetes mellitus.** Diabetes may cause incontinence due to autonomic neuropathy and polyuria.
- **Prostatectomy (men only).** Various mechanisms may lead to incontinence after prostatectomy.
- **Cardiovascular disease (CVD).** Diuretics used in the management of heart failure or hypertension commonly cause frequency of urine and may lead to incontinence.

Medication

- **Alpha blockers.** These can be useful in the symptomatic treatment of bladder instability and may improve continence. Ask about any adverse effects, particularly postural hypotension and problems with sexual function.
- **Anticholinergics.** Anticholinergics are useful for treating symptoms of overactive bladder and can also be used to treat storage symptoms associated with prostatic enlargement. The risk of precipitating urinary retention is much lower than was previously thought, provided the patient does not have severe voiding symptoms (e.g. markedly reduced flow).
- **5-α reductase inhibitors.** In men, these may help with reducing prostate volume. They can take up to 6 months to achieve a relatively small effect on urine flow and other urinary symptoms, but may be beneficial in the longer term. Ask about any sexual problems, which are a common adverse effect.
- **Diuretics.** Check whether the patient takes diuretics, which commonly cause urinary symptoms, particularly urinary frequency.

Allergies
- **Antibiotics.** Ask about any allergies to antibiotics, in case there is underlying urinary tract infection requiring treatment.

Family history
- **Renal disease.** Ask about a history of structural renal or other urogenital conditions.

Social history
- **Home and social life.** Social life is often affected by the symptoms. Patients with incontinence may be embarrassed about the smell of urine or by urinary frequency and urgency.
- **Domestic and marital relationships.** Have the problems affected close relationships or the patient's sex life?
- **Work.** Have there been any problems with work? Incontinence can be particularly troublesome if access to toilets is difficult (e.g. drivers).

Alcohol, smoking and recreational drugs
- **Alcohol.** Ask for details about past and present alcohol intake.
- **Caffeine.** Is there excessive caffeine intake?

Review of previous investigations
- **Bladder chart.** A bladder chart recording dates and times of continent and incontinent episodes, as well as fluid intake and urine output, can be useful.
- **Urea, creatinine, electrolytes and estimated glomerular filtration rate (eGFR).** Check whether renal function is normal.
- **Fasting blood glucose.** Has diabetes been excluded?
- **Peak urinary flow rate.** A reduced rate may indicate urinary outflow obstruction.
- **Urine dipstick and midstream specimen of urine (MSU).** Urine dipstick and microscopy/culture of MSU are useful first-line investigations.
- **Ultrasound.** This can be helpful in detecting and estimating any residual urine in the bladder.
- **Urodynamics.** This may be useful in selected cases.
- **PSA.** In men, a raised PSA may suggest benign prostatic hyperplasia or prostate cancer, but PSA can also be raised in urinary tract infection or prostatitis, or after digital rectal examination.

Examination

General
- **General condition.** Cachexia and pallor may suggest underlying malignancy or chronic illness.

- **Mental state.** Are there any obvious cognitive problems? Does the patient appear depressed?
- **Mobility.** Are there any obvious mobility problems?

Vital signs
- **Temperature.** A raised temperature suggests underlying infection.
- **Blood pressure.** Raised blood pressure may indicate renal disease or hypertension. Check for postural hypotension if there are problems with dizziness due to medication.

Abdomen
- **Masses.** Palpate carefully for any abdominal or renal masses.
- **Genitals.** In men, check carefully for any structural abnormalities, such as obvious meatal stenosis or phimosis.
- **Bladder.** Percuss and palpate for an enlarged bladder, which may indicate overflow incontinence. A tense bladder suggests high-pressure retention, whereas a non-irritable enlarged bladder may be caused by low-pressure chronic retention due to a failing detrusor muscle. An enlarged hypotonic bladder may have neurological causes.
- **Pelvic examination.** In women, check for atrophic vaginitis, prolapse and any pelvic masses.
- **Rectal examination.** In men, feel the prostate gland for enlargement and nodules, which may suggest benign prostatic hypertrophy or prostate cancer. Hard lumps of faeces may suggest faecal impaction or severe constipation.

Lower limbs
- **Neurology.** Check tone, power, sensation, coordination and reflexes if there is the possibility of an underlying neurological cause.

Bedside tests
- **Urine dipstick.** Check for glucose, blood, protein, nitrites and leucocytes (urinary tract infection).

Key references and further reading
1. Lavelle J, Karram M, Chu F et al. Management of incontinence for family practice physicians. *Am J Med* 2006;119:375–405.
2. Matza LS, Zyczynski TM, Bavendam T. A review of quality-of-life questionnaires for urinary incontinence and overactive bladder: which ones to use and why? *Curr Urol Rep* 2004;5:336–342.
3. National Institute for Health and Care Excellence (NICE). Urinary incontinence in women: management. NICE guidelines [CG171]. September 2013. Available from: http://www.nice.org.uk/guidance/cg171 (last accessed 29 April 2016).
4. National Institute for Health and Care Excellence (NICE). Incontinence – urinary, in women. Clinical knowledge summaries. 2015. Available from:

http://cks.nice.org.uk/incontinence-urinary-in-women (last accessed 29 April 2016).

5. Stoddart H, Donovan J, Whiteley E et al. Urinary incontinence in older people in the community: a neglected problem? *Br J Gen Pract* 2001;51:548–552.

6. Thüroff J, Abrams P, Andersson KE et al. EAU guidelines on urinary incontinence. November 2010. Available from: http://uroweb.org/wp-content/uploads/EurUrolarticle_31012011.pdf (last accessed 29 April 2016).

Urethral discharge in men

Key thoughts

Practical points
- **Diagnosis.** STIs (particularly chlamydia) are common and may only lead to mild and intermittent symptoms. Gonorrhoea is on the increase in some parts of the world.

Possible causes
- Physiological discharge.
- STI (e.g. chlamydia, gonorrhoea).
- Intraurethral infection.
- Physical or chemical injury.
- Urinary tract infection.
- Candidal balanitis.
- Urethral malignanc.

Important risk factors

- Human immunodeficiency virus (HIV) infection.
- Sexually activity.
- Unprotected vaginal sex.
- Multiple sexual partners.
- Diabetes mellitus.
- Age <35 years.
- Living in a city.
- Recent partner change.

RED FLAGS

- Systemic features
- Arthritis
- Fertility problems
- Testicular pain
- Exposure to HIV

History

Ideas, concerns and expectations
- **Ideas.** What does the patient think is the cause of the discharge?
- **Concerns.** Worries about STI or cancer are common.

The 10-Minute Clinical Assessment, Second Edition. Knut Schroeder.
© 2017 John Wiley & Sons, Ltd. Published 2017 by John Wiley & Sons, Ltd.

- **Expectations.** Why has the patient come to see you? Common reasons for consultation are reassurance and finding out the cause of symptoms.

History of presenting complaint

- **Nature of discharge.** Ask about the amount and colour of the discharge. Clear mucoid discharge is common on sexual arousal and is completely normal and benign. Yellow discharge may indicate gonococcal infection, whereas discharge due to chlamydia usually looks a bit thinner and clearer. Candidal discharge tends to be curd-like and white.
- **Risk of STI.** Carefully explore whether the patient is at risk of an STI. Find out whether he is sexually active and if he has had a recent change in sexual partner. Does he have more than one sexual partner? Are they male or female, or both? Do any of his sexual partners suffer knowingly from STI? Has he had sex with partner from a high-risk population (e.g. while abroad)? Does he use condoms? Does he engage in oral or anal sex? Has he ever or recently been seen at a genitourinary clinic?
- **Onset.** Discharge due to gonorrhoea occurs within about 7 days. In chlamydial infection, symptoms may take a few weeks to develop. Recurrent infections may be caused by herpes simplex infection or candidiasis, which is more common in people with diabetes.
- **Urinary symptoms.** Ask about any burning or pain when passing urine. This is often caused by urethritis, whereas candidal balanitis causes an itchy soreness of the foreskin or glans. Occasionally, urethral discharge may be caused by urinary tract infection, in which case other symptoms may be present, such as frequency of micturition, fever, suprapubic or loin pain and haematuria.
- **Origin of discharge.** Chlamydia and gonococcal infection typically lead to discharge directly from the urethra. A number of lesions around the glans penis may be considered to be 'discharge' by the patient; these can be caused by syphilis, herpes simplex or, rarely, penile carcinoma. Candidal balanitis can produce a clear exudate in addition to the typical white and creamy substance, particularly in men with an intact foreskin.
- **Testicular problems.** Ask about pain and inflammation in the scrotum, which may suggest orchitis or epididymo-orchitis resulting from gonococcal or chlamydial infection.
- **Rectum.** If there are anal symptoms, such as pain, itching and discharge, consider proctitis, particularly in homosexual men.
- **Urethral injury.** Ask whether any objects or substances have been inserted into the urethra. Intraurethral preparations may have been prescribed by a health professional. Consider the possibility of sex aids or foreign bodies having been inserted into the urethra.

Past and current medical problems

- **Diabetes.** Candida infections are more common in patients with diabetes.
- **Kidney disease.** Structural abnormalities of the urogenital tract may pose a higher risk of morbidity from infection.

Medication
- **Antibiotics.** Has the patient already received antibiotics for any of his symptoms?

Allergies
- **Antibiotics and antifungals.** Ask about any allergies to drugs that might be needed for the treatment of an underlying infection.

Review of previous investigations
- **Urethral swabs.** Have swabs been taken for chlamydia (enzyme-linked immunosorbent assay (ELISA) for chlamydial antigen) or gonorrhoea?
- **Urine for DNA amplification.** This may have been performed, as it is more sensitive and specific than ELISA.
- **Urine dipstick and MSU.** White cells, red cells and protein may be present in urethritis. Check for glucosuria if there is suspected candida infection, particularly if recurrent.

Examination

General
- **General condition.** Does the patient look unwell? Rarely, malaise may suggest sepsis due to urinary tract infection or septic arthritis in gonorrhoea.

Vital signs
- **Temperature.** A fever suggests urinary tract infection, orchitis or systemic infection. In rare cases, consider the possibility of septic arthritis if there is joint pain and stiffness.

Abdomen
- **Palpation.** Check for a palpable bladder. Tenderness in the suprapubic and/or loin regions suggests urinary tract infection.
- **Rectal examination.** Consider digital rectal examination if the history suggests proctitis or prostatitis.

Genitalia
- **Penis.** Check the penis carefully for any ulcers and rashes. Is any discharge visible at the urethral meatus? A clear or whitish urethral discharge may be caused by chlamydia, whereas the discharge in gonorrhoea tends to be slightly more yellow. Try and retract the foreskin fully to allow inspection of all parts of the glans. Single and painless ulcers occur in syphilis, whereas herpes simplex infection and Beçet's syndrome cause painful ulcers.
- **Scrotum.** A tender and hot testicle and/or epididymis suggests infection.
- **Groins.** Check for inguinal lymphadenopathy.

Skin
- **Rashes.** There may be skin rashes in advanced gonorrhoea or syphilis.

Head and neck
- **Eyes.** Look for conjunctivitis, which may be caused by gonorrhoea or chlamydia infection. Consider Reiter's syndrome if there is associated arthritis and urethritis.
- **Mouth.** Look for ulcers suggestive of Beçet's syndrome if the patient has genital ulcers, uveitis, arthropathy or skin lesions such as spots or bruises.

Upper and lower limbs
- **Arthritis.** A reactive arthritis may occur with chlamydial infection. Gonococcal infection may lead to bacterial arthritis, and one or more joints (commonly the knee joint) may be affected.

Bedside tests
- **Urine dipstick.** Check for glucose, blood, protein, nitrites and leucocytes. Send off for culture if results for nitrites and leucocytes are positive.

Key references and further reading

1. British Association for Sexual Health & HIV (BASHH). 2015 National guideline on the Management of non-gonococcal urethritis. Available from: http://www.bashh.org/documents/UK%20National%20Guideline%20on%20the%20Management%20of%20Non-gonococcal%20Urethritis%202015.pdf   (last accessed 29 April 2016).
2. British Association for Sexual Health & HIV (BASHH). 2015 UK national guideline for the management of infection with *Chlamydia trachomatis*. Available from: http://www.bashh.org/documents/2015_UK_guideline_for_the_management_of__Chlamydia_trachomatis_final_12....pdf   (last accessed 29 April 2016).
3. Miller KE. Diagnosis and treatment of *Chlamydia trachomatis* infection. *Am Fam Physician* 2006;73:1411–1416.
4. National Institute for Health and Care Excellence (NICE). Chlamydia – uncomplicated genital. Clinical knowledge summaries. 2011. Available from: http://cks.nice.org.uk/chlamydia-uncomplicated-genital (last accessed 29 April 2016).
5. Richens J. Main presentations of sexually transmitted infections in men. *BMJ* 2004;328:1251–1253.

Scrotal and testicular problems

Key thoughts

Practical points
- **Diagnosis.** Scrotal and testicular problems are frequently caused by benign conditions such as epididymal cyst or varicocele. Consider testicular cancer if a swelling is directly related or attached to the testicle.
- **Prognosis.** Testicular torsion and cancer are important diagnoses, not to be missed.

Differential diagnosis
- Hydrocele.
- Hernia.
- Testicular torsion.
- Epididymal cyst.
- Spermatocele.
- Varicocele.
- Haematocele.
- Testicular cancer.
- Epididymitis.
- Epididymo-orchitis.
- Trauma.
- Fibrotic nodules post vasectomy.

RED FLAGS

- Features suggesting testicular cancer (testicular lump)
- Patient being unwell
- General symptoms, such as weight loss, night sweats, fever, malaise, fatigue
- Sudden onset of severe pain (testicular torsion)

History

Ideas, concerns and expectations
- **Ideas.** What does the patient think is the underlying cause?
- **Concerns.** Concerns about future fertility, relationship problems and STI or cancer are common.

The 10-Minute Clinical Assessment, Second Edition. Knut Schroeder.
© 2017 John Wiley & Sons, Ltd. Published 2017 by John Wiley & Sons, Ltd.

- **Expectations.** Why has the patient come to see you? Symptom relief and reassurance are common reasons for consultation. Patients with a testicular lump may expect further investigation or referral.

History of presenting complaint

- **Quality of life.** Testicular pain can be very distressing. Many men will take a long time before consulting a health professional with testicular problems due to embarrassment or fear about a possible diagnosis of cancer.
- **Pain.** Pain in connection with scrotal swelling can have a number of causes. Consider epididymitis, epididymo-orchitis, testicular torsion, torsion of the testicular appendage, variocele, tumour, trauma and testicular hypersensitivity.
- **Onset and progression.** Particularly in adolescents and younger men, consider testicular torsion if there is acute onset of pain that radiates to the right iliac fossa. Torsion often occurs after exercise and requires emergency treatment to preserve testicular function. A haemorrhage associated with testicular tumour may also present acutely. Pain of more gradual onset over 24–48 hours is more likely to be due to inflammation or infection, and possible causes are epididymitis and epididymo-orchitis. Varicocele often causes intermittent pain or testicular 'heaviness', particularly after prolonged standing or exercise. Symptoms usually affect the left side. Also consider intermittent torsion if pain comes and goes, although this is relatively rare.
- **General symptoms.** Is the patient unwell? General malaise and fever point towards infection. Systemic features, such as low back pain, weight loss, loss of appetite and cough or shortness of breath, may rarely be caused by metastasis from a testicular tumour.
- **Age.** Malignant testicular tumours such as seminoma and teratoma commonly occur in men aged 20–40 years, while lymphomas are more frequent in the elderly. Testicular torsion can occur at any age but is much more common in boys, adolescents and younger men. In children, viral infection such as mumps may cause epididymo-orchitis (check immunisation status). Varicocele, epididymal cyst, hydrocele and inguinal hernia become more common with advancing age.
- **Additional unexplored issues.** Ask the patient whether there are any other problems or issues that you have not covered which might be important.

Common symptom patterns

- **Tumour.** Consider tumour if there is gradual onset of a painless and solid testicular swelling that does not transilluminate and affects the body of the testis. Pain may occur as a result of infarction or haemorrhage and does not exclude the possibility of a tumour, and patients often describe a feeling of 'heaviness'.
- **STI.** Is there a history of STI? Epididymo-orchitis may be caused by STI, such as chlamydia or gonorrhoea. Ask about urethral discharge, frequency of micturition, dysuria and symptoms of proctitis. Has there been a recent change of sexual partner, and has any partner shown signs of infection?

- **Epididymitis or epididymo-orchitis.** Testicular swelling and pain in connection with urinary tract infection in older men suggests orchitis. Does the patient complain of dysuria, frequency of urine or haematuria? Consider STI, such as chlamydia, particularly in younger men. Dysuria may also occur in testicular cancer. Consider development of an abscess if epididymitis has not settled with antibiotics.

Past and current medical problems
- **Cryptorchism.** Even if corrected by orchidopexy, cryptorchism carries an increased risk of testicular cancer.
- **Vasectomy.** This may result in the formation of granulomas, which may be palpable as small fibrotic nodules.
- **Cysts and hernias.** These may recur anytime.

Allergies
- **Antibiotics.** Ask about allergies to any antibiotics in case there is underlying infection that needs treatment.

Review of previous investigations
- **Urinalysis and MSU.** Are any previous urine results available? A 'first catch' is usually more helpful than MSU.
- **Ultrasound.** Look for any recent ultrasound reports, which can be very helpful in the diagnosis of scrotal symptoms.
- **Urethral swab.** This may help if urethral discharge or urethritis is present.

Examination

General
- **General condition.** Consider testicular torsion if the patient looks unwell or has collapsed. Severe infection may also cause general malaise. Cachexia may occur as a result of metastasis in late presentation of testicular tumour.
- **Gynaecomastia.** This may suggest the presence of an oestrogen-secreting testicular cancer.
- **Parotid swelling.** This may indicate mumps in children or non-immunised adults.

Vital signs
- **Temperature.** Fever suggests infection, such as epididymitis or epididymo-orchitis.
- **Pulse.** Tachycardia may be present in infection or due to pain in testicular torsion.
- **Respiratory rate.** Tachypnoea may rarely indicate metastasis if there is an underlying testicular cancer.

Groin
- **Hernia.** Look and feel for evidence of an indirect inguinal hernia. Is there a cough impulse? If there is a hernia, you will not be able to get above the swelling, and the 'hinge' will not be possible. Are there any scars indicating previous hernia operations, orchidopexy or removal of a varicocele?
- **Lymphadenopathy.** Check for inguinal lymphadenopathy, which may result from infection or tumour.

Scrotal examination
- **Inspection.** Any swellings of the size of a large orange are likely to be caused by hydrocele or inguino-scrotal hernia. Palpation and transillumination will usually distinguish between the two.
- **Location of the swelling.** Try to evaluate whether a swelling arises from the body of the testis, the epididymis or the cord. Assess the size, shape and consistency of the swelling.
- **Torsion.** The testis will be hot, tender and swollen and may have moved up in the scrotum. The axis of the affected testicle may have shifted to transverse. Nausea, vomiting and abdominal pain are common. A twist may be palpable in the spermatic cord, but examination is usually difficult due to the pain.
- **Prehn's sign.** Consider elevating the affected testicle. Pain usually decreases in epididymitis but remains the same or becomes worse in torsion.
- **Testicular tumour.** Any swelling arising from the body of the testis should be regarded as a tumour until proven otherwise – particularly if it is hard, fixed and adherent to the body of the testis. A lump separate from the testis is not a testicular tumour. Swellings of the epididymis are usually benign.
- **Hydrocele.** Compare the normal with the abnormal side. In a large hydrocele, you should be able to 'get above' the swelling and 'hinge' the mass upwards towards the abdominal wall. Hydroceles feel usually smooth and fluctuant and are not tender. Remember that hydroceles may develop secondary to testicular cancer.
- **Varicocele.** Elusive scrotal swellings may be caused by varicocele, which can feel like a 'bag of worms' in more severe cases, particularly on standing up.
- **Transillumination.** Use a powerful torch in a darkened room to confirm diagnoses of hydrocele, epididymal cyst or spermatocele. In young children, a hernial sac may also transilluminate, even if it contains intestine, but the hinge sign will be negative. A tumour or epididymo-orchitis may also present with a secondary hydrocele.
- **Infection.** Pain and tenderness in orchitis or epididymo-orchitis may also be located in the testis or epididymis.
- **Cysts.** Epididymal cysts are smooth, round and transilluminable.

Chest
- **Lungs.** Check for signs of metastatic spread if testicular cancer is suspected.

Abdomen
* **Palpation.** Check for organomegaly and any tenderness thereof.

Bedside tests
* **Urinalysis.** Protein, blood, nitrites and leucocyte cells may suggest urinary tract infection, orchitis or epididymitis.

Key references and further reading
1. Eaton S, Cendron M, Estrada C et al. Intermittent testicular torsion: diagnostic features and management outcomes. *J Urol* 2005;174:1532–1535.
2. National Institute for Health and Care Excellence (NICE). Scrotal swellings. Clinical knowledge summaries. 2010. Available from: http://cks.nice.org.uk/scrotal-swellings (last accessed 29 April 2016).
3. National Institute for Health and Care Excellence (NICE). Suspected cancer: recognition and referral. NICE guidelines [NG12]. June 2015. Available from: http://www.nice.org.uk/guidance/ng12 (last accessed 29 April 2016).
4. Scottish Intercollegiate Guidelines Network (SIGN). Management of adult testicular germ cell tumours. Guideline 124. March 2011. Available from: http://www.sign.ac.uk/pdf/sign124.pdf (last accessed 29 April 2016).

Erectile dysfunction

Key thoughts

Practical points
- **Diagnosis.** Erectile dysfunction is common. Many men find it difficult to talk about sexual issues and may present only long after the onset of problems with erections. Erectile dysfunction may be the first sign of underlying disease (e.g. diabetes, CVD).
- **Effect on life.** Establish how bothersome symptoms are for the patient and/or his partner. Loss of confidence, anxiety and depression are common.
- **Prognosis.** Many treatment options are available and they are often successful, particularly for non-organic causes of erectile dysfunction.

Possible causes
- Mental health problems (e.g. depression, anxiety).
- Endocrine conditions (e.g. hypothyroidism, diabetes, hypogonadism).
- CVD (e.g. peripheral vascular disease, heart failure).
- Neurological problems (e.g. spinal conditions).
- Drugs (e.g. antihypertensives, antidepressants).
- Malignancy (e.g. prostate cancer).
- Peyronie's disease.
- Trauma.
- Postoperative after urological operations (e.g. transurethral resection of the prostate).

> **RED FLAGS**
>
> - Prostate cancer
> - Back pain
> - Neurological symptoms
> - Undiagnosed diabetes
> - Undiagnosed CVD
> - Weight loss, fever, malaise, fatigue, night sweats
> - Complex psychological issues

History

Ideas, concerns and expectations
- **Ideas.** What does the patient think is causing the erectile dysfunction? What knowledge does he have about the factors that affect erections? What

The 10-Minute Clinical Assessment, Second Edition. Knut Schroeder.
© 2017 John Wiley & Sons, Ltd. Published 2017 by John Wiley & Sons, Ltd.

is his idea about 'normal' erectile function? Does he have any unusual beliefs?

- **Concerns.** Patients often fear that their relationship may break down.
- **Expectations.** Why has the patient come to see you, and what does he hope to gain? Many men find it very difficult to talk about erectile problems. Are expectations about the success of management realistic?

History of presenting complaint

- **Quality of life.** He may find it difficult to talk about sexual issues. How do symptoms affect his life and his relationship? How distressed is he by the problem? Try to conduct the consultation in comfortable surroundings, with privacy assured. Many men will wait for months or even years before consulting a health professional.
- **Define the problem.** Find out what exactly the problem is. Erection problems (initiation and/or maintenance), premature ejaculation, anorgasmia and lack of libido may all be described as 'impotence'. Erectile dysfunction can be defined as the inability to achieve and maintain an erection that is adequate for intercourse.
- **Onset.** Find out how long the problems have been present. Sudden onset may be psychogenic and linked to a particular life event. Erectile problems with an organic cause usually develop more gradually and tend to be progressive, with ejaculation not being affected. When was the last time the patient had sexual intercourse?
- **Circumstances.** A psychogenic cause is more likely if erections are affected only intermittently in certain situations and there are no problems when masturbating. Organic causes are more likely if erection problems occur all the time, on every occasion. If early-morning erections are present, then a purely organic cause is also unlikely.
- **Maintenance.** If there are good erections during foreplay or self-stimulation, which wane when attempting penetration or during intercourse, psychological or vascular factors may be responsible.
- **Libido.** Libido and ejaculatory function are usually maintained in organic erectile dysfunction. Consider psychological or relationship problems and endocrine conditions (see later) if there is loss of libido.
- **Relationship with partner.** How does the patient rate the state of his relationship with his partner? Have they discussed the problem, or have talks been prevented by embarrassment or a feeling of guilt? Does the partner have high expectations? Does he perceive his partner as being supportive?
- **Mental health.** Mental health problems, such as stress, anxiety and depression, are common causes or contributory factors.
- **Eye problems.** Ask about any eye problems. Nonarteritic anterior ischaemic optic neuropathy is a contraindication for phosphodiesterase inhibitors.
- **Treatment.** What has the patient tried so far? Has the couple considered psychosexual counselling?
- **Other symptoms.** Ask about general symptoms, such as tiredness, fever, malaise, sleep problems and depression, which may give clues about underlying conditions.

- **Local resources for referral.** Is the patient aware of local facilities and possibilities for referral, including psychosexual counselling?
- **Additional unexplored issues.** Ask whether there are any other unidentified problems or issues that you have not covered which might be important.

Past and current medical problems
- **Endocrine conditions.** Endocrine conditions, such as diabetes, hypothyroidism, hyperthyroidism, hypogonadism and hyperprolactinaemia, may all cause erectile dysfunction. Ask about specific symptoms, such as tiredness, lethargy, constipation and galactorrhoea.
- **Urological.** Erectile dysfunction or problems with ejaculation may occur after prostate or bladder surgery and irradiation. There is an aetiological link between erectile dysfunction and benign prostatic hyperplasia (endothelial dysfunction), with each condition more common when the other is present. Does the patient suffer from Peyronie's disease? Is there a diagnosis of prostate cancer? Are there any renal problems?
- **Cardiovascular.** Cardiovascular causes are also common, with arteriosclerosis/peripheral vascular disease and hypertension (and its treatment) being important. Hypotension, recent stroke, unstable angina and myocardial infarction are contraindications for prescribing phosphodiesterase inhibitors. Erectile dysfunction may be an early marker for CVD.
- **Neurological.** Check for a history of multiple sclerosis (MS), spinal cord compression, spina bifida, Parkinson's disease, poliomyelitis or pelvic surgery.

Medication
- **Drugs causing erectile dysfunction.** Erectile dysfunction is a common adverse effect of many drugs, including antihypertensives, antidepressants, cimetidine, LH-releasing hormone analogues and digoxin.
- **Drugs and appliances used to treat erectile dysfunction.** Have phosphodiesterase type-5 (PDE5) inhibitors already been prescribed or purchased without prescription? If so, how effective have they been? Are there any adverse effects? PDE5 inhibitors become more effective with use. Have other methods (e.g. intracavernous injections, urethral applications, pumps) been considered?
- **Nitrates.** Phosphodiesterase inhibitors are contraindicated in patients taking nitrates.

Alcohol, smoking and recreational drugs
- **Alcohol.** Alcohol may affect erections. Ask about past and present alcohol consumption.
- **Smoking.** Smoking is a risk factor for CVD. Heavy smoking may also have direct vascular effects on erections.
- **Drugs.** Use of recreational drugs or body-building preparations may affect erectile function.

Review of previous investigations
- **Full blood count.** Anaemia may be caused by chronic disease. A raised mean corpuscular volume (MCV) may be found in hypothyroidism or due to alcohol misuse.
- **Fasting blood glucose.** Is the patient diabetic?
- **Serum testosterone.** Testosterone levels should have been checked with an early-morning sample.
- **Serum prolactin.** Check for evidence of hyperprolactinaemia.
- **Thyroid function.** Check for both hypo- and hyperthyroidism.
- **Lipids.** A fasting lipid profile may be indicated to help assess cardiovascular risk, as there is increasing evidence of the link between erectile dysfunction and cardiovascular risk even in suspected psychological erectile dysfunction.
- **PSA.** A raised PSA may be caused by benign prostatic hyperplasia or prostate cancer. Prostate cancer can cause erectile dysfunction by invading the neurovascular bundles that run alongside the prostate.
- **Renal and liver function, including gamma-glutamyl transpeptidase (GGT).** Check for any abnormalities suggesting underlying disease.

Examination

General
- **General condition.** Does the patient look well? Are there any features of neurological or endocrine disease?
- **Face.** Does the patient look tired? Consider depression or hypothyroidism if there is reduced affect.
- **Weight.** Weight gain or weight loss may be caused by endocrine or other conditions.
- **Sexual characteristics.** Look for signs of hypogonadism (e.g. decreased body hair, development of breast tissue or decrease in muscle mass).

Vital signs
- **Blood pressure.** Hypotension with a systolic blood pressure of less than 90 mmHg is a contraindication for the prescription of phosphodiesterase inhibitors. Hypertension is a risk factor for CVD.

Chest
- **Heart and lungs.** Check for signs of heart disease.

Abdomen
- **Penis.** Look for any obvious abnormality of the penis. Cancer of the penis is rare but may not be mentioned by the patient. Look for evidence of Peyronie's disease (which may not be apparent in the non-erect penis), phimosis and hypospadias.
- **Scrotum.** Palpate both testes. Small testicles may be found in hypogonadism.

- **Prostate.** Perform a digital rectal examination to assess prostate size and consistency, particularly if there are associated lower urinary tract symptoms.

Lower limbs
- **Peripheral pulses.** Absent or reduced pulses suggest peripheral vascular disease.

Bedside tests
- **Blood glucose.** Check with a test strip to screen for diabetes.
- **Urine dipstick.** Check for signs of infection, glucosuria or possible renal disease.

Key references and further reading
1. British National Formulary. www.bnf.org.
2. Hackett G, Kell P, Ralph D et al. for the British Society for Sexual Medicine. British Society for Sexual Medicine guidelines on the management of erectile dysfunction. *J Sex Med* 2008;5:1841–1865.
3. Miller T. Diagnostic evaluation of erectile dysfunction. *Am Fam Physician* 2000;61:95–104.
4. National Institute for Health and Care Excellence (NICE). Erectile dysfunction. Clinical knowledge summaries. 2014. Available from: http://cks.nice.org.uk/erectile-dysfunction (last accessed 29 April 2016).
5. Rees J, Patel B. 10-minute consultation: erectile dysfunction. *BMJ* 2006; 332:593.

Renal or ureteric colic (kidney stones)

Key thoughts

Practical points
- **Diagnosis.** Renal stones are common and are often asymptomatic. Renal colic can be extremely painful and distressing. Search for underlying modifiable and nonmodifiable risk factors.

Differential diagnosis
- Idiopathic.
- Drugs.
- Insulin resistance and diabetes mellitus.
- Hypertension.
- Inflammatory bowel disease.
- Structural kidney abnormalities.
- Primary hyperparathyroidism.
- Gout.
- Abdominal aortic aneurysm (usually in later life).

Important risk factors
- Past or family history of kidney stones.
- Anatomical abnormalities of the urinary tract.
- Peripheral vascular disease.
- Hypercalciuria.
- Hyperuricosuria.
- Hyperoxaluria.
- Hot climates and dehydration.
- Low dietary intake of magnesium and calcium.

RED FLAGS

- Infection
- Urinary tract obstruction (especially in a solitary or transplanted kidney)
- Urosepsis
- Dehydration and inability to take oral fluids
- Intractable pain and/or vomiting
- Impending acute renal failure
- Bilateral obstructing stones

The 10-Minute Clinical Assessment, Second Edition. Knut Schroeder.
© 2017 John Wiley & Sons, Ltd. Published 2017 by John Wiley & Sons, Ltd.

- Abdominal aortic aneurysm
- Unclear diagnosis

History

Ideas, concerns and expectations
- **Ideas.** Find out what the patient believes to be the underlying cause.
- **Concerns.** Patients often worry about potential kidney damage and recurrence of pain.
- **Expectations.** Patients usually expect adequate analgesia and may ask for further investigation and/or referral.

History of presenting complaint
- **Quality of life.** How do symptoms affect activities of daily living? Renal colic can be extremely painful and distressing.
- **Pain.** The classic presentation is with acute severe colicky loin pain radiating to the groin, testicles in men or labia majora in women. Kidney stones may stay completely asymptomatic. Patients with renal colic are often restless and move about in distress, whereas those with peritonitis tend to lie still.
- **Systemic symptoms.** Fever and chills may occur if there is associated infection.
- **Urinary symptoms.** Dysuria, frequency, urgency and difficulty passing urine may occur once a stone has entered the ureter, bladder or urethra. Haematuria may result from minor damage to the walls of the renal calyceal system, ureter, bladder or urethra.
- **Gastrointestinal symptoms.** Nausea and vomiting are common because the renal capsule and the intestines share part of the innervation.
- **Gout.** A history of gout greatly increases the risk of kidney stones in men.
- **Enteric hyperoxaluria.** Increased intestinal absorption of oxalate may occur in ileal disease (e.g. Crohn's, ileal bypass), short-bowel syndrome or low calcium intake.
- **Increased ingestion of oxalate.** Consider foods such as rhubarb, spinach, nuts, chocolate, tea, beets, wheat bran, soya foods and strawberries if eaten in excess.
- **Stone prevention.** Has anything been tried to prevent stones in any previous episode? General measures include increasing fluid intake (single most important factor), reducing the intake of animal protein, restricting salt intake, maintaining normal calcium intake and decreasing dietary oxalate intake and intake of cranberry juice.
- **Other causes of pain.** Always consider the possibility of a ruptured abdominal aortic aneurysm in older men presenting with loin pain. Testicular torsion needs to be considered in (usually younger) men who present with testicular pain. Consider appendicitis in right-sided pain or diverticulitis in left-sided lower abdominal pain. Urinary tract infection is common in women.

Past and current medical problems
- **Significant past illnesses.** Ask about structural renal or urological abnormalities, a history of peripheral vascular disease or aneurysm, hypertension and previous stones.

Medication
- **Analgesics.** What has been tried and taken so far? Is analgesia effective? Are there any unwanted effects? Are there any contraindications or cautions (e.g. nonsteroidal anti-inflammatory drugs (NSAIDs), asthma, peptic ulcer disease, renal impairment)?
- **Drugs affecting stone disease.** Consider calcium with vitamin D, ephedrine or carboanhydrase inhibitors.

Other treatments
- **Stone removal.** Has shockwave lithotripsy ever been performed? Has the patient ever undergone ureteroscopy or percutaneous nephrolithotomy?

Allergies
- **Antibiotics.** Ask about allergies to any antibiotics that might need to be used for treatment of possible complicating urine infection.

Family history
- **Renal stones.** There may be a positive family history of renal stones.
- **Kidney disease.** Ask about any known family history of kidney disease.

Alcohol, smoking and recreational drugs
- **Alcohol.** Ask details about past and current alcohol consumption. Alcohol misuse can cause dehydration and is associated with gout.

Review of previous investigations
- **Full blood count.** Raised white cell count may suggest infection.
- **Urea, creatinine and electrolytes.** Check for underlying or complicating kidney disease (mandatory if there is only one functioning kidney).
- **Calcium, phosphate and bicarbonate.** Check in particular for hypercalcaemia.
- **Uric acid.** If raised, this may suggest gout, but normal values do not exclude this.
- **Parathyroid hormone.** This may be useful in the investigation of elevated serum calcium.
- **Stone analysis.** Have any previous stones been analysed for their contents?
- **Imaging.** Look out for previous imaging reports and evidence of structural abnormalities (e.g. kidney, ureter and bladder (KUB) X-ray, ultrasound scan, CT, intravenous urogram).
- **24-hour urine collection.** In recurrent stones, 24-hour urine assessment may be helpful, checking for urine volume, calcium, oxalate, uric acid, citrate, urine sodium and creatinine excretion.

Examination

General
- **General condition.** Renal colic can be extremely painful. Pain usually comes on in waves, with periods between acute exacerbations lasting up to about 30 minutes. Patients tend to be agitated and often pace around the room. If the patient looks unwell, consider kidney infection (e.g. pyelonephritis), which usually requires urgent action.

Vital signs
- **Temperature.** Raised temperature suggests associated urinary infection.
- **Pulse.** Tachycardia is often caused by pain and/or infection.
- **Blood pressure.** Blood pressure may be raised due to pain or underlying kidney disease. Raised blood pressure in itself may also be a risk factor for renal stones. Check for postural hypotension.

Abdomen
- **Tenderness.** Even severe renal colic will, in most cases, not cause significant tenderness, and tenderness in the renal angle and in the lower abdomen will suggest an alternative diagnosis. Check for evidence of a nephrectomy scar.
- **Masses.** Palpate for enlarged kidneys. Check the central abdomen for evidence of abdominal aortic aneurysm in older men (especially if there is a history of CVD).
- **Genitals.** Pain from renal colic may radiate into the labia or testicles. Check for testicular tenderness and swelling if there is a possibility of testicular torsion.

Lower limbs
- **Pulses.** Check peripheral pulses (peripheral vascular disease and abdominal aortic aneurysm).

Bedside tests
- **Urine dipstick.** Microscopic or macroscopic haematuria is common, but stones may occur in the absence of haematuria. The incidence of dipstick haematuria decreases with passing time in renal colic. Positive dipstick for leucocytes and nitrite may indicate urine infection. Dipstick is more sensitive than microscopy in detecting microscopic haematuria.
- **Urine microscopy.** This may show crystals, such as the classic hexagonal crystals seen in cystinuria.

Key references and further reading
1. British Association of Urological Surgeons (BAUS). Guidelines for acute management of first presentation of renal/ureteric lithiasis (excluding pregnancy). 2008. Available from: http://www.baus.org.uk/_userfiles/pages/files/Publications/RevisedAcuteStoneMgtGuidelines.pdf (last accessed 29 April 2016).

2. Miller NL, Lingeman JE. Management of kidney stones. *BMJ* 2007;334:468–472.

3. National Institute for Health and Care Excellence (NICE). Renal or ureteric colic – acute. Clinical knowledge summaries. 2015. Available from: http://cks.nice.org.uk/renal-or-ureteric-colic-acute (last accessed 29 April 2016).

4. Parmar MS. Kidney stones. *BMJ* 2004;328:1420–1424.

5. Teichman JM. Clinical practice. Acute renal colic from ureteral calculus. *N Engl J Med* 2004;350:684–693.

Haematuria

Key thoughts

Practical points

- **Diagnosis.** Urinary tract infection, urinary tract stones, urethritis, benign prostatic hypertrophy and bladder and prostate cancer are important causes of haematuria. Consider a renal cause if there is associated hypertension, abnormal renal function tests or proteinuria, particularly in patients with pre-existing renal conditions.
- **Prognosis.** In most cases, haematuria will require further investigation to rule out a serious underlying cause.

Possible causes

- **Infection.** Urinary tract infection, urethritis, prostatitis.
- **Malignancy.** Bladder or prostate cancer, renal carcinoma.
- **Trauma.** Accidents, foreign body, catheterisation.
- **Structural.** Urinary tract stones, polycystic kidney disease.
- **Haematological.** Anticoagulation therapy, coagulation disorder, sickle-cell disease.
- **Drugs.** Cyclophosphamide, sulphonamides, NSAIDs, rifampicin, nitrofurantoin.
- **Toxins.** Occupational chemicals or dyes.
- **Inflammatory.** Rarely, glomerulonephritis, Goodpasture's syndrome, post-irradiation.
- **Other.** Factitious, genital bleeding, menstruation, sexual abuse.

Differential diagnosis of dark or red urine

- Food (e.g. beetroot).
- Haemoglobinuria.
- Myoglobinuria.
- Bilirubinuria.
- Rarely, porphyria.

Important risk factors

- Age.
- Smoking.
- Occupational exposure to chemicals or dyes.

The 10-Minute Clinical Assessment, Second Edition. Knut Schroeder.
© 2017 John Wiley & Sons, Ltd. Published 2017 by John Wiley & Sons, Ltd.

RED FLAGS

- Frank haematuria
- Past history of cancer
- Systemic features, such as weight loss, fever, malaise, fatigue or night sweats
- Lower back pain
- Bone pain

History

Ideas, concerns and expectations
- **Ideas.** What does the patient believe is the underlying cause?
- **Concerns.** Haematuria can be a worrying symptom, and fears about cancer are common.
- **Expectations.** Patients often consult to rule out cancer. They will usually expect investigation and/or referral.

History of presenting complaint
- **Onset and progression.** How and when did the symptoms start? Is there an obvious explanation for the haematuria? Is there blood in the urine all the time, or are symptoms intermittent? Is the problem getting worse?
- **Pain.** Any severe intermittent loin pain is suggestive of renal colic, which may present with dipstick or frank haematuria. Malignancy typically presents with painless haematuria, but consider clot colic if there is significant bleeding from a tumour.
- **Asymptomatic dipstick haematuria.** Findings of '+' are significant and do not need to be confirmed on MSU specimens. Although routine dipstick testing is not recommended, urinalysis for blood may be performed as part of the workup for people with a reduced estimated glomerular filtration rate (eGFR) of <60 ml/min, newly identified proteinuria or suspected systemic disease with renal involvement.
- **Frank haematuria.** Find out whether the patient has had frank haematuria, which has prognostic implications in that a serious underlying cause is more likely. Blood present at the start of micturition suggests possible urethral bleeding, whereas blood at the end of the stream may originate from the bladder trigone. Blood present throughout the stream will have become mixed with the urine in the bladder and may be caused by a bladder or renal tumour.
- **Lower urinary tract symptoms.** An enlarged prostate is a common cause of dipstick haematuria in men. Ask about the presence of voiding symptoms, such as hesitancy, poor stream or terminal dribbling.
- **Previous urological problems.** Ask about any past urological history, such as renal stones, haematuria, prostate disease or bladder cancer. Has the patient had any urological investigations or operations?

Common symptom patterns
- **Urinary tract infection.** Ask about symptoms of urinary tract infection (e.g. dysuria, urinary frequency, nocturia, fever). Consider schistosomiasis or tuberculosis (TB) if the patient has travelled to or lived in endemic areas. Has the patient been exposed to TB?
- **Transitional cell carcinoma.** Ask about risk factors for bladder cancer, such as smoking (the most important risk factor by far) or exposure to carcinogens used in the textile, printing, cable and rubber industries. Diabetes mellitus may also increase the risk of bladder cancer.
- **Menstruation.** In women, consider the possibility of menstrual blood contaminating the urine sample.
- **Exercise and trauma.** Heavy exercise, such as long-distance running or swimming, may cause transient dipstick haematuria, which usually resolves within a day or two. Ask about any recent trauma.
- **General symptoms.** Ask about weight loss, arthralgia and recent throat infection, which may rarely point towards underlying kidney disease, such as glomerulonephritis.
- **Causes of red or dark urine.** Consider haemoglobinuria with a positive dipstick but no red cells on microscopy. Other causes include food, such as beetroot, and drugs, such as nitrofurantoin, rifampicin or senna. Think of porphyria if urine darkens on standing. Bilirubinaemia may occur in biliary obstruction.

Past and current medical problems
- **Bleeding diatheses.** Is there a history of clotting disorders?
- **Urological.** Look for details of any investigations and previous diagnoses with regard to conditions of the urinary tract (particularly bladder and kidneys).

Medication
- **Anticoagulants.** Patients on warfarin or, less commonly, aspirin may present with haematuria, particularly if there is underling urinary tract disease. Anticoagulants are more likely to provoke rather than cause haematuria.

Review of previous investigations
- **Full blood count.** Look for anaemia, which may be caused by chronic disease or chronic blood loss. Low platelets may contribute to bleeding problems.
- **Urea, creatinine and electrolytes.** Abnormal results may suggest underlying kidney disease.
- **Clotting screen.** Look for evidence of clotting disorders or abnormal values caused by the use of anticoagulants.
- **Urine dipstick and MSU.** Look for evidence of previous haematuria and infection. Normal results are significant in that the absence of infection should prompt further action.
- **Renal tract imaging.** Check the notes for reports of ultrasound, KUB X-ray or CT or intravenous urogram. Imaging aims to exclude structural lesions but may miss other renal causes (e.g. rare glomerulonephritis).

- **Urine cytology.** This is not a very good screening test, and a negative result does not exclude malignancy.
- **Cystoscopy.** Cystoscopy is helpful in excluding bladder cancer.

Examination

General
- **General condition.** Does the patient look unwell? Pallor and cachexia may suggest malignancy.

Vital signs
- **Temperature.** A raised temperature suggests urinary tract infection.
- **Pulse.** Tachycardia indicates infection or severe inflammation.
- **Blood pressure.** In most patients, this will be normal. Raised blood pressure may be caused by underlying kidney disease.

Abdomen
- **Palpation.** Check for renal masses and an enlarged bladder (urinary retention).
- **Rectal examination.** In men, consider rectal examination to check for signs of prostate cancer or benign prostatic hypertrophy.

Bedside tests
- **Urine dipstick.** A positive test for blood, protein, nitrites and/or leucocytes suggests infection. Proteinuria ± haematuria indicates possible underlying renal disease.

Key references and further reading
1. Buntinx F, Wauters H. The diagnostic value of macroscopic haematuria in diagnosing urological cancers: a meta-analysis. *Fam Pract* 1997;14:63–68.
2. Grossfeld GD, Wolf JS Jr, Litwan MS et al. Asymptomatic microscopic hematuria in adults: summary of the AUA best practice policy recommendations. *Am Fam Physician* 2001;63(6):1145–1154.
3. National Institute for Health and Care Excellence (NICE). Urological cancer – suspected. Clinical knowledge summaries. 2009. Available from: http://cks.nice .org.uk/urological-cancer-suspected (last accessed 29 April 2016).
4. Rees J, Patel B, Persad RA. Asymptomatic dipstick haematuria. *Trends Urol Gynaecol Sex Health* 2008;13:14–16.
5. Tomson C, Porter T. Review: asymptomatic microscopic or dipstick haematuria in adults: which investigations for which patients? A review of the evidence. *Br J Urol Int* 2002;90:185–198.
6. Vanholder R. Chronic kidney disease in adults: UK guidelines for identification, management and referral: full guidelines. *Nephrol Dial Transplant* 2006;21(7):1776–1777.

Chronic kidney disease

Key thoughts

Practical points

- **Diagnosis.** Chronic kidney disease (CKD) is common and is often diagnosed as part of screening in diabetes or hypertension. Patients with mild renal impairment are usually asymptomatic. Symptoms in more severe disease are usually nonspecific, with malaise and anorexia being common.
- **Prognosis.** Identify relevant complications, comorbidities and risk factors.

Possible causes

- **Prerenal.** Volume depletion, hypotension, heart failure, liver cirrhosis, sepsis, renal artery disease.
- **Renal.** Diabetes, drug-related (e.g. analgetics/NSAIDs), intrinsic renal disease, tubular injury, vascular conditions.
- **Postrenal.** Renal stones, prostate disease, bladder tumour, retroperitoneal fibrosis

Important risk factors

- Older age.
- Diabetes.
- CVD, including hypertension.
- Congestive heart failure.
- Pre-existing kidney or urological disease.
- Raised cholesterol.
- Rarely, chronic infection or myeloma.

RED FLAGS

- Refractory hyperkalaemia
- Intractable fluid overload
- Acute on chronic renal failure (oliguria and anuria, rising urea and creatinine over hours or days)

History

Ideas, concerns and expectations

- **Ideas.** Renal failure is often asymptomatic, and the patient may think there is nothing wrong. If there are symptoms, they are often nonspecific. Many people

The 10-Minute Clinical Assessment, Second Edition. Knut Schroeder.
© 2017 John Wiley & Sons, Ltd. Published 2017 by John Wiley & Sons, Ltd.

think that 'kidney disease' means that dialysis will be necessary and that they are at risk of dying prematurely. They may not know that CKD is a spectrum of disease, from mild renal impairment to severe kidney failure.

- **Concerns.** Concerns about progression and the possibility of developing kidney failure and the need for dialysis are common.
- **Expectations.** Patients may have unrealistic expectations about a cure and overall prognosis.

History of presenting complaint

- **Symptoms of CKD.** These are often nonspecific and commonly include malaise and anorexia in the early stages. In more severe kidney disease, patients may develop thirst, itching, twitching, nausea and vomiting. Oedema, dyspnoea, confusion and coma are late features.
- **Urinary symptoms.** Check for any urinary tract symptoms, such as frequency, hesitancy, dysuria, nocturia or haematuria, which might suggest a postrenal underlying cause.
- **Other symptoms.** Rarely, there may be underlying systemic disease, such as systemic lupus erythematosus (SLE), vasculitis or myeloma.
- **Chronic renal failure.** A long duration of symptoms suggests chronic renal failure, particularly if there are associated features, such as absence of acute illness, nocturia, anaemia, raised serum phosphate or hypocalcaemia.

Degree of renal failure

- **eGFR.** Check previous creatinine readings and eGFR. How rapidly did any changes occur?

CLASSIFICATION OF CKD

- **Stage 1 (normal):** GFR >90 ml/min/1.73 m^2 with other evidence of chronic kidney damage
- **Stage 2 (mild impairment):** GFR 60–89 ml/min/1.73 m^2 with other evidence of chronic kidney damage
- **Stage 3 (moderate impairment):** GFR 30–59 ml/min/1.73 m^2
- **Stage 4 (severe impairment):** GFR 15–29 ml/min/1.73 m^2
- **Stage 5 (established renal failure):** GFR <15 ml/min/1.73 m^2 or on dialysis

Risk factors and complications

- **Diabetes.** Is the patient diabetic? If so, are blood glucose levels well controlled? Check whether the patient is taking an angiotensin-converting enzyme (ACE) inhibitor.
- **Hypertension.** Is the patient on treatment for hypertension? Is medication being taken as prescribed?

- **Cardiovascular risk.** Check for risk factors of CVD, such as obesity, smoking, alcohol misuse, poor diet, lack of exercise, raised cholesterol, previous cardiovascular event and family history. Ask about symptoms of CVD, such as chest pain, intermittent claudication, breathlessness, tiredness and peripheral oedema.

Important presentations
- **Urinary tract obstruction.** Prostatic hypertrophy, prostate carcinoma, anatomical abnormalities of the urogenital tract or renal stone disease may lead to urinary tract obstruction and subsequent renal failure.
- **Renal disease.** Consider intrinsic renal disease if there are symptoms of underlying systemic disease, such as rashes, arthralgia, joint pains or muscle aches. Ask about recent introduction of new drugs, particularly chronic use of antibiotics and analgesics (e.g. NSAIDs, paracetamol).
- **Renal artery stenosis.** Acute loin pain and frank haematuria may be caused by occlusion of a normal renal artery, which can easily be misdiagnosed as renal colic. Renal function may deteriorate rapidly if patients with renal artery stenosis receive ACE inhibitors or diuretics, or if there is prolonged or severe hypotension. Also, consider aortic dissection as a possible underlying cause for renal hypoperfusion.
- **Metabolic and toxic causes.** Consider diabetic ketoacidosis, hyperosmolar coma, hyperuricaemia, hypercalcaemia or contrast media.

Past and current medical problems
- **Significant past illnesses.** Ask about a history of renal conditions, as well as diabetes and CVD. Does the patient suffer from cancer, chronic infection (e.g. HIV, hepatitis) or vascular disease?

Medication
- **Analgesics.** Analgesics may cause analgesic nephropathy, particularly if taken in larger than recommended doses and for prolonged periods of time.
- **Aminoglycosides.** These can be nephrotoxic, particularly if given at higher doses.
- **ACE inhibitors.** These may need to be stopped if there is a sudden rise in creatinine (>50%) or reduction in eGFR (>25%) after starting the drug or changing dose. Consider underlying renal artery stenosis.
- **Lipid-lowering medication.** Patients whose 10-year risk of CVD is over 20% should be considered for treatment with a statin.
- **Diuretics.** Are these already prescribed? Diuretics may cause significant dehydration and electrolyte disturbances, particularly at higher doses.

Family history
- **Polycystic kidneys.** A family history of polycystic kidneys or other renal disease may be relevant.
- **Cardiovascular risk factors.** Ask about a family history of CVD, diabetes, hyperlipidaemia, hypertension or peripheral artery disease.

Review of previous investigations

- **Electrolytes, urea and creatinine.** Hyperkalaemia and acidosis are common in renal failure. Dehydration may show up as a disproportionate rise in the urea/creatinine ratio. Serum urea is a poor indicator of renal function, as levels depend on many other factors. Serum creatinine also has limitations, in that it can remain relatively unchanged despite significant losses of renal function.
- **Full blood count.** Anaemia may be present in CKD. A raised white cell count may be caused by urinary or other infection. Eosinophilia can indicate acute interstitial nephritis. In microangiopathy, there may be thrombocytopenia and red cell fragments.
- **Blood glucose.** A raised fasting glucose suggests diabetes, and raised haemoglobin A1c (HbA1c) levels indicate poor control.
- **Calcium, phosphate and parathormone levels.** These may be indicated from stage 3 CKD.
- **Urine.** Urine osmolality over 500 mOsmol/l suggests a prerenal cause. Osmolality is usually under 300 mOsmol/l if there is a renal cause. Is there proteinuria? Has urine been tested for Bence–Jones proteins in suspected myeloma?
- **Urine protein/creatinine ratio.** This can be helpful in detecting proteinuria, which may be suspected from dipstick testing of an early-morning sample.
- **Renal tract ultrasound.** This may be indicated if there are lower urinary tract symptoms, treatment-resistant hypertension or an unexplained and progressive rapid fall in eGFR.
- **X-rays.** Stones may be visible on a plain abdominal X-ray showing the kidney, ureters and bladder. A chest X-ray may show up pulmonary oedema in more severe kidney disease if there is fluid overload.
- **Magnetic resonance imaging (MRI) or CT.** These allow more accurate assessment of the kidneys and renal vasculature. They must be used with caution in patients with severe renal impairment if contrast media are being used.

Examination

General

- **General condition.** Does the patient look unwell? Is there uraemic foetor or uraemic pigmentation (advanced disease only)?
- **Weight and height.** Measure and record weight and height, and calculate BMI.
- **Fluid status.** Check for signs of fluid depletion or overload.

Vital signs

- **Pulse.** Tachycardia may occur with heart failure, fluid depletion or overload.
- **Blood pressure.** Blood pressure is often elevated in CKD. Acute hypovolaemia may cause the blood pressure to drop. Postural hypotension indicates dehydration, particularly if there is no oedema.

Skin

- **Skin signs.** Look out for rashes, pallor, bruising, petechiae and purpura, which may rarely occur with vascular or inflammatory disease, disseminated intravascular coagulation, emboli and advanced kidney failure. Skin colour may turn to yellow-brown due to uraemia in advanced kidney disease.

Head and neck
- **Jugular venous pressure.** Check for signs of hypervolaemia and hypovolaemia.

Chest
- **Lungs.** Basal crackles suggest fluid overload and pulmonary oedema.
- **Heart.** Check for a pericardial rub (suggesting pericarditis).

Abdomen
- **Kidneys.** The kidneys are not usually palpable in most people, unless enlarged.
- **Bladder.** A large and painless bladder may be palpable in chronic urinary retention. If caused by acute retention, the bladder will usually be tender.

Lower limbs
- **Oedema.** Check for peripheral oedema, which may indicate renal, liver or heart failure.

Bedside tests
- **Urine dipstick and microscopy.** This may show blood, protein, leucocytes and nitrites in infection. Dysmorphic cells and red cell casts suggest glomerulonephritis in rare cases. Eosinophils may indicate rare acute interstitial nephritis.

Key references and further reading
1. Hilton R. Acute renal failure. *BMJ* 2006;333:786–790.
2. JBS 2: Joint British Societies' guidelines on prevention of cardiovascular disease in clinical practice. *Heart* 2005;91(Suppl. 5):v1–v52.
3. Lameire N, van Biesen W, Vanholder R. Acute renal failure. *Lancet* 2005;365:417–430.
4. Mitra PK, Tasker PRW, Ell MS. 10-minute consultation: chronic kidney disease. *BMJ* 2007;334:1273.
5. National Institute for Health and Care Excellence (NICE). Chronic kidney disease in adults: assessment and management. NICE guidelines [CG182]. July 2014. Available from: http://www.nice.org.uk/guidance/cg182 (last accessed 29 April 2016).
6. National Institute for Health and Clinical Excellence (NICE). Chronic kidney disease – not diabetic. Clinical knowledge summaries. 2015. Available from: http://cks.nice.org.uk/chronic-kidney-disease-not-diabetic (last accessed 29 April 2016).
7. Schrier RW, Wang W, Poole B, Mitra A. Acute renal failure: definitions, diagnosis, pathogenesis, and therapy. *J Clin Invest* 2004;114:5–14.
8. Vanholder R. Chronic kidney disease in adults: UK guidelines for identification, management and referral: full guidelines. *Nephrol Dial Transplant* 2006;21(7):1776–1777.

Mental health

Depression

Key thoughts

Practical points
- **Diagnosis.** Depression can present in many different ways and may be difficult to spot. Have a high index of suspicion and keep in mind physical causes, such as chronic diseases.
- **Prognosis.** Assess the severity of depression and the risk of suicide.

Differential diagnosis
- Psychosis.
- Postnatal depression.
- Seasonal affective disorder.
- Dementia.
- Anxiety.

Important risk factors
- Social problems.
- Past history of depression.
- Chronic disease (e.g. diabetes, heart disease, chronic obstructive pulmonary disease (COPD), cancer).
- Alcoholism.
- Bereavement.
- Old age.
- Vitamin D deficiency.

> **RED FLAGS**
>
> - Risk of suicide
> - Feeling of hopelessness
> - Chronic pain
> - Disabling symptoms
> - Severe and prolonged symptoms

History

Ideas, concerns and expectations
- **Ideas.** What is the patient's attitude to a diagnosis of depression? Many people continue to hold beliefs based on myths and irrational fears about mental health problems.

The 10-Minute Clinical Assessment, Second Edition. Knut Schroeder.
© 2017 John Wiley & Sons, Ltd. Published 2017 by John Wiley & Sons, Ltd.

- **Concerns.** Many people with depression feel they might be 'going mad'.
- **Expectations.** Those suffering from depression are often worried that 'nothing can be done' and need reassurance that treatment can be very effective.

History of presenting complaint

- **Quality of life.** How does the patient's current state of mind fit into the context of their life? What has been the story so far? A brief overview can help put symptoms into perspective. Questions like, 'How are things at home?' and 'Do you feel happy in yourself?' are often a good starting point.
- **Current functioning.** How do the symptoms affect daily life? Difficulties with ordinary activities, getting out of bed and going to work are common.
- **Symptoms of depression.** Depression can be diagnosed formally by using one of a number of standardised tools, such as the DSM-IV.
- **Precipitating factors.** Are there any obvious factors that have led to the development of depressive symptoms? Various crises and life events are common, including moving house, divorce, work issues and other family problems.
- **Additional symptoms of depression.** Consider asking about low self-confidence, reduced libido and sexual function, as well as any vague physical symptoms.
- **Physical illness.** Depression is common in chronic disease. Ask about neurological, respiratory, cardiological and abdominal symptoms.
- **Age.** Depression can present differently in different age groups. Young adults tend to sleep a lot, overeat, withdraw and show self-neglect. Older adults often present with insomnia, anxiety, anorexia, poor self-care and exacerbation of pre-existing physical conditions, such as painful arthritis, constipation, head and neck and back pain. Depression in dementia and Parkinson's disease is common, is easy to miss and can be hard to treat.
- **Psychosis.** Look for evidence of psychosis (e.g. hallucinations and delusions).
- **Risk of suicide.** Assess risk of suicide and consider asking the following questions:
  - Do you ever feel that you can't go on like this?
  - Have you ever made a suicide attempt?
  - Do you have any thoughts of harming yourself?
  - If so, have you made any plans?
  - Have you made any plans for putting your life in order?
  - Have you ever written a suicide note?
  - Has a family member ever committed suicide?

DIAGNOSTIC CRITERIA AND QUESTIONS TO USE IN ASSESSING MAJOR DEPRESSION

- **Depressed mood.** How has your mood been lately? Do you ever feel down, depressed or blue? How often does this happen? How long does it last?
- **Anhedonia.** Have you lost interest in your usual activities? Do you get less pleasure in things you used to enjoy?

- **Sleep disturbance.** How have you been sleeping? How does that compare with your normal sleep?
- **Appetite or weight change.** Has there been any change in your appetite or weight?
- **Decreased energy.** Have you noticed a decrease in your energy level?
- **Increased or decreases psychomotor activity.** Have you been feeling fidgety, or had problems sitting still? Have you slowed down, like you were moving in slow motion or stuck in mud?
- **Decreased concentration.** Have you been having trouble concentrating? Is it harder to make decisions than before?
- **Guilt or feelings of worthlessness.** Are you feeling guilty or blaming yourself for things? How would you describe yourself to someone who had never met you before?
- **Suicidal ideation.** Have you felt that life is not worth living or that you would be better off dead? Sometimes, when a person feels down or depressed they might think about dying: have you been having any thoughts like that?

The diagnosis of major depression requires five or more symptoms (including depressed mood or anhedonia) that have been present during a single 2-week period and have caused clinically significant distress or impairment in social, occupational or other important areas of functioning.

Source: Adapted from the *Diagnostic and Statistical Manual of Mental Disorders* (4th edition) (DSM-IV).

Past and current medical problems

- **Chronic conditions.** Depression can be triggered by or be a symptom of chronic physical illness, such as cancer, diabetes, COPD, cardiovascular disease (CVD) or hyperparathyroidism.
- **Psychiatric services.** Has the patient been referred to mental health services in the past? Depression is more common in severe mental illness (e.g. schizophrenia).

Medication and other treatments

- **Current medication.** Is the patient taking any drugs that can cause depressive symptoms, such as beta blockers or psychoactive medication?
- **Response to treatment.** Ask whether antidepressants have been effective in the past. If the patient is currently taking antidepressants, ask for details about dose, taking patterns and adverse effects. Try to find out whether the patient is taking the medication as prescribed, as suboptimal adherence is common.
- **Talking therapy.** Ask about previous counselling or cognitive behavioural therapy sessions. Have any of these been useful?

Social history

- **Education and work.** Depression is more common among people finishing education early and unemployed people.

- **Support.** Ask for details about social support networks.
- **Relationships.** Depression is common in separated or divorced patients and single parents. Ask about the state of the patient's relationships with a partner and with friends. Are there any conflicts? Is there bullying or abuse at home or work? Explore sensitively issues around any abuse in the past. Is there support from other family members?
- **Work.** Are there any problems at work? How have symptoms affected job performance? Is the patient unemployed or at risk of losing a job?
- **Finance.** Are there any financial problems?
- **Housing.** What is housing like? People in rented accommodation or living in urban areas are more likely to become depressed, particularly if living in neighbourhoods with social deprivation.
- **Loss.** Have there been any recent losses, such as a death in the family, family or relationship breakdown, redundancy or serious illness?
- **Crime.** Has there been any contact with the police? Have there been any previous offences? Is the patient on probation?

Alcohol and drugs
- **Alcohol and drug consumption.** Both may be triggers for depression or used as a coping mechanism. If an alcohol problem is present, it is often best to focus on this first.

Review of previous investigations
- **Bloods.** Blood tests are rarely necessary, but if additional symptoms or presentations are unusual, it may be worth checking for underlying disease. Common initial screening tests include full blood count, plasma viscosity, urea and electrolytes, liver function tests, glucose, thyroid-stimulating hormone (TSH) and calcium.

Examination

General
- **General state.** Does the patient look well? Is there evidence of personal neglect or physical abuse?
- **Mental state.** Is there evidence of psychosis or risk of suicide?
- **Alcohol.** Does the patient appear to be under the influence of alcohol? Are there obvious signs of alcoholic liver disease (e.g. spider naevi, jaundice, scratch marks, palmar erythema)?

Signs of depression
- **Appearance.** Does the patient look depressed? Is there evidence of self-neglect?
- **Communication.** Is there poor eye contact? Is speech normal or slowed down?
- **Behaviour.** Is there evidence of restlessness or apathy?

Key references and further reading

1. American Psychiatric Association (APA). *Diagnostic and Statistical Manual of Mental Disorders* (4th edition). American Psychiatric Association, Washington, DC; 1994.

2. National Institute for Health and Care Excellence (NICE). Depression: management of depression in primary and secondary care. NICE guidelines [CG23]. December 2004. Available from: http://www.nice.org.uk/guidance/cg23 (last accessed 29 April 2016).

3. National Institute for Health and Care Excellence (NICE). Depression in adults: recognition and management. NICE guidelines [CG90]. October 2009. Available from: http://www.nice.org.uk/guidance/cg90 (last accessed 29 April 2016).

4. National Institute for Health and Care Excellence (NICE). Depression. Clinical knowledge summaries. 2015. Available from: http://cks.nice.org.uk/depression (last accessed 29 April 2016).

5. Williams JW, Noël PH, Cordes JA et al. Is this patient clinically depressed? *JAMA* 2002;287:1160–1170.

Self-harm and harm to others

Key thoughts

Practical points

- **Safety and risks to health.** Ensure the patient's physical safety and assess the risk of further self-harm. Also ensure your own personal safety during the assessment.
- **Management.** Determine whether a patient needs medical or psychiatric admission, psychiatric assessment as an outpatient or counselling. Any decisions about future management should be based on a comprehensive psychiatric, psychological and social assessment after the initial assessment. Fuller assessment should usually take place in the emergency department, with adequate treatment facilities.
- **Acknowledge your own feelings.** Caring for people who self-harm is challenging. Recognising the personal and professional feelings that self-harm invokes in us is important. You may feel negative, angry, frustrated, challenged, stressed or insufficiently skilled.

Differential diagnosis

- Physical self-harm.
- Impulsive self-harm.
- Attempted suicide.

RED FLAGS

- Ongoing thoughts of suicide
- Suicide note
- Previous self-harm
- Act planned in advance
- Severe depression
- Acute psychosis
- Cognitive impairment

History

Ideas, concerns and expectations

- **Ideas.** Assume in all patients presenting with self-harm that there might be a genuine intent of self-destruction. Even if an act seems trivial, the intent may have been serious. Try to ask about and acknowledge feelings such as

---

The 10-Minute Clinical Assessment, Second Edition. Knut Schroeder.
© 2017 John Wiley & Sons, Ltd. Published 2017 by John Wiley & Sons, Ltd.

self-dislike, social isolation, embarrassment, shame, helplessness, anger and frustration.
- **Concerns.** Ask about any particular current worries that the patient may have about health, effect on others, finance or the future in general.
- **Expectations.** Ask about expectations in terms of what should happen now and in the future.

History of presenting complaint
- **Reason for self-harm.** Ask open questions about the story behind the episode of self-harm. Why now? What were the circumstances? Try and appear calm and unhurried, and communicate clearly. Be patient and give the patient time to express their feelings.
- **Method of self-harm.** Some patients may use more than one method to harm themselves (e.g. someone with a cut wrist may also have taken an overdose).
- **Suicidal risk.** Suicidal risk is not static and can change at any time, in either direction.
- **Emotional distress.** Emotional distress is associated with self-harm, both before and after the event. Showing respect and understanding in a calm and private environment will help the patient to relax.
- **Seriousness of the act.** Was the act planned in advance? Was the patient likely to be found? Was there a suicide note? Was the patient alone? Did the patient think the act would result in death? Did the patient want to die, and do they still?
- **Type of event.** Physical self-injury involves cutting or burning the skin in response to emotional distress. Impulsive self-harm commonly presents in the form of an overdose precipitated by alcohol consumption and arguments. Attempted suicide is associated with suicidal thoughts, which often have been present for weeks or months. They may not always have been verbalised and can take the form of thoughts such as 'Others will be better off without me'. Self-mutilation may be associated with psychosis.
- **Overdose.** Find out exactly what has been taken, when and in what dose. Suspected overdose will usually require urgent action.
- **Home and social circumstances.** Most acts of self-harm are performed by vulnerable people in response to a social crisis. Discuss the reasons for any self-harm and the effect it has had on the patient. Does the patient live alone? If not, who else is at home?
- **Risk factors for self-harm.** The following factors increase the risk of self-harm:
  o **Past attempts.** Has the patient attempted suicide in the past?
  o **Depression.** Is there evidence of severe depression, such as ideas of guilt, hopelessness or low mood?
  o **Suicidal ideation.** Has the patient had any thoughts of suicide?
  o **Plans.** Is there a plan of action? If so, have any preparations been made?
  o **Weapons.** Does the patient have the weapons and skills needed to carry out any plan?

- ○ **Auditory hallucinations.** Are there any voices commanding and encouraging self-harm? Are there any delusions?
- ○ **Hospital admission.** Has the patient been discharged from hospital recently?
- ○ **Illegal drugs.** Are illegal drugs being used?
- ○ **Other illness.** Is there chronic pain or other chronic illness?
- ○ **Bereavement.** Has there been a recent death in the family, especially of a partner?
- • **Risk of harm to others.** Consider the following in assessing the risk of harm to others:
  - ○ **Past history.** Is there any past history of impulsive behaviour or violence towards others?
  - ○ **Blame.** Is anyone else blamed for the patient's problems?
  - ○ **Punishment.** Does the patient believe anyone should be punished?
  - ○ **Hallucinations.** Do any hallucinatory voices encourage the patient to harm others?
  - ○ **Drugs.** Are any illegal drugs being used or traded?
  - ○ **Plan.** Does the patient have any plan or intent to harm others?
  - ○ **Weapons.** Does the patient have the weapons and skills needed to carry out any plan?
  - ○ **Suicide pact.** Has the patient made a suicide pact (e.g. an exhausted carer looking after a demented spouse)?
  - ○ **Homicide.** Does the patient want to 'save' a loved one from the horrors of this world or end a disabled child's life?
- • **Pregnancy and puerperium.** Depression is common during pregnancy and in the puerperium. Have a low threshold for hospital admission in women presenting with ideas of self-harm prior to or following delivery, when immediate psychiatric and social assessment may be needed.

Medication
- • **Antidepressants.** Is the patient taking antidepressants?
- • **Drugs dangerous in overdose.** Consider whether the patient is taking any drugs that would be dangerous to health if taken as an overdose (e.g. paracetamol, tricyclic antidepressants, sedatives, opiates).

Social history
- • **Home.** Ask for details about housing and home life. Are others around for support?

Alcohol and drugs
- • **Alcohol.** Find out whether alcohol has been taken in the preceding 24 hours; this might affect the assessment.
- • **Drugs.** Financial issues are common in drug users, which can lead to suicidal intentions, particularly if the situation seems hopeless.

Examination

General
- **General state.** Does the patient look unwell?
- **Airway, breathing and circulation (ABC).** Check ABC if there is reduced consciousness.
- **Physical injuries.** Look for any obvious physical injuries that need urgent attention.

Vital signs
- **Temperature.** There may be fever in acute overdose. Hypothermia may occur if the patient has been exposed to the cold after an overdose with sedating drugs.
- **Pulse.** Tachycardia may occur after overdose of centrally stimulating substances.
- **Blood pressure.** Low blood pressure may suggest impending shock; for example, after opioid overdose.

Preliminary psychosocial assessment
- **Risk of incomplete assessment.** Is there a risk that the patient will leave before the assessment is completed and treatment is provided?
- **General state.** Look for marked restlessness or extremely variable mood.
- **Mental capacity.** Determine the patient's mental capacity to make decisions about treatment or care needs. Decide whether a formal mental health assessment is required. Assume mental capacity unless there is evidence to the contrary.
- **Risk of suicide.** Is the patient actively suicidal?
- **Willingness to be assessed.** Is the patient happy to undergo more extensive psychosocial assessment?
- **Level of distress.** Is the patient still distressed and/or suicidal?
- **Mental illness.** Look for signs of mental illness.

Skin
- **Scars and injection marks.** Look for any evidence of physical self-harm or drug misuse.

Head and neck
- **Pupils.** Pinpoint pupils indicate opioid overdose. Mydriasis suggests overdose with central stimulants or brain damage if there is hypoxia in comatose patients.

Key references and further reading
1. Department of Health. *National Suicide Prevention Strategy for England: Annual Report on Progress.* DoH Publications, London; 2003.
2. Harrison A. A guide to risk assessment. *Nurs Times* 2003;99:44–45.
3. National Institute for Health and Care Excellence (NICE). Self-harm in over 8s: short-term management and prevention of recurrence. NICE guidelines

[CG16]. July 2004. Available from: http://www.nice.org.uk/guidance/cg16 (last accessed 29 April 2016).

4. National Institute for Health and Care Excellence (NICE). Self-harm. Clinical knowledge summaries. 2014. Available from: http://cks.nice.org.uk/self-harm (last accessed 29 April 2016).

5. Royal College of Psychiatrists. Assessment following self-harm in adults. Council report CR122. October 2004. Available from: http://www.rcpsych.ac.uk/pdf/Assessment%20following%20SH%20CR122.pdf (last accessed 29 April 2016).

Anxiety, phobias and panic disorder

Key thoughts

Practical points
- **Diagnosis.** Anxiety and related disorders can present in various ways. The main types of anxiety disorder are generalised anxiety disorder, panic disorder and phobias (e.g. agoraphobia, social phobia and simple phobias). Identify any underlying medical causes or complications.
- **Prognosis.** Assess the impact of symptoms on daily life and whether there is a need for urgent action.

Differential diagnosis
- **Medical.** Heart disease, hyperthyroidism.
- **Mental health.** Depression, psychosis, alcohol misuse.

> ### RED FLAGS
>
> - Suicidal ideas
> - Severe alcohol misuse
> - Depression
> - Social isolation
> - Coronary heart disease

History

Ideas, concerns and expectations
- **Ideas.** What are the patient's ideas about the condition? Patients commonly feel that there may not be a cure and that they are 'going mad'. Patients with anxiety and panic disorder often present late for fear of any stigma that might be attached to the diagnosis. 'Anxiety' has a medical meaning, and many people would prefer describing themselves as 'suffering from anxiety' to being labelled as 'anxious'.
- **Concerns.** Many patients suspect that physical symptoms are caused by anxiety but do not want a physical diagnosis to be missed. Pain often suggests tissue damage to patients, who are often not aware that emotional illness can cause physical symptoms without physical damage. Many people get very worried about their health. Panic attacks can be disabling and frightening and may lead to social isolation due to avoidance behaviour.
- **Expectations.** Explore expectations about management and prognosis.

The 10-Minute Clinical Assessment, Second Edition. Knut Schroeder.
© 2017 John Wiley & Sons, Ltd. Published 2017 by John Wiley & Sons, Ltd.

History of presenting complaint

- **Screening and severity.** Consider using a formal questionnaire to screen and assess the severity of generalised anxiety disorder, such as the GAD-7, which considers the frequency and severity of a number of anxiety-related symptoms (see box).
- **Quality of life.** Ask open questions about how and in what context the symptoms started. How has day-to-day life been affected?
- **Timing of seeking help.** Why is the patient presenting now? Has a normal concern become so overwhelming and so severe that they are seeking medical attention? A person can respond differently to the same stressor on different occasions. Effects of stress can build up, so that minor worries may suddenly tip the balance.
- **Life events.** Is the patient's mental state reasonable, given the circumstances? Bereavement, stress at work and relationship or financial problems can all cause anxiety and panic.
- **Worry.** Find out what the patient is worried about. Is there concern about trivial problems? Worry is often described as an unreasonable or exaggerated response to personal circumstances and seen as a 'mental weakness'.
- **Sleep.** Have there been difficulties going to sleep or sleeping through the night?
- **Stress.** Stress is usually seen as being caused by environmental factors that cause anxiety. 'Suffering from stress' may be accepted as part of a busy lifestyle.
- **Tension.** Is there a feeling of inner tension or doom?
- **Autonomic symptoms.** Does the patient suffer from headaches or neck ache? Find out whether there are symptoms such as trembling, tingling, dizzy spells, sweating, urinary frequency, dyspepsia, diarrhoea, blurred vision, tremor or dry mouth.
- **Indications for secondary care referral.** Consider specialist referral if there are severe disabling symptoms or if there are physical, social or psychological complications. Also consider referral if there is little or no response to treatment or if the necessary treatment is unavailable in the community.

GAD-7

- Feeling nervous or on edge
- Not being able to stop or control worrying
- Trouble relaxing
- Being so restless that it is hard to sit still
- Becoming easily annoyed or irritable
- Feeling afraid, as if something awful might happen

Source: Spitzer RL, Kroenke K, Williams JB, Löwe B. A brief measure for assessing generalised anxiety disorder: the GAD-7. *Arch Intern Med* 2006;166:1092–1097.

Common symptom patterns
- **Depression.** A number of questions can be helpful in identifying depression: Do you feel low? Do you suffer from low energy? Do you still have interest in doing things that you normally enjoy? Has your confidence gone down? How do you feel about the future? Do you find it difficult at times to think straight and make decisions? Do you eat too little or too much? Have you lost or put on weight? Do you feel you have generally slowed down?
- **Phobias.** Does the patient suffer from phobias? Anxiety about death or general health is common. Ask about situations such as being in open spaces, attending public events, flying, being in an elevator and engaging in public speaking. Also check whether there are any fears about specific objects, such as needles or spiders. The fear is usually an overestimated and irrational fear of the real danger (e.g. a plane crashing).
- **Panic attacks.** Check whether disabling panic attacks have occurred. Are there symptoms such as dizziness, palpitations, shortness of breath, tingling, shaking, feelings of unreality, feelings of being detached, fear of losing control or chest pain? These symptoms may be perceived as being life-threatening and serious. Ask about frequency and any precipitating factors. Do attacks come unexpectedly? Is there evidence of avoidance behaviour? If so, how does it affect the patient's life?

Past and current medical problems
- **Cardiovascular.** Ask about hypertension and cardiac disease.
- **Neurological.** Check for a history of migraine or vestibular abnormalities.
- **Mental health.** Have there been any previous episodes of anxiety or depression? Have community or hospital mental health services been involved at any time?

Medication and other treatments
- **Drug treatment.** Does the patient use any prescription drugs to treat anxiety? Withdrawal from sedatives can cause symptoms of anxiety. What has been the response to treatment so far? Ask whether medication is taken as prescribed.
- **Drugs causing anxiety.** Consider thyroid hormone overdose in patients with hypothyroidism. Theophylline, beta agonists and steroids may cause symptoms of anxiety in patients with asthma. Many antidepressants can cause symptoms of anxiety at the start of treatment (especially selective serotonin reuptake inhibitors (SSRIs)).
- **Over-the-counter medication.** Ask whether any over-the-counter medication is being taken.
- **Talking therapy.** Have any talking therapies been tried (e.g. counselling, cognitive behavioural therapy, group workshops)?

Alcohol and drugs
- **Alcohol.** Anxiety (particularly social phobia) can contribute to alcohol misuse. Anxiety is a common feature of alcohol withdrawal, although the patient

may not recognise and realise this. Generalised anxiety and panic disorder can emerge from alcohol misuse and improve with 6–8 weeks of abstinence; in depression, improvement may be noticed within 1 month.

- **Drugs.** Ask about drugs like cannabis, opioids, hallucinogens and stimulants such as amphetamines, which can cause severe anxiety on withdrawal or after longer-term use.
- **Caffeine.** Increased caffeine intake can cause or contribute to anxiety.

Social history
- **Home.** Are there any activities that the patient cannot take part in? Ask about symptoms of agoraphobia and any effects they have on socialising.
- **Work.** Have there been any problems with work?

Examination

General
- **General appearance.** Does the patient look anxious or depressed?

Vital signs
- **Pulse.** Tachycardia may result from anxiety or another underlying cause, such as heart or lung disease. Hyperthyroidism may cause sinus tachycardia or an irregularly irregular pulse due to atrial fibrillation.
- **Blood pressure.** Symptoms of anxiety may cause or be caused by raised blood pressure.
- **Respiratory rate.** An increased respiratory rate may lead to hyperventilation.

Endocrine assessment
- **Thyroid status.** Palpate the thyroid for size and lumps. Look for a fine tremor and sweaty palms

Key references and further reading

1. Barr Taylor C. Panic Disorder. *BMJ* 2006;332:951–955.
2. Hogfe EA, Ivkovic AN, Fricchione GL. Generalized anxiety disorder: diagnosis and treatment. *BMJ* 2012;345:e7500.
3. National Institute for Health and Care Excellence (NICE). Generalised anxiety disorder and panic disorder in adults: management. NICE guidelines [CG113]. January 2011. Available from: http://www.nice.org.uk/guidance/cg113 (last accessed 29 April 2016).
4. National Institute for Health and Care Excellence (NICE). Generalized anxiety disorder. Clinical knowledge summaries. 2015. Available from: http://cks.nice.org.uk/generalized-anxiety-disorder (last accessed 29 April 2016).
5. Spitzer RL, Kroenke K, Williams JB, Löwe B. A brief measure for assessing generalised anxiety disorder: the GAD-7. *Arch Intern Med* 2006;166:1092–1097.

Alcohol screening

Key thoughts

Practical points
- **Diagnosis.** Alcohol misuse is common and is often under-reported. Patients may present with various physical and emotional problems caused by excess alcohol consumption.
- **Prognosis.** Mental health-related problems, gastrointestinal symptoms and alcoholic liver disease are important complications.

Important risk factors
- Depression.
- Social isolation.
- Family problems.

> **RED FLAGS**
>
> - Lack of control
> - Concern about alcohol intake expressed by the patient or others
> - Signs of liver disease
> - Gastrointestinal problems in conjunction with depression
> - Alcohol dependency
> - Suicidal ideas
> - Loss of employment
> - Mental health problems, including depression, anxiety and insomnia

History

Ideas, concerns and expectations
- **Ideas.** The potential harm that can result from alcohol misuse is often under-estimated. Many people are unaware of safe drinking limits or the number of units in different types of alcohol.
- **Concerns.** A feeling of guilt is common. Have others raised any concerns?
- **Expectations.** If the patient recognises that an alcohol problem exists, are there any expectations with regard to further management? Many will have unrealistic hopes for a 'quick fix'. What is the patient's readiness to change their drinking (the answer will influence the goals to be set, the timing of the next follow-up appointment and the urgency of referral, if necessary)?

The 10-Minute Clinical Assessment, Second Edition. Knut Schroeder.
© 2017 John Wiley & Sons, Ltd. Published 2017 by John Wiley & Sons, Ltd.

History of alcohol intake

- **Suspect alcohol misuse.** Alcohol misuse can cause multiple symptoms, including dyspepsia, abdominal pain, insomnia, anxiety, panic disorder and depression. Ask about alcohol consumption whenever this might be a cause for any presenting problem.
- **Denial.** Some people find it difficult to talk about their average alcohol intake or are even in denial about the amount of alcohol they consume.
- **Type of alcohol.** Ask about the type of alcohol product being consumed and its alcohol content (information on calculating units of alcohol is available at www.drinkaware.co.uk).

Levels of drinking

- **At-risk consumption.** To keep health risks to a minimum, it is recommended to drink no more than 14 units per week.
- **Problem drinking.** Problem drinking occurs when alcohol causes problems for the drinker, for the drinker's friends and family or for society as a whole.
- **Dependence and addiction.** In alcohol dependence, there is intermittent periodic intoxication, which affects the drinker's life. There is usually severe and uncontrollable craving and the dose consumed usually increases as a result of tolerance.
- **Support.** Has the patient ever contacted an agency that supports people with alcohol problems or attended alcohol support groups, such as Alcoholics Anonymous (AA)? Ask about telephone counselling and access to information on the Internet.

SCREENING QUESTIONS

- **Frequency.** How often do you have a drink containing alcohol?
- **Quantity.** How many drinks containing alcohol do you have on a typical day when you are drinking? What size of glass is being used? How long does a bottle last? Is this being shared with others? What is the most you have had to drink on any one day in the past month? Heavy drinking sessions are not always taken into account when estimating the weekly average, even if they occur fairly frequently.
- **Heavy drinking.** How often do you have six or more drinks on a single occasion?
- **Stopping to drink.** How often during the last year have you failed to do what is normally expected from you because of drinking?
- **Increased drinking.** Have others noticed or commented on your drinking?
- **Morning drinking.** How often during the last year have you needed a first drink in the morning to get yourself going after a heavy drinking session?
- **Guilt.** How often during the last year have you had a feeling of guilt or remorse after drinking?

- **Memory and blackouts.** How often during the last year have you been unable to remember what happened the night before because you had been drinking?
- **Injuries.** Have you or someone else been injured as a result of your drinking?
- **Concerns.** Has a relative or friend, or a doctor or another health worker been concerned about your drinking or suggested you cut down?

Source: Babor TF, de la Fuente JR, Saunders J, Grant M. AUDIT: the alcohol use disorders identification test. Guidelines for use in primary health care (2nd edition). Available from: http://whqlibdoc.who.int/hq/2001/WHO_MSD_MSB_01.6a.pdf (last accessed 29 April 2016).

Effects of alcohol problems on daily life

- **Social life.** Have there been any problems with relationships, employment or finance? Has the patient stopped taking part in certain activities because of alcohol?
- **Responsibilities.** Is the patient able to go to work or school and keep up with responsibilities? Have there been any problems with the police? Does the patient drive? It is easy to still be over the limit the morning after drinking.

Questions to ask if answers are vague

- **Clarification.** Find out what patients mean if they say, 'I am just a social drinker' or 'I only drink with meals'.
- **Giving choices.** By asking, 'Would you think you drink about one or two glasses of wine per night, or more like eight to ten?', you show that you will not be shocked by any answers.
- **Offer excuses.** Offer a medical or social excuse for drinking: 'Do you drink to help you go to sleep? Many people have a glass or two if they cannot go to sleep' or 'Do you ever drink wine with your meals? Many people find this helps them digest their food.'
- **Drinking pattern.** Are there any episodes of binge or heavy regular drinking? For how long have these occurred?
- **Timing.** Ask whether the patients drinks during the day or only in the evening?
- **Associated behaviours.** Does the patient drink alone? Are there particular situations in which they drink?
- **Associated symptoms.** Does the patient suffer from hangovers, withdrawal symptoms or night sweats? Gastrointestinal symptoms such as anorexia, nausea and vomiting are common.
- **Fits.** Has the patient ever had a fit or passed out in connection with alcohol?

Mental health

- **Psychiatric history.** Is there a history of substance misuse? Are there any previous contacts with mental health services?

- **Current mental health problems.** Are there any current mental health problems that need addressing, or is there input from the mental health team? Are there any suicidal thoughts or plans?

Social history

- **Home.** Who else is at home? Alcohol problems are common in homeless people.
- **Social background.** Ask about social background, in terms of family, schooling and work. Are support networks in place? Is there a child at risk?
- **Family.** Is there a family history of heavy drinking? Are any other members of the current household drinkers?
- **Driving.** Have there been any driving incidents or drunken-driving offences? Guidelines on drinking and driving are available from the Driver and Vehicle Licensing Agency (DVLA) (https://www.gov.uk/drink-driving-penalties).
- **Other substances:** Does the patient use other substances, such as tobacco, cannabis or illicit drugs?

SIGNS OF ALCOHOL DEPENDENCE

- **Lack of control.** This is the most important feature.
- **Increasing amounts.** There is a need to use increased amounts of alcohol to achieve the desired effect.
- **Urge.** There is a strong urge to drink despite harmful effects.
- **Detoxification.** There may have been repeated attempts to cut down or stop alcohol.
- **Withdrawal symptoms.** There may be withdrawal symptoms when the patient is not drinking.

Examination

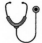

General

- **Breath.** Is there a smell of alcohol or a sweeter smell of metabolites?
- **Speech.** Is speech normal or dysarthric (suggesting either alcohol intoxication or cerebellar involvement)?
- **Eye contact.** Poor eye contact and reduced affect suggest depression.
- **Signs of alcohol withdrawal.** The patient may appear anxious, shaky and sweaty.

Signs of liver disease

- **Skin.** Look for spider naevi, jaundice, scratch marks and palmar erythema.

Abdominal examination

- **Palpation.** Is the liver palpable? Are there any obvious signs of liver failure?

Key references and further reading

1. Babor TF, de la Fuente JR, Saunders J, Grant M. AUDIT: the alcohol use disorders identification test. Guidelines for use in primary health care (2nd edition). Available from: http://whqlibdoc.who.int/hq/2001/WHO_MSD_MSB_01.6a.pdf (last accessed 29 April 2016).

2. Coulton S, Drummond C, James D et al. Opportunistic screening for alcohol use disorders in primary care: comparative study. *BMJ* 2006;332:511–517.

3. National Institute for Health and Care Excellence (NICE). Alcohol-use-disorders: diagnosis, assessment and management of harmful drinking and alcohol dependence. NICE guidelines [CG115]. February 2011. Available from: http://www.nice.org.uk/guidance/cg115 (last accessed 29 April 2016).

4. National Institute for Health and Care Excellence (NICE). Alcohol – problem drinking. Clinical knowledge summaries. 2015. Available from: http://cks.nice.org/alcohol-problem-drinking (last accessed 29 April 2016).

5. Saunders JB, Aasland OG, Babor TF et al. Development of the alcohol use disorders identification test (AUDIT): WHO collaborative project on early detection of persons with harmful alcohol consumption – II. *Addiction* 1993;88:791–804.

6. Department of Health. Alcohol Guidelines Review – Report from the Guidelines development group to the UK Chief Medical Officers. Available from: https://www.gov.uk/government/uploads/system/uploads/attachment_data/file/489797/CMO_Alcohol_Report.pdf (last accessed 24 May 2016).

Alcohol dependence

Key thoughts

Practical points

- **Diagnosis and prognosis.** Alcohol dependence is common. Alcohol-related problems affect individual patients, their families and society as a whole. Alcohol dependence can be difficult to spot and may often go undiagnosed. Assessment of health problems and mental health is important to allow targeted treatment.
- **Detoxification.** In heavy drinkers, detoxification medication is likely to be necessary in achieving abstinence. Establish whether you are able to prescribe or need the support of a specialist agency. Detoxification can be carried out at home or in a hospital, if available.

Important risk factors

- Depression.
- Anxiety.
- Social isolation.
- Bereavement.
- Family history of alcoholism.

RED FLAGS

- Lack of control
- Concern about alcohol intake expressed by the patient or others
- Signs of liver disease
- Gastrointestinal problems in conjunction with depression
- Alcohol dependency
- Suicidal ideas
- Loss of employment
- Mental health problems, including depression, anxiety and insomnia

History

Ideas, concerns and expectations

- **Ideas.** The potential harm that can result from alcohol misuse is often underestimated. Many people, including those with established alcohol problems, are unaware of safe limits of alcohol consumption.
- **Concerns.** Many patients with established health problems due to alcoholism (e.g. alcoholic liver disease, gastrointestinal problems, depression) will become

The 10-Minute Clinical Assessment, Second Edition. Knut Schroeder.
© 2017 John Wiley & Sons, Ltd. Published 2017 by John Wiley & Sons, Ltd.

concerned about their health. Partners and other family members will often be even more worried and may have encouraged the patient to seek medical help.

- **Expectations.** What are the expectations and preferences with regard to further management? Why is the patient presenting now?

History of alcohol-related problems

- **Alcohol history.** Ask open questions around alcohol consumption. How did it all start? How does alcoholism fit into the context of the patient's life? How has quality of life been affected, for both the patient and those close to them?
- **Physical problems.** Common problems are dyspepsia, CVD, alcohol-related injury and pancreatitis.
- **Diet.** Many people with alcohol problems have a poor diet and may be missing meals.
- **Mental health.** Anxiety, loss of confidence, depression and aggression are common. Alcohol is frequently used as self-medication for insomnia, distress or mental problems. Have the patient's partner or family complained about their drinking? Have there been any criminal offences (e.g. drunk driving or being involved in a fight)? Have there been any suicide attempts? Are there current thoughts of suicide?
- **Motivation.** What is the level of motivation for cutting down or stopping alcohol consumption?

Signs and complications of alcohol dependence

- **Increasing amounts.** Is there a need to use increasing amounts of alcohol to achieve the desired effect?
- **Urge.** Is there a strong urge to drink despite harmful effects?
- **Detoxification.** Have there been repeated attempts to cut down or stop drinking?
- **Withdrawal symptoms.** Does the patient suffer from withdrawal symptoms when not drinking? Check for symptoms such as loss of appetite, nausea, vomiting, restlessness, agitation, tachycardia, sweating, hallucinations, confusion, tremor and seizures.
- **Sexual dysfunction.** Sexual difficulties, such as loss of libido and erectile dysfunction, are common.
- **Wernicke–Korsakoff syndrome.** In Wernicke's encephalopathy, poor diet, missing meals or gastrointestinal disturbance lead to low levels of thiamine intake and absorption. Wernicke's encephalopathy is a medical emergency. It may present with confusion, ataxia and nystagmus, but these signs may be absent, and it is important to maintain a high index of suspicion. At-risk patients will need to be considered for parenteral intramuscular Pabrinex.

Past and current medical problems

- **Alcohol-related problems.** Ask about any past serious medical problems or problems that have resulted from alcohol consumption.

- **Current medical problems.** Are there any urgent or chronic medical problems that need further assessment, investigation or treatment?
- **Liver.** Ask about a history of hepatitis or cirrhosis.
- **Cardiovascular.** Check for a history of high blood pressure, stroke and cardiomyopathy.
- **Gastrointestinal.** Consider gastritis and pancreatitis if there are problems with nausea, vomiting, dyspepsia or abdominal pain.
- **Neurological.** Ask about symptoms of blackouts, neuropathy, myopathy, brain damage or impaired cognition. Have there been any fits?
- **Mental health.** Depression and anxiety are common, either as a cause of increased alcohol consumption or as a result of misuse. Ask about any changes in personality. Have there been any hallucinations during periods of withdrawal?

Social history
- **Background.** Ask about social background, including family, schooling and work. What is the current life situation? Are there any support networks?
- **Family problems.** Are there any marital problems or partner abuse? Consider child abuse and neglect.
- **Social.** Are there any social or financial problems? Ask about any problems with work, including absenteeism. Is there a need for a sick note? Ask about any episodes of public drunkenness.
- **Crime.** Have there been any conflicts with the law, including traffic offences and fights?

Assessment of readiness for detoxification
- **Timing.** Is this the best time? Detoxification should take place at a time that is convenient and suitable for the patient, whenever possible. They must have a relapse-prevention plan. If they do not have an answer to the question, 'What are you going to do instead of drinking?', then they are not ready and need more support for preparation, preferably with the help of an alcohol agency.
- **Motivation.** Is there self-motivation for detoxification or is there pressure from others?
- **Withdrawal state.** Is there evidence of withdrawal symptoms, such as agitation, confusion, fits, hallucinations, disorientation or memory problems?
- **Past attempts.** Has community detoxification been attempted before? If so, why did it fail? Was it due to lack of motivation or a lack of a relapse-prevention plan?
- **Social support.** Are any friends or relatives available to supervise?

Indications for asking specialist services for advice or support
- **Mental health.** Confusion, hallucinations and risk of suicide.
- **Social.** Lack of support at home.
- **Medical.** Severe vomiting or diarrhoea, malnourishment, metabolic problems, epilepsy or fits.
- **Severity**. Severe dependence and multiple substance misuse.

- **Other.** History of previous complicated withdrawal (including uncontrollable withdrawal symptoms and an unwillingness to be seen on a daily basis).

Review of recent investigations
- **Full blood count.** Check for macrocytosis.
- **Liver function tests.** Alcohol can cause abnormal liver function tests and a raised gamma-glutamyl transpeptidase (GGT).
- **Vitamin B12 and folate.** A poor diet may lead to vitamin deficiencies.
- **Ultrasound.** If liver function tests are abnormal, has an abdominal ultrasound scan been performed?

Examination

General
- **Breath.** Does breath smell of alcohol?
- **Balance.** Abnormalities may suggest intoxication or neuropathy. Truncal ataxia may be present.
- **Confusion.** Confusion and memory problems are features of Wernicke–Korsakoff syndrome.

Vital signs
- **Temperature.** This may be raised in infection and acute withdrawal. Hypothermia may occur in Wernicke–Korsakoff syndrome.
- **Pulse.** Check for atrial fibrillation.
- **Blood pressure.** Alcohol is a risk factor for hypertension.

Skin
- **Skin.** Look for palmar erythema, spider naevi, scratch marks and jaundice. Rosacea is also common.

Head and neck
- **Eyes.** Ophthalmoplegia and nystagmus are rare signs of Wernicke–Korsakoff syndrome.

Abdomen
- **Liver.** Check the liver for enlargement.
- **Epigastrium.** Epigastric tenderness may suggest gastritis or, less commonly, pancreatitis.

Key references and further reading
1. Burge SK, Schneider FD. Alcohol-related problems: recognition and intervention. *Am Fam Physician* 1999;59:361–370, 372.
2. National Institute for Health and Care Excellence (NICE). Alcohol-use-disorders: diagnosis, assessment and management of harmful drinking and alcohol dependence. NICE guidelines [CG115]. February 2011. Available from: http://www.nice.org.uk/guidance/cg115 (last accessed 29 April 2016).

3. National Institute for Health and Care Excellence (NICE). Alcohol – problem drinking. Clinical knowledge summaries. 2015. Available from: http://cks.nice.org/alcohol-problem-drinking (last accessed 29 April 2016).
4. Royal College of Psychiatrists (RCP). Roles and responsibilities of doctors in the provision of treatment for drug and alcohol misusers. Council report CR131. January 2005. Available from: http://www.drugsandalcohol.ie/17841/1/RCP_RCGP_Roles_and_responsibilities_of_doctors.pdf (last accessed 29 April 2016).

Illicit drug misuse

Key thoughts

Practical points
- **Diagnosis.** Drug users are at risk from complications such as human immunod-eficiency virus (HIV), hepatitis, social problems and mental illness. It is important to provide general medical care to drug users, as for any other patient.

Important risk factors
- Homelessness.
- Mental health problems.
- Social problems.
- Peer use of drugs.

> **RED FLAGS**
>
> - Sharing of needles or other equipment
> - High drug use
> - Using cocktails of drugs or polydrug use
> - Suicidal ideation
> - Hepatitis B or C infection
> - HIV infection
> - Opioid users who have been abstinent (increased risk of overdose-related death)

History

Ideas, concerns and expectations
- **Ideas.** Many drug users are wary about health professionals. Try to engage them by using a particularly emphatic and nonjudgemental approach.
- **Concerns.** Worries about future health, employment, personal safety and finance are common.
- **Expectations.** Find out what preferences the patient has in terms of treatment. Common reasons for consultation include a prescription for a drug substitute and treatment of complications such as infection or constipation. The patient may rightly expect confidentiality, but if they are about to tell you about any illegal activities, you may warn them of your right to disclose information in the public interest.

The 10-Minute Clinical Assessment, Second Edition. Knut Schroeder.
© 2017 John Wiley & Sons, Ltd. Published 2017 by John Wiley & Sons, Ltd.

History of presenting complaint

- **History of drug misuse.** What is the story behind the drug use in the context of the patient's life?
- **Onset.** Is this an acute or longstanding problem?
- **Main problems.** What are the main problems at the moment? For which of these problems does the patient need help? What are the main withdrawal effects, if any? Which problems contribute most to a reduction in quality of life at the moment?
- **Motivation.** Is the patient motivated to come off drugs?

Drug-taking behaviour

- **Reasons and circumstances.** Why and when does the patient take drugs? Common reasons for taking drugs are to combat insomnia and to reduce withdrawal effects. Alcohol is often used to alleviate heroin withdrawal. Ask about drug-taking routines in terms of times, places and people. Where are the drugs obtained, and at what cost?
- **Past and current drug-taking.** Ask about the age when drug taking began and get details about periods of drug-taking. When did drug-taking first become a problem? Establish details of all illicit drugs taken in the past month, including cannabis. Record types of drug taken, the quantity and frequency of use and the route of administration. What is the minimum amount needed for comfort? Have there been any periods of abstinence? What has been the period of heaviest drug use so far? Are cocktails of drugs being used? Are multiple drugs being taken at different times? Always ask about alcohol, which is particularly harmful to drug users who suffer from hepatitis B or C.
- **Past treatments.** Ask whether the person has ever tried to stop previously. Have they taken part in any previous drug-abstinence programmes or rehabilitation?
- **Injecting history.** Has the patient ever injected drugs? If so, how recently? Past injectors are at higher risk of hepatitis B and C, HIV and other needle-borne infections. Obtain details about needle supply and whether equipment has been shared.
- **Finance.** How much money is spent on drugs on average? Where does the money come from? If appropriate, consider asking women if they have been accepting money for sex, as prostitution puts them at higher risk of sexually transmitted infections (STIs), physical and emotional abuse and pregnancy.
- **Cognitive impairment.** Drug use may affect cognitive impairment. There is a risk of psychosis in young cannabis users, particularly if there is a family history. Check for possible stimulant-induced psychosis and paranoia.
- **Respiratory symptoms.** Smoking drugs such as cannabis can cause chronic bronchitis and increases the risk of lung carcinoma.
- **Risky behaviours.** Ask about overdosing, mixing drugs, driving habits, frequency of intoxication and unsafe sex. Guidance on driving-related issues is available from the DVLA (https://www.gov.uk/drink-driving-penalties).
- **Tolerance.** Is more of the substance needed now than before?

- **Mental health problems.** These are common among drug users. Is there a history of overdose, self-harm or contact with mental health services? Are there any symptoms of depression, anxiety or drug-induced psychosis? Have friends or relatives noticed a personality change? Is there a lack of interest in usual activities?
- **Overdoses.** Have there been any deliberate or accidental overdoses in the past?
- **Withdrawal symptoms and signs.** In opioid users, ask about sneezing, sleep problems, runny nose, sweating, agitation and vomiting.

EFFECTS AND ADVERSE EFFECTS OF IMPORTANT DRUG CLASSES

- **Amphetamines.** Lead to heightened alertness, concentration and confidence. Adverse effects include dehydration, difficulty concentrating, jaw clenching, cardiac arrhythmias, psychosis and sudden death.
- **Opiates.** Produce sedative effects, euphoria and increased well being. Adverse effects are abscesses, venous collapse, heart and other organ damage, opiate dependence, respiratory depression and death.
- **Cocaine.** Causes positive mood and euphoria. Can lead to psychiatric symptoms, such as anxiety and paranoia, dizziness and muscle twitching. Violent behaviour and aggression are common. May also cause cardiac problems, such as cardiomyopathy and arrhythmias.
- **Ecstasy.** Leads to positive mood, feelings of intimacy and increased energy. Adverse effects are similar to those of amphetamines.

Past and current medical problems
- **Chronic conditions.** Ask about any chronic conditions that might be relevant for further management, such as diabetes, asthma or heart disease.
- **Infection.** Ask about hepatitis B and C and HIV infection. Has the patient been vaccinated against hepatitis B?
- **Organ damage as a result of drug use.** Ask about evidence of liver disease, seizures during use or withdrawal and cardiac problems. Have there been any overdoses?
- **Deep venous thrombosis.** Ask about past deep venous thrombosis and any treatments.

Medication
- **Medication.** Is any other medication (e.g. sedatives, hypnotics) being prescribed or taken without prescription? Ask about contraception in women.

Alcohol
- **Alcohol.** Alcohol has specific additional health risks.

Social history
- **Social problems.** Has there been a decline in school or work performance, conduct or attendance? Have there been any complaints about irresponsible behaviour? Ask about other social, legal and interpersonal difficulties.
- **Housing.** Ask about the current home situation. Is homelessness an issue? What is the living environment like?
- **Support.** Is there a supporting family or partner? Are the partner or other family members also drug users? Ask about friends and other social relationships.
- **Employment.** Ask about educational background, previous jobs and current employment or unemployment. Are work colleagues aware? Has the patient ever lost a job as a result of drug use?
- **Contact with criminal justice system.** Have there been any convictions? Is the drug habit financed by illegal activities?
- **Financial situation.** Is there an increased need for money?
- **Child protection.** Are there any dependent children? What are the effects of drug use on their well being?

Review of previous investigations
- **Infectious diseases.** Check any virology test results and immunisation history. In women, ask about cervical screening. Has the patient ever had an HIV test?
- **Liver function.** Hepatitis commonly causes abnormal liver function tests, as does excessive alcohol use.

Examination

General
- **General condition.** Does the patient look unwell? Restlessness, rapid speech, agitation and large pupils are common with psychostimulants.
- **Gait.** Is gait unsteady? Are there any obvious neurological features?
- **Evidence of drug use.** Look for paint stains on clothes and skin. Is there any evidence of inhalant misuse? Does the patient seem intoxicated?
- **Mouth.** Check oral health. Does the breath smell of chemicals?
- **Nutritional status.** Is there evidence of malnutrition?
- **Neglect.** Look for signs of neglect in terms of personal hygiene or clothing.

Vital signs
- **Temperature.** This may be raised in infection and acute withdrawal. Always consider the possibility of endocarditis in intravenous drug users.
- **Pulse.** Tachycardia is commonly caused by infection, drug withdrawal or intoxication. Some drugs may cause arrhythmias.
- **Blood pressure.** This may be raised in withdrawal or low in opioid overdose.

Skin
- **Injection sites.** Check the orearms, groins, lower limbs and neck for injection marks and signs of infection. There may be track marks, and drug users may wear long sleeves even on hot days to cover them up.

- **Scars.** Are there any other scars indicating self-harm?
- **Lymph glands.** Check for lymphadenopathy (HIV, other infections).

Head and neck
- **Nose.** Inspect the nasal mucosa and septum, which may be damaged as a result of cocaine misuse.
- **Pupils.** Pinpoint pupils occur in opioid intoxication and become mydriatic in withdrawal. Psychostimulants lead to large pupils.
- **Sclerae.** Jaundice may indicate hepatitis.

Chest
- **Heart.** Listen for murmurs. Endocarditis and valve problems may result from unsafe injections.
- **Lungs.** Listen for any signs of infection. Pneumonia is common.

Abdomen
- **Liver.** Check for hepatomegaly (hepatitis, alcoholic liver disease).

Mental state
- **Behaviour.** Focus on mood and thought content. Are there any abnormal beliefs or experiences?

Key references and further reading
1. Department of Health (England) and the devolved administrations. *Drug Misuse and Dependence: UK Guidelines on Clinical Management.* Department of Health (England), the Scottish Government, Welsh Assembly Government and Northern Ireland Executive, London; 2007. Available from: http://www.nta.nhs.uk/uploads/clinical_guidelines_2007.pdf (last accessed 29 April 2016).
2. National Institute for Health and Care Excellence (NICE). Drug misuse: psychosocial interventions. NICE guidelines [CG51]. July 2007. Available from: http://www.nice.org.uk/guidance/cg51 (last accessed 29 April 2016).
3. Tashkin DP. Airway effects of marijuana, cocaine, and other inhaled illicit agents. *Curr Opin Pulm Med* 2001;7:43–61.

Obsessive–compulsive disorder

Key thoughts

Practical points
- **Diagnosis.** Diagnosis is often delayed due to secrecy and shame associated with symptoms, or because characteristic symptoms are not recognised.
- **Prognosis.** Early diagnosis is important, because effective treatments are available to reduce symptoms and suffering.
- **Impact.** Assess the impact of symptoms on daily life. Obsessive–compulsive disorder can be very disabling and distressing.

Differential diagnosis
- Other mental health problems, including panic disorder, depression, psychosis.
- Tourette's syndrome.

Associated conditions
- Alcoholism.
- Depression.

> **RED FLAGS**
>
> - Suicidal risk
> - Social isolation
> - Severely disabling symptoms

History

Ideas, concerns and expectations
- **Ideas.** What does the patient know about obsessive–compulsive disorder?
- **Concerns.** What are the main worries? Fears about losing a job or social isolation are common.
- **Expectations.** What is the reason for attendance? Are there any particular expectations with regard to treatment?

The 10-Minute Clinical Assessment, Second Edition. Knut Schroeder.
© 2017 John Wiley & Sons, Ltd. Published 2017 by John Wiley & Sons, Ltd.

History of presenting complaint

- **Quality of life.** Allow the patient time to tell you their story in their own words. What is the impact of obsessive–compulsive behaviour on their day-to-day life?
- **Screening questions.** The following questions may help with identifying obsessive–compulsive disorder:
  - Do you wash or clean a lot?
  - Do you check things a lot?
  - Is there any thought that keeps bothering you that you would like to get rid of but can't?
  - Do your daily activities take a long time to finish?
  - Are you concerned about orderliness and symmetry?
  - Do these problems trouble you?
- **Age of onset.** Obsessive–compulsive disorder can occur at any age, but most patients will present in childhood or adolescence.
- **Insight.** People with obsessive–compulsive disorder are usually aware of their senseless symptoms, such as intrusive, recurrent thoughts or unwanted repetitive behaviours.
- **Obsessions.** Obsessions are unwanted impulses, ideas or images that occupy the mind. The key feature of these ideas is that they are 'ego-dystonic': they do not fit in with the patient's view of themselves and are experienced as unpleasant. Ask about fear of making a mistake, fear of contamination, need for exactness or symmetry, fear of harm coming to the self, fear of behaving unacceptably and sexual or religious obsessions.
- **Compulsions.** Ask patients whether they have any rituals that they carry out. Compulsions consist of unwanted and repetitive behaviours or mental acts. Ask about cleaning, hand-washing, ordering and arranging, hoarding and frequent checking. Mental acts include repeating words silently, rumination and counting. Symptoms such as hoarding may not be perceived as a problem.
- **Disability.** Is there any loss of function? Ask about ability to go to school or work. Adults can become housebound.
- **Avoiding behaviours.** Patients often try to avoid situations where obsessive thoughts or behaviours may occur.

Past and current medical problems

- **Pregnancy or puerperium.** Symptoms of obsessive–compulsive disorder can manifest themselves or become worse during pregnancy or puerperium.
- **Psychiatric conditions.** Ask about depression, specific and social phobias, eating disorders, alcohol problems, panic disorder, Tourette's syndrome and schizophrenia. Check whether there are features of body dysmorphic disorder, hypochondriasis or anorexia nervosa.

Social history

- **Home.** Ask about home circumstances and available support. Is housing a problem? Does the patient live in a deprived area? Are there any problems within their family?
- **Sexuality.** Are there thoughts or behaviours that interfere with sexual acts?

Examination

General condition

* **Mental state.** Is there evidence of depression or anxiety? Observe general behaviour, speech, eye contact and facial expression.

Skin
* **Skin.** Is there hand eczema, due to frequent washing?
* **Hair.** Is there evidence of trichotillomania?

References
1. National Institute for Health and Care Excellence (NICE). Obsessive-compulsive disorder and body dysmorphic disorder: treatment. NICE guidelines [CG31]. November 2005. Available from: http://www.nice.org.uk/guidance/cg31 (last accessed 29 April 2016).
2. Watson HJ, Rees CS. Meta-analysis of randomized, controlled treatment trials for pediatric obsessive–compulsive disorder. *J Child Psychol Psychiatry* 2008;49:489–498.

Mania

Key thoughts

Practical points

- **Diagnosis.** Mania is usually part of bipolar disorder, as most people will also suffer from depressive episodes. Differentiate between full, minor manic or mixed episodes with or without major depressive episodes (bipolar I disorder) and hypomania with at least one episode of major depression but where criteria for full mania are not met (bipolar II disorder).
- **Prognosis.** Bipolar I disorder often leads to problems with day-to-day life and hospital admissions, whereas in bipolar II disorder there are no psychotic features and there is less impact on function. Always consider the risk of suicide, which is relatively high in people with bipolar disorder.

Differential diagnosis

- Alcohol intoxication.
- Drug ingestion.
- Drug withdrawal.
- Hyperthyroidism.
- Hypothyroidism.
- Dementia.
- Schizophrenia.
- Cerebrovascular event.

Risk factors

- Family history.
- Drug misuse.

RED FLAGS

- Suicidal or homicidal ideas
- Personal neglect
- Significant financial or work problems

History

Ideas, concerns and expectations

- **Ideas.** Does the patient have insight into the diagnosis? Is mania perceived as a problem? How does the patient feel about a diagnosis of mania? It is common

The 10-Minute Clinical Assessment, Second Edition. Knut Schroeder.
© 2017 John Wiley & Sons, Ltd. Published 2017 by John Wiley & Sons, Ltd.

for those in the manic or hypomanic phase to be lacking in insight, and they may become very defensive or irritable if questioned about the rationality of their beliefs.

- **Concerns.** The main concerns are usually put forward by other people close to the patient, who are worried about their physical health or about financial problems resulting from mania.
- **Expectations.** Why has the patient (or those close to them) come to see you? What are their expectations with regard to further management?

History of presenting complaint

- **Quality of life.** Allow the patient (or those close to them) to tell you about the main problems in their own words. How does mania affect activities of daily living? If possible, ask the patient for consent to obtain further information from other people.
- **Onset and progression.** When did the patient or other people first notice that their behaviour had changed? How many episodes of mania and depression have there been? Frequency and duration of episodes can be variable. The severity of symptoms may vary within a single day and from day to day. Patients may lead a completely normal life and function normally at work between episodes. Some patients have so-called 'rapid cycling', with four or more episodes of mania and depression a year, without returning to normal in between.
- **Symptoms of mania.** Patients may be extremely happy or suffer from irritability or anger. Physical and mental activity is usually increased, often accompanied by grandiose ideas and self-important views. Appetite may be increased or, more usually, become disordered. An altered sleep pattern is very common, and both mania and hypomania can lead to exhaustion. Without treatment, the impact on physical health can be severe. Recklessness with money can be problematic for the patient and their family. They may feel unstoppable or out of control, and their sexual drive may be increased. It is very common for patients in their manic phase to believe that their ideas and thoughts are of great importance and brilliance.
- **Grandiose ideas.** Consider grandiose delusions if people believe themselves to have extraordinary abilities, powers or privileges for which there is no evidence. Explore whether there are also auditory hallucinations or delusions of persecution. Lack of insight is often the main problem, as patients may not see a need to change their behaviour.
- **Hypomania.** In hypomania, there is increased energy and activity with persistently elevated mood, without delusion or hallucinations.
- **Depression.** During the depressive phase, thoughts will be more negative and patients will not enjoy daily activities. There is reduced energy and low mood, which is often worse in the morning. Patients may feel guilty or have low self-esteem without any obvious reason. Ask about associated symptoms, such as reduced appetite, weight loss, loss of libido and sleep problems. Delusions of impending death, severe illness or persecution may occur in severe cases, with patients losing the will to live and neglecting themselves.

- **Activities.** Ask whether there are difficulties completing projects. People with mania are often easily distracted, leaving many activities unfinished.
- **Suicidal or homicidal thoughts.** Carefully explore whether the patient has any thoughts of harming themselves or others, or has made any plan to do so.
- **Exacerbating and relieving factors.** The pattern of cycles in bipolar disorder may be negatively influenced by drinking, stress, illicit drugs and other medical conditions. Appropriate drug treatment, group sessions and other therapies may improve the course of the illness.
- **Past management.** Has the patient ever received treatment for bipolar disorder? Is the patient aware of the diagnosis, treatment options and drug adverse effects? Do the patient and those close to them know how to contact self-help and support groups? Have the patient and those close to them developed any coping strategies, and are they aware of warning symptoms and triggers?
- **Additional unexplored issues.** Ask whether there are any other problems or issues that you have not covered but which the patient or those close to them would like to discuss.

Past and current medical problems

- **General physical health.** Ask about any significant current or past medical problems (especially HIV infection, syphilis and epilepsy), which can may cause symptoms of mania through their effects on the brain.

Medication

- **Antipsychotics.** These are often given first-line in the acute phase of mania if the patient is not taking any other psychoactive medication. In the medium and longer term, mood stabilisers are used. Valproate and lithium are sometimes given if there has been a good response to these drugs in the past.
- **Antidepressants.** These should usually be stopped during manic phases.
- **Benzodiazepines.** These are sometimes used for the treatment of severe agitation.
- **Steroids.** Systemic steroids may result in secondary mania or depression.

Family history

- **Bipolar disorder.** Ask about a family history of bipolar disorder.

Social history

- **Home.** Ask specifically about any relationship problems. Has the patient and any partner ever sought help (e.g. relationship counselling)? Are there any financial problems, as patients may incur debts during the manic phase?
- **Work.** Problems at work are common. Ask about any particular issues that may have arisen during manic phases.

Alcohol, smoking and recreational drugs

- **Alcohol.** Ask for details about past and current alcohol consumption.

- **Illicit drugs.** Bipolar disorder may be precipitated or exacerbated by consumption of recreational drugs or acute drug withdrawal. Ask for details about the type and amount of drugs consumed.

Review of previous investigations

- **Urea and electrolytes.** These are useful in detecting renal or electrolyte disturbances if there is severe dehydration due to personal neglect.
- **Thyroid function.** Both hyper- and hypothyroidism can precipitate or exacerbate symptoms of bipolar disorder.
- **Electroencephalogram.** This may be helpful in the diagnosis of epilepsy.
- **Head computerised tomography (CT) or magnetic resonance imaging (MRI) scan.** This may help exclude brain lesions in selected cases.

Examination

General

- **Clothing.** The patient may appear unkempt or present in bizarre clothes.
- **Signs of self-harm.** Look for any obvious signs of self-harm, such as cuts and bruises.
- **Dehydration.** Look for evidence of dehydration if self-neglect is evident.

Mental state

- **Speech.** Pressure of speech will usually be obvious during the manic phase. Slowed speech is characteristic of the depressive phase.
- **Thoughts.** Thoughts may be racing and flight of ideas will be present. Grandiose ideas may come up during the consultation.
- **Energy.** The patient will usually appear very energetic, and hyperactivity is common.
- **Eye contact.** In the depressive phase, eye contact may be reduced.
- **Affect.** Patients may be tearful and apathetic during the depressive phase.

Key references and further reading

1. National Institute for Health and Care Excellence (NICE). Bipolar disorder: assessment and management. NICE guidelines [CG185]. September 2014. Available from: http://www.nice.org.uk/guidance/cg185 (last accessed 29 April 2016).
2. National Institute for Health and Care Excellence (NICE). Bipolar disorder. Clinical knowledge summaries. 2015. Available from: http://cks.nice.org.uk/bipolar-disorder (last accessed 29 April 2016).
3. Swann AC, Geller B, Post RM et al. Practical clues to early recognition of bipolar disorder: a primary care approach. *Prim Care Companion J Clin Psychiatry* 2005;7:15–21.

Schizophrenia

Key thoughts

Practical points

- **Diagnosis.** Presentations can be subtle. Many people with schizophrenia may not present at all or present very late. The main diagnostic features are delusions, hallucinations, thought disorder and lack of insight. Consider intoxication (e.g. cannabis, alcohol, amphetamines) or drug overdose (accidental or suicidal) in first presentation of psychosis or in an acute exacerbation in a patient with established schizophrenia.
- **Impact on life.** Assess the impact of the condition on the patient, their relatives and their carers.

Differential diagnosis (organic and psychiatric)

- Delirium (e.g. infection, toxic, metabolic, endocrine, neurological).
- Metabolic disorders.
- Acute drug-related psychoses.
- Alcoholic hallucinations.
- Mania.
- Encephalitis.
- Panic disorder.
- Psychotic depression.
- Temporal lobe epilepsy.
- Dementia.
- Cerebral syphilis.

Risk factors

- Family history.
- Social isolation.
- Migrants.
- Family problems.
- Heavy cannabis use in adolescence.
- Intrauterine and perinatal complications.
- Intrauterine infection, particularly viral.
- Abnormal early cognitive/neuromuscular development.

Associated conditions

- Other mental health problems, such as depression.
- Drug and alcohol misuse.

The 10-Minute Clinical Assessment, Second Edition. Knut Schroeder.
© 2017 John Wiley & Sons, Ltd. Published 2017 by John Wiley & Sons, Ltd.

RED FLAGS

- Suicidal thoughts
- Severe social problems
- Self-neglect
- Hallucinations

History

Ideas, concerns and expectations
- **Ideas.** If a diagnosis of schizophrenia has already been made, ask what this means to the patient and those close to them. A sense of shame is common, and patients may feel stigmatised.
- **Concerns.** Psychotic symptoms can be extremely frightening. Patients may be worried about losing their job or social isolation.
- **Expectations.** Why is the patient presenting now?

History of presenting complaint
- **Context.** Ask about onset and progression of symptoms. How does the illness fit into the context of the patient's life?
- **Quality of life.** What is the impact of symptoms on the quality of life? Psychotic episodes can be extremely distressing for the patient and those close to them. Are there any problems with day-to-day activities, including personal care, finances, household management and work?
- **Pattern of psychotic episodes.** There may have been one or more psychotic episodes, with or without persistent deficits. The commonest pattern is one of prolonged illness with recurrent acute episodes. Difficulties at work and in the social sphere are often present. Some patients will recover completely, but others may never improve. Relapsing illness also occurs, with people being well between psychotic episodes.
- **Problems in connection with psychosis.** Ask what are the main problems and symptoms at the moment. Self-esteem is often low. Partial lack of insight is common, and symptoms are often not seen as part of an illness needing treatment. Useful questions are, 'Do you feel that something funny might be going on?', 'Have you heard any strange or unusual voices or noises?' and 'Do you feel that people are getting at you or that there is a plot against you?'.
- **Delusions.** These are bizarre beliefs, firmly adhered to in the face of the evidence. They are not shared by other members of the culture, and tend to be highly individualistic in schizophrenia. They often reflect fears of being harmed and may be associated with elaborate ideas of conspiracies against the patients (paranoia). Are normal perceptions being interpreted in an unusual way and regarded as being highly significant?
- **Thought disturbance.** This can be difficult to assess but may become apparent if speech is incoherent or does not seem to convey any meaningful information.

Language may be peculiar, and the patient may have coined new words (neologisms). Is there a reduced quantity or content of speech? Look out for erroneous or absurd beliefs that are held with an unusual conviction and do not respond to logic; this suggest delusions.

- **Passivity phenomena.** These are present if the patient believes their thoughts and perceptions are being influenced by others (delusions of control or thought broadcasting).
- **Auditory hallucinations.** Third-person auditory hallucinations (the patient hearing at least two voices talking about them) are characteristic. Other auditory hallucinations include voices giving a running commentary and voices arguing with one another. These may all feel like a normal experience to the patient. Try to identify the content of any hallucinations and any past and potential responses to them.
- **Decision-making.** Ask about recent decisions the patient has made. Have any of these been impulsive or foolish? Have they endangered the patient or others?
- **Drive.** Is there a lack of drive or ambition? This may have a serious impact on a patient's daily life. Even when they recover from an acute episode of illness, patients with schizophrenia can be apathetic and disengaged from the world.
- **Negative symptoms.** Underactivity may affect speech. There may be emotional flattening and low motivation, leading to self-neglect and social withdrawal.
- **Third-party information.** Relatives and friends can often help if there is incomplete information or a lack of insight. The family may also confirm whether certain beliefs are cultural, and therefore not delusions. Talking to family members can help identify negative symptoms, such as apathy, emotional withdrawal and a lack of attention to personal hygiene or appearance.

Past and current medical problems
- **Mental health.** Are letters from other mental health professionals available that contain further information? What was the response to any previous treatments? Have there been any previous suicide attempts? Are any support services involved at the moment?

Medication
- **Current and past medication.** Ask for details about current medication. Is this used to treat the acute episode or maintain remittance? Is there already a lead person who coordinates care? Are the drugs effective?
- **Adverse effects.** Antipsychotic medication is often poorly tolerated. Ask specifically about extrapyramidal adverse effects, such as bradykinesia, dystonia and menstrual disturbances caused by hyperprolactinaemia. There may also be anticholinergic adverse effects, such as dry mouth, blurred vision, postural hypotension or constipation. Weight gain (which can be massive) and sedation can also occur.
- **Adherence.** Is medication being taken regularly? Are there any problems remembering to take tablets? How does the patient feel about taking medication? Because many drugs have unpleasant adverse effects, patients are often

reluctant to take them. Patients may agree to have weekly or fortnightly depot injections for their antipsychotic medication.

Social history

- **Housing.** Ask for details about housing and find out who else lives with the patient. Are there any problems with regard to accommodation?
- **Finance.** Are there any financial concerns?
- **Relationships.** Ask about support and social networks, including a partner, friends and family. Loss of ambition is common, and activities and social interactions may be reduced.
- **Health professionals.** Are any other health professionals or other multidisciplinary team members involved (e.g. community mental health team, charities, social worker)? Has there been any psychosocial input? It is essential that patients with a first-episode psychosis are referred to a psychiatrist or community mental health team and have expert advice on long-term management.

Alcohol and drugs

- **Drugs.** Drug misuse is common in people with schizophrenia.
- **Alcohol.** Ask about past and current use of alcohol.

Examination

General

- **Appearance.** Is there evidence of neglect or abuse? Assess the general nutritional state.
- **Dystonia.** Acute dystonias and severe systemic reactions to antipsychotics may occur.
- **Alcohol.** Look for signs of alcoholic liver disease (e.g. scratch marks, jaundice, palmar erythema, spider naevi).
- **Drugs.** Check for signs of drug misuse (e.g. needle marks).
- **Organic psychosis.** Check for physical signs of organic psychosis.

Mental state

- **Behaviour.** Does the patient appear withdrawn? Are there any obvious mannerisms or stereotypical behaviour?
- **Cognition.** Assess orientation, attention, concentration and memory. Is there any evidence of delirium or dementia?
- **Blunting of affect.** How does the patient respond to emotional issues? There may be a subjective feeling of reduced emotion or a degree of indifference to emotional disturbances. Alternatively, emotion may be expressed inappropriately in the form of senseless laughter or giggling. The patient may appear 'flat' or 'odd'.
- **Depression.** Look for signs of depression, which is common in schizophrenia.

- **Speech.** Speech may be flat, and there may be reduced facial expressions, both of which can be very distressing and disabling. Patients may also be guarded in their responses, and some may appear to be responding to internal voices. Are there any interruptions to the flow of speech (thought blocking)? There may be loss of normal thought structure, and speech may appear bizarre.
- **Beliefs.** Are there any obvious delusions with regard to thought control or broadcasting?
- **Abnormal experiences.** Are there any hallucinations (especially auditory)?
- **Rapport.** Rapport may be poor, which can show as reduced eye contact and nonverbal communication. There may be lack of spontaneity and reduced flow of conversation.

Key references and further reading

1. National Institute for Health and Care Excellence (NICE). Psychosis and schizophrenia in adults: prevention and management. NICE guidelines [CG178]. February 2014. Available from: http://www.nice.org.uk/guidance/cg178 (last accessed 29 April 2016).
2. National Institute for Health and Care Excellence (NICE). Psychosis and schizophrenia. Clinical knowledge summaries. 2015. Available from: http://cks.nice.org.uk/psychosis-and-schizophrenia (last accessed 29 April 2016).
3. Picchioni MM, Murray RM. *Schizophrenia. BMJ* 2007;335:91–95.
4. White T, Anjum A, Schulz SC. The schizophrenia prodrome. *Am J Psychiatry* 2006;163:376–380.

Skin

Moles and malignant melanoma

Key thoughts

Practical points
- **Diagnosis.** Most moles are harmless, but new, growing or changing moles should raise suspicion of melanoma.
- **Prognosis.** Melanoma can be cured if diagnosed early and treated quickly.

Risk factors for melanoma
- Excessive exposure to the sun.
- Severe sunburn, particularly in childhood.
- Long-term exposure to the sun.
- Fair or freckled skin.
- Red or fair hair.
- Skin that does not tan or that burns before it tans.
- Multiple moles (>100 in younger people and >50 in the elderly).
- Dysplastic moles.
- Life in sunny countries.
- Family history of melanoma.
- Outdoor occupation.
- Previous melanoma.
- Immunosuppression.

Differential diagnosis
- Benign naevus.
- Seborrhoeic wart.
- Blue naevus.
- Dermatofibroma.
- Pyogenic granuloma.
- Pigmented basal cell carcinoma.
- Squamous cell carcinoma.

RED FLAGS

- New mole or a change in appearance/size
- Irregular shape or border
- Irregular colour
- Bleeding or crusting
- Inflammation

The 10-Minute Clinical Assessment, Second Edition. Knut Schroeder.
© 2017 John Wiley & Sons, Ltd. Published 2017 by John Wiley & Sons, Ltd.

- Increase in size
- Largest diameter ≥7 mm
- Pain, itching or change in sensation

History

Ideas, concerns and expectations

- **Ideas.** Does the patient know about red-flag features of malignant melanoma? Is the patient aware of measures to prevent melanoma, such as avoiding direct sun exposure between 11 am and 3 pm, covering up skin, using sunscreens and avoiding sunburn?
- **Concerns.** Patients often worry that a mole could be a melanoma but present late because of fear that the diagnosis will be confirmed.
- **Expectations.** Although in many cases a melanoma can be confidently ruled out by the non-specialist, patients will often expect specialist referral.

History and features of melanoma

- **Quality of life.** Some patients are very worried about the possibility of malignant melanoma, particularly if there is a positive family history or if they have had cancer in the past. Excessive concerns often reduce the quality of life substantially.
- **Site.** Melanomas can grow anywhere, even in areas that are not usually exposed to the sun, such as the buttocks and the sole of the foot. In women, they are most common on the leg, whereas in men, they often occur on the back. In the elderly, melanomas commonly appear on the face.
- **Growth.** Any newly growing or enlarging mole should raise suspicion of melanoma.
- **Outline.** Ordinary moles have a smooth outline, whereas the edges of a melanoma often appear irregular.
- **Pigmentation.** Irregular pigmentation within a mole suggests possible melanoma.
- **Inflammation.** New and unprovoked inflammation of a mole may be a sign of malignancy.
- **Bleeding.** Ask about any bleeding, oozing or crusting.
- **Sensation.** New-onset itch or pain in a mole may be found in melanoma.
- **Size.** A mole that is larger than any other mole on the body is suggestive of melanoma, particularly if its diameter is >7 mm.
- **Previous melanoma.** Consider recurrence if there is a personal history of melanoma.
- **Features of metastatic spread.** Ask about systemic features, such as fever, night sweats, weight loss, loss of appetite, cough, dyspnoea, bone pain and swollen lymph nodes.

Family history

- **Melanoma.** Check for a family history of melanoma in a first-degree relative.

Social history
- **Life or travel in sunny places.** Ask for details about any longer-term stays in sunny countries.
- **Hobbies.** Ask about any outdoor hobbies. Melanomas commonly occur on the calves in cyclists.

Examination

General
- **Lymph nodes.** Search for regional lymphadenopathy, which may indicate metastatic spread.

Skin
- **Skin lesion.** Describe the site, size (in millimetres, measured in at least two dimensions) and appearance. Particularly note whether there are irregular margins, irregular pigmentation, surrounding erythema or ulceration. Seborrhoeic keratoses have a regular round border, a wart-like surface and a 'stuck-on' appearance. A hard, round, even lesion that feels like a dried pea is usually a dermatofibroma. Squamous cell carcinoma may present as a non-healing lesion with significant induration.

Chest
- **Lungs.** Search for any clinical evidence of lung metastases, if indicated by the history, although these are often asymptomatic.

Abdomen
- **Liver.** A hard and nodular liver may suggest metastases (only if extensive – this will often be difficult or impossible to detect clinically).

Key references and further reading
1. Bishop JN, Bataille V, Gavin A et al. The prevention, diagnosis, referral and management of melanoma of the skin: concise guidelines. *Clin Med* 2007;7:283–290.
2. National Institute for Health and Care Excellence (NICE). Melanoma and pigmented lesions. Clinical knowledge summaries. 2011. Available from: http://cks.nice.org.uk/melanoma-and-pigmented-lesions (last accessed 29 April 2016).
3. National Institute for Health and Care Excellence (NICE). Melanoma: assessment and management. NICE guidelines [NG14]. July 2015. Available from: http://www.nice.org.uk/guidance/ng14 (last accessed 29 April 2016).
4. Roberts DLL, Anstey AV, Barlow RJ et al. UK guidelines for the management of cutaneous melanoma. *Br J Dermatol* 2002;146:7–17.

Pressure ulcers

Key thoughts

Practical points

- **Diagnosis.** Pressure ulcers are common, especially in patients with reduced mobility and other risk factors. Identify possible causes for pressure ulcers (e.g. vascular conditions, reduced sensation or reduced mobility). Search for modifiable risk factors, such as diabetes. Consider the possibility of neglect if there are new deep pressure sores in nursing home residents. All those vulnerable to pressure ulcers should receive initial and ongoing pressure ulcer assessment.

Potential causes

- Vascular conditions.
- Dementia and acute confusional state.
- Loss of mobility due to trauma or surgery.

Important risk factors

- Obesity.
- Pressure, shearing and friction.
- Reduced mobility.
- Sensory impairment.
- Incontinence.
- Acute, chronic and terminal illness.
- Significant comorbidity (e.g. diabetes, cardiovascular disease (CVD)).
- Poor posture.
- Reduced cognition.
- Previous pressure ulcers.
- Extremes of age.
- Poor nutrition status and dehydration.
- Moist skin.
- Inadequate equipment (e.g. bed, seating) that does not provide adequate pressure relief.

RED FLAGS

- Infection
- Delirium
- Dementia
- Poor mobility

The 10-Minute Clinical Assessment, Second Edition. Knut Schroeder.
© 2017 John Wiley & Sons, Ltd. Published 2017 by John Wiley & Sons, Ltd.

- Failure of conservative management
- Poor general health
- Signs of malignancy

History

Ideas, concerns and expectations
- **Ideas.** What does the patient or their carer think is causing the ulcer? What do they know about preventive measures?
- **Concerns.** Patients with cognitive impairment who develop pressure sores may show a lack of concern for ulcer prevention. Fears about infection and subsequent sepsis are common.
- **Expectations.** Expectations with regard to the speed of healing may be unrealistic.

History of presenting complaint
- **Quality of life.** How does the pressure ulcer affect the quality of life? Pain is common, and pressure ulcers can become very uncomfortable, particularly if there is associated infection.
- **Onset and progression.** When did the ulcer first develop, and how has it progressed? If there is deterioration, how quickly has it occurred? Does the ulcer continue to grow in size?
- **Site.** Pressure ulcers in adults often develop over bony prominences (e.g. hip, sacrum or ankles).
- **Pain.** Ascertain the level of pain and whether it is controlled by analgesia. Even if they are not in pain, patients may feel uncomfortable in their chair, bed or elsewhere. Ask for details about sitting and sleeping positions.
- **Posture.** Are there any postural problems that predispose to pressure ulcers (e.g. fractures, spasticity)? How often is the patient repositioned?
- **Pressure change.** Has there been any recent pressure change or change in equipment?
- **Predisposing factors.** Reduced level of consciousness and impaired mobility are important risk factors for pressure ulcers. Is there evidence of an acute illness, either metabolic or infectious? Malnutrition and dehydration are other important factors to consider. Urinary or faecal incontinence and excessive sweating may contribute. Is there a recent onset of dementia or memory loss? Is there a possibility of neglect?
- **External factors.** Consider moist skin, external pressure, friction and shearing due to clothes or bedding. Tolerance to pressure varies between individuals.
- **Infection.** Are there symptoms or signs of infection (pus, odour, fever, raised skin infection, erythema)? Has a swab been taken? Has wound-cleaning and debridement taken place? In non-healing ulcers or ulcers that are particularly difficult to treat, consider the possibility of underlying osteomyelitis (an X-ray may be indicated) or, rarely, malignancy.

Effects of problem on daily life
- **Home.** How does the pressure ulcer affect day-to-day life? Ask about all relevant daily activities, from getting up in the morning to dressing, shopping, cooking and personal care.

Past and current medical problems
- **Risk factors.** People undergoing surgery or in critical care are at high risk. Other risk factors include vascular disease, terminal or chronic illness (e.g. diabetes or chronic obstructive pulmonary disease (COPD)), orthopaedic conditions, sensory impairment in stroke or diabetes and decreased conscious level (see also Important Risk Factors at start of chapter). Is there a history of pressure ulcers?
- **Surgery.** Has the patient undergone surgery for pressure ulcers in the past?

Medication
- **Prescribed medication.** In particular, ask about sedatives and opioids that might cause increased sedation and reduced perception of pain and discomfort in pressure ulcer-prone areas, particularly during sleep. Diuretics may lead to dehydration.
- **Over-the-counter medicines.** Ask about any over-the-counter medications that might potentially decrease or increase plasma concentrations of prescribed drugs.
- **Nonsteroidal anti-inflammatory drugs (NSAIDs).** These may increase peripheral oedema and should therefore be used for analgesia only with much caution.
- **Antibiotics.** Does the patient currently take antibiotics for treatment of an infected pressure ulcer? If so, has a swab been obtained prior to starting treatment?
- **Dressings.** What, if any, dressings have been used so far? Who has been treating the pressure ulcer until now?
- **Devices.** Are any pressure-relieving devices being used?

Allergies
- **Antibiotics.** Check for any allergies to antibiotics in case these are needed for the treatment of infected ulcers.

Social history
- **Home.** Does the patient live alone? Who is the main carer? Can adequate nursing care be provided in the community to help with the dressing of ulcers? Are other services involved, such as a physiotherapist or occupational therapist? Are there particular risk factors for pressure ulcers due to the home situation, such as poor seating or an inadequate mattress?
- **Social life.** What limitations are there to going out and socialising? Who visits?

Alcohol
- **Alcohol intake.** Alcohol misuse may reduce sensation in pressure areas and thereby contribute to the development of pressure ulcers.

Review of recent investigations
- **Full blood count and plasma viscosity.** Check for signs of infection.
- **Renal and liver function.** Impaired renal or liver function may prolong wound-healing.
- **Thyroid function.** Consider the possibility of hypothyroidism, which may contribute to the development of pressure ulcer.
- **Glucose.** Would-healing may be slow in patients with diabetes.

Examination

General
- **General condition.** Consider nutritional status and look for evidence of neglect. Does the patient look unwell?
- **Mobility.** Assess general mobility.
- **Circumstances.** Is there any obvious cause for the pressure ulcer? Look at both the patient (nutrition, self-neglect, signs of systemic illness, clothing) and their surroundings (chair, mattress, cushions, clothes, empty alcohol or medicine bottles).

Vital signs
- **Temperature.** Always consider the possibility of wound infection in patients who develop an otherwise unexplained fever.
- **Pulse.** Tachycardia suggests infection or heart failure.
- **Blood pressure.** Check for hypertension.
- **Respiratory rate.** Tachypnoea suggests chest infection or heart failure.

Skin inspection
- **Pressure ulcer sites.** Inspect sacrum, ischial tuberosity and heels. Also look at all other parts of the body where pressure is exerted as part of daily living and other activities (e.g. elbows, temporal region of skull, shoulders, back of head and toes). Are there external forces from furniture, equipment or clothing?
- **Features of raised pressure ulcer risk.** Assess the skin regularly and make sure you inspect all vulnerable areas (e.g. over bony prominences, such as the hips or sacrum). Look for persistent erythema, non-blanching hyperaemia, localised heat, blisters, localised swelling and oedema, induration, purplish or bluish discoloration and localised coolness of the skin.
- **Size.** Assess the size of the ulcer, measuring in at least two dimensions.
- **Description.** Assess the amount and appearance of exudate and look for signs of infection. Is there pain or tenderness? Describe the appearance of the wound

and the surrounding skin. Look for underlying tracking, sinus or fistula. Offensive odour or slough suggests infection.

- **Grading.** Grade an ulcer according to the European Pressure Ulcer Classification System (see box).
- **Sensation.** Test sensation around pressure ulcers. Sensory problems may suggest diabetes or vitamin B12 deficiency.

EUROPEAN PRESSURE ULCER CLASSIFICATION SYSTEM

- **Grade 1.** Non-blanchable skin, warmth, oedema, some induration or hardness of skin.
- **Grade 2.** Partial thickness loss involving epidermis, dermis or both. Ulcer is superficial and may present as an abrasion or blister.
- **Grade 3.** Full-thickness skin loss. May involve necrosis or subcutaneous tissue. Can extend to, but not through, underlying fascia.
- **Grade 4.** Extensive destruction and damage to muscle, bone or supporting structures. Extensive tissue necrosis with or without full skin loss.

Source: European Pressure Ulcer Advisory Panel (EPUAP). Pressure ulcer treatment guidelines. 2003. Available from: http://www.epuap.org/guidelines/ (last accessed 29 April 2016).

Lower limbs

- **Mobility.** Check general mobility and ability to get up from a lying or sitting position.
- **Power.** Assess power of hip and foot flexors.

Beside tests

- **Glucose.** Check blood glucose for evidence of diabetes.
- **Urine.** Dipstick for protein, blood, nitrites and leucocytes. Urinary incontinence due to urinary tract infection is an important precipitating factor in the development of pressure ulcers.

Key references and further reading

1. Bergstrom N, Braden B, Kemp M et al. Predicting pressure ulcer risk: a multisite study of the predictive validity of the Braden Scale. *Nurs Res* 1998;47:261–269.
2. Defloor T, Schoonhoven L. Inter-rater reliability of the EPUAP pressure ulcer classification system using photographs. *J Clin Nurs* 2004;13:952–959.
3. European Pressure Ulcer Advisory Panel (EPUAP). Pressure ulcer treatment guidelines. 2003. Available from: http://www.epuap.org/guidelines/ (last accessed 29 April 2016).
4. National Institute for Health and Care Excellence (NICE). Pressure ulcers: prevention and management. NICE guidelines [CG179]. April 2014. Available from: http://www.nice.org.uk/guidance/cg179 (last accessed 29 April 2016).

Ophthalmology

Eye injuries

Key thoughts

Practical points
- **Diagnosis.** Eye injuries are common in clinical practice. Corneal injuries are common, and most will heal quickly. Penetrating eye injuries can easily be missed.
- **Prognosis.** Look for serious complications, such as penetrating eye injury, blowout fracture or a foreign body embedded in the eye. Estimate the risk of future visual loss to decide whether to refer or admit urgently.

Differential diagnosis
- Corneal abrasion.
- Foreign body.
- Contusion.
- Arc eye.
- Chemical injuries due to acid or alkali.
- Radiation damage (e.g. ultraviolet (UV) light).
- Lid laceration.
- Penetrating eye injury.
- Blowout fracture.
- Ruptured globe.

Important risk factors
- Failing to wear eye protection when appropriate.
- Occupations such as welding or grinding.
- Skiing or snowboarding (UV damage).

RED FLAGS

- Only one functioning eye (risk to overall vision and risk of injury when the other eye is amblyopic)
- Loss of vision
- High-speed injury
- Severe pain
- Penetrating injury
- Distorted pupil
- Retinal damage on fundoscopy
- Possibility of blowout fracture

The 10-Minute Clinical Assessment, Second Edition. Knut Schroeder.
© 2017 John Wiley & Sons, Ltd. Published 2017 by John Wiley & Sons, Ltd.

History

Ideas, concerns and expectations

- **Ideas.** What does the patient believe has happened to the eye? Do not always assume a given cause–effect relationship to be true.
- **Concerns.** Fears about losing sight are common.
- **Expectations.** Does the patient expect any compensation payments from a third party?

History of presenting complaint

- **Quality of life.** Pain, discomfort and reduced vision can severely impair the quality of life and day-to-day activities. Check what routine activities the patient is now unable to do.
- **Symptoms.** Is there any pain? Where exactly is the pain? Has vision been affected? Floaters in association with trauma suggest vitreous haemorrhage due to ocular penetration. Double vision indicates swelling within the orbit or cranial nerve damage.
- **Time and mode of injury.** Find out what exactly happened, and when. Many injuries only become apparent some time after the original incident, due to an inflammatory response. Differentiate between physical and chemical trauma. Is the injury likely to be superficial or deep? Distinguish between blunt and perforating injuries. Was there a high-speed injury, such as hammer-and-chisel trauma? Consider blowout fracture in case of a forceful blunt injury. Be sure to record all your findings carefully for both clinical and medicolegal reasons.
- **Type of foreign body.** If a foreign body has entered the eye, find out whether it is glass, metal or another material. There is a risk of fungal infection with organic matter. Ferrous metals can rapidly form a rust ring if missed, and then cause long-term damage.
- **Other injuries.** Have there been any other injuries to the head or other areas of the body? What treatment has been received so far?
- **Previous vision.** Ask for details about previous visual acuity. Does the patient suffer from any ongoing eye problems? Has there been any other eye trauma in the past?
- **Eye protection.** Were goggles or glasses worn at the time of the injury?
- **Non-accidental injury.** Consider the possibility of non-accidental injury in any eye trauma, particularly in injuries that are unusual or inconsistent with the history.

Review of previous investigations

- **Imaging.** Has the patient already had any radiological investigations, such as X-ray, ultrasound or computerised tomography (CT)? Magnetic resonance imaging (MRI) is usually avoided if there is a possibility of a metal foreign body within the eye.

Past and current medical problems
- **Significant past illnesses.** Ask about any significant chronic medical problems, such as diabetes or hypertension, which can affect the eyes and vision.
- **Immunisation status.** Check whether the patient is up to date with tetanus immunisation.

Medication
- **Analgesics.** What has been taken so far? Has medication been effective?
- **Eye drops.** Have any eye drops of any sort been used?

Allergies
- **Antibiotics.** Ask about allergies to any antibiotics that may need to be used.

Examination

General
- **General condition.** Does the patient look unwell? Is there any obvious evidence of trauma to other parts of the body, such as airway involvement? If there is blepharospasm, local anaesthetic drops may need to be given prior to examination of the affected eye (e.g. proxymethacaine 0.5% or benoxinate 0.4%).

Eye inspection
- **General inspection.** Look carefully at the injured area. Check for tenderness, bruising, subcutaneous emphysema and conjunctival haemorrhages. Examine the eye front to back, including lids, conjunctiva, cornea, sclera, anterior chamber, pupil shape, vitreous body and retina.
- **Eye lids.** Are the lids intact or damaged? Evert the lid with the aid of a cotton bud and look for foreign bodies, which can easily be missed. Infraorbital anaesthesia suggests blowout fracture.
- **Conjunctiva.** Subconjunctival haemorrhage can conceal a penetrating injury.
- **Cornea.** Check the cornea for abrasions using fluorescein and blue light. Corneal scarring and opacification may occur as a result of chemical burns. Arc eye may present with painful foreign-body sensation, blepharospasm and watering of the eye.
- **Sclera.** Penetrating injuries may be difficult to spot.
- **Anterior chamber.** Check the anterior chamber with a portable slit lamp or with direct ophthalmoscopy set at +10 dioptres.
- **Pupils.** Check the size, reactivity and shape.
- **Fundoscopy.** Check the vitreous body and retina for any abnormalities.

Eye tests
- **Visual acuity.** Measure visual acuity in both eyes (with and without glasses) using a Snellen chart. If this is worse than 6/60, ask the patient to count fingers

at 1 m distance. Normal vision does not exclude serious eye injury, such as penetrating trauma. Use a pinhole if the vision is decreased. If vision is poor, use finger and hand movements and perception of light at a distance of 1 m.
- **Red reflex.** If this is absent, consider serious intraocular damage, such as vitreous haemorrhage or hyphaema.
- **Eye movements.** Is there diplopia or abnormal gaze?
- **Visual fields.** Check visual fields.

Head and neck
- **Infraorbital nerve.** Loss of sensation in the infraorbital region or anaesthesia of the maxillary teeth and upper lip suggests injury to the infraorbital nerve due to blowout fracture. There may be associated double vision due to tethering of the inferior rectus and inferior oblique muscles, leading to reverse diplopia on both downgaze and upgaze.

Key references and further reading
1. Kay-Wilson LG. Localisation of corneal foreign bodies. *Br J Ophthalmol* 1992; 76:741–742.
2. Khaw PT, Shah P, Elkington AR. ABC of eyes: injury to the eye. *BMJ* 2004;328 (7430):36–38.
3. National Institute for Health and Care Excellence (NICE). Red eye. Clinical knowledge summaries. 2012. Available from: http://cks.nice.org.uk/red-eye (last accessed 29 April 2016).

The acute red eye

Key thoughts

Practical points
- **Diagnosis.** Conjunctivitis is very common. Trauma and iritis are other important causes.
- **Prognosis.** Differentiate between benign and serious conditions (e.g. chemical burns or penetrating injuries), which require urgent referral or admission. Serious causes are usually associated with pain or trauma.

Serious and sight-threatening causes
- Acute glaucoma.
- Uveitis.
- Keratitis.
- Scleritis.
- Blunt and penetrating eye injury.
- Foreign body.
- Chemical burns.

Differential diagnosis and associated conditions
- **Painful red eye.** Conjunctivitis, episcleritis, scleritis, keratitis, corneal ulcer, iritis, intraocular infection, acute glaucoma.
- **Uveitis.** Ankylosing spondylitis, Reiter's syndrome, ulcerative colitis, Crohn's disease, Still's disease, sarcoidosis, toxoplasmosis, tuberculosis, syphilis, herpes zoster.
- **Trauma.** Subconjunctival haematoma, corneal and conjunctival foreign body, corneal abrasion, corneal flash burn.
- **Other.** Dry eye, blepharitis.
- **Projection of pain from other areas.** Migraine, cluster headache, temporal arteritis, sinusitis, zoster ophthalmicus, trigeminal neuralgia.

Important risk factors
- Rheumatological/autoimmune conditions (episcleritis, scleritis, peripheral ulcerative keratitis, keratoconjunctivitis sicca).
- Chlamydial infection (conjunctivitis).
- Long-sightedness (glaucoma).

The 10-Minute Clinical Assessment, Second Edition. Knut Schroeder.
© 2017 John Wiley & Sons, Ltd. Published 2017 by John Wiley & Sons, Ltd.

RED FLAGS

- Visual loss
- Severe pain
- Photophobia
- Coloured halos around points of light in the patient's vision
- Corneal opacity
- Chemical burns
- Ciliary flush
- Blunt or penetrating injury
- Suspected acute glaucoma
- Suspected temporal arteritis
- Deep foreign bodies in the cornea
- Smaller pupil in the affected eye

History

Ideas, concerns and expectations
- **Ideas.** What does the patient believe is the cause of the eye problem?
- **Concerns.** Worries about potential loss of vision are common.
- **Expectations.** Patients may expect a 'quick fix' and not realise the potential seriousness of certain eye conditions.

History of presenting complaint
- **Quality of life.** Eye problems can seriously affect patients' quality of life. How bothersome are the symptoms? Are there any activities that the patient cannot do, or can do only with difficulties?
- **Onset and progression.** Establish the time and speed of onset. How have symptoms progressed since then?
- **Pain.** Is there associated pain or discomfort? Pain may originate from the eye itself or from periorbital structures. Pain may also be projected to the eye from other areas, such as in headache or sinusitis. Common causes of pain are abnormalities in the eye lids, ocular muscles, cornea, sclera, uvea or optical nerve. Preceding pain and tingling suggest herpes zoster of the ophthalmic division of the trigeminal nerve. A severe throbbing pain associated with nausea and vomiting, visual loss and halos around lights suggests acute glaucoma.
- **Trauma.** Is there a history of preceding trauma? Obtain details about the exact mechanism of any eye trauma. Corneal abrasions may occur as a result of direct injury by a finger, stick or piece of paper. Is there a history of flash burn or chemical injury? Any potentially serious blunt or penetrating eye trauma needs careful assessment by a specialist. Consider foreign bodies such as pieces of grit or eye lashes if there is a feeling of a foreign body. Always consider the potential of eye injury in any facial trauma.
- **Distribution.** Are symptoms unilateral or are both eyes affected?

- **Symptom pattern.** A seasonal or recurrent occurrence suggests allergic reactions, hay fever or iritis.
- **Contact lenses.** Does the patient wear contact lenses? Check how long contact lenses have been left in situ and whether they are being cleaned appropriately. Corneal abrasions may occur if contact lenses are left in for too long, particularly overnight. Wearers of soft contact lenses are more prone to infection.
- **Rash.** Consider herpes zoster if there is an associated vesicular rash on the face, which may extend beyond the hairline. Complications can include blepharitis, conjunctivitis, keratitis, uveitis, secondary glaucoma, ophthalmoplegia and optic neuritis. A rash on the tip of the nose increases the risk of corneal involvement (Hutchinson sign).
- **Discomfort and discharge.** Common symptoms of conjunctivitis include gritty discomfort with mild photophobia and discharge. Vision is usually preserved. Mucopurulent discharge suggests bacterial infection. Consider chlamydia conjunctivitis if usual topical antibiotics fail, and in particular if there is associated urethritis or salpingitis. Crusty, red and itchy eyelids suggest blepharitis, which may be associated with styes and chalazion.
- **Eye lid.** Are there any problems with the eye lid, such as blepharitis, contact dermatitis, mucus membrane pemphigoid, symblepharon (conjunctival adhesions) or ocular rosacea?
- **Eye drops.** Are eye drops being used for glaucoma or dry eye? Dry eyes may be found in Sjögren's syndrome. Eye drops may also cause allergic reactions.

Review of previous investigations
- **Full blood count and inflammatory markers.** Blood tests are not usually needed. The white cell count and inflammatory markers such as plasma viscosity may be raised in episcleritis and scleritis.
- **Rheumatoid factor.** Rheumatoid arthritis may be associated with episcleritis and scleritis.

Past and current medical problems
- **Significant past illnesses.** Ask about chronic diseases such as hypertension or rheumatological conditions.
- **Eye problems.** Is there a history of eye disease? Has the patient had any eye operations or suffered from eye trauma in the past?

Medication
- **Anti-inflammatory drugs.** Have nonsteroidal anti-inflammatory drugs (NSAIDs) been taken? If not, check whether there are any contraindications, such as a history of allergy, asthma or active peptic ulcer.
- **Drugs precipitating glaucoma.** Anticholinergics, antidepressants, adrenergic agonists and selective serotonin reuptake inhibitors (SSRIs) may precipitate acute angle closure glaucoma.
- **Steroid eye drops.** Have these been given previously? Significant visual complications may occur as a result of inappropriate use of topical steroids, and these preparations should not normally be initiated by non-specialists in primary care.

Allergies
- **Eye drops.** Ask about allergies to any eye drops that might need to be given for the treatment of the underlying condition.

Examination

General
- **General condition.** Does the patient appear unwell? General malaise, fever and nausea suggest acute glaucoma or systemic disease.

Head and neck
- **Pre-auricular lymph nodes.** These may be enlarged in acute viral conjunctivitis.

Eye inspection
- **Location of redness.** Establish the exact location of the redness and whether eyelids, conjunctiva, cornea, sclera, episclera or intraocular structures are affected. Is the redness unilateral or are both eyes affected?
- **Eye lids.** Look for signs of blepharitis and foreign bodies. Look for purulent discharge (suggesting conjunctivitis), watering, blepharospasm and lagophthalmus.
- **Conjunctiva.** Large cobblestone papillae under the upper lid and conjunctival swelling suggest allergic conjunctivitis. In bacterial conjunctivitis, there is usually conjunctival redness with mucopurulent discharge, glued eyes, itch and a history of conjunctivitis. Viral conjunctivitis may present with an often bilateral watery discharge associated with swollen pre-auricular and submandibular lymph nodes. Keratitis may develop after 1 week. Uniocular involvement associated with dermatitis in distribution of the trigeminal nerve suggests herpes zoster conjunctivitis. Subconjunctival haematoma may present without trauma and may be associated with hypertension or bleeding diatheses. In scleritis, the whole eyeball is red and inflamed, and there is usually some visual loss and pain. Typically, pain disturbs sleep in scleritis.
- **Cornea.** Examine with fluorescein and blue light, if indicated; any lesions will appear green. Corneal lesions can be distinguished from conjunctivitis with the presence of pain and, often, loss of vision by a central ulcer or exudate (hypopyon) in the anterior chamber. An ulcer may be visible as a white infiltrate. A central or marginal ulcer may be seen with fluorescein staining. A branching or dendritic ulcer suggests herpes simplex keratitis, particularly if corneal sensation is decreased. A hazy cornea suggests acute glaucoma.
- **Iris.** Ciliary injection in association with blurred vision, photophobia and pain radiating to the brow or temple suggests acute iritis. The pupil usually contracts, and in severe cases, an exudate (hypopyon) may form in the anterior chamber. Posterior synechiae may be visible because the iris adheres to the anterior lens surface, causing an irregularly shaped cornea.

- **Pupil.** A fixed, semi-dilated oval pupil in association with a red eye, hazy cornea and tender hard eye ball may occasionally suggest acute glaucoma. Miosis may be found in anterior uveitis.

Eye tests

- **Photophobia.** The penlight test for photophobia can be useful for distinguishing between benign and serious eye pathology.
- **Vision.** Measure visual acuity in both eyes with and without glasses using a Snellen chart, which will establish a baseline and may point towards particular problems. If visual acuity is worse than 6/60, ask the patient to count fingers at a distance of 1 m. Normal vision does not exclude serious eye injury, such as penetrating trauma. Use a pinhole if the vision is decreased. If vision is poor, use finger and hand movements at a distance of 1 m and then perception of light.
- **Visual fields.** Visual-field defects may be found in chronic glaucoma.
- **Eye movements.** Suspect anterior uveitis if pain worsens when the eyes converge and pupils constrict (Talbot's sign). Pain on reading is one of the first symptoms of anterior uveitis when the ciliary body (part of the uveal tract) contracts during accommodation.
- **Eye ball.** Gently palpate the eye ball in suspected glaucoma. The eye ball will feel hard in significantly raised intraocular pressure.

Vital signs

- **Blood pressure.** Hypertension may be implicated in subconjunctival haemorrhage. High blood pressure may also result from pain or acute glaucoma.

Skin

- **Facial rash.** Check the face and scalp areas beyond the hairline for any vesicular rashes, indicating herpes zoster infection.

Key references and further reading

1. Leibowitz HM. The red eye. *NEJM* 2000;343:345–351.
2. McCluskey P, Powell R. The eye in systemic inflammatory conditions. *Lancet* 2004;364(9451):2125–2133.
3. National Institute for Health and Care Excellence (NICE). Red eye. Clinical knowledge summaries. 2012. Available from: http://cks.nice.org.uk/red-eye (last accessed 29 April 2016).
4. Rietveld RP, ter Riet G, Bindels PJE et al. Predicting bacterial cause in infectious conjunctivitis: cohort study on informativeness of combinations of signs and symptoms. *BMJ* 2004;329:206–208.
5. Wirbelauer C. Management of the red eye for the primary care physician. *Am J Med* 2006;119:302–306.
6. Yaphe J, Pandher KS. The predictive value of the penlight test for photophobia for serious eye pathology in general practice. *Fam Practice* 2003;20:425–427.

Gradual painless visual disturbance

Key thoughts

Practical points
- **Diagnosis.** Gradual painless loss of vision is common. Findings from the initial assessment are important in deciding on the urgency of referral. The final diagnosis of the underlying condition is usually made by opticians or ophthalmologists.
- **Prognosis.** Treatable causes such as diabetic retinopathy may need swift referral to avoid irreversible loss of vision.

Possible causes
- Refractive errors.
- Cataract.
- Glaucoma.
- Age-related macular degeneration.
- Diabetic or hypertensive retinopathy.
- Neurological conditions.

Important risk factors
- Cardiovascular risk factors, such as diabetes, hypertension and hyperlipidaemia.
- Age.

RED FLAGS

- Bilateral loss of vision
- Rapid deterioration of vision
- Suspected serious pathology
- Threat to loss of independence
- Neurological symptoms
- Visual-field defects
- Human immunodeficiency virus (HIV) infection

History

Ideas, concerns and expectations
- **Ideas.** What does the patient think is causing the visual problems? What is the perceived level of visual impairment?

The 10-Minute Clinical Assessment, Second Edition. Knut Schroeder.
© 2017 John Wiley & Sons, Ltd. Published 2017 by John Wiley & Sons, Ltd.

- **Concerns.** Loss of vision and the possibility of blindness can be extremely frightening and disabling. There are potentially huge implications for family and social life, as well as for work and driving. Older people are at risk of losing their independence and may worry about becoming isolated. Chronic loss of vision may go unnoticed and is often only picked up on routine eye screening.
- **Expectations.** Why has the patient come to see you now? Which issue(s) should be the focus of the consultation?

History of presenting complaint
- **Quality of life.** How far do the visual problems affect the quality of life and activities of daily living? During which activities are the visual symptoms most obvious or bothersome? Does the patient already use visual or mobility aids?
- **Description of eye symptoms.** What are the main eye symptoms? Blurred vision and loss of vision are common and often occur as a result of cataract or refractive errors (due to changes in the shape or size of the eye). Myopia (short-sightedness) and astigmatism are common. Presbyopia due to hardening of the lens and reduced ciliary muscle function may cause difficulty in reading. Glares in bright light and cloudy or misty vision suggest cataract, which may develop faster in uncontrolled diabetes.
- **Onset and progression.** When did the symptoms start and how did they progress? Consider uncontrolled diabetes if cataract worsens over weeks rather than months or years.
- **Pattern of visual loss.** Consider neurological causes if loss of vision is bilateral. A gradual visual-field loss in association with distortion of straight lines suggests age-related macular degeneration. There may also be abnormal blue–yellow colour perception. A progressive peripheral visual-field loss suggests glaucoma.
- **Associated symptoms or conditions.** Endocrine abnormalities suggest possible optic-nerve compression, in rare cases due to intracranial tumour, particularly if associated with bitemporal visual-field defects.
- **Double vision.** Intermittent double vision may occasionally be caused by myasthenia gravis.

Past and current medical problems
- **Previous eye problems.** People with macular degeneration or diabetes are at higher risk of macular haemorrhage. When was the last eye check done?
- **Diabetes.** Diabetes can accelerate the development of cataract and is a risk factor for vascular eye disease. Transient refractive symptoms may occasionally be caused by fluctuating blood sugar levels in people with diabetes.
- **Other vascular risk factors.** Hypertension and hyperlipidaemia also increase the risk of vascular eye disease, such as central/branch retinal vein or artery occlusion.
- **Neurological disease.** A number of neurological conditions may present with eye problems.
- **HIV and acquired immunodeficiency syndrome (AIDS).** Eye problems such as retinitis should be considered in HIV infection.

Medication

- **Anticoagulants and antiplatelet drugs.** Is the patient already taking aspirin or warfarin for the prevention of embolic events? Are there any contraindications to these drugs, should they be needed for the treatment of vascular disease?
- **Drugs causing visual problems.** Hydroxychloroquine may cause maculopathy. Systemic steroids may contribute to the development of cataracts and glaucoma.

Family history

- **Retinal dystrophies.** Some retinal dystrophies are hereditary; these are usually rare. Reduced night vision and poor perception of movement in the periphery may be presenting symptoms.

Social history

- **Home.** Ask for details about home life. Is there a threat to independent living? Who is at home to provide support? Has the patient been advised not to drive and to contact the relevant driving authority? Ask about daily activities, such as reading and household chores. Visual loss is an important risk factor for falls in the elderly.
- **Work.** Are there any problems with work (e.g. driving)?
- **Travel.** Consider the possibility of trachoma in people who have lived or worked in countries where this is endemic.

Alcohol, smoking and recreational drugs

- **Alcohol.** Heavy drinking increases the risk of cardiovascular problems.
- **Smoking.** A smoking history increases the risk of cardiovascular disease (CVD) and retinopathy. Has smoking-cessation advice been offered?

Review of previous investigations

- **Fasting lipids and glucose.** Raised values increase the risk of CVD.
- **Liver function.** Liver function should be checked in cases where a statin might be required.

Examination

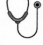

General

- **General condition.** Does the patient look well? Look for signs of depression, which may occur as a result of visual loss (e.g. reduced eye contact, lack of facial expression, low-volume voice, tearfulness).

Eye inspection

- **Eye lids.** Ptosis may rarely occur in connection with intracranial tumours or due to myasthenia gravis.
- **Eye movements.** Check eye movements if you suspect a neurological cause.

- **Pupils.** Unilateral pupil dilation may rarely suggest an intracranial cause, such as tumour.
- **Fundus.** Pathological cupping implies glaucoma. Look for microvascular problems, such as exudates and haemorrhages, indicating diabetic retinopathy. Hyperpigmentation at the macula with surrounding atrophic areas suggests dry age-related macular degeneration.

Eye tests
- **Visual acuity.** Measure visual acuity in both eyes (with and without glasses) using a Snellen chart. If visual acuity is worse than 6/60, ask the patient to count fingers at a distance of 1 m. Normal vision does not exclude serious eye injury, such as penetrating trauma. Use a pinhole if the vision is decreased. If vision is poor, use finger and hand movements and then perception of light at a distance of 1 m. Using a pinhole will improve visual acuity in refractive errors, but will not make a difference if there is an underlying macular cause.
- **Visual fields.** Try to establish the pattern of visual-field loss by doing a confrontational field examination. Consider macular degeneration if there is a central field loss. In glaucoma, peripheral vision tends to be affected.
- **Red reflex.** An absent red reflex or a dark shadow across the red reflex indicates an opacity within the media of the eye (e.g. cataract).

Head and neck
- **Carotid bruit.** Although a carotid bruit is not a reliable sign and is not diagnostic, it may be indicative of CVD.

Bedside tests
- **Urine dipstick.** Check for blood and protein, which may indicate renal involvement in hypertension. Glycosuria suggests diabetes.

Key references and further reading

1. Miller NR, Newman NJ. The eye in neurological disease. *Lancet* 2004;364: 2045–2054.
2. National Institute for Health and Care Excellence (NICE). Red eye. Clinical knowledge summaries. 2012. Available from: http://cks.nice.org.uk/red-eye (last accessed 29 April 2016).
3. Quillen DA. Common causes of vision loss in elderly patients. *Am Fam Physician* 1999;60:99–108.
4. Vu HTV, Keefe JE, McCarthy CA, Taylor HR. Impact of unilateral and bilateral vision loss on quality of life. *Br J Ophthalmol* 2005;89:360–363.

Sudden painless visual disturbance

Key thoughts

Practical points
- **Diagnosis.** The main presenting symptoms are sudden onset of flashes and floaters, loss of vision and double vision. Establishing the underlying cause for acute visual problems can be challenging, and usually requires specialist assessment. Painless visual loss may be associated with pain at other sites (e.g. headache in temporal arteritis or meningitis).
- **Prognosis.** Important conditions not to be missed are amaurosis fugax, temporal arteritis and intraorbital tumour.

Possible causes
- **Eye.** Retinal vein thrombosis, retinal detachment, glaucoma, vitreous or macular haemorrhage, retrobulbar neuritis (although this may be painful), disciform macular degeneration, intraorbital tumour.
- **Vascular.** Amaurosis fugax due to transient ischaemia, migraine, hypertension, temporal arteritis, central retinal artery occlusion, autoimmune arteritis, intracranial arteriovenous malformation.
- **Systemic.** Meningitis, meningococcal septicaemia.

Important risk factors
- Previous flashes and floaters.
- Cardiovascular risk factors, such as diabetes, hypertension and hyperlipidaemia.

RED FLAGS

- Loss of vision, particularly in association with previous flashes and floaters
- Sudden loss of central visual acuity only
- Sudden loss of vision associated with features of temporal arteritis
- Missing area of vision (scotoma)
- Severe floaters and flashes
- Dark curtain in the periphery of vision
- Sudden onset of double vision associated with pain, ptosis and a dilated pupil
- Signs of infection (e.g. meningitis)

The 10-Minute Clinical Assessment, Second Edition. Knut Schroeder.
© 2017 John Wiley & Sons, Ltd. Published 2017 by John Wiley & Sons, Ltd.

History

Ideas, concerns and expectations
- **Ideas.** What does the patient think is causing the visual problems?
- **Concerns.** Sudden loss of vision can be extremely frightening, and people often fear they may lose their eyesight.
- **Expectations.** What expectations are there with regard to the level of visual acuity (e.g. drivers, pilots and any other occupations that need good vision)?

History of presenting complaint
- **Quality of life.** How do symptoms affect the quality of life and activities of daily living? Visual impairment can be very distressing and disabling.
- **Description of eye symptoms.** What are the main eye symptoms? Common presenting problems are flashes and floaters, sudden loss of vision and double vision.
- **Onset and progression.** When did the symptoms start, and how did they progress? If symptoms are transitory, how long do they last? If lasting for about 20 minutes, migraine is a likely cause.
- **Pattern of visual loss.** Find out which part of vision is affected (i.e. central vision, the whole of the visual field or just the top or bottom half). Loss of central vision that is associated with vague pains behind the eye, particularly in younger people, may be caused by optic neuritis in multiple sclerosis. Also consider neurological causes if loss of vision is bilateral. Transient refractive symptoms may occasionally be caused by fluctuating blood sugar levels in people with diabetes.
- **Associated symptoms or conditions.** Neurological symptoms such as facial or limb weakness may indicate a transient ischaemic attack (TIA). Preceding floaters may indicate retinal detachment. Vitreous haemorrhage is more common in diabetes. Always consider the possibility of temporal arteritis if there is headache, particularly in the elderly (ask about jaw claudication, scalp tenderness, loss of appetite, sweats and proximal muscle weakness).
- **Flashes and floaters.** These are common and usually benign, but may be caused by posterior vitreous detachment. In vitreous detachment, floaters may appear as cobwebs or be spider-shaped. There may also be flashes of light. Flashes and floaters may be caused by the formation of a hole in the retina. This can result in retinal detachment, which may present with floaters appearing as a spider's web moving in and out of the visual pathway. Patients may have the urge to clean their glasses frequently and wipe the floaters away.
- **Sudden loss of vision.** Important causes are retinal detachment, temporal arteritis and macular haemorrhage. If half the vision in both eyes is affected, consider homonymous hemianopia due to occlusion of one of the posterior cerebral arteries.
- **Double vision.** Sudden onset of double vision may be caused by trauma in younger people or microvascular infarcts in older people, particularly those with diabetes and hypertension. Intermittent double vision may be caused by myasthenia gravis and tends to become more pronounced as the day goes by, due to increasing fatigue of the ocular muscles.

Common symptom patterns
- **Migraine.** Ocular symptoms in migraine may include flashes of light, loss of central vision, scintillating holes in the vision or rhythmically flashing zigzag lines, which usually present together with other typical features of migraine, such as headache, nausea and vomiting. Attacks usually last for about 20 minutes and may present without any other features of migraine.
- **Amaurosis fugax.** Temporary loss of vision (usually in one eye) may be caused by TIA. Attacks last for less than 24 hours (usually 10–15 minutes).
- **Temporal arteritis.** This usually occurs in older people (>60 years of age), with total loss of vision secondary to anterior ischaemic optic neuropathy, often with preceding episodes of amaurosis fugax. If left untreated, there is a high risk of the other eye being affected over the next 1–2 weeks. Additional features include temporal or generalised headache, pain on chewing or talking (jaw claudication) and systemic symptoms such as fever, anorexia, weight loss and malaise.
- **Macular haemorrhage.** There is usually central loss of vision and an underlying diagnosis of macular degeneration. Patients may state that straight lines such as doorways or tiles appear bent (metamorphosia).
- **Subarachnoid haemorrhage.** Sudden onset of double vision associated with pain, pupil dilation and ptosis suggests subarachnoid haemorrhage.

Past and current medical problems
- **Significant past illnesses.** Ask about significant risk factors for CVD, such as hypertension, diabetes and hyperlipidaemia.
- **Stroke or TIA.** If there is a history of stroke or TIA, has the patient been referred to a stroke unit (if available) for rapid-access workup?
- **Previous eye problems.** People with macular degeneration are at higher risk of macular haemorrhage.

Medication
- **Anticoagulants and antiplatelet drugs.** Is the patient already taking aspirin or warfarin for the prevention of embolic events? Are there any contraindications to these drugs if they are needed for the treatment of vascular disease?

Social history
- **Home.** Ask for details about home life. Is there a threat to independent living resulting from the eye problems? Who is at home to provide support? Has the patient been advised not to drive and to contact the relevant driving authority?
- **Work.** What level of vision is required at the workplace (consider especially pilots, drivers and people having to cope with small details on a computer screen)?

Review of previous investigations
- **Full blood count.** Polycythaemia and thrombocytosis increase the risk of thrombotic events.

- **Inflammatory markers.** C-reactive protein (CRP) or plasma viscosity will usually be raised in temporal arteritis.
- **Fasting lipids and glucose.** Raised values increase the risk of CVD.
- **Haemoglobin A1c (HbA1c).** Check the level of diabetic control if the patient is diabetic.
- **Liver function.** This should be checked in case a statin is required.
- **Electrocardiogram (ECG).** Look for evidence of atrial fibrillation (AF) or other arrhythmia, which may cause cardiac thrombi and resulting embolism.
- **Echocardiogram.** Look for intracardiac thrombi (embolic stroke/TIA).
- **CT brain.** Intracranial lesions may present with visual problems.
- **Carotid Doppler.** Has this been performed to look at the patency of the carotid arteries?

Examination

General
- **General condition.** Does the person look well? People with migraine may look unwell and avoid bright light. Elderly people with temporal arteritis may show signs of weight loss and generally look unwell.

Vital signs
- **Pulse.** Check for evidence of arrhythmia. Consider embolism resulting from AF.
- **Temperature.** There may be a low-grade fever in temporal arteritis.
- **Blood pressure.** Arterial hypertension is a risk factor for arteriosclerosis.

Eye inspection
- **Eye lids.** Unilateral ptosis may occur with subarachnoid haemorrhage.
- **Pupils.** A painful third-nerve palsy with pupil involvement is highly suspicious of a posterior communicating artery aneurysm.
- **Fundus.** Fundoscopy has limited value in the assessment of acute visual loss. Check the size and colour of the optic disc. A yellow–grey disc with blurred margins and haemorrhages suggests papilloedema. Pathological cupping implies glaucoma. Also check for venous pulsation, although this may be difficult to see.

Eye tests
- **Visual acuity.** Measure visual acuity in both eyes (with and without glasses) using a Snellen chart. If visual acuity is worse than 6/60, ask the patient to count fingers at a distance of 1 m. Normal vision does not exclude serious eye injury such as penetrating trauma. Use a pinhole if the vision is decreased. If vision is poor, use finger and hand movements and then perception of light at a distance of 1 m. If visual acuity improves with use of a pinhole, a macular cause is less likely.
- **Visual fields.** Try to establish the pattern of visual-field loss by doing a confrontational field examination. A central field defect indicates optic neuritis or

macular haemorrhage. A unilateral half-field defect may be caused by ischaemic optic neuropathy, temporal arteritis or retinal vein occlusion.

• **Red reflex.** An absent red reflex or a dark shadow across the red reflex indicates an opacity within the media of the eye.

Head and neck

• **Temporal arteries.** Pulseless and tender temporal arteries suggest temporal arteritis.
• **Carotid bruit.** This is not a reliable sign and is not diagnostic, but it may point towards vascular disease.

Key references and further reading

1. Bots ML, van der Wilk EC, Koudstaal PJ et al. Transient neurological attacks in the general population. Prevalence, risk factors, and clinical relevance. *Stroke* 1997;28:768–773.

2. Hayreh SS, Podhajsky PA, Raman R, Zimmerman B. Giant cell arteritis: validity and reliability of various diagnostic criteria. *Am J Ophthalmol* 1997;123:285–296.
3. Kang HK, Luff AJ. Management of retinal detachment: a guide for non-ophthalmologists. *BMJ* 2008;336:1235–1240.
4. National Institute for Health and Care Excellence (NICE). Retinal detachment. Clinical knowledge summaries. 2015. Available from: http://cks.nice.org.uk/retinal-detachment (last accessed 29 April 2016).

Eye problems in older people

Key thoughts

Practical points
- **Diagnosis.** Visual problems are common in older people and can have serious effects on the quality of life. Identify treatable or modifiable causes, such as refractive errors and cataract. Assess the effect of eye problems on day-to-day life.
- **Prognosis.** Exclude serious causes (e.g. temporal arteritis) that will need urgent action. Eye problems in older people may put their independence at risk. Look for evidence of complications resulting from poor vision, such as depression and falls.

Possible causes
- Refractive errors.
- Cataract.
- Age-related macular degeneration (ARMD).
- Glaucoma.
- Diabetes.
- Amaurosis fugax due to TIA.
- Temporal arteritis (rare).

> ### RED FLAGS
>
> - Sudden-onset visual loss
> - Headache
> - Confusion
> - Eye pain with visual loss

History

Ideas, concerns and expectations
- **Ideas.** Many elderly people wrongly believe loss of vision is a normal part of ageing and that 'nothing can be done'.
- **Concerns.** The prospect of losing vision can be very frightening and may lead to a reduction in confidence.
- **Expectations.** Many patients need adequate vision in order to be able to continue to drive, read, work around the house and take part in leisure activities.

The 10-Minute Clinical Assessment, Second Edition. Knut Schroeder.
© 2017 John Wiley & Sons, Ltd. Published 2017 by John Wiley & Sons, Ltd.

History of presenting complaint

- **Quality of life.** Gradual visual loss may be underestimated by the patient or accepted as part of ageing, especially if there is loss of visual acuity and night vision. Find out how the eye problems affect the quality of life and daily activities. Ask about activities such as cooking, watching television, housework, reading and driving.
- **Onset.** Was the onset of eye problems sudden or gradual? Gradual deterioration suggests refractive errors, ARMD or possible diabetic changes. Acute loss of vision and visual-field loss may occur with conditions such as TIA, temporal arteritis or retinal vein thrombosis.
- **Use of visual aids.** The role of the optometrist in the community is vital. When were the eyes last checked? Has the patient been prescribed glasses? Are they being worn? Has there been any change in visual acuity? The cost of new glasses may lead elderly patients to use family members' glasses or to stick with glasses that have become inappropriate. They may even wear two pairs at once to try and improve vision.
- **Exposure.** Is there a history of ectropion or other eyelid malposition?
- **Nutrition.** Poor nutrition can affect vision through vitamin A deficiency (xerophthalmia), which fortunately has now become rare in many countries.
- **Associated problems.** Has visual loss led to any falls, accidents or other problems?

Common symptom patterns

- **ARMD.** Ask about distorted vision of straight edges (e.g. book shelves or door frames). Is vision blurred? Are there any visual-field defects (blind spots)?
- **Cataract.** Ask about risk factors, which include UVB radiation, age, diabetes, alcohol, smoking, vitamin-deficient diet and corticosteroid use. Symptoms include glare in bright light or during night driving and difficulty in distinguishing objects in low light.
- **Dry eye.** Dry eye can present as grittiness, reflex tearing and redness.
- **Chronic glaucoma.** Chronic glaucoma is often asymptomatic. Ask about any visual-field defects, which patients will often not notice until late ('thief of sight').
- **Acute glaucoma.** Acute glaucoma is rare and may present with eye pain and blurred vision. Occasionally, rainbow-coloured rings occur around white lights.
- **Thyroid eye disease.** This may cause lid retraction, dry eyes, tissue swelling, proptosis, corneal problems and ophthalmoplegia.

Past and current medical problems

- **Diabetes.** Diabetes is a common cause of eye problems (particularly diabetic retinopathy). As a rule of thumb, diabetic retinopathy usually presents more than 10 years after the initial diagnosis of diabetes. Fluctuations in blood sugar may lead directly to acute visual problems.
- **CVD.** This increases the risk of visual loss due to stroke or TIA.

- **Thyroid disease.** Consider thyroid eye disease in all patients with abnormal thyroid function.
- **Connective-tissue disorders.** Ask about joint pains and symptoms of vasculitis if there is evidence of iritis.

Medication
- **Dry eyes.** Drugs that can lead to dry eyes include NSAIDs, diuretics, preservatives in eye drops, decongestants, beta blockers and antidepressants.

Social history
- **Home.** Ask about home circumstances and level of support. If the patient lives alone, assess the threat to independent living due to visual problems.
- **Driving.** Drivers with eye problems are at greater risk of accidents and need early investigation and management.

Examination

General
- **General status.** Assess nutritional state and look for evidence of self-neglect.

Vital signs
- **Blood pressure.** Raised blood pressure is a risk factor for hypertensive retinopathy.

Eyes
- **Visual acuity.** Assess visual acuity formally with a Snellen chart. Refractive errors are common. If vision is improved with pinhole testing, consider lens opacity due to cataract and refractive errors.
- **Eye lids.** Chronic inflammation and ectropion can cause excess evaporation of tears, leading to dry eye.
- **Schirmer test.** If appropriate, check for reduced tear production.
- **Fluorescein staining.** Look for evidence of epithelial loss and reduced marginal tear strip.
- **Fundoscopy.** This can be difficult but may be worth attempting. Consider dilating the pupil with 1% tropicamide eye drops if there are no symptoms or signs of acute glaucoma. Check for elevation of the macula due to fluid, blood or drusen around the macula (suggesting ARMD). Look for signs of diabetic retinopathy, such as microaneurysms, haemorrhages, exudates and proliferative retinopathy. Fundoscopy should be complemented by an optician's eye check, which is far more wide-ranging and specific than fundoscopy alone. Eye checks are often free to the elderly and include certain assessments (e.g. pressure testing for glaucoma) that may not be available to non-specialists.
- **Range of movement.** Check eye movements and the presence of double vision.

Neurological
- **Seventh nerve.** Impaired seventh nerve function due to stroke or Bell's palsy may cause exposure keratopathy.

Key references and further reading

1. Moeini HA, Masoudpour H, Ghanbari H. A study of the relation between body mass index and the incidence of age related macular degeneration. *Br J Ophthalmol* 2005;89:964–966.
2. National Institute for Health and Care Excellence (NICE). Giant cell arteritis. Clinical knowledge summaries. 2014. Available from: http://cks.nice.org.uk/giant-cell-arteritis (last accessed 29 April 2016).
3. National Institute for Health and Care Excellence (NICE). Glaucoma. Clinical knowledge summaries. 2014. Available from: http://cks.nice.org.uk/glaucoma (last accessed 29 April 2016).
4. National Institute for Health and Care Excellence (NICE). Cataracts. Clinical knowledge summaries. 2015. Available from: http://cks.nice.org.uk/cataracts (last accessed 29 April 2016).
5. Smeeth L, Iliffe S. Community screening for visual impairment in the elderly. *Cochrane Database Syst Rev* 2006;(3):CD001054.

Ear, nose and throat

Neck swelling

Key thoughts

Practical points
- **Diagnosis.** Benign conditions, such as lymphadenopathy due to pharyngitis or tonsillitis, are common. In persistent neck swelling (>3 weeks), consider alternative causes (e.g. head and neck cancer, tuberculosis (TB) in at-risk groups, human immunodeficiency virus (HIV)).

Possible causes
- Goitre.
- Infective lymphadenopathy (e.g. nonspecific viral infections, Epstein–Barr virus (EBV), TB, HIV).
- Malignant lymphadenopathy (e.g. lymphoma, metastasis).
- Thyroglossal cyst.
- Rarely, carotid aneurysm, salivary gland infection or malignancy, superior vena cava obstruction.

> **RED FLAGS**
>
> - Persistent unexplained swellings (>3 weeks)
> - Persistent sore throat
> - Unilateral unexplained pain in the head and neck area for more than 4 weeks associated with ear ache but normal otoscopy
> - Persistent mouth ulcers
> - Red and white patches of the oral mucosa
> - Systemic symptoms, such as fever, night sweats, malaise and weight loss

History

Ideas, concerns and expectations
- **Ideas.** What does the patient believe is the underlying cause?
- **Concerns.** Worries about underlying cancer or TB are common.
- **Expectations.** Patients will often expect further investigation or referral.

History of presenting complaint
- **Quality of life.** Persistent neck lumps often cause significant concern and anxiety, and patients may present late because of anxieties that their fear about possible underlying cancer might be confirmed.

The 10-Minute Clinical Assessment, Second Edition. Knut Schroeder.
© 2017 John Wiley & Sons, Ltd. Published 2017 by John Wiley & Sons, Ltd.

- **Onset.** Lymphadenopathy due to throat infections is common and is usually accompanied by a sore throat. An unexplained swelling of recent onset or a change over 3–6 weeks in a previously undiagnosed lump should raise suspicions of cancer.
- **Site.** Where is the lump? Any unexplained and persistent swellings of the parotid or submandibular glands or elsewhere on the head and neck may indicate malignancy.
- **Pain.** Ask about any unexplained or persistent sore throat and pain in the head or neck. Ear ache with normal otoscopy is particularly suspicious.
- **Mouth ulcers.** Have there been any unexplained mouth ulcers or unusual changes of the oral mucosa persisting for more than 3 weeks?
- **Hoarseness and voice changes.** Hoarseness due to benign conditions usually settles within 6 weeks. If symptoms persist, consider possible metastasis from laryngeal cancer, thyroid tumour or recurrent laryngeal nerve palsy due to lung cancer (Pancoast tumour).
- **Dysphagia.** Ask about swallowing problems, particularly if these have lasted for more than 3 weeks.
- **Nasal symptoms.** Nasal symptoms are commonly caused by acute upper respiratory infections. Any persistent unilateral nasal obstruction, particularly if associated with purulent discharge, should raise concerns about malignancy.
- **Teeth.** Unexplained tooth mobility not associated with periodontal disease may rarely be caused by an underlying tumour.
- **Eyes.** Have the eyes changed in appearance? Orbital masses can cause proptosis of the eyes, particularly if unilateral.
- **Breathing.** Stridor may occur due to tracheal compression in advanced thyroid cancer.
- **Smoking and alcohol.** Have a high level of suspicion in heavy smokers and drinkers who present with symptoms suggestive of head and neck cancer. Also consider other uses of tobacco, including chewing pan, gutkha and betel.
- **Age.** Head and neck cancers are more common in people over 45 years of age. Any neck swelling in a prepubertal child lasting for more than 3 weeks should also raise concerns and prompt further investigation/referral.
- **General symptoms.** Ask about unintentional weight loss, sleep problems, fatigue, malaise, night sweats and lymphadenopathy, which may indicate malignancy or chronic infection (e.g. TB).

Past and current medical problems
- **Significant past illnesses.** Ask particularly about a past history of cancer or TB.
- **Irradiation.** A history of neck irradiation raises the possibility of thyroid cancer.

Family history
- **Endocrine tumour.** Ask about a family history of thyroid tumours.

Social history
- **Home.** Has home life been affected by any of the symptoms?
- **Contact with infectious diseases.** Has the patient travelled to a hot country lately or had contact with TB?

Review of previous investigations

- **Full blood count and plasma viscosity.** Look for evidence of inflammation or infection. The differential blood cell count may be abnormal in haematological cancer, such as lymphoma.
- **Imaging.** A chest X-ray is useful for ruling out cancer in patients presenting with hoarseness for more than 3 weeks, particularly in smokers over the age of 50 and heavy drinkers.
- **Biopsy.** Have any biopsies been taken from neck lesions in the past?

Examination

General

- **General condition.** Does the patient look unwell? Cachexia may point to underlying malignancy.
- **Pallor.** Look for signs of anaemia.
- **Lymph nodes.** Generalised lymphadenopathy suggests systemic illness.

Head and neck

- **Oral mucosa.** Look out for swellings or ulcers. Any red and white patches of the oral mucosa should be regarded as suspicious.
- **Neck lump.** An intradermal lump suggests sebaceous cyst (if there is a central punctum) or lipoma.
- **Anterior triangle.** Tender and mobile lymph nodes suggest infection. Consider malignancy if lumps or swellings are non-tender, hard or fixed to the underlying structures. A swelling that moves with tongue protrusion may be caused by a thyroglossal cyst. If the submandibular glands are swollen, inspect and palpate the salivary glands carefully, looking for sources of infection or malignancy. Tumours from the head and neck often metastasise into the submandibular region. Other possible diagnoses are carotid aneurysm and carotid body tumour.
- **Posterior triangle.** Consider lymphadenopathy due to glandular fever, HIV, TB, metastases or lymphoma if there are multiple lumps. Other causes include a pharyngeal pouch, subclavian artery aneurysm and cervical rib. Tumours of the chest and abdomen often metastasise to the lower aspect of the posterior triangle. If indicated, look for Virchow's node, which lies on the left side, deep in the angle between the sternocleidomastoid muscle and the clavicle.
- **Parotid swelling.** If the parotid gland is swollen, inspect the orifice of the parotid duct and palpate the gland with the head tilted backwards.
- **Facial nerve.** Check the function of the facial nerve if there is a possibility of a lesion within the parotid gland.
- **Thyroid gland.** Palpate the thyroid gland, which should move upwards on swallowing. Check for goitre and nodules.

Abdomen

- **Liver and spleen.** Check for hepatosplenomegaly, which may rarely indicate haematological cancer or metastasis (usually difficult or impossible to detect clinically).

Key references and further reading

1. National Institute for Health and Care Excellence (NICE). Suspected cancer: recognition and referral. NICE guidelines [NG12]. June 2015. Available from: http://www.nice.org.uk/guidance/ng12 (last accessed 29 April 2016).
2. Siminosky K. The rational clinical examination: does this patient have a goiter? *JAMA* 1995;273:813–817.
3. Smith OD, Ellis PD, Bearcroft PW et al. Management of neck lumps – a triage model. *Ann R Coll Surg Engl* 2000;82:223–226.
4. Tromp D, Brouha X, Hordijk G-J et al. Patient factors associated with delay in primary care among patients with head and neck carcinoma: a case-series analysis. *Fam Pract* 2005;22:554–559.

Sore throat

Key thoughts

Practical points
- **Diagnosis.** Viral upper respiratory infection is the most common cause. Consider glandular fever or even malignancy in unusual presentations or if symptoms are prolonged.

Possible causes
- Viral (common cold, infectious mononucleosis).
- Bacterial (streptococcal, also consider rarer causes such as gonococcal infection or diphtheria).
- Allergy.
- Acid reflux.
- Malignancy.
- Reactions to medication.
- Irritation.

RED FLAGS

- General symptoms (e.g. weight loss, malaise, night sweats and fever)
- Possibility of sexually transmitted infection (STI)
- Immunosuppression from infection (HIV) or from drugs such as carbimazole or steroids
- Patient systemically unwell
- Unilateral peritonsillitis and peritonsillar abscess
- History of rheumatic fever
- Stridor
- Swallowing problems
- Difficulty breathing
- Dehydration
- More than five episodes in the past 12 months

History

Ideas, concerns and expectations
- **Ideas.** Patients often think sore throat must be caused by bacterial infection.

The 10-Minute Clinical Assessment, Second Edition. Knut Schroeder.
© 2017 John Wiley & Sons, Ltd. Published 2017 by John Wiley & Sons, Ltd.

- **Concerns.** Sore throat can be very unpleasant, and patients commonly worry that it might cause damage to the throat. Fears about possible throat cancer are also common.
- **Expectations.** Patients will often expect reassurance or a prescription for antibiotics (which will usually not be indicated).

History of presenting complaint
- **Quality of life.** Sore throat can impair the quality of life considerably.
- **Onset.** Acute onset usually results from upper respiratory tract infection or, less commonly, glandular fever (infectious mononucleosis). Exposure to other people with streptococcal throat infection makes strep throat more likely. Slow and gradual onset, particularly in the elderly, may rarely be caused by a tumour, particularly if there is unilateral throat swelling.
- **Pain and fever.** Pain on swallowing associated with fever and cervical lymphadenopathy is often caused by viral infection (which will not respond to antibiotics).
- **Throat irritation.** Dry and cold air, tobacco smoke or mouth breathing at night commonly cause throat irritation and dryness.
- **Neck swelling.** Consider lymphadenopathy and peritonsillar abscess if there is acute throat and neck swelling. Gradually increasing neck swelling may rarely indicate tumour, particularly in the elderly.
- **Voice changes.** Consider laryngeal malignancy if throat symptoms are associated with a persistent hoarse voice, especially in current and past smokers.
- **Rash.** Consider scarlet fever due to streptococcal throat infection or infectious mononucleosis if the patient has a rash.
- **Systemic illness.** Antibiotics may be needed if the patient is systemically unwell, particularly if there is unilateral peritonsillitis and immunosuppression. Antibiotics in uncomplicated acute throat infections are rarely required in the initial phase.
- **Likelihood of group A streptococcal infection.** The presence of fever >38 °C, the absence of cough, tender anterior cervical lymphadenopathy and tonsillar swelling or exudates make group A streptococcal infection more likely (Centor criteria).
- **Sexual history.** Ask about a history of STI. Consider gonococcal, chlamydial or treponemal infection if there has been oral sex with a partner with overt or possible infection.
- **Other symptoms.** Consider lymphoma or leukaemia (rare) if there are night sweats, fever, weight loss or bruising.

Past and current medical problems
- **Diabetes.** Patients with diabetes are at higher risk of infection.
- **Rheumatic fever.** A past history of rheumatic fever is an indication for antibiotics.
- **Immunosuppression.** Have a lower threshold for giving antibiotics in immunocompromised patients (e.g. leukaemia, lymphoma, HIV infection, steroids).

- **Hyperthyroidism.** A sore throat in a patient on carbimazole, for hyperthyroidism, may indicate agranulocytosis.
- **Allergy.** Is there a personal history of allergies?
- **Acid reflux.** This commonly causes sore throat in the morning.

Medication

- **Antibiotics.** Have antibiotics already been prescribed for this episode? Ask for details about the type of antibiotic (penicillin V is usually the first choice) and whether it was taken as prescribed. Ampicillin and amoxicillin may cause a rash in glandular fever and are best avoided for the treatment of sore throat.
- **Oral contraceptive.** Ask women of child-bearing age whether they are taking the combined oral contraceptive pill, as antibiotics may reduce its effect and increase the risk of pregnancy. Is the woman aware of the need for extra protection for the duration of treatment plus another 7 days (7-day rule)?
- **Carbimazole.** Symptoms of sore throat should be taken very seriously in patients taking carbimazole because of possible neutropenia. An urgent full blood count is usually required, and the drug should be stopped until results are available.
- **Chemotherapy.** Also consider the possibility of neutropenia in patients on chemotherapy.
- **Over-the-counter preparations.** Paracetamol and antiseptic mouthwashes for the treatment of sore throat can usually be bought without prescription.

Allergies

- **Antibiotics.** Check for and record the type and severity of any past reactions to antibiotics, particularly penicillin.

Social history

- **Home.** Have symptoms affected home and family life in any way?
- **School and work.** Has the patient had to take time off school or work due to throat symptoms? If problems are recurrent, how many days have been lost in the past 12 months?

Review of previous investigations

- **Throat swab.** Throat swabs are not required in uncomplicated acute sore throat. A throat swab may help identify infection in high-risk patients, if an STI or other uncommon infection is suspected or if there is no response to treatment. Carriage of beta-haemolytic streptococcus is common and does not necessarily indicate active infection. Swabs may not always pick up an infection.
- **Full blood count.** This will only be required in selected cases. Atypical mononuclear cells are commonly found in glandular fever, and an infectious mononucleosis test may be positive. Look for agranulocytosis in patients taking immunosuppressive drugs or carbimazole. The full blood count may also be abnormal in malignancy (e.g. leukaemia).
- **Inflammatory markers.** Raised inflammatory markers suggest infection or, rarely, malignancy.

Examination

General
- **General condition.** Does the patient look unwell? Antibiotics are not usually needed for uncomplicated suspected viral infection, but have a lower threshold for giving antibiotics in patients with systemic upset.

Vital signs
- **Temperature.** Fever is common in acute upper respiratory infection.
- **Airway and breathing.** Be aware that throat inspection may in rare cases lead to acute deterioration, especially if there are signs of upper airway obstruction.

Skin
- **Rash.** Look for the typical scarlatiniform rash of scarlet fever, which usually begins with fine erythematous papules on the trunk and then spreads to the extremities, sparing the palms and soles. The rash blanches on pressure and can feel like sandpaper.

Head and neck
- **Tongue.** Look for the typical 'strawberry tongue' of scarlet fever, which may be associated with perioral pallor.
- **Throat inspection.** Small blisters on the palate and fauces may indicate coxsackie virus infection. Severe erythema or a grey–white tonsillar and pharyngeal exudate is common with streptococcal throat infection and infectious mononucleosis. In addition, white patches in the throat of children may be caused by candidiasis or, less commonly, immunodeficiency or diphteria (in non-immunised patients). Consider diabetes or immunodeficiency if there is white exudate in adults. Do not examine the throat if you are considering epiglottitis.
- **Lymphadenopathy.** The anterior cervical lymph glands tend to be markedly enlarged and tender in infectious mononucleosis and other throat infections. Consider malignancy, such as lymphoma or leukaemia, if the lymph nodes are enlarged but non-tender.
- **Neck swelling.** Unilateral swelling below the mandible points is a sign of peritonsillar abscess.
- **Ears.** Look for evidence of associated otitis media.

Abdomen
- **Spleen.** Splenomegaly may occur with infectious mononucleosis.

Key references and further reading

1. Centor, RM, Witherspoon, JM, Dalton, HP et al. The diagnosis of strep throat in adults in the emergency room. *Med Decis Making* 1981;1:239.
2. Ebell MH, Smith MA, Barry HC et al. The rational clinical examination: does this patient have strep throat? *JAMA* 2000;284:2912–2918.

3. Ford C. Evaluation and management of laryngopharyngeal reflux. *JAMA* 2005;294:1534–1540.
4. Little P, Williamson I. Sore throat management in general practice. *Fam Pract* 1996;13:317–321.
5. National Institute for Health and Care Excellence (NICE). Sore throat. Clinical knowledge summaries. 2015. Available from: http://cks.nice.org.uk/sore-throat-acute (last accessed 29 April 2016).
6. National Prescribing Centre (NPC). The management of common infections in primary care – key points. Available from: http://www.isdbweb.org/documents/file/798_15.pdf (last accessed 29 April 2016).
7. Wagner FP, Mathiason MA. Using centor criteria to diagnose streptococcal pharyngitis. *Nurse Pract* 2008;33:10–12.

Ear pain

Key thoughts

Practical points

- **Diagnosis.** Otitis externa and media are common causes of ear pain. Ear pain can be very distressing and may seriously impair the quality of life. Rarely, serious causes such as cholesteatoma, meningitis or cerebral abscess may present with ear pain.

Possible causes

- Otitis externa.
- Acute otitis media.
- Otitis media with effusion.
- Furuncle in posterior canal wall.
- Postauricular lymphadenopathy.
- Rarely, cholesteatoma, meningitis, sigmoid sinus thrombosis, cerebral abscess, mastoiditis and Bezold's abscess (pus tracking along the digastric muscles in the direction of the chin or along the sternocleidomastoid muscle), parotitis.

RED FLAGS

- Only one hearing ear
- Vertigo
- Hoarseness
- Dysphagia
- Facial weakness
- Meningism
- Persistent discharge, perforation or effusion
- Recurrent attacks of otitis media in adults

History

Ideas, concerns and expectations

- **Ideas.** What does the patient believe is causing the ear pain?
- **Concerns.** Common concerns are permanent loss of hearing and the possibility of underlying malignancy.
- **Expectations.** Many patients expect antibiotics for the treatment of ear pain, which may or may not be indicated.

The 10-Minute Clinical Assessment, Second Edition. Knut Schroeder.
© 2017 John Wiley & Sons, Ltd. Published 2017 by John Wiley & Sons, Ltd.

History of presenting complaint
- **Quality of life.** Ear pain can seriously affect the quality of life. Ask how daily activities are affected (e.g. school, work).
- **Otorrhoea.** Pain that eases with the onset of purulent discharge suggests acute otitis media with perforation. Chronic discharge in a painful ear indicates otitis media. Offensive discharge in connection with reduced hearing and tinnitus may be caused by cholesteatoma.
- **Fever.** Fever is common with acute otitis media. Consider the possibility of mastoiditis in rare cases.
- **Respiratory infection.** Otitis media is likely if ear pain develops in connection with upper respiratory infection.
- **Swimming.** Ear pain in swimmers or after a beach holiday suggests infective otitis externa.
- **Associated ear symptoms.** Ask about tinnitus, discharge and hearing loss, which may rarely suggest cholesteatoma. Facial weakness, vomiting, headache or dizziness suggests a more serious underlying cause.
- **Previous ear problems or surgery.** Ask about past problems with the affected and non-affected ear and any previous ear surgery, such as tympanoplasty or tympanostomy tubes ('grommets').
- **Referred pain.** Associated neck pain may indicate problems with the cervical spine (C2), wisdom teeth or sinuses (V) or the pharynx or larynx (IX, X). Other common sources for referred pain are dental disease, tonsillitis and temporomandibular joint disorders.
- **Headache.** Consider mastoiditis (rare) if the pain radiates to the area behind the ear or if there is localised or generalised headache.
- **Gradenigo's triad.** Petrositis (infection of the petrous temporal bone) may develop in rare cases, presenting with subacute otitis media, retro-orbital pain and abducens nerve palsy.
- **Recent antibiotics.** Symptoms and signs of mastoiditis may be more subtle if the patient has been taking antibiotics in the preceding few weeks, particularly if inappropriate antibiotics were used for too short a period or if they were taken incorrectly. Consider mastoiditis or an abscess if pain and fever persist despite appropriate antibiotic treatment.

Past and current medical problems
- **Diabetes.** Diabetes predisposes to infection.
- **Immunodeficiency.** Ear infections may become serious if there is underlying immunodeficiency (e.g. HIV infection).

Medication
- **Analgesics.** Ask what has been taken and what has worked. Have there been any adverse effects?
- **Steroids.** Symptoms in patients on regular and high-dose steroids may be masked.

Allergies
- **Antibiotics.** Ask about allergies to any antibiotics that may need to be used for treatment.

Social history
- **Home.** How far has home life been affected by the ear problems?
- **Work.** Is there a need for a sick note? Does the patient work in an environment where a particularly high level of auditory function is required (e.g. teacher, pilot, diver)?
- **Travel.** Ask whether any air travel is planned, as this may lead to further barotrauma (especially if middle-ear ventilation is impaired).

Examination

General
- **General state.** Does the patient look unwell? Rarely, reduced consciousness may suggest intracranial involvement or meningitis following mastoiditis.

Vital signs
- **Temperature.** Fever suggests acute otitis media or other infection.

Head and neck
- **Ear inspection.** Look for signs of infection (tender and red tragus or pinna, obvious purulent discharge).
- **Area behind the ear.** Inspect the postauricular area for oedema, swelling or erythema (mastoiditis). From behind, check whether the external ear has been displaced down and outwards. Feel for a fluctuant swelling behind the ear and tenderness over the mastoid antrum (McEwen's triangle) or over the mastoid tip, which also suggests mastoiditis.
- **Otoscopy.** An inflamed tympanic membrane or a change in colour suggests acute otitis media. Additional signs are bulging of the tympanic membrane with loss of landmarks and perforation with discharge of pus. The external auditory meatus may be narrowed in mastoiditis due to pressure on to the posterior–superior meatal wall. Debris, discharge and an inflamed swollen external auditory meatus suggest otitis externa. Look for ulcers or polyps on the canal floor with exposed bone, which indicates malignant otitis externa.
- **Hearing.** Assess hearing either informally with finger rubbing or, if hearing loss has been reported by the patient, with Weber and Rinne testing.
- **Neck.** If indicated, check for neck stiffness as a sign of meningitis. Pain on neck movements may indicate cervical spine pathology.
- **Eyes.** Look for oedema of the upper eye lid if local spread of infection is suspected. Check for diplopia, which suggests rare abducens nerve involvement (Gradenigo's triad: abducens paralysis, pain and otitis).
- **Cranial nerves.** Examine the cranial nerves carefully if mastoiditis is a possibility. Subtle neurological signs may be the only findings in masked mastoiditis.

Key references and further reading

1. Charlett SD, Coatesworth AP. Referred otalgia: a structured approach to diagnosis and treatment. *Int J Clin Pract* 2007;61:1015–1021.
2. Ely JW, Hansen MR, Clark EC. Diagnosis of ear pain. *Am Fam Physician* 2008; 77:621–628.
3. Jaber JJ, Leonette JP, Lawrason AE, Feustel PJ. Cervical spine causes for referred otalgia. *Otolaryngol Head Neck Surg* 2008;138:479–485.
4. Jensen PM, Lous J. Criteria, performance and diagnostic problems in diagnosing acute otitis media. *Fam Pract* 1999;16:262–268.
5. National Institute for Health and Care Excellence (NICE). Otitis externa. Clinical knowledge summaries. 2015. Available from: http://cks.nice.org.uk/otitis-externa (last accessed 29 April 2016).
6. National Institute for Health and Care Excellence (NICE). Otitis media – acute. Clinical knowledge summaries. 2015. Available from: http://cks.nice.org.uk/otitis-media-acute (last accessed 29 April 2016).

Hearing loss in adults

Key thoughts

Practical points
- **Diagnosis.** Hearing loss is a common presentation, particularly in older people. Try to distinguish between problems in the outer, middle and inner ear. Impacted ear wax and presbyacusis are frequent causes. Rarely, more serious conditions such as acoustic neuroma or cholesteatoma may present with hearing loss.

Possible causes
- Impacted wax in the external ear canal.
- Presbyacusis (cochlear degeneration).
- Otitis media.
- Diffuse otitis externa.
- Menière's disease.
- Acute sensorineural hearing loss.
- Otosclerosis.
- Rarely, cholesteatoma, acoustic neuroma, nasopharyngeal tumour.

> **RED FLAGS**
>
> - Neurological symptoms
> - Rapid onset (<72 hours)
> - Progressive unilateral hearing loss and tinnitus
> - Onset after trauma
> - Cerebrospinal fluid (CSF) otorrhoea
> - Increasing pain
> - Persistent offensive discharge
> - Chronic bleeding

History

Ideas, concerns and expectations
- **Ideas.** Many people feel that hearing loss will be irreversible and that not much can be done to improve symptoms. There is often a great reluctance to consider wearing a hearing aid.
- **Concerns.** Social interaction can be severely impaired, and hearing loss can increase fears about social isolation and induce loss of self-confidence.
- **Expectations.** Ask about expectations with regard to further investigation and management.

The 10-Minute Clinical Assessment, Second Edition. Knut Schroeder.
© 2017 John Wiley & Sons, Ltd. Published 2017 by John Wiley & Sons, Ltd.

History of presenting complaint

- **Quality of life.** Hearing loss can severely impair the quality of life. Find out what the patient thinks is the main problem at the moment (e.g. going to work, talking on the phone, taking part in conversations).
- **Previous ear problems.** Ask about ear infections, ear injury, ear surgery and previous difficulties with hearing. Tympanic membrane perforation may have occurred as a result of ear trauma, surgery or chronic otitis media.
- **Age.** Older age is a risk factor for hearing loss. Age-induced hearing loss (presbyacusis) is usually progressive and bilateral, initially affecting the higher frequencies. The worst environment for people with this condition in terms of hearing is a crowded room.
- **Onset.** How long has the hearing loss been present? Painless gradual onset of hearing loss in younger people suggests ear wax or adenoids. Presbyacusis usually starts gradually in older people. Consider otosclerosis if there is painless progressive hearing loss in middle-aged women.
- **Progression.** Progressive hearing loss may indicate serious underlying disease, particularly if symptoms are unilateral.
- **Site.** Unilateral hearing loss occurs in otitis media, but always consider acoustic neuroma if symptoms are persistent, progressive or associated with headache.
- **Discharge and ear ache.** Discharge and debris in the ear canal in otitis externa can cause conductive hearing loss. Ask about risk factors for otitis externa, such as a history of eczema in the ear canal, swimming and using cotton buds to 'clean' the ear. Ear discharge, ear ache and hearing loss are common symptoms of chronic suppurative otitis media. There is usually a sudden improvement of pain once the ear drum has perforated.
- **Waxy occlusion.** Cerumen may block the external ear canal, particularly if cotton-tipped buds are used. Foreign bodies occur particularly in children and in patients with mental health problems or learning difficulties. Oedema and exostosis may occur in frequent swimmers.
- **Tinnitus and vertigo.** Associated tinnitus and vertigo suggest Ménière's disease, particularly if increasing in severity. Attacks are usually recurrent. Similar symptoms occur as a result of ischaemic events, so ask about cardiovascular risk factors such as diabetes, smoking, hypertension, raised cholesterol and previous cardiovascular events. Also consider the possibility of acoustic neuroma.
- **Nasal and breathing problems.** Ask about nasal problems, including congestion and discharge, snoring, mouth breathing and sinus pains, which may cause temporary loss of hearing due to swelling of the Eustachian tube.
- **Noise.** Ask about a history of noise exposure, either at work or in connection with leisure (e.g. rock concerts). Sudden changes in noise, such as explosions or barotrauma in pilots or divers, may cause ear damage.
- **Treatments.** What treatments have been tried and what has worked in the past? Betahistine can be useful in the treatment of Ménière's disease.
- **Hearing aid.** Has the patient ever been formally assessed for a hearing aid? What did the audiometry results show? Is any hearing aid working and being used correctly?

Past and current medical problems
- **Cardiovascular disease (CVD).** Consider vascular causes of hearing loss if there is a past history of stroke or heart disease.
- **Diabetes.** Recurrent infections are more common in people with diabetes. Diabetes is also a risk factor for vascular causes of hearing loss.

Family history
- **Otosclerosis.** Otosclerosis tends to run in families.

Medication
- **Ototoxic drugs.** Ototoxicity is a recognised adverse effect of a number of drugs, including aminoglycosides, salicylates, some loop diuretics and quinine. Consider ear damage, particularly if drugs have been given at high doses over a prolonged period of time.
- **Ear drops.** Has any treatment for otitis externa been effective in the past?
- **Steroids.** Patients on steroids may be at higher risk of infection. Symptoms and signs of mastoiditis may be masked.

Allergies
- **Antibiotics.** Ask about allergies to any antibiotics that might need to be used for the treatment of ear infections.

Social history
- **Home.** Have there been any problems at home as a result of the hearing loss? Marital problems are not uncommon. Have phone calls been missed?
- **Work.** How far do the hearing problems affect work? Good hearing is important for many professions (e.g. pilots, teachers, musicians).
- **Social life.** Hearing loss can be very disabling and carries a risk of social isolation. Inability to take part in group conversations is an early problem with hearing loss.

Review of previous investigations
- **Ear swabs.** If there is ear discharge, are any swab results available in case there is little or no response to antibiotic treatment?
- **Glucose.** Consider diabetes in recurrent infection.

Examination

General
- **Gait.** If gait is unsteady, consider vestibular or cerebellar involvement.

Vital signs
- **Temperature.** A fever suggests otitis media or mastoiditis (rare).

Ears
- **External ear.** Look for deformity, obvious discharge and signs of eczema. Look behind the pinna for signs of mastoiditis.
- **Tenderness.** Check for tenderness on pressing the tragus or pulling the pinna, which suggests otitis externa.
- **Ear canal.** Check for wax and foreign bodies. A scaly, inflamed, swollen or macerated ear canal may be caused by otitis externa. Describe the odour, quantity and nature of any discharge. Cysts and benign and malignant tumours may occur within the ear canal.
- **Ear drum.** Look for any inflammation, indrawing or perforation. Perforations are consistent with chronic suppurative otitis media. Defects in the superior atticoantral aspect of the tympanic membrane may be caused by a cholesteatoma, in which case a white mass may also be visible. Look for a fluid level or bubbles (indicating effusion).
- **Hearing.** Do a simple whisper test (ask the patient to repeat words or numbers while gently placing and moving a finger on the tragus of the opposite ear to mask any noise). If the patient wears a hearing aid, make sure it is working properly and inserted correctly.
- **Rinne and Weber.** If patients fail the whisper test, perform Rinne's and Weber's tuning fork tests to differentiate between conductive and sensorineural hearing loss. These tests do not need to be used for general screening.

Head and neck
- **Oropharynx.** Look for any swellings or signs of infection that might cause problems with ventilation of the inner ear (e.g. tonsillitis).
- **Lymph nodes.** Check for cervical lymphadenopathy.
- **Facial tenderness.** Tenderness over the sinuses suggests sinusitis.
- **Cranial nerves.** Examine cranial nerves as suggested by the history, particularly if mastoiditis is a possibility.

Key references and further reading
1. Bagay A, Thavendiranathan P, Detsky A. The rational clinical examination: does this patient have hearing impairment? *JAMA* 2006;295:416–428.
2. Edmiston R, Mitchell C. 10-minute consultation: hearing loss in adults. *BMJ* 2013;346:f2496.
3. Isaacson JE, Vora NM. Differential diagnosis and treatment of hearing loss. *Am Fam Physician* 2003;68:1125–1132.
4. Yueh B, Shapiro N, MacLean CH, Shekelle PG. Screening and management of adult hearing loss in primary care: scientific review. *JAMA* 2003;289:1976–1985.

Tinnitus

Key thoughts

Practical points
- **Diagnosis.** Try to distinguish between otological causes and conditions affecting the central nervous system (CNS). Tinnitus may also be caused by other conditions, such as anaemia or heart murmurs.
- **Quality of life.** Tinnitus can be very disabling and may range from mild symptoms to severe disability. Associated depression and even self-harm are not uncommon.

Possible causes
- Idiopathic.
- Otitis media.
- Exposure to loud noise.
- Menière's disease.
- Ototoxic medication.
- Intracranial malignancy.
- Brainstem lesions.
- Head injury.
- Rarely, anaemia, hyper- or hypothyroidism, renal failure, heart murmur.

> **RED FLAGS**
> - Gradually worsening tinnitus
> - Chronic ear discharge
> - Headache
> - Depression and risk of self-harm
> - Associated hearing problems
> - Neurological symptoms

History

Ideas, concerns and expectations
- **Ideas.** What does the patient think is causing the tinnitus?
- **Concerns.** Patients are often worried that their symptoms might not be taken seriously. Fears about cancer and lasting disability are common.
- **Expectations.** Patients will often expect specialist referral or further investigation, which may or may not be indicated depending on the underlying cause.

The 10-Minute Clinical Assessment, Second Edition. Knut Schroeder.
© 2017 John Wiley & Sons, Ltd. Published 2017 by John Wiley & Sons, Ltd.

History of presenting complaint

- **Quality of life.** Tinnitus can be very distressing and disabling. Find out what effects the symptoms have on the quality of life and day-to-day activities. If tinnitus is severe or persistent, patients may become depressed or even suicidal.
- **Site.** Is the tinnitus unilateral or bilateral? Consider local causes, such as acoustic neuroma or cholesteatoma, if symptoms are unilateral. Systemic causes (e.g. heart murmur, anaemia) usually lead to bilateral tinnitus. Bilateral tinnitus may be worse on one side, and the distinction may be difficult in practice.
- **Onset.** Consider ear infection (especially otitis media), exposure to loud noise or head injury if symptoms have started suddenly. Subacute onset is more common in dental or jaw problems, after whiplash injury or in acoustic neuroma (rare).
- **Character.** A pulsatile tinnitus suggests a vascular cause. Intermittent and variable low-pitch tinnitus occurs with Menière's disease (often described as 'rumbling like a machine'). Higher-frequency tinnitus may be sensorineural in origin.
- **Hearing loss.** If there is associated hearing loss, consider eighth-nerve damage. Concomitant vertigo and 'fullness' of the ear suggest otitis media or, less commonly, Menière's disease.
- **Hyperacusis.** Are quieter environments preferred? Patients with hyperacusis may try to avoid loud noises which can in turn exacerbate tinnitus.
- **Pain.** Associated pain may suggest ear infection, tumour or trauma. Pain may be referred, such as in nasopharyngeal carcinoma (rare).
- **Ear discharge.** Painless mucoid discharge is common with chronic otitis media or otitis externa, whereas a foul-smelling creamy discharge suggests cholesteatoma.
- **Depression.** Tinnitus can lead to depression and even self-harm.
- **Sleep.** Sleep problems are common with tinnitus, may aggravate depression and can be very troublesome.
- **Injury.** Has there been any trauma or surgery?
- **Neurological symptoms.** Consider brain-stem disease if there are other neurological symptoms, such as double vision or gait problems, suggesting ataxia.

Past and current medical problems

- **Systemic disease.** Ask about hyper- and hypothyroidism, renal failure, heart problems and anaemia, all of which may cause or exacerbate tinnitus.
- **Neurological conditions.** Is there a history of neurological disease, such as multiple sclerosis (MS)?
- **Cancer.** Consider metastatic disease or primary tumour if there is a history of cancer.

Medication

- **Ototoxic medication.** Consider aspirin and other nonsteroidal anti-inflammatory drugs (NSAIDs), quinine and antibiotics (especially aminoglycosides, erythromycin and tetracycline).

Other treatments
- **Holistic approach.** Have other health professionals been involved in the past, including ear, nose and throat (ENT) specialists, audiologists, hearing therapists, counsellors and clinical psychologists?

Family history
- **Ear problems.** Ask about a family history of any ENT problems. Otosclerosis typically causes bilateral tinnitus and conductive hearing loss.

Social history
- **Home.** Tinnitus may lead to marital problems due to associated depression and insomnia.
- **Work.** Has work been affected in any way? Tinnitus is common in musicians and other people exposed to chronic noise at work.

Review of previous investigations
- **Full blood count.** Blood tests are rarely needed. Look for underlying anaemia.
- **Urea and electrolytes.** Check for evidence of renal disease.
- **Thyroid-stimulating hormone (TSH).** A normal TSH excludes hyper- or hypothyroidism.
- **Magnetic resonance imaging (MRI).** Brain scanning is indicated if malignancy needs to be excluded. MRI can be helpful in ruling out acoustic neuroma or cholesteatoma.

Examination

General
- **Gait.** Obvious gait ataxia suggests an underling neurological cause.

Vital signs
- **Pulse.** Tachycardia or atrial fibrillation may occur in hyperthyroidism (a rare cause of tinnitus).
- **Blood pressure.** Raised blood pressure may rarely cause tinnitus (usually only if very high).

Head and neck
- **Throat.** Examine the throat and look for any obvious causes of eustachian tube dysfunction (e.g. enlarged tonsils or rare tumour), which may cause or contribute to tinnitus.
- **External ear.** Look for evidence of chronic middle-ear infection or otitis externa.
- **Neck swelling.** A goitre suggests underlying thyroid disease.
- **Hearing.** Briefly assess hearing using the whisper test. Weber's and Rinne's tests may be helpful in differentiating between unilateral and bilateral hearing loss and between conductive and sensorineural causes.

- **Eye movements.** Check for diplopia and pupillary responses.
- **Fundoscopy.** Papilloedema may occur in raised intracranial pressure (rare).
- **Cranial nerves.** Examine the cranial nerves in detail if you suspect acoustic neuroma, cholesteatoma or a neurological cause.
- **Carotids.** Auscultation may suggest carotid stenosis, which can cause tinnitus.

Chest
- **Heart.** Listen to the heart for a venous hum or any bruits.

Key references and further reading
1. Halford JBS, Anderson SD. Tinnitus severity measured by a subjective scale, audiometry and clinical judgement. *J Laryngol Otol* 1991;105:89–93.
2. Luxon LM. Tinnitus: its causes, diagnosis, and treatment. *BMJ* 1993;306:1490–1491.
3. National Institute for Health and Care Excellence (NICE). Tinnitus. Clinical knowledge summaries. 2010. Available from: http://cks.nice.org.uk/tinnitus (last accessed 29 April 2016).
4. Sindhusake D, Golding M, Wigney D et al. Factors predicting severity of tinnitus: a population-based assessment. *J Am Acad Audiol* 2004;15:269–280.

Sinusitis and facial pain

Key thoughts

Practical points
- **Diagnosis.** There are many potential causes of facial pain. Rhinosinusitis often presents with purulent nasal discharge, facial pressure, postnasal drip and mid-facial pain.

Differential diagnosis

- Rhinosinusitis.
- Tension headache.
- Trigeminal neuralgia.
- Referred dental pain.
- Migraine.
- Temporomandibular joint dysfunction.
- Cluster headache.
- Malignancy.
- Atypical facial pain.

RED FLAGS

- Periorbital cellulitis
- Unilateral features (e.g. mass or polyp)
- Reduced consciousness
- Neck stiffness
- Double vision and reduced visual acuity
- Swelling or paraesthesia over any facial bone
- Focal neurological signs
- Nasal bleeding
- Immunosuppression
- Suspected intracranial or intraorbital complication

History

Ideas, concerns and expectations
- **Ideas.** What does the patient think is causing the symptoms?
- **Concerns.** Worries about chronicity or underlying cancer are common.
- **Expectations.** A common reason for consultation is a request for antibiotics (which may or may not be indicated) and symptom relief. Some patients will only expect explanation and reassurance after a thorough examination.

The 10-Minute Clinical Assessment, Second Edition. Knut Schroeder.
© 2017 John Wiley & Sons, Ltd. Published 2017 by John Wiley & Sons, Ltd.

History of presenting complaint
- **Quality of life.** How have the quality of life and day-to-day activities been affected? Facial pain can be distressing and disabling.
- **Onset and duration.** Rhinosinusitis often starts after a cold or some other upper respiratory tract infection. Acute rhinosinusitis may last for 3 months, with full recovery, whereas in chronic rhinosinusitis, symptoms persist for more than 3 months, without full recovery. Bacterial infection is more likely if acute rhinosinusitis lasts for more than 7 days and if there is a history of initial improvement followed by deterioration of symptoms.
- **Nasal blockage.** A history of nasal blockage is common in rhinosinusitis.
- **Nasal discharge.** Purulent green or yellow discharge makes bacterial infection more likely and is a good predictor of rhinosinusitis.
- **Facial pain.** Bacterial infection is more likely if there is unilateral or asymmetrical facial pain and tenderness. Headache is common (and is often worse on bending forward) in rhinosinusitis, particularly over the sinus areas. The site of the pain may give clues about other underlying causes.
- **Facial swelling.** Consider osteomyelitis of the frontal sinus or a tumour with breach of bone boundaries if there is a swelling or mass over any of the facial bones.
- **Systemic symptoms.** Fever and malaise make bacterial infection more likely.
- **Atopy.** Hay fever and other allergies may play some role in the development of rhinosinusitis.
- **Eye symptoms.** Consider periorbital cellulitis (rare) if there is eye swelling and oedema, fever, pain, chemosis and erythema around the eye. An orbital abscess (also rare) may be present if there is additional proptosis in association with double vision and reduced visual acuity. Rarely, tumour invasion of the orbit shows similar features.
- **Neurological symptoms.** Reduced consciousness, headache, visual problems, seizures, ataxia and other focal neurological symptoms and signs suggest rare cerebral abscess.
- **Toothache.** Ask about previous tooth problems, which may cause symptoms that resemble rhinosinusitis.

Past and current medical problems
- **ENT problems.** Ask about any previous throat, ear and nose problems. Has the patient had any ENT operations in the past?
- **Diabetes.** Patients with diabetes are at higher risk of infection.
- **Immunosuppression.** HIV infection, cancer, granulomatous disease and congenital immunodeficiency are rare risk factors for the development of rhinosinusitis and may lead to a reduced response to treatment.

Medication
- **Analgesics.** Ask what has been taken and how much. This will give an indication of the severity of the symptoms.
- **Decongestants.** Have any been tried, and have they worked?

- **Steroids.** Intranasal topical steroids may be useful in rhinitis, recurrent acute rhinosinusitis and chronic rhinosinusitis.
- **Antibiotics.** These may have been given if there is suspected bacterial infection. A prolonged course over at least 2 weeks is often needed to allow for reduced drug delivery within the nasal sinuses.

Allergies
- **Antibiotics.** Ask about allergies to any antibiotics that might be needed for the treatment of rhinosinusitis.

Social history
- **Home.** Has home life been affected by the symptoms? Insomnia is common.
- **Work.** Has the patient had to take time off work? Is a sick note needed?

Review of previous investigations
- **Full blood count and plasma viscosity.** These are rarely needed, but may be abnormal in infection.
- **Computerised tomography (CT).** This is rarely necessary, but is the imaging investigation of choice for the investigation of chronic sinusitis.

Illicit drugs
- **Cocaine.** Cocaine may damage the nasal mucosa.

Examination

General
- **General condition.** Suspect bacterial and more severe infection if the patient is unwell.
- **Drowsiness.** Consider meningitis if the patient is drowsy.

Vital signs
- **Temperature.** A fever suggests bacterial infection.
- **Pulse.** Tachycardia can result from fever, pain or use of oral decongestants.
- **Blood pressure.** Oral decongestants may lead to raised blood pressure and must be taken with caution in people with hypertension.

Head and neck
- **Eyes.** Look for signs of periorbital cellulitis or abscess (e.g. oedema, swelling, reduced visual acuity, double vision, ophthalmoplegia or proptosis). Photophobia suggests possible meningitis.
- **Neck stiffness.** Neck pain and stiffness may occur in meningitis.
- **Sinus palpation.** Palpate over all sinuses for tenderness, evidence of osteitis and loss of bone contour. In addition, tap the maxillary teeth with a tongue depressor, as some cases of rhinosinusitis may be caused by dental root infection.

- **Nose.** Look for any obvious obstruction due to septum deviation or polyps. Prolonged use of topical decongestants may lead to rebound rhinitis. Intranasal cocaine use can cause severe damage to the nasal mucosa.

Key references and further reading

1. Ah-See K, Young A. Clinical review: sinusitis and its management. *BMJ* 2007;334:358–361.
2. Lindbaek M, Hjortdahl P. The clinical diagnosis of acute purulent sinusitis in general practice – a review. *Br J Gen Pract* 2002;52:491–495.
3. National Institute for Health and Care Excellence (NICE). Sinusitis. Clinical knowledge summaries. 2013. Available from: http://cks.nice.org.uk/sinusitis (last accessed 29 April 2016).
4. Williams JW, Simel DL. The rational clinical examination: does this patient have sinusitis? *JAMA* 1993;270:1242–1246.

Problems in older people

General health assessment in older people

Key thoughts

Practical points
- **Diagnosis.** Reasons for consultation are often multifactorial, and comprehensive assessment is the key. Obtain views from the patient, carers, family and other members of the multidisciplinary team to get a fuller picture.
- **Prognosis.** Careful functional and medical assessment is essential to improving function, relieving symptoms and improving the quality of life. Establish which problems need active treatment and which require observation or palliation.

Common reasons for initial presentation
- Cognitive impairment.
- Incontinence.
- Reduced mobility.
- Falls.
- Deafness.
- Breathlessness.
- Constipation.
- Diarrhoea.
- Pain.
- Depression and social isolation.
- Weight loss.
- Adverse drug reactions.

RED FLAGS
- Cognitive problems
- Weight loss, malaise, fever, sweats, anorexia
- Sensory deficit
- High number of active medical problems
- Depression
- Recent or frequent health service use
- Falls

The 10-Minute Clinical Assessment, Second Edition. Knut Schroeder.
© 2017 John Wiley & Sons, Ltd. Published 2017 by John Wiley & Sons, Ltd.

History

Ideas, concerns and expectations

- **Ideas.** Find out how the patient and their carers feel about current and future health.
- **Concerns.** Are there any particular health concerns or other worries? Fears about losing independence or developing serious illness are common.
- **Expectations.** What does the patient expect from you and from life in general?

History of presenting complaint

- **History taking.** If communication is difficult when taking a history, find out why. If hearing is a problem, make sure the hearing aid works. Common problems with hearing aids include a flat or absent battery, a tube blocked with wax, the device not being switched on or a hearing aid not being worn at all. If there is cognitive impairment, obtain information from other sources, such as family and carers, or other health professionals.
- **Quality of life.** Allow the patient and their carers to tell you about any problems in their own words. Ask about current quality of life and identify any unmet needs.
- **Unmet needs.** Areas to consider are:
  - Physical and mental health.
  - Medication.
  - Access to services and information about medical conditions.
  - Eyesight, hearing and communication difficulties.
  - Social isolation and caring for others.
  - Poverty and housing.
  - Falls.
  - Self-care.
  - Relationships.
  - Alcohol.
- **Tiredness.** Tiredness is common in older people. Consider mental health problems (e.g. depression) or organic causes (e.g. anaemia, heart failure), especially if accompanied by other relevant symptoms.

Functional assessment

- **Daily activities.** Consider asking about daily activities, such as getting out of bed, washing, toileting, getting dressed, using the stairs, preparing a meal and eating it, walking outside, using the car or public transport, shopping, doing the laundry, watching television and any hobbies and leisure activities.
- **Falls.** Ask about falls. There may be retrograde amnesia, so if the patient says they 'must have tripped', do not necessarily assume that they had a fall for purely mechanical reasons. Episodic unconsciousness can cause falls and may result from cardiovascular causes, such as arrhythmia, vasovagal syncope or postural hypotension. Transient ischaemic attacks (TIAs) usually do not cause episodic

unconsciousness. If the patient is at risk of falls, consider a formal falls assessment (see NICE 2014).
- **Incontinence.** Ask about any lower urinary tract symptoms (urinary tract infection) and problems with constipation (may lead to urinary and overflow incontinence).
- **Social isolation.** Risk factors include living alone, being male and mood or cognitive problems.
- **Nutrition.** Enquire about any change in weight or dietary intake and gastrointestinal symptoms such as anorexia, nausea or vomiting.
- **Independence.** Has managing personal affairs become a problem? Consider health and safety and whether the patient might be at risk or has been subject to harm, abuse or neglect. Establish the level of autonomy and how far the patient is able to make their own choices and decisions. How involved is the patient in family and community life? Are aids to maintain independence available (e.g. helpline alarms, key safes, monetary benefits, sheltered accommodation, carer support or respite care)?

Past and current medical problems
- **Chronic conditions.** Ask about a history of cardiovascular disease (CVD) (e.g. stroke, atrial fibrillation (AF), heart failure), respiratory conditions (e.g. asthma, chronic obstructive pulmonary disease (COPD)), diabetes and neurological conditions (dementia, Parkinson's disease).
- **Predictors for poor outcome.** Memory problems, weight loss, sensory deficit, a high number of active medical problems, depression, recent health service use and falls indicate poorer prognosis.
- **Prognostic factors for disability.** Disability is more likely to become a problem if there is loss of cognitive function, poor self-rated health or visual impairment.

Medication
- **Multiple drugs.** Many problems in older people are associated with drug interactions or adverse drug reactions. Older people are likely to be on multiple drugs and often have impaired resistance to toxicity if there is age- or disease-related deterioration of renal or liver function. Postural hypotension from diuretics will often be more problematic if a patient also has arthritis or cerebral vascular disease.
- **Over-the-counter medicines.** Over-the-counter medicines are commonly used. They may help with symptom relief, but can also cause problems via adverse effects. For example, laxatives may cause diarrhoea, dehydration and electrolyte imbalances, antihistamines may lead to confusion or drowsiness and codeine-containing medications may cause constipation.

Alcohol and smoking
- **Alcohol misuse or dependence.** Alcohol misuse may be hidden in older people who have retired or who have few social contacts. Has the patient always been drinking or did this start later in life? Risk factors include bereavement,

retirement, financial problems, poor sleep, family issues and concerns about the patient's own health. Suspect alcohol misuse if a patient presents with variable moods, malnutrition, memory loss, depression, diarrhoea or recurrent falls or injuries.

- **Smoking.** Current and past smoking increases the risk of lung cancer and CVD, as well as COPD. Record past and current smoking status and calculate the number of pack years (= (number of cigarettes smoked per day × number of years smoked)/20).

Review of previous investigations

- **Full blood count and plasma viscosity.** Look for evidence of anaemia. A raised mean corpuscular volume (MCV) may point towards alcohol problems, hypothyroidism or vitamin B12/folate deficiency. A raised plasma viscosity suggests infection, inflammation or malignancy.
- **Blood glucose.** Diabetes is common and may be undiagnosed or poorly controlled.
- **Urea, electrolytes and liver function tests.** Renal function may be impaired in older people, and abnormal tests may make some drugs unsuitable for prescription.
- **Thyroid-stimulating hormone (TSH).** Hypothyroidism is often underdiagnosed and can produce often subtle symptoms such as tiredness and depression.

Examination

General assessment

- **Nutritional status.** Malnourishment may result from reduced intake or from an underlying medical condition. Look for loss of subcutaneous fat (triceps, chest), muscle wasting (quadriceps, deltoid), oedema (ankle or sacral) and ascites.
- **Delirium.** If history-taking has been difficult, look for evidence of delirium (e.g. the patient sitting quietly, looking bewildered or picking at their clothes).

Signs of abuse

- **Physical abuse.** Consider the possibility of physical abuse if there are unexplained injuries. Important signs to look for are cuts, burns, bruises, fractures, lacerations, poorly managed wounds, poor skin and hygiene, dehydration, poor nutritional status, low weight and broken glasses.
- **Psychological abuse.** Suspect psychological abuse if there is hesitation to talk openly in front of a carer or about a carer, if there is anger without obvious cause in a carer, if the carer or patient tells implausible stories, if there is unexplained fearfulness or if there is unusual behaviour such as biting, rocking or sucking.
- **Financial abuse.** Consider financial abuse if there are unexplained withdrawals from bank accounts, changes of will or unpaid bills.

- **Sexual abuse.** Suspect sexual abuse if there are bruises around breasts or genital areas, genital infections, stained or torn underwear or a reluctance to be washed around genital areas.
- **Neglect.** Look out for signs of neglect, such as poor personal hygiene, poor skin condition, lack of help with eating or drinking and the presence of safety hazards.

Vital signs
- **Temperature.** Check for fever (infection) and hypothermia (e.g. inadequate heating or clothing).
- **Pulse.** AF is common and often underdiagnosed.
- **Blood pressure.** Check lying and standing blood pressure (postural hypotension). Arterial hypertension is common.

Head and neck
- **Carotids.** Auscultate the carotids to check for carotid bruits. Although this is not a particularly sensitive or specific sign, it may prompt further investigations to exclude carotid stenosis.

Chest
- **Heart.** Check for murmurs suggesting valvular lesions. AF can more accurately be diagnosed by cardiac auscultation than by palpation of the radial pulse.
- **Lungs.** Check for basal crackles (indicating heart failure).

Abdomen
- **Palpation.** Feel the abdomen for any masses or signs of organomegaly. Is there clinical evidence of an abdominal aortic aneurysm?
- **Rectal examination.** Constipation may cause urinary incontinence and can lead to agitation. Also check for rectal masses (rectal carcinoma) and assess the prostate gland in men for enlargement and nodularity.

Musculoskeletal
- **Vertebral fracture.** Look for any evidence of vertebral fracture. Important signs are height loss, vertebral tenderness, kyphosis, decreased lumbar lordosis, protuberant abdomen, reduced lung function and reduced weight.
- **Gait.** Observe the patient getting up from a chair, walking through the room, turning and sitting down again. If indicated, you may also observe them walking up and down a staircase.
- **Cerebellar signs and balance.** Ask the patient to stand with their eyes closed (while being ready to support them in case there is imbalance) to check for cerebellar problems and ataxia.

Bedside tests
- **Urine.** Inspect and smell the urine and perform a dipstick test for protein, glucose, blood, leucocytes and ketones.

Key references and further reading
1. Detsky AS, Smalley PS, Chang J. Is this patient malnourished? *JAMA* 1994;271: 54–58.
2. Drennan V, Walters K, Lenihan P et al. for the SPICE Research Group. Priorities in identifying unmet need in older people attending general practice: a nominal group technique study. *Fam Pract* 2007;24:454–460.
3. Iliffe S, Kharicha K, Harari D et al. Health risk appraisal in older people 2: the implications for clinicians and commissioners of social isolation risk in older people. *Br J Gen Pract* 2007;57:277–282.
4. National Institute for Health and Care Excellence (NICE). Falls – risk assessment. Clinical knowledge summaries. 2014. Available from: http://cks.nice.org.uk/falls-risk-assessment (last accessed 29 April 2016).
5. Papaioannou A, Watts NB, Kendler DL et al. Diagnosis and management of vertebral fractures in elderly adults. *Am J Med* 2002;113:220–228.
6. Tas Ü, Verhagen AP, Bierma-Zeinstra SMA et al. Prognostic factors of disability in older people: a systematic review. *Br J Gen Pract* 2007;57:319–323.

Cognitive problems and dementia

Key thoughts

Practical points
- **Diagnosis.** Cognitive problems are common in the elderly and may have remediable causes. It is important to assess function and the impact of memory loss on day-to-day life.

Possible causes
- Depression.
- Delirium.
- Alzheimer's disease.
- Multi-infarct dementia.
- Lewy body dementia.

Important risk factors
- CVD.
- Diabetes mellitus.
- Family history of dementia.

RED FLAGS

- Falls
- Head injury
- Bereavement
- History of cancer
- Rapidly progressing symptoms
- Severe disability and risk to independence
- Confusional state
- Systemic symptoms, such as fever, night sweats or weight loss

History

Ideas, concerns and expectations
- **Ideas.** What does the patient or their carer believe is the cause of the memory loss? Enquire carefully and tactfully, particularly if there is little insight.
- **Concerns.** Memory loss can be very distressing and disabling. Fears about loss of independence and confidence and the need for further social or community input are common.

The 10-Minute Clinical Assessment, Second Edition. Knut Schroeder.
© 2017 John Wiley & Sons, Ltd. Published 2017 by John Wiley & Sons, Ltd.

- **Expectations.** Explore expectations with regard to prognosis, further investigation and management.

History of presenting complaint
- **Context.** Allow the patient and their carer time to give you an account of developments over the past 12 months.
- **Onset.** Acute onset of cognitive problems may indicate possible delirium due to medical illness (e.g. infection). If symptoms are chronic, consider possible dementia, depression or malignancy. Stepwise deterioration may result from multi-infarct dementia.
- **Description of cognitive problems.** Find out exactly what the current problems are and how they affect day-to-day life (e.g. loss of short-term memory, concentration, issues around personal safety, wandering). Ask about behavioural problems, such as agitation, shouting, aggression and sexual inhibition, which can cause considerable problems for carers.
- **Hallucinations.** These are common in delirium and prolonged alcohol misuse.
- **Movement.** Does the patient have problems with walking or tremor (suggesting Parkinson's disease or Parkinsonism)?

Effects of memory loss on daily life
- **Relevant factors.** Check for factors that might affect performance, including educational level and general skills.
- **Prior functioning.** Establish the prior level of functioning and attainment, language and sensory impairment, as well as main occupation.
- **Daily function.** Ask about eating, sleeping, shopping, washing, transport, social life, ability to handle finances and ability to use the telephone.
- **Driving.** Find out whether the patient still drives and whether there have been any accidents or near misses.
- **Comorbidity.** Check for a history of psychiatric illness and other physical or neurological problems.
- **Global assessment.** Enquire about attention and concentration, orientation, memory, praxis, language and problem-solving.
- **Other needs.** Enquire about unmet needs around sex, spirituality, religion and personal care.

Features of underlying disease
- **Symptoms of acute illness.** Check for symptoms of infection (e.g. chest, urinary tract or gastrointestinal symptoms). Chest pain and shortness of breath may be caused by cardiac ischaemia.
- **Depression.** Depression in the elderly may present as memory loss. Ask about other symptoms of depression, such as tearfulness, irritability, appetite, sleep and diurnal variation of symptoms. Assess risk of suicide.
- **Alcohol history.** Ask about past and current levels of alcohol intake. Has there been a recent change in drinking pattern? Prolonged excessive alcohol consumption can affect cognitive function.

- **Symptoms of thyroid disease.** Ask about cold intolerance, tiredness and loss of energy.

Past and current medical problems
- **Chronic conditions.** CVD, neurological disorders such as Parkinson's, multiple sclerosis, epilepsy and endocrine conditions such as diabetes or hypothyroidism may all be associated with memory loss.

Medication
- **Polypharmacy.** Is the patient taking multiple drugs? Are there any difficulties with taking medication? Ask about adverse effects, swallowing problems and what the patient does to remember to take drugs. Are any compliance aids being used?
- **Psychotropic drugs.** Antidepressants, sedatives and other psychotropic medications may all cause memory problems.
- **Over-the-counter medication.** Ask about any over-the-counter or herbal preparations that might interact with regular medication.
- **Contraindications to cholinesterase inhibitors.** These are used for the treatment of Alzheimer's disease. Check for contraindications to their use, such as vascular problems, prostatic symptoms and active peptic ulceration.

Social history
- **Home.** Does the patient live alone? Do family members and neighbours visit? Are there any dangers to the patient due to memory loss? Do support services need to be involved?
- **Carers.** How do the carers cope? Their health is important, and early detection of depression can prevent family breakdowns. Memory loss can negatively affect relationships.

Review of previous investigations
- **Full blood count.** Look for anaemia and signs of infection. A raised MCV may suggest excess alcohol, vitamin B12 or folate deficiency or hypothyroidism.
- **Inflammatory markers.** Raised plasma viscosity may indicate infection or malignancy.
- **Biochemistry.** Low sodium and high calcium can cause cognitive impairment. Check results of renal and liver function, bone profile (hyperparathyroidism, bone metastases), lipids and serum glucose.
- **Thyroid function.** Hypothyroidism can cause memory problems.
- **Serum B12 and folate.** Vitamin B12 and folate deficiency may cause neurological problems.
- **Chest X-ray.** Look for evidence of infection or malignancy.
- **Electrocardiogram (ECG).** Check for atrial fibrillation (AF) or signs of cardiac disease.
- **Computerised tomography (CT) head.** Is there any evidence of cerebral atrophy not explained by age, small or large vessel disease or brain tumour?

- **Urine dipstick and midstream specimen of urine (MSU).** Check for infection, which may be incidental.

Examination

General
- **General appearance.** Does the patient look unwell? Self-neglect suggests difficulty coping at home.
- **Cachexia.** Causes of cachexia may include difficulty preparing or eating food, diabetes, malignancy and malnourishment.

Vital signs
- **Temperature.** Check for infection if there is fever.
- **Pulse.** Check for an irregularly irregular pulse (AF), which can lead to embolic brain infarcts.
- **Blood pressure.** Check for postural hypotension and hypertension.
- **Respiratory rate.** Tachypnoea indicates possible respiratory infection, malignancy, anaemia or heart failure.

Cognitive function
- **Year.** Ask what year it is. Score 4 if incorrect.
- **Month.** Ask what month it is. Score 3 if incorrect.
- **Address phrase.** Give the patient a fictitious address phrase with five components to remember (e.g. John Smith, 42 High Street, Bedford).
- **Time.** Ask what time it is (to within 1 hour). Score 3 if incorrect.
- **Count backwards.** Ask the patient to count backwards from 20 to 1. Score 2 if there is one error, score 4 if there is more than one.
- **Reverse months.** Ask the patient to name the months of the year in reverse. Score 2 if there is one error, score 4 if there is more than one.
- **Repeat address.** Ask the patient to repeat the address phrase. Count the number of errors and score 2 for each, up to a maximum of 10.
- **Scoring.** Any score over 7 suggests dementia.

Head and neck
- **Fundoscopy.** Papilloedema indicates raised intracranial pressure.

Chest
- **Carotids.** Carotid bruits are neither a specific nor a sensitive sign but may give clues about underlying vascular disease.
- **Heart.** Check for aortic stenosis. Check the heart rate by auscultation, as this may be different from the radial pulse (especially in AF).
- **Lungs.** Check for signs of infection and heart failure.

Abdomen
- **Ascites.** The presence of intra-abdominal fluid may suggest liver failure, heart failure, malignancy or malabsorption.
- **Palpation.** Check for tenderness and masses (e.g. possible malignancy).

Bedside tests
- **Urine dipstick.** Test for glucose, ketones, nitrites, leucocytes and protein. Is there evidence of urinary infection?
- **Glucostix.** Check for hyper- or hypoglycaemia.

Key references and further reading

1. Alzheimer's Society. www.alzheimers.org.uk.
2. Brooke P, Bullock R. Validation of the 6 item cognitive impairment test. *Int J Geriatr Psychiatry* 1999;14:936–940.
3. De Lepeleire J, Heyrman J, Baro F, Buntinx F. A combination of tests for the diagnosis of dementia had a significant diagnostic value. *J Clin Epidemiol* 2005;58:217–225.
4. Holsinger T, Deveau J, Boustani M, Williams JW Jr. The rational clinical examination: does this patient have dementia? *JAMA* 2007;297:2391–2404.
5. Katzman R, Brown T, Fuld P et al. Validation of a short orientation-memory-concentration test of cognitive impairment. *Am J Psychiatry* 1983;140(6):734–739.
6. National Institute for Health and Care Excellence (NICE). Dementia: supporting people with dementia and their carers in health and social care. NICE guidelines [CG42]. November 2006. Available from: http://www.nice.org.uk/guidance/cg42 (last accessed 29 April 2016).
7. National Institute for Health and Care Excellence (NICE). Dementia. Clinical knowledge summaries. 2015. Available from: http://cks.nice.org.uk/dementia (last accessed 29 April 2016).

Falls in older people

Key thoughts

Practical points

- **Diagnosis.** Falls are common in older people and are a cause of significant morbidity and mortality.
- **Prognosis.** Identification of risk factors and falls prevention can save lives, as over 50% of people who fall will fall again.

Potential causes

- **Cardiovascular.** Arrhythmia, postural hypotension, ischaemic heart disease, vertebrobasilar insufficiency, micturition syncope, carotid sinus hypersensitivity.
- **Sensory problems.** Loss of vision, hearing loss.
- **Neurological.** Stroke/TIA, dementia, peripheral neuropathy (e.g. diabetes), Parkinson's disease and Parkinsonism, epilepsy, labyrinthitis.
- **Environmental.** Thick carpets with risk of tripping, steep stairs, lack of hand rails, slippery floors, poor lighting, difficult access to toilet, bath tub instead of shower, cluttered rooms, inadequate footwear.
- **Drugs.** Sedative/psychotropic drugs, diuretics, antihypertensives (especially alpha blockers), over-the-counter medication.
- **Toxic.** Alcohol excess.
- **Musculoskeletal.** Osteoarthritis, foot problems.
- **Infection.** Urinary tract infection (urgency and frequency of urine).

RED FLAGS

- Recurrent falls
- Difficulty coping at home
- Poor mobility
- Bone pain (especially hip, wrist and spine)
- Head injury
- Confusion
- Loss of consciousness
- Risk factors for osteoporosis and fractures (e.g. smoking, early menopause, height loss/kyphosis, low body mass index (BMI), long-term steroid use, family history of hip fracture)

The 10-Minute Clinical Assessment, Second Edition. Knut Schroeder.
© 2017 John Wiley & Sons, Ltd. Published 2017 by John Wiley & Sons, Ltd.

History

Ideas, concerns and expectations
- **Ideas.** The patient may not remember the fall or may not want to mention it for fear of having to move into alternative accommodation. What does the patient or their carer think has caused the fall?
- **Concerns.** How do the patient and/or their carer feel about the fall? Falls can be extremely frightening and often reduce confidence. Anxiety about falling increases the risk of further falls.
- **Expectations.** What are the expectations with regard to future mobility?

History of presenting complaint
- **Quality of life.** How has the quality of life been affected? Are there any limitations to daily activities as a result of the fall(s)?
- **Circumstances around the fall.** Try to get the full story about the fall and ask the patient to describe in detail what happened. Where did the fall take place? What was the patient doing at the time (sitting, rising from a chair, walking, running)? Why did the patient fall? Was there loss of consciousness? Was there preceding dizziness on getting up? Ask about vision, neck problems and general mobility. Are there preventable risk factors, such as environmental causes? Ask for details of fall initiation, descent and impact. Was the patient able to get up again unaided? Are there any injuries? Were there any witnesses?
- **Previous falls.** If falls are recurrent or unexplained, specialist referral for further assessment might be indicated (e.g. falls service, if available). Find out whether the circumstances of the current fall were different from those of previous falls.
- **Loss of consciousness.** Has there been loss of consciousness? If so, how long did it last? Is there amnesia? If there was loss of consciousness or amnesia (e.g. due to epilepsy), 24-hour ECG and brain imaging will usually be indicated.
- **Balance problems.** Balance problems due to postural hypotension, stroke, diuretics or labyrinthitis make future falls more likely.
- **Associated symptoms.** Shortness of breath or chest pain may indicate cardiovascular or respiratory problems. Incontinence or urinary symptoms suggest urinary infection. People may fall because they have to rush to the toilet. Was there any dizziness or blurred vision? Are there any symptoms of acute infection? Is there any pain or stiffness due to joint problems?
- **Eye problems.** Ask about recent eye checks and visual problems. Simple tripping over unnoticed objects is an important cause to consider.
- **Previous mobility and function.** Is input from other services needed, such as physiotherapy or occupational therapy? Are mobility aids being used? Is a pendant alarm available? Are rooms cluttered?
- **Mental health.** Ask about symptoms of depression (feeling down, depressed or hopeless, taking little interest or pleasure in doing things) and sleep problems.
- **Abuse.** If the story is inconsistent or does not make sense, consider the possibility of abuse.

- **Other problems.** Ask the patient and their carer if there are any other issues that you have not covered but which might be important.

Past and current medical problems
- **Conditions increasing the risk of falling.** Conditions that can cause or contribute to the risk of falls include cardiovascular (arrhythmia, postural hypotension), neurological (stroke, epilepsy, Parkinson's disease, dementia, peripheral neuropathy) and endocrine (diabetes, hypothyroidism) problems. Ask specifically about any history of arthritis and joint problems.

Medication
- **Prescribed medication.** Psychotropic medication, antihypertensives and diuretics may cause falls, especially in older people. In case of polypharmacy, reducing the number of drugs can prevent falls. Are there any drug side effects, such as change in bladder or bowel function, dizziness or drowsiness? Antihypertensives may cause postural hypotension.
- **Over-the-counter medication.** Ask about any additional drugs and herbal medicines that have been bought over the counter, as some may interact with prescribed medicines or increase the risk of falling in their own right.

Social history
- **Home situation.** Is the patient living alone? Are there any carers? Is the home suitable in terms of number of levels, access to toilets and transport? What is normal mobility like? Are there any problems with lighting or floors? Are there difficulties in accessing the kitchen and bathroom? Are there problems with climbing stairs? Have any adaptations been made to the home already? Are clothes appropriate and fitting well? Are any services already involved?

Alcohol
- **Alcohol.** Alcohol misuse is common in the elderly and increases the risk of falls.

Review of previous investigations
- **Full blood count.** Look for signs of anaemia, infection or systemic disease. A raised MCV may indicate vitamin B12 or folate deficiency, hypothyroidism or alcohol misuse.
- **Inflammatory markers.** Raised plasma viscosity may suggest infection, inflammation or malignancy.
- **Urea and elctrolytes.** Check that the renal function is normal. Urea may be raised in dehydration.
- **Liver function tests and gamma-glutamyl transpeptidase (GGT).** Albumin may be low if nutrition is poor or in malignant disease. GGT is often raised in alcohol misuse, but this is neither specific nor sensitive.
- **Glucose and haemoglobin A1c (HbA1c).** Is there a history of diabetes? If so, how well is this controlled?
- **Thyroid function.** Is there evidence of hypothyroidism?

- **Vitamin B12 and folate.** Deficiencies may be due to poor diet or malabsorption and may cause neurological problems.
- **ECG.** Is there evidence of an arrhythmia (e.g. AF or heart block)?
- **Chest X-ray.** Are there signs of infection, cardiomegaly or malignancy?
- **Carotid dopplers.** These can be helpful in identifying carotid artery stenosis if symptoms suggest TIA.
- **CT or magnetic resonance imaging (MRI) head.** These are useful for the investigation of a suspected intracranial cause.

Examination

General
- **General appearance.** Does the patient look unwell? Look for evidence of self-neglect, which suggests difficulty coping at home.
- **Environment.** Check footwear, clothing and walking aids for suitability.
- **Obvious injuries.** Look in particular for injuries of the head, neck, wrists and hips. Signs of old bruising suggest previous falls. Are injuries consistent with the mechanism of the fall? If not, consider the possibility of abuse.
- **Nutrition and hydration.** Is the patient dehydrated or malnourished? There may be difficulties with food preparation or eating. Think of other underlying causes, such as malignancy and dementia.
- **General mobility.** Check whether the patient is able to get up unaided from a lying and a sitting position. Assess walking on the flat and up stairs, if appropriate. Ask whether there are any problems turning in bed.
- **Parkinson's disease.** Are there any obvious features of Parkinson's disease?

Vital signs
- **Temperature.** The temperature may or may not be raised in infection. Hypothermia may indicate inadequate clothing or heating.
- **Pulse.** Look for an irregular pulse (suggesting atrial fibrillation). Tachycardia may be caused by infection or fluid depletion. Heart block may cause a slow heart rate.
- **Blood pressure.** Check blood pressure lying and standing for postural hypotension (e.g. adverse effects from antihypertensive or psychotropic medication, volume depletion, autonomic dysfunction, cardiovascular compromise or venous pooling). Is there hypertension?
- **Respiratory rate.** Tachypnoea may suggest chest infection, heart disease, anaemia or chronic pulmonary disease.

Skin
- **Bruising.** Look in detail for any bruising and assess underlying structures for any damage.

Head and neck
- **Conjunctiva and sclerae.** If these are pale, it may suggest anaemia. Look for jaundice.

- **Mucus membranes.** Look for anaemia and cyanosis.
- **Eyes and vision.** Check current vision with and without glasses and compare with the results of any previous eye tests. Look for cataract and diabetic retinopathy. Check visual fields.
- **Hearing.** Impacted ear wax can lead to hearing and balance problems.
- **Muscle weakness.** Look for any facial weakness, indicating the possibility of a stroke.
- **Spinal movement.** Are there any problems with neck movements that would suggest cervical spondylosis?

Upper limbs
- **Range of movement.** Is movement in any way restricted?
- **Muscle strength and bulk.** Are the upper limbs strong enough to support the patient when getting up after a fall?

Chest
- **Heart.** Cardiac murmurs may suggest valvular disease or a flow murmur in anaemia. Auscultate the heart rate and rhythm to identify AF, which may go undetected on palpation of the radial pulse alone.
- **Lungs.** Check for signs of infection and heart failure.

Lower limbs
- **Deformities.** Look for any deformities at the knee or hip, such as turning out of the foot. Consider hip fracture if there is hip pain with an externally rotated and shortened leg.
- **Feet.** Look for any calluses, deformities, ulcers or bunions.
- **Power.** Test the power of hip and foot flexors.
- **Sensation.** Assess sensation in the feet, particularly in patients with diabetes. Diabetic neuropathy may impair sensation and balance.
- **Range of movement.** Check the hips and knees in particular for any obvious problems.
- **Timed 'up and go' screening test.** Ask the patient to get up from the chair and walk across the room over a distance of about 3 metres, turn, walk back to the chair and sit down again (normal time is between 7 and 10 seconds). A patient taking more than 20 seconds or who is unable to complete the test is at increased risk of falling. Look for subtle signs of hemiparesis or Parkinson's disease.
- **Romberg's test.** A brief, modified Romberg's test can predict future falls better than complicated tests. Ask the patient to stand on the right and left foot with the eyes open and closed (making sure to stand very close to the patient to catch them before they fall). Record the time until balance is lost (maximum 30 seconds). Less than 5 seconds is abnormal. Allow three trials per test.
- **Footwear.** Inspect shoes and look for even wear. Flat shoes are usually safer.

Cognitive function
- **Year.** Ask what year it is. Score 4 if incorrect.
- **Month.** Ask what month it is. Score 3 if incorrect.
- **Address phrase.** Give the patient a fictitious address phrase with five components to remember (e.g. John Smith, 42 High Street, Bedford).
- **Time.** Ask what time it is (to within 1 hour). Score 3 if incorrect.
- **Count backwards.** Ask the patient to count backwards from 20 to 1. Score 2 if there is one error, score 4 if there is more than one.
- **Reverse months.** Ask the patient to name the months of the year in reverse. Score 2 if there is one error, score 4 if there is more than one.
- **Repeat address.** Ask the patient to repeat the address phrase. Count the number of errors and score 2 for each, up to a maximum of 10.
- **Scoring.** Any score over 7 suggests dementia or delirium requiring further assessment.

Bedside tests
- **BM stick.** Check for hypo- and hyperglycaemia.
- **Urine dipstick.** Proteinuria, haematuria, leucocytes and nitrites suggest urinary tract infection.

Key references and further reading
1. American Geriatrics Society, British Geriatrics Society and American Academy of Orthopaedic Surgeons Panel on Falls Prevention. Guideline for the prevention of falls in older persons. *J Am Geriatr Soc* 2001;49:664–672.
2. Fuller G. Falls in the elderly. *Am Fam Physician* 2000;61:2159–2168, 2173–2174.
3. Ganz DA, Bao Y, Shekelle PG, Rubenstein LZ. Will my patient fall? *JAMA* 2007;297:77–86.
4. Gerdham P, Ringsberg KAM, Akesson K, Obrant K. Clinical history and biologic age predicted falls better than objective functional tests. *J Clin Epidemiol* 2005;58:226–232.
5. Kannus P, Sievänen H, Palvanen M et al. Prevention of falls and consequent injuries in elderly people. *Lancet* 2005;366:1885–1893.
6. Katzman R, Brown T, Fuld P et al. Validation of a short orientation-memory-concentration test of cognitive impairment. *Am J Psychiatry* 1983;140(6):734–739.
7. National Institute for Health and Care Excellence (NICE). Falls in older people: assessing risk and prevention. NICE guidelines [CG161]. June 2013. Available from: http://www.nice.org.uk/guidance/cg161 (last accessed 29 April 2016).
8. National Institute for Health and Care Excellence (NICE). Falls – risk assessment. Clinical knowledge summaries. 2014. Available from: http://cks.nice.org.uk/falls-risk-assessment (last accessed 29 April 2016).
9. Podsiadlo D, Richardson S. The timed up and go: a test of basic functional mobility for frail elderly people. *J Am Geriatr Soc* 1991;9:142–148.

Delirium and acute confusional state

Key thoughts

Practical points

- **Diagnosis.** The diagnosis largely rests on clinical skills, as useful tests do not exist. Identifying an underlying cause can be challenging.
- **Prognosis.** Early detection of delirium is important because potentially treatable serious causes such as metabolic disturbances or subdural haematoma may easily go unnoticed.

Possible causes

- Infection (e.g. pneumonia, urinary tract infection).
- Alzheimer's disease.
- Subdural haematoma.
- Metabolic (e.g. diabetic emergencies).
- Hypothermia.
- TIA and stroke (e.g. dysphasia presentation).
- Transient global amnesia.

RED FLAGS

- Sodium <128 mmol/l or >145 mmol/l
- Raised calcium
- Severe headache
- Sudden onset of symptoms such as dysphasia
- Rapid deterioration
- Poor clinical state
- Fever or hypothermia
- Seizure
- Features of raised intracranial pressure
- Introduction of new medication (e.g. overdose, adverse effects)
- Alcohol misuse
- Recent surgery

History

Ideas, concerns and expectations

- **Ideas.** Find out what the patient and their carer think might be wrong. Understanding the patient's perspective will help guide clinical management. Visual

The 10-Minute Clinical Assessment, Second Edition. Knut Schroeder.
© 2017 John Wiley & Sons, Ltd. Published 2017 by John Wiley & Sons, Ltd.

hallucinations are common and patients often try to make sense of them by developing false beliefs or delusions.
- **Concerns.** Delirium can be extremely frightening and may cause agitation.
- **Expectations.** What is the main reason for consultation? Do the patient and their carer expect additional support at home?

History of presenting complaint
- **Quality of life.** Ask for details about how the patient is coping and how daily activities have been affected. Delirium can be very distressing for both patient and carers.
- **Onset.** Acute onset of confusion may occur in relation to drug withdrawal or drug excess or with a vascular event. Acute-on-chronic confusion indicates delirium superimposed on dementia or another pre-existing mental disorder. A more gradual deterioration may suggest dementing illnesses, such as Alzheimer's disease.
- **Precipitating factors.** Check whether there is a history suggestive of alcoholism or depression. Could symptoms be due to overdose?
- **Changes in mental state.** 'Delirium' describes a state of organic and fluctuating mental confusion. Ask family and carers about what changes they have noticed and how they have affected the patient. Delirium can easily be missed if patients are generally withdrawn. It is common in physically old people, particularly in those with pre-existing dementia, and causes are often multifactorial.
- **Progression.** If confusion is fluctuating, consider subdural haematoma or dementia with Lewy bodies, which may present with fluctuating confusion, hallucinations and extrapyramidal signs.
- **Cognitive function.** Are there problems with memory and attention?
- **Sleep.** Disturbance of the sleep–wake cycle can cause confusion. Are there any disturbing dreams or nightmares that keep the patient awake at night or cause undue anxieties? Also ask about daytime sleepiness.
- **Additional unexplored issues.** Ask the patient and their carer whether there are any other problems or issues that you have not covered which might be important.

Common symptom patterns
- **Sensory deprivation.** Hearing and visual impairment, as well as deterioration in sensory function, can cause confusion.
- **Hypo- or hyperthermia.** Temperature regulation may be impaired in the elderly. Ask about problems with heating or recent exposure to cold or heat.
- **Acute illness.** Check for symptoms of urinary or respiratory infection or dehydration. Is a catheter in place?
- **Metabolic causes.** Could symptoms be caused by dehydration, liver failure, electrolyte disturbances, hypoglycaemia, thyrotoxicosis or hypothyroidism?
- **Nutrition.** Vitamin deficiencies may be present if the diet is poor.
- **Mental health.** Ask about symptoms of depression, psychosis, anxiety, fear, irritability, euphoria and apathy. Any of these may fluctuate during the day. Are

there any empty bottles or a note indicating that the patient has taken excessive amounts of sedatives or psychotropic medication?

Past and current medical problems
- **Poor physical state.** General physical frailty is a risk factor.
- **Central nervous system (CNS) lesions.** Is there a history of CNS trauma, space-occupying lesions, epilepsy, neurodegenerative disorders or cerebral ischaemia?
- **Hospital admissions or operations.** Confusion is relatively common after emergency surgery, such as orthopaedic or abdominal operations.
- **Dementia.** A history of dementia predisposes to acute confusion.
- **Multimorbidity.** Diabetes and CVD are common and may contribute to the development of confusion.

Medication
- **Drug toxicity.** Polypharmacy in the elderly is common and may lead to confusion. Look out for psychotropic drugs and those with anticholinergic effects or resulting in hyponatraemia. Opiates may cause drowsiness and confusion. Consider other drugs, such as sedatives, antihistamines, antiarrhythmics (e.g. digoxin), oxybutynin and bronchodilators (e.g. theophylline).
- **Over-the-counter medication.** Ask whether any over-the-counter or herbal medicines are taken in addition to prescribed drugs, as these may be toxic or might interact with regular medication.
- **Withdrawal syndromes.** Consider withdrawal from alcohol, benzodiazepines, selective serotonin reuptake inhibitors (SSRIs) or opiates.

Social history
- **Home.** Hospital admission will be required in many cases. As a basis for planning future care, check details about the home situation. Is the patient generally coping? Is additional care or a more permanent care package needed in the future?
- **Relationships.** Ask about family and friends. Are there any relationship problems that might need to be addressed?
- **Carers.** Are family or professional carers involved in the care of the patient? Get their contact details and try to obtain additional information from third parties, if possible. Ask about depression, which is common and underdiagnosed in carers.
- **Finance.** Financial problems are not uncommon and may affect decisions about future care.

Alcohol and drugs
- **Alcohol.** Alcohol misuse is a frequent cause of confusion, both through direct toxic effects and due to complications (e.g. alcoholic liver disease).
- **Smoking.** Consider lung cancer and CVD in patients with a smoking history.

Review of previous investigations
- **Full blood count.** Look for anaemia. A raised white cell count may point to infection. Raised MCV may indicate hypothyroidism, vitamin B12/folate deficiency or alcohol misuse.
- **Inflammatory markers.** Raised plasma viscosity suggests infection or inflammation.
- **Biochemistry.** Look for hyponatraemia, commonly caused by drugs or infection. Hypernatraemia suggests that the patient is probably not drinking enough. Check past results of urea and electrolytes, glucose, liver function tests, thyroid function and calcium in case there is a metabolic disorder.
- **Chest X-ray.** Is there evidence of infection or malignancy?
- **Electrocardiogram.** Look for signs of arrhythmia or ischaemia.
- **Urine culture and sensitivity.** Look for evidence of previous urinary tract infection.
- **CT or MRI head.** Normal scans make an intracranial cause less likely.
- **Drug screen and alcohol levels.** If relevant, check whether these have been done in the past.

Examination

General
- **General state.** Does the patient look unwell? Consider malignancy or another serious condition if there is cachexia. Check for signs of dehydration and malnourishment. Acute physical illness increases the risk of delirium.
- **Behaviour.** Are there any obvious abnormalities in terms of general appearance and behaviour (e.g. picking at bed clothes or reaching out for objects that aren't there)?

Mental state
- **Disorganised thinking.** Is speech disorganised or incoherent (e.g. rambling or irrelevant conversation)? Are ideas illogical? Is there unpredictable switching between topics?
- **Altered level of consciousness.** Describe as alert (normal), vigilant (hyperaroused), lethargic (drowsy, easily aroused), stupor (difficult to rouse) or coma (cannot be roused).

Vital signs
- **Temperature.** Fever suggests infection, but temperature may not always be raised. Hypothermia may be caused by inadequate clothing or heating or a CNS-related problem with temperature regulation.
- **Pulse.** Check for tachycardia and arrhythmias. AF is common and is an important risk factor for stroke.
- **Blood pressure.** Check for hypertension and postural hypotension (fluid depletion).

- **Respiratory rate.** Tachypnoea indicates chest infection, anaemia or heart failure.

Head and neck
- **Ears.** Ensure there is no ear wax that might affect hearing. Reduced hearing may exacerbate an acute confusional state.
- **Cranial nerves.** Check vision and pupil responses. Look out for facial weakness. Check the fundi for papilloedema (raised intracranial pressure).

Cognitive function
- **Year.** Ask what year it is. Score 4 if incorrect.
- **Month.** Ask what month it is. Score 3 if incorrect.
- **Address phrase.** Give the patient a fictitious address phrase with five components to remember (e.g. John Smith, 42 High Street, Bedford).
- **Time.** Ask what time it is (to within 1 hour). Score 3 if incorrect.
- **Count backwards.** Ask the patient to count backwards from 20 to 1. Score 2 if there is one error, score 4 if there is more than one.
- **Reverse months.** Ask the patient to name the months of the year in reverse. Score 2 if there is one error, score 4 if there is more than one.
- **Repeat address.** Ask the patient to repeat the address phrase. Count the number of errors and score 2 for each, up to a maximum of 10.
- **Scoring.** Any score over 7 suggests dementia.

Chest
- **Heart.** Check the heart rhythm, as AF and other arrhythmias may go unnoticed on assessment of the radial pulse alone.
- **Lungs.** Check for crackles (heart failure, respiratory infection).

Abdomen
- **Palpation.** Feel for tenderness and masses (e.g. malignancy). A palpable bladder may indicate urinary retention.
- **Rectal examination.** Check for faecal impaction and rectal carcinoma. An enlarged and nodular prostate may raise suspicions about prostatic carcinoma in men.

Lower limbs
- **Oedema.** Peripheral oedema suggests possible heart failure.

Bedside tests
- **Urinalysis.** Proteinuria, haematuria, leucocytes and nitrites suggest urinary infection.
- **Blood glucose stick.** Check for hypo- and hyperglycaemia.
- **Pulse oximetry.** Is there evidence of hypoxia?

Key references and further reading
1. British Geriatric Society. Guidelines for the prevention, diagnosis and management of delirium in older people in hospital. Clinical guideline 170. January 2006. Available from: http://www.bgs.org.uk/index.php/clinicalguides/170-clinguidedeliriumtreatment (last accessed 29 April 2016).
2. Brooke P, Bullock R. Validation of the 6-item cognitive impairment test. *Int J Geriatr Psychiatry* 1999;14:936–940.
3. Leentjens AFG, van der Mast RC. Delirium in older people: an update. *Curr Opin Psychiatry* 2005;18:325–330.
4. National Institute for Health and Care Excellence (NICE). Delirium. Clinical knowledge summaries. 2015. Available from: http://cks.nice.org.uk/delirium (last accessed 29 April 2016).
5. Royal College of Physicians (RCP). Prevention, diagnosis and management of delirium in older people. Concise guideline to good practice 6. June 2006. Available from: https://www.rcplondon.ac.uk/guidelines-policy/prevention-diagnosis-referral-and-management-delirium-older-people (last accessed 29 April 2016).
6. Young J, Inouye SK. Delirium in older people. *BMJ* 2007;334:842–846.

Depression in older people

Key thoughts

Practical points

- **Diagnosis.** Depression is common in older people and is often missed. Chronic conditions (e.g. heart disease, stroke, diabetes) and life events (e.g. bereavement) often contribute to low mood and may result in additional social and physical problems.

Potential causes

- Bereavement.
- Endogenous depression.
- Hypothyroidism.
- Chronic disease (heart disease, diabetes, stroke, epilepsy, cancer).
- Dementia.
- Parkinson's disease.
- Loneliness.
- Loss of independence.
- Vitamin D deficiency.

RED FLAGS

- Suicidal thoughts
- Serious physical illness
- Feelings of hopelessness
- Low weight (BMI<18)
- Self-neglect

History

Ideas, concerns and expectations

- **Ideas.** What does the patient or their carer believe is causing their low mood? Try to explore the patient's attitude to depression, as mental illness still carries a lot of stigma. Many older people do not see depression as an illness in the same way as a physical condition. They may not be aware that effective treatment options are available.
- **Concerns.** Many patients have seen relatives or friends with depression, and they may be worried about the future. Patients may feel they are 'going mad' and that they will never improve.

The 10-Minute Clinical Assessment, Second Edition. Knut Schroeder.
© 2017 John Wiley & Sons, Ltd. Published 2017 by John Wiley & Sons, Ltd.

- **Expectations.** Some patients with depression and their relatives may hope for a 'quick fix'. They may not be aware that treatment will usually need to be continued for months, and that an effect will not be noticeable straight away.

History of presenting complaint

- **Quality of life.** Allow the patient time to describe their problems or symptoms in their own words. Loneliness, loss (e.g. bereavement, loss of independence), financial problems, poor social stimulation and poor health and mobility can affect the quality of life considerably. Which day-to-day activities are mainly affected? Disability and depression are risk factors for each other.
- **Symptoms of depression.** Ask directly about low mood, as older people often do not complain about this. Lack of energy and extreme tiredness without obvious reason are common. Ask about loss of interest or pleasure in doing things, loss of self-esteem and confidence and feelings of low self-worth, hopelessness and helplessness. Are there feelings of excessive or inappropriate guilt? Are there any problems with memory or concentration? Has appetite changed? Are there any sleep problems?
- **Socialising.** Has the patient started to avoid going out or engaging in social activities?
- **Personal background.** Is there a reason for the patient's being depressed? If there is time, get an overview of the patient's life story and normal mental state. Are they single? Do they have many (or any) friends or family? Try to differentiate between depression and understandable sadness.
- **Symptom fluctuation.** In depression, symptoms are present on most days most of the time.
- **Duration.** For a diagnosis of depression, symptoms should have been present for at least 2 weeks.
- **Somatic symptoms.** Ask about somatic symptoms, such as chest pain, shortness of breath, abdominal pain, a lump in the throat, back ache and indigestion.
- **Sexual function.** Sexual problems such as erectile dysfunction and reduced libido are common in depression and can make the condition worse. Many older people lead an active and fulfilling sex life, and addressing this issue openly can help relieve anxiety.
- **Suicidal thoughts.** Ask whether there are any thoughts of self-harm or if the patient has written a suicide note. Ask for details about any ideas of how to carry out self-harm. How common and intense are any thoughts of self-harm? Obtain details of any previous suicide attempts.

Past and current medical problems

- **Depression.** Ask about any previous episodes of depression, their duration, their effect on life and the response to treatment.
- **Endocrine conditions.** Endocrine diseases such as thyroid disorders, hyper- and hypocalcaemia and diabetes may all cause depression.
- **Neurological conditions.** Consider Parkinson's disease, stroke, brain tumour and dementia.

- **Other conditions.** Conditions that may cause or exacerbate depressive symptoms include occult malignancy, metastatic cancer, chronic heart or lung conditions, polymyalgia rheumatica, folate deficiency and pernicious anaemia.

Personal history

- **Overview of personal situation.** A brief personal history can help put symptoms into context. Consider asking for details about the different stages in life.
- **Childhood.** Ask when and where the patient was born, and whether there were any complications around delivery. What was their family like? What did their parents do for a living? Was the patient well and happy as a child? Was any special schooling needed?
- **Work.** What education did the patient have, and what jobs did they hold?
- **Interests.** Does the patient have any special interests or hobbies, and do they now?
- **Relationships.** Ask about personal relationships, marriage and any children.
- **Retirement.** Ask about the timing of retirement and whether retirement is enjoyable.
- **Difficulties in life.** Are there any things that the patient has found difficult to deal with in life?

Medication

- **Current medication.** Are there any adverse drug effects that might contribute to depression? Examples are codeine, levodopa, amantadine, corticosteroids and beta blockers.
- **Drug taking.** Is the patient able to take medication independently? If not, is a carer able to help? This is important when discussing drug treatment of depression or if there is risk of suicide.

Social history

- **Home.** Who else, if anyone, is at home? Living alone is a risk factor for depression.
- **Family problems.** Ask about any social or family problems that might contribute to depression.
- **Losses or bereavement.** Ask about bereavement, breakdown of relationships, sudden inability to carry out hobbies, loss of income, loss of independence and loss of physical health or sex life.
- **Use of medical or social services.** Depression is a common and often undiagnosed reason for frequent attendance.
- **Carers.** Ask about symptoms of depression in older people who care for others.

Alcohol

- **Excessive alcohol intake.** Alcohol misuse can cause depression and may need to be addressed before other treatments are started.
- **Smoking.** Smoking is a risk factor for lung cancer, COPD and CVD, all of which may contribute to the development of depression.

Review of previous investigations
- **Full blood count.** Acute and chronic infections, as well as anaemia and inflammatory conditions, can all present with depression. A raised MCV may indicate vitamin B12 or folate deficiency, alcohol misuse or hypothyroidism.
- **Inflammatory markers.** Raised plasma viscosity may indicate infection, inflammation or malignancy.
- **Urea, electrolytes, live function tests and GGT.** Look for any significant abnormalities. A raised GGT points towards alcohol misuse.
- **Glucose and HbA1c.** These are useful in assessing glycaemic control in patients with diabetes.
- **Thyroid function test.** Look for evidence of hypothyroidism.

Examination

General
- **General impression.** Check facial expression, posture and mannerisms. Does the patient look depressed? Is there eye contact during conversation, or do they look down most of the time?
- **Hydration.** Is there evidence of dehydration?

Cognitive function
- **Year.** Ask what year it is. Score 4 if incorrect.
- **Month.** Ask what month it is. Score 3 if incorrect.
- **Address phrase.** Give the patient a fictitious address phrase with five components to remember (e.g. John Smith, 42 High Street, Bedford).
- **Time.** Ask what time it is (to within 1 hour). Score 3 if incorrect.
- **Count backwards.** Ask the patient to count backwards from 20 to 1. Score 2 if there is one error, score 4 if there is more than one.
- **Reverse months.** Ask the patient to name the months of the year in reverse. Score 2 if there is one error, score 4 if there is more than one.
- **Repeat address.** Ask the patient to repeat the address phrase. Count the number of errors and score 2 for each, up to a maximum of 10.
- **Scoring.** Any score over 7 suggests dementia.

Skin
- **Inspection.** Inspect the skin for evidence of self-neglect. Are there faeces stains under the finger nails, indicating dementia or self-neglect?

Head and neck
- **Fundoscopy.** Check the fundi for evidence of papilloedema (e.g. raised intracranial pressure due to rare brain tumour).

Abdomen
- **Palpation.** Feel the abdomen for any masses or organomegaly.

Bedside tests

- **Urinalysis.** Check for proteinuria, haematuria, leucocytes and nitrites (urinary tract infection), as well as glucose (diabetes).

Key references and further reading

1. Katzman R, Brown T, Fuld P et al. Validation of a short orientation-memory-concentration test of cognitive impairment. *Am J Psychiatry* 1983;140(6):734–739.
2. National Institute for Health and Care Excellence (NICE). Depression in adults with chronic physical health problem: recognition and management. NICE guidelines [CG91]. October 2009. Available from: http://www.nice.org.uk/guidance/cg91 (last accessed 29 April 2016).
3. National Institute for Health and Care Excellence (NICE). Depression. Clinical knowledge summaries. 2015. Available from: http://cks.nice.org.uk/depression (last accessed 29 April 2016).
4. Sheikh JI, Yesavage JA. Geriatric Depression Scale (GDS): recent evidence and development of a shorter version. *Clin Gerontol* 1986;5:265.
5. van Marwijk HW, Wallace P, de Bock GH et al. Evaluation of the feasibility, reliability and diagnostic value of shortened versions of the geriatric depression scale. *Br J Gen Pract* 1995;45:195–199.
6. Yesavage JA, Brink TL, Rose TL et al. Development and validation of a geriatric depression screening scale: a preliminary report. *J Psychiatr Res* 1983;17:37–49.

Palliative and end-of-life care

Key thoughts

Practical points

- **Diagnosis.** Terminally ill patients often have social issues, complex needs and multiple comorbidities. Assessment should include physical, psychological, social, practical and spiritual needs. Common underlying medical conditions include cancer, heart failure and chronic obstructive airway disease.
- **Patient preferences.** Talking about death and dying can be difficult, but asking patients about their wishes and how they would like to be cared for at an early stage increases the chances that their wishes will be fulfilled. Consider addressing these issues over several consultations.
- **Prognosis.** Patients and carers often ask about the prognosis. In the case of cancer, a rule of thumb is that if patients worsen by the month, then they have months to live; if by the week, then weeks; if day by day, then death is likely to happen fairly soon.

RED FLAGS

- Severe depression
- Severe physical symptoms, such as vomiting, diarrhoea or constipation
- Uncontrolled pain
- Bone pain
- Living alone and social isolation
- Rapid deterioration

History

Ideas, concerns and expectations

- **Ideas.** What does the patient understand about any underlying medical conditions? Many people have little knowledge about modern chemotherapy and radiotherapy, and discussing these can help alleviate fears. People may also be unaware of the types of symptomatic relief that are available.
- **Main concerns.** People at the end of their lives often have a number of concerns. Consider asking the following questions:
  - What is the most important issue for you right now?
  - How do you feel about the future?
  - What is your biggest concern or worry?

The 10-Minute Clinical Assessment, Second Edition. Knut Schroeder.
© 2017 John Wiley & Sons, Ltd. Published 2017 by John Wiley & Sons, Ltd.

o Should you feel worse, how and where would you like to be cared for?
o Is there any unfinished business that you would like to attend to?
o Are there any financial worries?
o Are there problems with sleeping?

- **Expectations.** Are there any particular expectations about future care and the course of the illness? Also explore carers' expectations.

Current problems

- **Constipation.** Is passing stool difficult? Consider terminally ill patients to be constipated until proven otherwise. Check that sufficient amounts of appropriate laxatives are prescribed, particularly if the patient takes high-dose opioids.
- **Mood.** Depression is common and can mimic other conditions. Maintain a high index of suspicion of possible mental health problems.
- **Nausea and vomiting.** Try to identify specific and treatable causes. Nausea may be caused by opioids or chemotherapy, direct pressure from a tumour, gastrooesophageal reflux or anxiety.
- **Pain.** Where is the pain? Is it controlled by analgesia? Try and identify the underlying problem.
- **Tiredness.** Excessive tiredness is common. Look for any obvious treatable underlying cause (e.g. high doses of opioids, sedatives). Has anything been tried to help with tiredness? Hypnotics may help with sleep at night and reduce daytime fatigue. Corticosteroids may also be useful.
- **Secretions.** Ask about oral thrush and increased secretions.
- **Neurological problems.** Are there problems with sphincter or bladder control? Ask about sensory loss or weakness in the lower limbs. Spinal cord compression often presents as back pain with or without radiation.

Past and current medical problems

- **Chronic conditions.** Check for any chronic conditions that need to be managed, in addition to problems associated with terminal care. Discussing treatment options and the management plan is important to optimising drug treatment and avoiding prescription of drugs that are no longer necessary or appropriate.

Medication

- **Symptom relief.** Are relevant drugs available for pain control (e.g. paracetamol, nonsteroidal anti-inflammatory drugs (NSAIDs), opioids), terminal agitation (e.g. benzodiazepines, haloperidol), nausea and vomiting (e.g. antiemetics) or increased secretions (e.g. hyoscine)? Consider supplying these in a box for use by the patient, the community team or the out-of-hours service. Is medication being taken as prescribed? If not, find out why.
- **Allergies.** Ask about allergies to any drugs that might be needed for symptom control.
- **Steroids.** Steroid overuse can cause agitation, thrush, muscle wasting, bed sores, diabetes and cushingoid symptoms.

Prognosis
- **Chronic illness.** The clinical course is different for different chronic and terminal illnesses. In heart failure or respiratory disease, deterioration may occur rapidly.
- **Markers of poor prognosis.** Markers of poor prognosis in heart or respiratory failure are:
  - Breathlessness at rest.
  - Depression.
  - Weight loss.
  - Frequent hospital admissions.
  - Reduced overall activity.
  - **COPD only.** Deteriorating lung function, episodes of confusion, cor pulmonale, reduced arterial oxygen saturation.
  - **Heart failure only.** Tachycardia >100 beats per minute, deteriorating renal function.

Social history
- **Home.** What is the home situation like? Are any services in place to help the patient cope with daily life?
- **Relationships.** Ask about partners, children, friends and relatives. Are there relationship issues that are unresolved and may need addressing?
- **Carer.** Is a carer involved in looking after the patient? If so, what is their relationship? Does the carer have enough support, or are there any unidentified health needs?
- **Agencies involved.** Are any other health professionals involved in the patient's care? Are they communicating effectively? Do they use aids such as home packs, patient-held records, handover forms or medication cards? Is there a nominated coordinator of care?

Review of previous investigations
- **Full blood count and plasma viscosity.** Anaemia is common in chronic disease and malignancy. Blood transfusion may provide symptomatic relief if tiredness from anaemia is a problem. The plasma viscosity may give an indication of disease activity.
- **Urea, electrolytes and liver function tests.** Deteriorating function of major organs may require additional therapy and can affect prognosis.
- **Chest X-ray.** Is there evidence of lung metastasis or infection?
- **Other imaging.** Abdominal ultrasound and CT/MRI scans may reveal intra-abdominal spread of malignancy.

Examination

General inspection
- **Nutritional status.** Look for evidence of malnutrition and dehydration.
- **Respiratory distress.** Cyanosis and difficulty in breathing may indicate a need for oxygen treatment, particularly if there is associated heart failure.

- **Alertness.** Drowsiness might be caused by general deterioration or by high doses of opioids.
- **Depression.** Look for facial expression, slow actions, poor eye contact and tearfulness.

Skin

- **Inspection.** Check for scratch marks (which may suggest itching, for example from eczema or liver disease), excessive sweating, pressure sores in areas of high pressure, fungating wounds and lymphoedema.

Head and neck

- **Anaemia.** Look for pale conjunctivae and mucus membranes.
- **Fundoscopy.** Check for papilloedema in case there is headache, vomiting or a change in behaviour (possibility of raised intracranial pressure).
- **Superior vena cava obstruction.** Search for dilated veins in the neck (may present unilaterally).

Chest

- **Heart.** Listen for any abnormalities (e.g. fourth heart sound in heart failure).
- **Lungs.** Crackles may be heard in infection and heart failure.

Abdomen and back

- **Inspection.** Stained underwear or bedclothes may suggest loss of sphincter or bladder control, increasing the risk of skin ulceration.
- **Palpation.** Palpate the abdomen and search for any masses and organomegaly. Is ascites present?
- **Lower back.** Check for sacral oedema.

Limbs

- **Legs.** Look for oedema and check perfusion. Check for ulcers and fungal infection.

Key references and further reading

1. Murray SA, Boyd K, Sheikh A. Palliative care in chronic illness. *BMJ* 2005; 330:611–612.
2. National Institute for Health and Care Excellence (NICE). End of life care for adults. NICE quality standard [QS13]. November 2011. Available from: http://www.nice.org.uk/guidance/qs13 (last accessed 29 April 2016).
3. National Institute for Health and Care Excellence (NICE). Palliative care – general issues. Clinical knowledge summaries. 2015. Available from: http://cks.nice.org.uk/palliative-care-general-issues (last accessed 29 April 2016).

Parkinson's disease

Key thoughts

Practical points

- **Diagnosis.** Diagnosis is clinical, and there is no specific test. Consider alternative diagnoses that present in a similar way.
- **Comorbidity.** Identify mental health problems, such as dementia and depression, which are common in patients with Parkinson's disease.
- **Prognosis.** Assess the degree of disability and effects on quality of life resulting from both motor and non-motor symptoms.
- **Management.** In patients with established Parkinson's disease, assess response to treatment.

Differential diagnosis and important comorbidities

- Drug-induced.
- CVD.
- Dementia.
- Essential tremor.

> **RED FLAGS**
>
> - Falls
> - Depression
> - Social isolation
> - Severe disability
> - Lack of response to treatment

History

Ideas, concerns and expectations

- **Ideas.** Ask the patient and their carer about their understanding of Parkinson's disease. A common misconception is that Parkinson's disease is directly associated with dementia.
- **Concerns.** Find out about any fears or concerns about the future. Many people with Parkinson's disease are worried about the impact that the disease has on their lives and the effects on carers and families.
- **Expectations.** Find out about the patient's needs and preferences with regard to management.

The 10-Minute Clinical Assessment, Second Edition. Knut Schroeder.
© 2017 John Wiley & Sons, Ltd. Published 2017 by John Wiley & Sons, Ltd.

Quality of life
- **Quality of life.** How do symptoms affect the quality of life of both patient and carer? Which day-to-day activities have become problematic?

Motor symptoms
- **Tremor.** This is the main presenting symptom in many cases. There is usually unilateral tremor that is worse at rest and has a 'pill-rolling' rotary component. Over time, the tremor may spread to other limbs. Essential tremor is not associated with hypokinesia or rigidity. It improves with alcohol, is related to posture, worsens with movement and usually affects both hands.
- **Hypokinesia.** Ask whether initiating and maintaining repetitive movements is difficult. If already on treatment, has movement improved with medication such as levodopa? Ask whether gait has become more shuffling and whether handwriting has changed (e.g. micrographia). Have others noticed a loss of facial expression? Is there difficulty rising from a chair? Are there any problems doing up or undoing buttons?
- **Swallowing.** Dribbling suggests swallowing problems, which many people with Parkinson's disease find very embarrassing.
- **Postural instability.** Ask about balance and whether there have been any falls. Have there been any injuries? Are changes to the home necessary in order to prevent future falls (e.g. installation of hand rails, removal of obstructions)?
- **Abnormal movements.** In advanced Parkinson's disease, dyskinesias can develop together with other unpredictable movements as a result of reduced drug efficacy.

Non-motor symptoms
- **Sleep.** Rapid eye movement (REM) sleep problems and vivid dreams are common in early Parkinson's disease, and sleep problems can be very distressing. Are there any difficulties rolling over in bed? Is getting out of bed a problem during the night?
- **Dizziness.** Postural hypotension is a frequent accompanying symptom that can be very troublesome.
- **Mood.** Depression is an early feature of Parkinson's disease, and early recognition and treatment have the potential to improve the quality of life considerably.
- **Memory.** Ask about early symptoms and signs of dementia, which may complicate Parkinson's disease, but is not necessarily associated with it.
- **Neuropsychiatric symptoms.** Ask about hallucinations, agitation, apathy, anxiety, delusions, irritability and disinhibition, all of which can have severe implications for day-to-day life.
- **Autonomic disturbance.** Ask about bowel dysfunction (e.g. constipation), weight loss, bladder dysfunction and any sexual problems (which may affect relationships). Having an opportunity to talk about these issues can be therapeutic in itself for the patient and/or their carer.

Past and current medical problems
- **Other chronic conditions.** Look out for cardiovascular risk factor such as diabetes, hypertension and raised cholesterol.

Medication
- **Drugs that may cause motor symptoms.** Check for drugs that can induce Parkinsonism (e.g. neuroleptics, antidepressants and some antiemetics).
- **Treatment of Parkinson's disease.** Ask which drugs the patient is taking. Are they effective? Are there any adverse effects? Ask about motor fluctuations and dyskinesias (which occur with levodopa), as well as neuropsychiatric effects (common with ropinirole and pramipexole). Ask whether drugs are taken as prescribed.

Involvement of other health professionals
- **Other health professionals.** Ask for details about past and current involvement of other health professionals.
- **Physiotherapy.** Physiotherapy can help improve gait and movement initiation and may result in increased independence.
- **Occupational therapy.** Occupational therapy assessment can be helpful in assessing needs regarding home care and family roles. Occupational therapists may provide advice on how to improve transfers and mobility, and they will also look at safety issues.
- **Speech and language therapy.** Speech therapists can improve vocal loudness, pitch range and speech intelligibility in order to improve communication. They may also be able to address swallowing problems.

Review of previous investigations
- **Full blood count.** Macrocytosis may suggest alcohol misuse, hypothyroidism or vitamin B12/folate deficiency.
- **Thyroid function tests.** Thyroid disease can present with general 'slowing down'.
- **Liver function tests.** Is there evidence of liver failure or alcohol misuse?
- **Urea and electrolytes.** Check for evidence of renal failure, which will influence decisions about choice of medication.

Examination

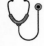

General
- **Sweating.** Excessive sweating may suggest hyperthyroidism or anxiety as an alternative cause of tremor.
- **Smell of alcohol.** Alcohol may cause postural tremor.

Signs of Parkinson's disease
- **Lack of facial expression.** Look for drooling and monotonous speech. Dysarthria may suggest cerebellar disease.
- **Tremor.** Look for tremor with a 'pill-rolling' component, which is usually unilateral and worse at rest. Check for intention tremor by performing the finger–nose test.

- **Rigidity.** Move the upper limbs passively at the wrist and elbow to check for the typical 'cog-wheel' rigidity.
- **Posture.** Check for postural instability, which can lead to poor balance and falls.
- **Gait.** Is the gait shuffling? Is there a delay or difficulty in initiation of movements? Cerebellar dysfunction can also cause abnormal gait and coordination. Look for loss of arm swing.

Vital signs
- **Pulse.** Make sure there is no undiagnosed arrhythmia, such as AF. Tachycardia may be present in alternative causes of tremor (e.g. hyperthyroidism, anxiety and drug withdrawal).
- **Blood pressure.** Is there evidence of uncontrolled hypertension? Check lying and standing blood pressure for postural hypotension.

Cognitive function
- **Year.** Ask what year it is. Score 4 if incorrect.
- **Month.** Ask what month it is. Score 3 if incorrect.
- **Address phrase.** Give the patient a fictitious address phrase with five components to remember (e.g. John Smith, 42 High Street, Bedford).
- **Time.** Ask what time it is (to within 1 hour). Score 3 if incorrect.
- **Count backwards.** Ask the patient to count backwards from 20 to 1. Score 2 if there is one error, score 4 if there is more than one.
- **Reverse months.** Ask the patient to name the months of the year in reverse. Score 2 if there is one error, score 4 if there is more than one.
- **Repeat address.** Ask the patient to repeat the address phrase. Count the number of errors and score 2 for each, up to a maximum of 10.
- **Scoring.** Any score over 7 suggests dementia.

Key references and further reading

1. Clarke CE. Clinical review: Parkinson's disease. *BMJ* 2007;335:441–445.
2. Katzman R, Brown T, Fuld P et al. Validation of a short orientation–memory–concentration test of cognitive impairment. *Am J Psychiatry* 1983;140(6):734–739.
3. National Institute for Health and Care Excellence (NICE). Parkinson's disease in over 20s: diagnosis and management. NICE guidelines [CG35]. June 2006. Available from: http://www.nice.org.uk/guidance/cg35 (last accessed 29 April 2016).
4. National Institute for Health and Care Excellence (NICE). Parkinson's disease. Clinical knowledge summaries. 2014. Available from: http://cks.nice.org.uk/parkinsons-disease (last accessed 29 April 2016).
5. Parkinson's UK. www.parkinsons.org.uk.
6. Rao G, Fisch L, Srinivasan S et al. The rational clinical examination: does this patient have Parkinson disease? *JAMA* 2003;289:347–353.

Index

The 10-Minute Clinical Assessment, Second Edition. Knut Schroeder.
© 2017 John Wiley & Sons, Ltd. Published 2017 by John Wiley & Sons, Ltd.

Printed and bound by CPI Group (UK) Ltd, Croydon, CR0 4YY

09/06/2025

14685989-0001